I0063690

TRP Channels in Health and Disease

TRP Channels in Health and Disease

Special Issue Editor

Alexander Dietrich

MDPI • Basel • Beijing • Wuhan • Barcelona • Belgrade

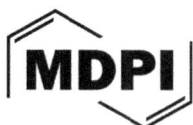

MDPI

Special Issue Editor
Alexander Dietrich
Ludwig-Maximilians-Universitat Muenchen
Germany

Editorial Office
MDPI
St. Alban-Anlage 66
4052 Basel, Switzerland

This is a reprint of articles from the Special Issue published online in the open access journal *Cells* (ISSN 2073-4409) from 2018 to 2019 (available at: https://www.mdpi.com/journal/cells/special_issues/TRP)

For citation purposes, cite each article independently as indicated on the article page online and as indicated below:

LastName, A.A.; LastName, B.B.; LastName, C.C. Article Title. *Journal Name* **Year**, *Article Number*, Page Range.

ISBN 978-3-03921-082-4 (Pbk)
ISBN 978-3-03921-083-1 (PDF)

© 2019 by the authors. Articles in this book are Open Access and distributed under the Creative Commons Attribution (CC BY) license, which allows users to download, copy and build upon published articles, as long as the author and publisher are properly credited, which ensures maximum dissemination and a wider impact of our publications.

The book as a whole is distributed by MDPI under the terms and conditions of the Creative Commons license CC BY-NC-ND.

Contents

About the Special Issue Editor

Alexander Dietrich, Prof. Dr. at the Walther-Straub-Institute of Pharmacology and Toxicology, LMU-Munich, Germany, worked on TRP channels since 1997, received his Ph.D. degree from the University of Heidelberg/Germany. A postdoctoral fellow at the University of California Los Angeles (UCLA)/USA, Habilitation at the University of Marburg/Germany, he was also the winner of the Galenus-von-Pergamon Prize for basic Science 2007 and has published more than 90 peer-reviewed manuscripts, book chapters, and invited reviews. Editorial Board Member of *Cells*.

cells

MDPI

Editorial

Transient Receptor Potential (TRP) Channels in Health and Disease

Alexander Dietrich

Walther-Straub-Institute of Pharmacology and Toxicology, Member of the German Centre for Lung Research (DZL), Medical Faculty, LMU Munich, Nussbaumstr. 26, D-80336 Munich, Germany; Alexander.Dietrich@lrz.uni-muenchen.de

Received: 29 April 2019; Accepted: 2 May 2019; Published: 4 May 2019

Almost 25 years ago, the first mammalian transient receptor potential (TRP) channel, now named TRPC1, was cloned and published (reviewed in [1]). Although the exact function of TRPC1 is still elusive [1], TRP channels now represent an extended family of 28 members, fulfilling multiple roles in the living organism [2]. Their identified functions include control of body temperature, transmitter release, mineral homeostasis, chemical sensing, and survival mechanisms in a challenging environment. The TRP channel superfamily covers six families: TRPC, with C for "canonical"; TRPA, with A for "ankyrin"; TRPM, with M for "melastatin"; TRPML, with ML for "mucolipidin"; TRPP, with P for "polycystin"; and TRPV, with V for "vanilloid" (see Figure 1). They all share a structure of six transmembrane (TM) regions, with a pore domain between TM5 and 6 and cytoplasmic amino- and carboxyl-termini. Functional nonselective, Ca^{2+} permeable TRP channels are tetramers, which consist of the same or different TRP monomers preferentially from the same family [3].

Eleven mutant TRP channels cause a spectrum of 16 human diseases, additionally emphasizing their essential role in vivo [2]. Moreover, TRP channels are important pharmacological targets for specific novel therapeutic treatment options for patients. Along these lines, specific TRP modulators have been identified in recent years and are now tested in vitro and in vivo against symptoms caused by dysfunctional TRP proteins or pathophysiological processes (such as pain, chronic inflammation, fibrosis, and edema), which occur if normal physiological responses are out of control [2,4].

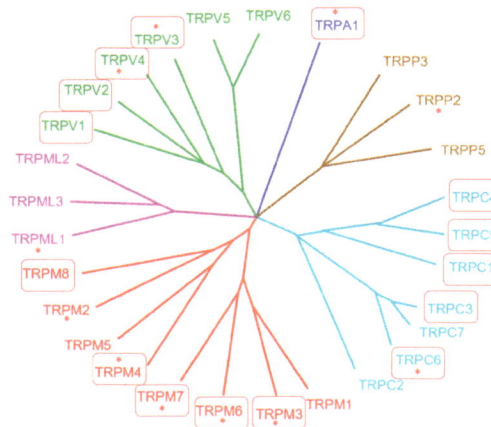

Figure 1. Phylogenetic tree of the transient receptor potential (TRP) superfamily in vertebrates. Boxed TRP channels are highlighted in the manuscripts of this special section. Stars (*) indicate the mutant TRP channels that cause human diseases. Picture modified from [5].

Over the last few years, new findings on TRP channels confirm their exceptional function as cellular sensors and effectors. This special issue of Cells features a collection of eight reviews and seven original articles summarizing the current state-of-the-art research on TRP channels, with a focus on TRP channel activation, their physiological and pathophysiological function, and their roles as pharmacological targets for future therapeutic options.

Returning to the roots of the mammalian TRP channel discovery, TRPC1 may preferentially work as a regulator of heterotetrameric **TRPC1/4/5** channels rather than of a homomeric TRPC1 ion channel (reviewed in [1]). Dr. Minard and colleagues present an excellent overview on the function of these heteromeric channel complexes in different tissues and pathologies, and they introduce specific small molecular modulators that are important for future research and as therapeutic options in pathophysiological processes [6].

Belonging to the same family of canonical TRPC channels, **TRPC3** controls specific functions in the cardiovascular system, the brain, the immune system, during cancer progression, and tissue remodeling, which are summarized in the comprehensive review by Drs. Tiapko and Groschner. They also present new therapeutic approaches, such as photopharmacology and optochemical genetics, to manipulate the action of TRPC3 for the intervention of its tissue-specific tasks [7].

Along the same lines, Drs. Tian and Zhu present evidence in their original article for a specific and exclusive role of **TRPC3** for the metabotropic glutamate receptor 1 (mGluR1)-mediated augmentation of slow excitatory postsynaptic currents (sEPSC) by type B γ-aminobutyric acid (GABA$_B$) receptors in the Purkinje cells of the cerebellum. This molecular mechanism is essential in long-term depression, as well as synapse elimination, and may regulate motor coordination and learning [8].

A characteristic feature of TRPC3, TRPC6, and TRPC7 is their activation by diacylglycerol (DAG) as a product of receptor-induced phospholipase-C activity (reviewed in [9]). Recent evidence, however, suggests that **TRPC4** and **TRPC5** channels are also activated by DAG [10]. The much more complex molecular mechanism includes the C-terminal interaction with the scaffolding proteins Na$^+$/H$^+$ exchange regulatory factors 1 and 2 (NHERF1 and NHERF2), which dynamically regulate the DAG sensitivity of TRPC4 and TRPC5. These cellular events are summarized by Drs. Mederos y Schnitzler, Gudermann, and Storch [11].

The role of ion channels and transporters, especially that of **TRPC6** in inflammation, is the topic of a review by Dr. Ramirez and colleagues. They present an overview on TRPC6 channel activity in leucocytes, transendothelial migration, chemotaxis, phagocytosis, and cytokine release [12]. The importance of channel function is underlined by the very recent identification of a single nucleotide polymorphism (SNP) in the TRPC6 gene in patients with the autoimmune disease lupus erythematosus by the same authors [13].

TRPA1 is the only member of the TRPA family, carrying a higher amount of ankyrin repeats (16 for human TRPA1) at the amino-terminus than other TRP proteins (usually four). Chemical modification of its cysteine residues makes TRPA1 an attractive candidate as a toxicant sensor (reviewed in [14]). Dr. Lüling and coauthors in their original article identified heat shock 70 kDa protein 6 as an effector regulated by the activation of TRPA1 by sulfur mustard (SM), a chemical warfare agent used during the civil war in Syria. The authors of this manuscript used a proteomic approach to identify differentially regulated proteins in TRPA1-expressing HEK293 and A549 cells after SM treatment. The selective TRPA1 inhibitor AP18 was used to distinguish the TRPA1-mediated effect from unspecific effects [15].

Moving to the TRPM family, Drs. Liu, Ong, and Ambudkar introduce an exciting role of **TRPM2** in salivary glands. Xerostomia, also known as dry mouth, is an irreversible side effect after therapeutic irradiation of head and neck cancers. TRPM2-deficient mice showed only a transient loss of salivary gland exposure with more than 60% recovery after irradiation [16]. Moreover, there is evidence for a role of this channel in inflammatory processes and inducing the autoimmune disease Sjögren's syndrome. The involvement of TRPM2 and other TRP channels in salivary gland excretion is discussed in this comprehensive review [17].

Patients carrying a mutation in their **TRPM4** protein suffer from cardiac conduction disease, emphasizing TRPM4's key role in the heart [18]. Drs. Wang, Naruse, and Takahashi highlight the functions of this channel in cardiovascular pathophysiology, e.g., ischemia-reperfusion injury causing myocardial infarction [19].

The kinase-coupled **TRPM7** channel is expressed in multiple cells of the immune system, such as lymphocytes, mast cells, neutrophils, and macrophages. Recently, it was demonstrated that the enzymatic activity of TRPM7 is required for the gut homing of intra-epithelial lymphocytes [20]. Mrs. Nadolni and Dr. Zierler shed light on how the TRPM7 channel, and/or kinase activity, is essential for pathologies, such as allergic hypersensitivity, arterial thrombosis, and graft versus host disease [21].

Menthol, as a cooling compound from peppermint, has been used for hundreds of years without the molecular basis of its action being revealed. Soon after cloning the eighth member—**TRPM8**—of the melastatin family of TRP channels, several laboratories have reported that natural and synthetic cooling mimetics, such as icilin, eucalyptol, and menthol, activate this channel (reviewed in [22]). Dr. Khare and colleagues now provide evidence that the application of menthol may induce a so-called "browning" effect in subcutaneous adipose tissue, although a direct involvement of TRPM8 has not been identified yet [23].

Two original contributions analyze the distribution of TRPV channels in human tissues using immunohistochemistry. Dr. Del Fiacco and colleagues present evidence for the expression of **TRPV1** channels in a region of the human brain, which they name Locus Karalis (Locus K). Most interestingly, TRPV1-like immunoreactivity partially overlaps with that of neuropeptides calcitonin gene-related peptide (CGRP) and substance P [24].

Drs. Rizopoulos, Papadaki-Petrou, and Assimakopoulou analyze the expression of TRPV1, TRPV2, TRPV3, and TRPV4 proteins in the mucosal epithelium of colitis ulcerosa patients in comparison to healthy volunteers. In their research, they identified a decreased expression of **TRPV1**, while **TRPV4** channels were found to be upregulated in tissues of patients. For **TRPV2** and **TRPV3**, no changes in expression levels were observed [25].

Many different TRP channel structures were recently resolved by cryo-electron microscopy (reviewed in [26]). In each case a large amount of pure protein material is required, which cannot be easily produced in *E. coli*, as eukaryotic post-translational processing is required for channel maturation. Therefore, another cheap eukaryotic expression system for TRP channels is presented by Dr. Zhang and colleagues. They recombinantly produced **11 human TRP members** in the yeast *Saccharomyces cerevisiae* and confirmed retained functionality for TRPM8 as the model target [27]. *S. cerevisiae* on its own also expresses a TRP channel called **TRPY1**, which is activated by increased cytosolic levels of Mn^{2+} in response to oxidative stress, as outlined in an original manuscript by Drs. Ruta, Nicolau, Popa, and Farcasanu [28].

Last but not least, Dr. Steinritz and colleagues systematically screened available literature to identify the role of TRP channels as chemical sensors in the human body. **TRPA1**, **TRPM8**, and **TRPV1** proteins are coexpressed in many tissues and are most frequently associated with toxicity sensing. **TRPV4** channels are cited less often, with other TRP channels (TRPC1, TRPC4, and TRPM5) being expressed to a lesser extent [29].

In summary, this special issue of Cells presents a comprehensive overview of the latest data on four TRP channel families and will hopefully convince readers of the importance of these proteins for human physiology and as drug targets for future therapeutics.

Acknowledgments: I thank all the authors for their hard work to produce up-to-date and comprehensive manuscripts in a timely manner, as well as the publisher BMC for permission to re-use Figure 1. The editorial help given by Jacky Zhang is greatly appreciated, and I am also grateful to the editorial board of Cells for giving me the opportunity to serve as guest editor for this special issue.

Conflicts of Interest: The author declares no conflict of interest.

References

1. Dietrich, A.; Fahlbusch, M.; Gudermann, T. Classical Transient Receptor Potential 1 (TRPC1): Channel or Channel Regulator? *Cells* **2014**, *3*, 939–962. [CrossRef]
2. Nilius, B.; Szallasi, A. Transient receptor potential channels as drug targets: From the science of basic research to the art of medicine. *Pharmacol. Rev.* **2014**, *66*, 676–814. [CrossRef] [PubMed]
3. Hofmann, T.; Schaefer, M.; Schultz, G.; Gudermann, T. Subunit composition of mammalian transient receptor potential channels in living cells. *Proc. Natl. Acad. Sci. USA* **2002**, *99*, 7461–7466. [CrossRef] [PubMed]
4. Dietrich, A. Modulators of Transient Receptor Potential (TRP) Channels as Therapeutic Options in Lung Disease. *Pharmaceuticals* **2019**, *12*, 23. [CrossRef]
5. Nilius, B.; Owsianik, G. The transient receptor potential family of ion channels. *Genome Biol.* **2011**, *12*, 218. [CrossRef] [PubMed]
6. Minard, A.; Bauer, C.C.; Wright, D.J.; Rubaiy, H.N.; Muraki, K.; Beech, D.J.; Bon, R.S. Remarkable Progress with Small-Molecule Modulation of TRPC1/4/5 Channels: Implications for Understanding the Channels in Health and Disease. *Cells* **2018**, *7*, 52. [CrossRef]
7. Tiapko, O.; Groschner, K. TRPC3 as a Target of Novel Therapeutic Interventions. *Cells* **2018**, *7*, 83. [CrossRef]
8. Tian, J.; Zhu, M.X. GABAB Receptors Augment TRPC3-Mediated Slow Excitatory Postsynaptic Current to Regulate Cerebellar Purkinje Neuron Response to Type-1 Metabotropic Glutamate Receptor Activation. *Cells* **2018**, *7*, 90. [CrossRef] [PubMed]
9. Dietrich, A.; Kalwa, H.; Rost, B.R.; Gudermann, T. The diacylglycerol-sensitive TRPC3/6/7 subfamily of cation channels: Functional characterization and physiological relevance. *Pflug. Arch.* **2005**, *451*, 72–80. [CrossRef] [PubMed]
10. Storch, U.; Forst, A.L.; Pardatscher, F.; Erdogmus, S.; Philipp, M.; Gregoritza, M.; Mederos, Y.S.M.; Gudermann, T. Dynamic NHERF interaction with TRPC4/5 proteins is required for channel gating by diacylglycerol. *Proc. Natl. Acad. Sci. USA* **2017**, *114*, E37–E46. [CrossRef]
11. Mederos, Y.S.M.; Gudermann, T.; Storch, U. Emerging Roles of Diacylglycerol-Sensitive TRPC4/5 Channels. *Cells* **2018**, *7*, 218. [CrossRef]
12. Ramirez, G.A.; Coletto, L.A.; Sciorati, C.; Bozzolo, E.P.; Manunta, P.; Rovere-Querini, P.; Manfredi, A.A. Ion Channels and Transporters in Inflammation: Special Focus on TRP Channels and TRPC6. *Cells* **2018**, *7*, 70. [CrossRef]
13. Ramirez, G.A.; Coletto, L.A.; Bozzolo, E.P.; Citterio, L.; Delli Carpini, S.; Zagato, L.; Rovere-Querini, P.; Lanzani, C.; Manunta, P.; Manfredi, A.A.; et al. The TRPC6 intronic polymorphism, associated with the risk of neurological disorders in systemic lupus erythematous, influences immune cell function. *J. Neuroimmunol.* **2018**, *325*, 43–53. [CrossRef]
14. Dietrich, A.; Steinritz, D.; Gudermann, T. Transient receptor potential (TRP) channels as molecular targets in lung toxicology and associated diseases. *Cell Calcium* **2017**, *67*, 123–137. [CrossRef]
15. Luling, R.; John, H.; Gudermann, T.; Thiermann, H.; Muckter, H.; Popp, T.; Steinritz, D. Transient Receptor Potential Channel A1 (TRPA1) Regulates Sulfur Mustard-Induced Expression of Heat Shock 70 kDa Protein 6 (HSPA6) In Vitro. *Cells* **2018**, *7*, 126. [CrossRef]
16. Liu, X.; Cotrim, A.; Teos, L.; Zheng, C.; Swaim, W.; Mitchell, J.; Mori, Y.; Ambudkar, I. Loss of TRPM2 function protects against irradiation-induced salivary gland dysfunction. *Nat. Commun.* **2013**, *4*, 1515. [CrossRef]
17. Liu, X.; Ong, H.L.; Ambudkar, I. TRP Channel Involvement in Salivary Glands-Some Good, Some Bad. *Cells* **2018**, *7*, 74. [CrossRef]
18. Kruse, M.; Schulze-Bahr, E.; Corfield, V.; Beckmann, A.; Stallmeyer, B.; Kurtbay, G.; Ohmert, I.; Brink, P.; Pongs, O. Impaired endocytosis of the ion channel TRPM4 is associated with human progressive familial heart block type I. *J. Clin. Investig.* **2009**, *119*, 2737–2744. [CrossRef]
19. Wang, C.; Naruse, K.; Takahashi, K. Role of the TRPM4 Channel in Cardiovascular Physiology and Pathophysiology. *Cells* **2018**, *7*, 62. [CrossRef]
20. Romagnani, A.; Vettore, V.; Rezzonico-Jost, T.; Hampe, S.; Rottoli, E.; Nadolni, W.; Perotti, M.; Meier, M.A.; Hermanns, C.; Geiger, S.; et al. TRPM7 kinase activity is essential for T cell colonization and alloreactivity in the gut. *Nat. Commun.* **2017**, *8*, 1917. [CrossRef]
21. Nadolni, W.; Zierler, S. The Channel-Kinase TRPM7 as Novel Regulator of Immune System Homeostasis. *Cells* **2018**, *7*, 109. [CrossRef]

22. Almaraz, L.; Manenschijn, J.A.; de la Pena, E.; Viana, F. Trpm8. *Handb. Exp. Pharm.* **2014**, *222*, 547–579. [CrossRef]
23. Khare, P.; Chauhan, A.; Kumar, V.; Kaur, J.; Mahajan, N.; Kumar, V.; Gesing, A.; Chopra, K.; Kondepudi, K.K.; Bishnoi, M. Bioavailable Menthol (Transient Receptor Potential Melastatin-8 Agonist) Induces Energy Expending Phenotype in Differentiating Adipocytes. *Cells* **2019**, *8*, 383. [CrossRef]
24. Del Fiacco, M.; Serra, M.P.; Boi, M.; Poddighe, L.; Demontis, R.; Carai, A.; Quartu, M. TRPV1-Like Immunoreactivity in the Human Locus K, a Distinct Subregion of the Cuneate Nucleus. *Cells* **2018**, *7*, 72. [CrossRef]
25. Rizopoulos, T.; Papadaki-Petrou, H.; Assimakopoulou, M. Expression Profiling of the Transient Receptor Potential Vanilloid (TRPV) Channels 1, 2, 3 and 4 in Mucosal Epithelium of Human Ulcerative Colitis. *Cells* **2018**, *7*, 61. [CrossRef]
26. Madej, M.G.; Ziegler, C.M. Dawning of a new era in TRP channel structural biology by cryo-electron microscopy. *Pflug. Arch.* **2018**, *470*, 213–225. [CrossRef]
27. Zhang, L.; Wang, K.; Klaerke, D.A.; Calloe, K.; Lowrey, L.; Pedersen, P.A.; Gourdon, P.; Gotfryd, K. Purification of Functional Human TRP Channels Recombinantly Produced in Yeast. *Cells* **2019**, *8*, 148. [CrossRef]
28. Ruta, L.L.; Nicolau, I.; Popa, C.V.; Farcasanu, I.C. Manganese Suppresses the Haploinsufficiency of Heterozygous trpy1Delta/TRPY1 Saccharomyces cerevisiae Cells and Stimulates the TRPY1-Dependent Release of Vacuolar Ca(2+) under H(2)O(2) Stress. *Cells* **2019**, *8*, 79. [CrossRef]
29. Steinritz, D.; Stenger, B.; Dietrich, A.; Gudermann, T.; Popp, T. TRPs in Tox: Involvement of Transient Receptor Potential-Channels in Chemical-Induced Organ Toxicity-A Structured Review. *Cells* **2018**, *7*, 98. [CrossRef]

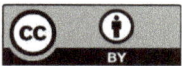

© 2019 by the author. Licensee MDPI, Basel, Switzerland. This article is an open access article distributed under the terms and conditions of the Creative Commons Attribution (CC BY) license (http://creativecommons.org/licenses/by/4.0/).

cells

MDPI

Review

Remarkable Progress with Small-Molecule Modulation of TRPC1/4/5 Channels: Implications for Understanding the Channels in Health and Disease

Aisling Minard [1,†], Claudia C. Bauer [2,†], David J. Wright [2,†], Hussein N. Rubaiy [3], Katsuhiko Muraki [4], David J. Beech [2] and Robin S. Bon [2,*]

1   School of Chemistry, University of Leeds, Leeds LS2 9JT, UK; cm10a3m@leeds.ac.uk
2   Department of Discovery and Translational Science, Leeds Institute of Cardiovascular and Metabolic
     Medicine, University of Leeds, Leeds LS2 9JT, UK; c.bauer@leeds.ac.uk (C.C.B.);
     d.j.wright1@leeds.ac.uk (D.J.W.); d.j.beech@leeds.ac.uk (D.J.B.)
3   Centre for Atherothrombosis and Metabolic Disease, Hull York Medical School, Hull HU6 7RX, UK;
     h.rubaiy@hull.ac.uk
4   Laboratory of Cellular Pharmacology, School of Pharmacy, Aichi-Gakuin University, 1-100 Kusumoto,
     Chikusa, Nagoya 464-8650, Japan; kmuraki@dpc.agu.ac.jp
*   Correspondence: r.bon@leeds.ac.uk
†   These authors contributed equally to this work.

Received: 27 April 2018; Accepted: 23 May 2018; Published: 1 June 2018

Abstract: Proteins of the TRPC family can form many homo- and heterotetrameric cation channels permeable to Na^+, K^+ and Ca^{2+}. In this review, we focus on channels formed by the isoforms TRPC1, TRPC4 and TRPC5. We review evidence for the formation of different TRPC1/4/5 tetramers, give an overview of recently developed small-molecule TRPC1/4/5 activators and inhibitors, highlight examples of biological roles of TRPC1/4/5 channels in different tissues and pathologies, and discuss how high-quality chemical probes of TRPC1/4/5 modulators can be used to understand the involvement of TRPC1/4/5 channels in physiological and pathophysiological processes.

Keywords: ion channel; TRPC; small molecules; calcium; chemical probes

1. Introduction

Transient Receptor Potential (TRP) proteins form tetrameric, non-selective ion channels permeable to Na^+, K^+ and—in most instances—Ca^{2+} [1–4]. The 28 mammalian TRP homologues are divided into six subclasses (TRPM, TRPV, TRPA, TRPP, TRPML and TRPC) according to distinctions at the sequence level [3,5], while TRPN (NOMPC) proteins (present in, for example, fruit flies, nematodes and zebrafish) have no mammalian homologues [3]. Four monomers are needed to form a functional ion channel; more than 28 different mammalian TRP channels can form because channels may consist of homomers or heteromers of subunits (Figure 1), each with their own characteristics and functions. Although there is differential expression of TRPs in different cells, tissues, and in different pathologies, most TRP proteins are broadly expressed in both excitable and non-excitable cells, where they enable coupling of relatively slow chemical and physical events to cellular signalling, either directly or indirectly [1,6,7]. The regulation of some TRP channels by many modulators has led to the idea that the channels are complex integrators of multiple chemical and physical factors [1,8].

There are seven members of the TRPC subfamily, of which TRPC2 is not expressed in humans and the great apes because it is encoded by a pseudogene in these species [9]. TRPC proteins are especially prone to formation of heterotetrameric channels within subgroups (Figure 1), one consisting of TRPC3, TRPC6 and TRPC7 and the other of TRPC1, TRPC4 and TRPC5 [5]. TRPC4 and TRPC5 are the most closely related TRPC proteins [10], with 69% sequence identity (BLAST search [11]). TRPC1, which can interact with proteins from other TRP channel families [12,13], may not form functional homomeric channels, but is an important contributor to heteromeric channels with TRPC4 and/or TRPC5 [1,14–18].

This review focuses on channels composed of TRPC1, TRPC4 and TRPC5 (Section 2), their small-molecule modulators (Section 3) and their roles in health and disease (Section 4), to highlight examples and opportunities for the use of small-molecule TRPC1/4/5 modulators to study the role of these channels in physiology and disease. We have used the following notations (Figure 1B): TRPC1, TRPC4 and TRPC5 (etc.) denote the different proteins or any channels incorporating them; TRPC1/4/5 denotes channels composed of TRPC1, TRPC4 and/or TRPC5 (homo- or heteromeric; any ratio); TRPC4:C4 and TRPC5:C5 (etc.) denote specific homomeric channels; TRPC1:C5, TRPC1:C4, TRPC4:C5 and TRPC1:C4:C5 denote specific heteromeric channels (any ratio); and TRPC4–C1 and TRPC5–C1 denote (channels composed of) recombinant, concatemeric proteins (fusions of TRPC1 at the C-terminus of either TRPC4 or TRPC5 through a short linker) that have been developed in our lab to control channel stoichiometry [15,19,20]. The majority of TRPC1/4/5 channels discussed in this review are human and rodent homologues, and where relevant to the discussion, species have been annotated.

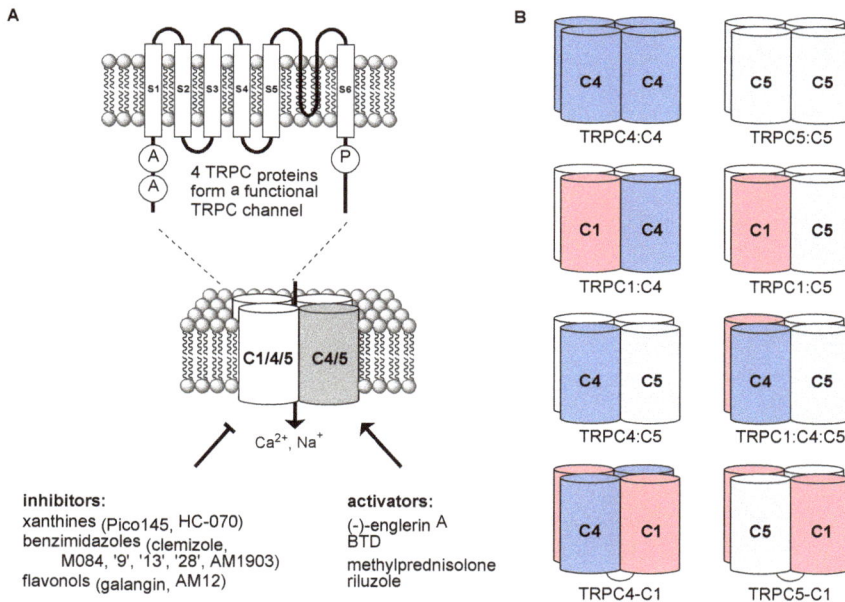

Figure 1. (**A**) Formation of tetrameric TRPC1/4/5 cation channels by TRPC1/4/5 proteins and recently discovered small-molecule modulators discussed in this review. Domains "A" are the ankyrin repeat domains present in all TRPC proteins, and "P" is the PDZ binding domain present in TRPC4 and TRPC5. (**B**) Composition of different TRPC1/4/5 channels discussed in this review. Native channels are believed to exist predominantly as heteromers, but their exact compositions and stoichiometries are often unknown (as depicted by white subunits, which may be TRPC1/4/5 proteins or other TRP(C) proteins). Linked subunits depict recombinant TRPC4–C1 and TRPC5–C1 concatemeric proteins that can be used to control channel stoichiometry.

2. Composition of TRPC1/4/5 Tetrameric Channels

The tetrameric nature of TRPC channels was originally predicted from their homology to voltage-gated potassium channels such as $K_V1.2$, for which a crystal structure is available [21]. Current data suggest that TRPC proteins form a variety of homo- and heterotetrameric channels (see below). The recent "resolution revolution" in cryo-electron microscopy [22] has led to the determination of a wide variety of high resolution ion channel structures, providing novel insights into ion channel function. There are examples of TRP channel high resolution structures from each TRP subfamily, which confirm their tetrameric structures [23–27]. Recently, cryo-EM structures of of several TRPC channels, including human TRPC3:C3 [28], human TRPC6:C6 [29], mouse TRPC4:C4 [30] and zebrafish TRPC4:C4 [31] have been reported. hTRPC3 and hTRPC6 share limited homology with hTRPC1, hTRPC4 and hTRPC5 proteins (approximately 40% sequence identity). It is noteworthy that the hTRPC6/C6 channel structure was determined in the presence of a small molecule inhibitor, BTDM, which is bound at a similar position to resiniferatoxin and capsaicin in TRPV1 structures [32,33], between the pore-forming region of one subunit and the voltage sensing-like domain (VSLD) of another. mTRPC4 shares 97% sequence identity with hTRPC4, 70% identity with hTRPC5 and 48% identity with hTRPC1 and so mTRPC4:C4 is the closest homologue to hTRPC1/4/5 channels that has been structurally characterised. It is interesting that in both the mouse and zebrafish TRPC4:C4 structures, a disulfide bond is observed between Cys549 and Cys554 (numbered according to the mouse gene); these disulfides have been previously implicated in channel gating in TRPC5 [34,35] and are conserved only in TRPC1, TRPC4 and TRPC5. Both TRPC4:C4 structures were solved in their closed state in the absence of modulators, so more structural information is required to understand the gating mechanisms of these channels. Additionally, there are only three unique heteromeric structures of any ion channels [36–38] and none of these contain TRP proteins. Therefore, to probe the heteromerisation of TRPC channels, we must rely on indirect measurements of their interaction. In this section, we describe evidence for the formation of different TRPC1/4/5 channels, in both overexpression systems and as native channels.

2.1. Channels Formed by Overexpressed TRPC1/4/5 Proteins

There is some evidence to suggest that TRPC1, when overexpressed, is retained in the endoplasmic reticulum (ER) but is found at the plasma membrane when co-expressed with TRPC4 or TRPC5 [39]. Förster Resonance Energy Transfer (FRET) experiments using TRPC1 labelled with Cyan Fluorescent Protein (CFP) and Yellow Fluorescent Protein (YFP) suggest that there are at least two TRPC1 monomers in the tetrameric complex at the ER. The authors suggest the formation of a homotetrameric TRPC1 channel; however, these data do not explicitly rule out a TRPC1 interaction with other natively expressed ion channel monomers, such as Orai1, which has been implicated in the formation of heteromeric channels with TRPC1 [40]. Additionally, it was observed that TRPC4 and TRPC5, when co-expressed with TRPC1, showed different I–V relationships (for examples, see Figure 2), a lower calcium flux, and increased selectivity to sodium ions compared with TRPC4:C4 or TRPC5:C5 homomeric channels [41]. Another study, involving FRET and co-transfected HEK293 cells, demonstrated that TRPC1, TRPC4 and TRPC5 were able to form homomers, that TRPC1 could interact with either TRPC4 or TRPC5, and that TRPC4 and TRPC5 could interact with each other. In this study, co-immunoprecipitation also suggested each homomeric interaction and the same heteromeric interactions between TRPC4 and TRPC5, and TRPC4 and TRPC1 [42]. However, these FRET and co-immunoprecipitation data do not provide direct insight into stoichiometries of heteromeric channels. In addition, stoichiometries may vary depending on expression levels of different TRPC proteins.

Atomic Force Microscopy (AFM) was used to probe TRPC1 tetrameric structure when overexpressed in and purified from HEK293 cells [43]. The authors measured the angles between antibodies binding to TRPC1 (approximately 90 and 180 degrees), which suggested that TRPC1 forms tetramers. Considering TRPC1 was transiently overexpressed, it is surprising that observed tetramers were only seen with two or fewer antibodies bound, which could suggest the formation of heterotetramers with other natively expressed channel proteins from the TRP and other families. The majority of particle sizes were, however, consistent with monomeric TRPC1, suggesting that tetramers were broken up during purification in 3-[(3-cholamidopropyl) dimethylammonio]-1-propanesulfonate (CHAPS) detergent.

We have recently demonstrated that recombinant, concatemeric TRPC4–C1 or TRPC5–C1 proteins can be overexpressed to form functional channels, the I–V relationships and reduced Ca^{2+} permeability of which closely resemble those of native heteromeric TRPC1:C4 and TRPC1:C5 channels [15,19,20]. These concatemers allow the functional analysis of TRPC heterotetramers with fixed stoichiometry, which will be critical to the development of small molecules specific to homo- or heterotetramers [20].

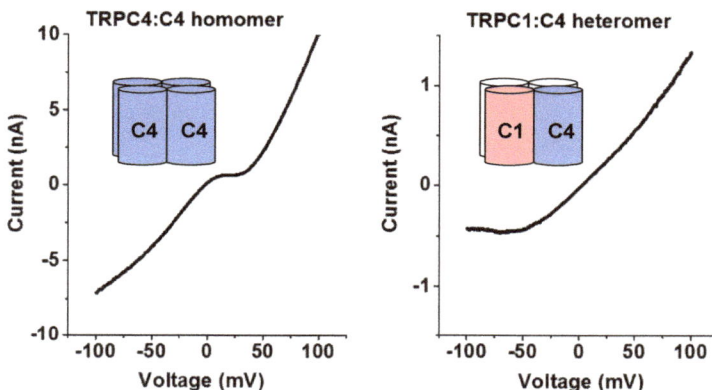

Figure 2. Example I–V plots of homomeric (**left**) and heteromeric/concatemeric (**right**) TRPC1/4/5 channels. Recordings from overexpressed TRPC4:C4 and TRPC1:C4 channels are shown. For examples of native I–V plots, see references [14,16].

2.2. Native TRPC1/4/5 Channels

It has been observed that TRPC proteins show differential tissue expression [44]. Since TRPC1 is expressed in a wide variety of tissues and native I–V plots [14,16] resemble overexpressed heteromeric or concatemeric channels (Figure 2), it is likely that TRPC1 is predominantly observed in heterotetrameric channels in vivo. Additionally, there are several examples of detecting TRPC heterotetramerisation ex vivo that largely agree with the above overexpression studies. For example, TRPC1, TRPC4 or TRPC5 were purified from mouse hippocampal cells using antibodies specific to any one isoform [18]. These data suggest the formation of a tetramer containing TRPC1, TRPC4 and TRPC5; however, alternatively there could be populations of TRPC1/4, TRPC1/5 and TRPC4/5 channels, which would result in similar co-immunoprecipitation results. In a second example, TRPC4 and TRPC5, after formaldehyde crosslinking, were co-immunoprecipitated from bovine aortic endothelial cells [45]. These results suggest that different tetrameric TRPC1/4/5 channels are formed in vivo.

Further complicating the field of TRPC heterotetramerisation is the existence of splice isoforms of TRPC proteins; two have been reported for TRPC1 [46,47], and seven for TRPC4 [48,49]. Of the TRPC4 isoforms, TRPC4α and TRPC4β have been studied in most detail. TRPC4α and TRPC4β (which lacks 84 residues towards the C terminus) show differential tissue expression. TRPC4β:C4β channels no longer respond to phosphatatidylinositol 4,5-bisphosphate [50], but are still activated by (−)-englerin A [51]. These splice variants are likely to result in even more heterogeneity in TRPC1/4/5 channels.

In summary, there has been much progress in the field of TRPC1/4/5 heterotetramer identification. It should be noted that interactions found in co-immunoprecipitation experiments with detergent-solubilised TRPC1/4/5 proteins may not accurately reflect interactions in native membranes, and even in experiments that involve formaldehyde crosslinking before cell lysis, it may be difficult to exclude interactions between different homomeric channels during co-immunoprecipitations. However, the combination of co-immunoprecipitation results and the fact that I–V plots of native channels closely resemble those of cells that either co-express TRPC4/5 and TRPC1, or express TRPC4–C1 or TRPC5–C1 concatemers, strongly suggests that TRPC1, TRPC4 and TRPC5 form functional heterotetrameric channels in different tissues. There is currently no firm evidence to suggest the native stoichiometry—or, more probably, stoichiometries—of these multimers though.

3. Recent Progress with Small-Molecule Modulators of TRPC1/4/5 Channels

TRPC1/4/5 channels are modulated by a wide range of physiological factors, and physical and chemical stimuli, including temperature, redox status, G-protein signalling, endogenous lipids, heavy metal ions, dietary lipids, natural products and synthetic small molecules. We and others have previously reviewed the development of small-molecule modulators of TRP(C) channels [1,52]. Traditionally, TRPC1/4/5 channels have often been activated with lanthanide ions (La^{3+}, Gd^{3+}), GPCR agonists such as carbachol, or small molecules such as rosiglitazone (which is non-specific and has low potency), and inhibited with the non-specific small molecules such as 2-APB or SFK96365. In addition, for most traditional small-molecule TRPC1/4/5 modulators, little is known about their mode-of-action, and cellular targets of these molecules are likely diverse. Although some TRPC1/4/5 modulators are thought to bind directly to the channels, no small-molecule binding sites have been identified so far.

In 2011, Miller et al. reported ML204 (Figure 3) as a low micromolar inhibitor of TRPC4 and TRPC5 channels that did not inhibit other TRP channels and lacked binding to a panel of 68 receptors [53], leading to use in several studies of the roles of TRPC1/4/5 channels (see Section 4). However, recent studies suggest that ML204 is a relatively poor inhibitor of TRPC1:C4 and TRPC1:C5 channels, at least when channels are activated by (−)-englerin A [16,19]. Because most native TRPC1/4/5 channels are thought to be heteromeric, this needs to be taken into account when using ML204 for functional studies.

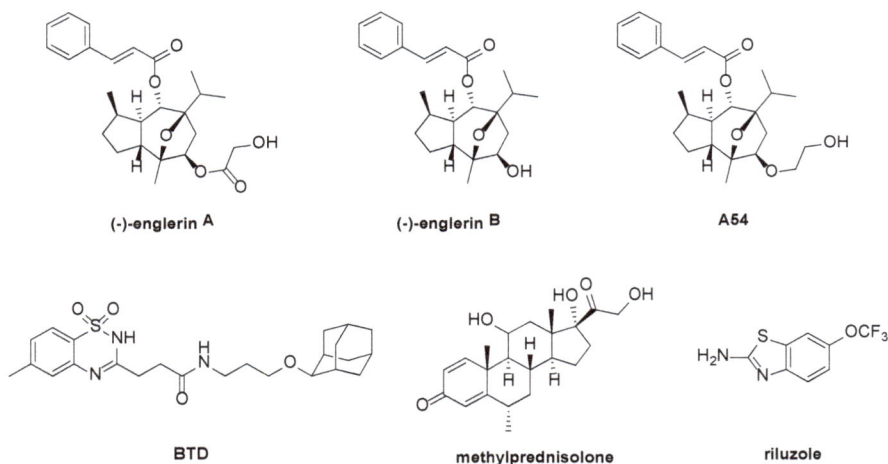

Figure 3. Structures of recently reported TRPC1/4/5 activators, the (−)EA metabolite (−)EB, and the (−)EA antagonist A54.

Since 2013, remarkable progress has been made with the discovery and development of potent and efficacious small-molecule modulators with unique selectivity profiles and improved pharmacological properties. In this section, we highlight selected small-molecule TRPC1/4/5 modulators reported since our previous review of the field [1].

3.1. Activators

3.1.1. Englerins

Screening of organic extracts from the East African plant *Phyllanthus engleri* against the NCI 60 cancer cell panel, followed by bioactivity-guided fractionation, led to the identification of the sequiterpene natural product $(-)$-englerin A $((-)$EA; Figure 3) as a compound with highly selective cytotoxicity against renal carcinoma cell lines [54,55]. Independent target identification approaches by the groups of Waldmann, Christmann and Beech [14,15] and by Novartis [51] revealed that $(-)$EA is a potent and efficacious activator (EC$_{50}$ = 10 nM) of native TRPC1:C4 channels in A498 renal cancer cells (see Section 4.3 for more detail about its relevance to cancer cell death).

Subsequent experiments revealed that $(-)$EA activates TRPC4:C4 and TRPC5:C5 channels with low nanomolar EC$_{50}$ values (11 and 7 nM, respectively) and a strong stimulatory effect on both intracellular Ca^{2+} levels and TRPC4:C4 and TRPC5:C5 ionic currents [14]. $(-)$EA has similar activating effects on heteromeric TRPC1:C4 and TRPC1:C5 channels, but TRPC6, TRPM2 and TRPV4 channels, 10 other ion channels, and 59 GPCRs lack responses to $(-)$EA [14,51]. $(-)$EA has been proposed to affect protein kinase C isoform θ (PKCθ) [56] and L-type calcium channels as well [57], although at higher concentrations (most experiments were done with 1–10 μM of $(-)$EA). Despite extensive target identification campaigns, no further targets have been found [14,51]. This suggests that $(-)$EA is a highly selective activator of TRPC1/4/5 channels.

The molecular mechanism by which $(-)$EA selectively activates TRPC1/4/5 channels is not understood. Excised membrane patch recordings in the presence or absence of G protein blockade suggest that $(-)$EA activates TRPC4/5 channels directly via a site exposed extracellularly or accessible only via the external leaflet of the bilayer [12]. The recent identification of A54 (Figure 3), a competitive antagonist of $(-)$EA-induced (but not Gd^{3+}-induced) TRPC4/5 activation, suggests the presence of a well-defined $(-)$EA binding site in TRPC4/5 channels [58]. Carson et al. found $(-)$EA to be stable in human and canine plasma. However, in plasma from rats and mice, $(-)$EA converts to the inactive metabolite $(-)$-englerin B $((-)$EB; resulting from glycolate ester hydrolysis; Figure 3) [51]. These effects were recapitulated in vivo upon oral dosing of 5 mg/kg in rodents: $(-)$EA blood levels did not rise above 12 nM, but $(-)$EB levels of >50 nM were detected. $(-)$EB neither activates TRPC1/4/5 channels nor is a potent A498 killer and also glycolic acid is inactive [51,59]. $(-)$EA is acutely toxic to rodents, although higher doses are tolerated upon intraperitoneal or subcutaneous injection than upon intravenous administration and toxicity may depend on drug formulation [51,60]. In contrast, $(-)$EB does not show toxicity to rodents [51].

3.1.2. BTD and Methylprednisolone

Through a screen of a ChemBioNet compound library against (mouse) TRPC5, Beckmann et al. found two novel TRPC5 activators: the glucocorticoid methylprednisolone (EC$_{50}$ = 12 μM) and N-[3-(adamantan-2-yloxy)propyl]-3-(6-methyl-1,1-dioxo-2H-1λ^6,2,4-benzothiadiazin-3-yl)propanamide (BTD; EC$_{50}$ = 1.4 μM) (Figure 3) [61]. The TRPC5 activation by these compounds is long-lasting, reversible, and sensitive to the recently published TRPC5 inhibitor clemizole (see Section 3.2.2). The more potent compound in this study, BTD, was studied in most detail. Although far less potent than $(-)$EA, BTD has remarkable selectivity on TRPC1/4/5 channel subtypes: patch clamp recordings revealed that BTD activates homomeric TRPC5:C5 channels as well as heteromeric TRPC1:C5 and (putative) TRPC4:C5 channels, but not TRPC4:C4 and TRPC1:C4 channels. The fact that BTD does not affect phospholipase C signalling, and activates TRPC5:C5 channels in inside-out excised membrane patches when applied from the intracellular side, suggests that the compound has a direct effect on TRPC5 channels. BTD has no effect on channels formed by TRPC3, TRPC6, TRPC7, TRPA1, TRPV1, TRPV2, TRPV3, TRPV4, TRPM2 and TRPM3. Methylprednisolone also showed selectivity for TRPC5 channels over other TRP channels, but can potentiate carbachol-induced TRPC4 activation.

3.1.3. Riluzole

Riluzole (Figure 3) is a marketed drug that delays the progression of amyotrophic lateral sclerosis (ALS) [62], and it also has anti-depressant properties [63]. Its wide-ranging effects on neural activity—in particular the neuromotor system—are thought to result from its effect on multiple ion channels; a review of the neural mechanisms of action of riluzole in ALS has been published by Bellingham [64]. Through a medium-throughput screen on mTRPC5-expressing HEK293 cells, Richter et al. found that riluzole activates TRPC5 channels with an EC_{50} of 9.2 μM [65]. Riluzole also activates overexpressed heteromeric TRPC1:C5 channels and endogenous TRPC5 channels in the U-87 glioblastoma cell line. The riluzole-induced TRPC5 activation is mechanistically different from La^{3+}-mediated activation. TRPC5 activation by riluzole is reversible upon washout, independent of G protein signalling and PLC activity, and occurs in both inside-out and cell-attached patches. These data suggest a relatively direct mechanism of action on TRPC5 channels.

3.2. Inhibitors

3.2.1. Xanthines

A patent by Hydra Biosciences and Boehringer-Ingelheim claims substituted xanthines and their use as TRPC5 inhibitors [66]. Circa 20% of the 621 compounds therein were reported to have IC_{50} values <100 nM, and eight compounds were further tested in rodent models of anxiety/depression. Studies from two different groups on the effects of the two most promising compounds in the patent have now been published. Our lab reported Pico145 (later called HC-608 by its inventors; Figure 4) as the most potent inhibitor of TRPC1/4/5 channels known to date [19,20]. In calcium recordings, Pico145 inhibits TRPC4 and TRPC5 with IC_{50} values of 349 pM and 1.3 nM, respectively. However, the highest potencies were measured against heteromeric channels (formed by TRPC4–C1 or TRPC5–C1 concatemers; IC_{50} values of 33 pM and 199 pM, respectively) and (−)EA-activated, endogenous TRPC1:C4 channels in A498 renal carcinoma cells (IC_{50} = 49 pM). In whole-cell recordings, Pico145 inhibits both inward and outward currents of TRPC4–C1 with picomolar IC_{50} values, upon activation with either (−)EA or the physiological TRPC4/C5 agonist sphingosine-1-phosphate (S1P). In contrast, 100 nM Pico145 does not affect activities of TRPC3, TRPC6, TRPV1, TRPV4, TRPA1, TRPM2, TRPM8 or store-operated Ca^{2+} entry mediated by Orai1.

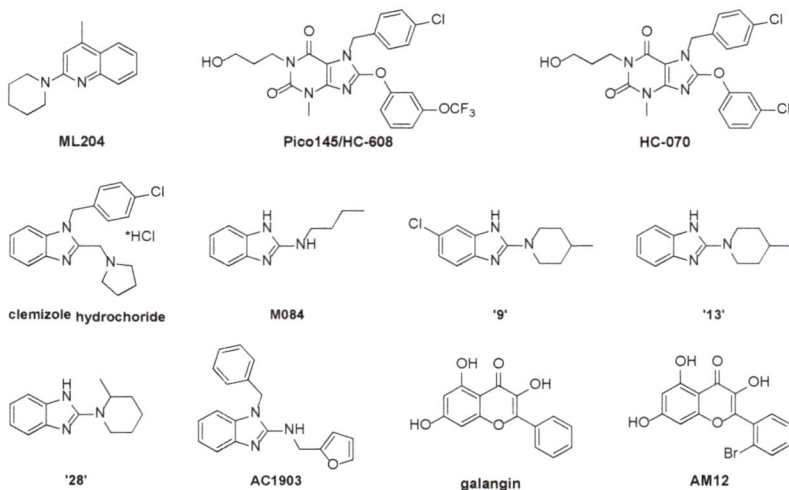

Figure 4. Structures of ML204 and recently reported TRPC1/4/5 inhibitors.

The molecular mechanism by which Pico145 selectively inhibits TRPC1/4/5 channels—and distinguishes between specific tetramers—is not understood. Excised outside-out membrane patch recordings suggest that Pico145 inhibits TRPC4 channels directly via a site exposed extracellularly or accessible only via the external leaflet of the bilayer, in a manner independent of cellular signalling mechanisms or Ca^{2+} concentrations, and that the potency of Pico145 depends partially on the concentration of the agonist $(-)$EA [19]. In addition, the rather mild voltage-dependence of the block does not support the idea of blockage deep inside the ion pore and electric field. Pico145 can also inhibit TRPC4 channels activated with the direct agonist Gd^{3+}, although at low concentrations (10 pM), Pico145 can also potentiate Gd^{3+}-induced currents mediated by TRPC4 [19]. These data, in combination with the ability of Pico145 to distinguish between closely related channels, suggest that Pico145 occupies a well-defined binding site essential to TRPC4/5 channel gating.

Recently, Just et al. reported the anxiolytic and antidepressant effects in mice of HC-070 (Figure 4), a close analogue of Pico145/HC-608 (for details, see Section 4.1.1) [67]. As part of this study, the activities of HC-070 were tested against TRPC1/4/5 channels (including human, mouse and rat versions) activated by La^{3+} or carbachol (the latter in combination with overexpression of muscarinic receptors), giving IC_{50} values between 0.3 and 2 nM. In addition, both Pico145/HC-608 and HC-070 were subjected to substantial selectivity profiling against a large set of ion channels, receptors, enzymes, kinases and transporters. At 1–2 μM (their solubility limit in Ringer's buffer), both compounds showed less than 50% inhibition of almost all tested targets. In addition, HC-070 [67] and Pico145 [66] have suitable pharmacokinetic properties for oral dosing. The excellent potency and selectivity of Pico145 and HC-070, in combination with their pharmacokinetic profiles and ready availability—both compounds can be synthesised in three steps from commercially available precursors—make these compounds highly suitable for functional studies of TRPC1/4/5 channels in cells and animals. These data also suggest that small molecules can be pharmacologically distinctive (by almost 40-fold for Pico145) for specific members of the TRPC1/4/5 subfamily, and that the development of multimer-specific inhibitors may be feasible.

3.2.2. Benzimidazoles

Several derivatives of benzimidazole and 2-aminobenzimidazole have been reported as TRPC1/4/5 inhibitors. Clemizole hydrochloride (Figure 4) was originally developed as a histamine H_1-receptor agonist [68]. However Richter et al. identified it as a novel inhibitor of (mouse) TRPC5:C5 channels with an IC_{50} of 1.1 μM [69]. Clemizole inhibits TRPC5:C5 channels reversibly and inhibition is irrespective of activation mode. TRPC4β:C4β channels are also inhibited by clemizole with an IC_{50} of 6.4 μM. In whole-cell patch-clamp recordings, 10 μM clemizole inhibits heteromeric TRPC1:C5 channels, and 50 μM clemizole partially inhibits riluzole-activated currents in the U-87 glioblastoma cell line. However, clemizole has limited selectivity, as it also inhibits channels formed by TRPC3 (IC_{50} = 9.1 μM), TRPC6 (IC_{50} = 11.3 μM) and TRPC7 (IC_{50} = 26.5 μM).

Following a high-throughput screen of 305,000 compounds (the same campaign that afforded the TRPC4/5 inhibitor ML204), M084 (Figure 4) was identified as a reversible inhibitor of (mouse) TRPC4 and TRPC5 with better stability and inhibitory kinetics than ML204 [70]. Because of relatively low potency of M084 against TRPC4:C4 (IC_{50} = 3.7–10.3 μM), TRPC5:C5 (IC_{50} = 8.2 μM) and TRPC1:C4 (IC_{50} = 8.3 μM), and its slight inhibition of TRPC3 (IC_{50} ~50 μM) and TRPC6 (IC_{50} ~60 μM), a series of 28 further 2-aminobenzimidazoles was generated and tested, suggesting that 2-aminobenzimidazoles and 2-aminoquinolines (such as ML204) have similar structure-activity relationship (SAR) profiles, and leading to three compounds ("9", "13" and "28"; Figure 4) with slightly higher potency than M084 (IC_{50} values between 3.1 and 6.6 μM) that do not inhibit TRPC3 and TRPC6. At 30 μM, M084 and its analogues "9", "13" and "28" do not activate or inhibit Ca^{2+} influx mediated by TRPA1, TRPM8, TRPV1 or TRPV3. The compounds inhibit TRPC4-mediated currents when applied from the extracellular side, and inhibition is not dependent on activation mode. In addition, at 30–100 μM, these compounds block the plateau potential mediated by TRPC4-containing channels in mouse lateral septal neurons.

A recent report on the use of small-molecule TRPC5 inhibitors to suppress progressive kidney disease (see Section 4.2) included the identification of AC1903 (Figure 4) as a selective TRPC5 inhibitor [71]. AC1903 shares structural similarities with both clemizole and M084 (Figure 4), and is equipotent to ML204 against riluzole-evoked TRPC5-mediated currents in whole-cell patch recordings (IC_{50} values of 13.6 and 14.7 μM, respectively). AC1903 is a weak inhibitor of TRPC4 ($IC_{50} > 100$ μM) and does not inhibit TRPC6 (no inhibition at 100 μM). In standard kinase profiling assays, AC1903 did not show off-target effects. No further selectivity assays on ion channels and receptors were reported, and it is not clear what the effect of AC1903 is on heteromeric TRPC1/4/5 channels.

3.2.3. Flavonols

Several dietary factors, including lipids and polyphenols, are known to inhibit TRPC channels [1]. More recently, we reported the identification of galangin (Figure 4), a natural product from *Alpinia officinarum* and other members of the ginger family, as a TRPC5 inhibitor [72]. Galangin inhibits homomeric TRPC5:C5 with an IC_{50} of 0.45 μM. In addition, galangin inhibits the basal (IC_{50} = 1.9 μM) and La^{3+}-evoked (IC_{50} = 6.1 μM) Ca^{2+} responses of differentiated 3T3-L1 cells (a model of mature adipocytes), which are thought to be mediated by heteromeric TRPC1:C5 channels. Subsequent structure-activity relationship (SAR) studies of 48 natural and synthetic flavonols led to the discovery of the more potent analogue AM12 (Figure 4), which inhibits TRPC5:C5 with an IC_{50} of 0.28 μM but is a relatively weak inhibitor of TRPC1:C5 channels. AM12 has no significant inhibitory effect on TRPC3, TRPV4, TRPM2 and store-operated Ca^{2+} release. The reversible inhibition by AM12 of (−)EA-evoked currents of TRPC4:C4 and TRPC5:C5 in outside-out excised membrane patches suggest a relatively direct effect on the channels. However, the effect of AM12 is dependent on the mode of activation; AM12 potentiates TRPC5 when stimulated with S1P or lysophosphatidylcholine (LPC) rather than (−)EA or Gd^{3+}. The SAR of the flavonol series also revealed that subtle changes to the flavonol structure can have major impacts on TRPC5 modulatory activity.

3.3. Choosing TRPC1/4/5 Modulators for Studies in Cells, Tissues and Animals

The effects of selected small-molecule TRPC1/4/5 modulators have been summarised in Tables 1 and 2. These compounds (and others described in this review) were profiled by different research groups using a variety of assays (e.g., fluorometric Ca^{2+} and Tl^+ measurements, calcium imaging, whole-cell patch recordings, excised membrane patch recordings, single channel recordings) in a variety of cell lines, and against TRPC1/4/5 channels from different species (usually the closely related human or mouse homologues). In addition, in inhibition assays, a wide range of activation mechanisms was used, including (−)EA, lanthanides, carbachol (often with overexpression of muscarinic receptors), and riluzole. Such differences need to be taken into account during the design of studies in cells or animals that make use of TRPC1/4/5 modulators.

Table 1. Overview of selected TRPC1/4/5 activators.

Compound Name	Targets (EC_{50})	Potential Off-Targets	Comments	References
(−)-englerin A	TRPC1/4/5 (1–10 nM)	PKCθ, $Ca_V1.2$ (μM concentrations needed)	High selectivity and efficacy; unstable in rodent plasma/GI tract	[14,15,51,56,57]
BTD	TRPC5:C5 (1.3 μM) TRPC1:C5, TRPC4:C5	TRPM8 (EC_{50} = 20.6 μM)	No effect on TRPC4:C4, TRPC1:C4, or other tested TRP channels	[61]
Riluzole	TRPC5:C5 (9.2 μM), TRPC1:C5	Multiple ion channels	Marketed drug	[64,65]

Table 2. Overview of selected TRPC1/4/5 inhibitors.

Compound Name	Targets (IC$_{50}$; Activator)	Potential Off-Targets	Comments	References
Pico145/HC-608	TRPC1/4/5 (0.03–1.3 nM; (−)EA)	Not known	Highly selective; suitable for in vivo use	[19,66,67]
HC-070	TRPC1/4/5 (0.3–2 nM; La^{3+} or carbachol/muscarinic receptors)	Not known	Highly selective; suitable for in vivo use	[66,67]
AC1903	TRPC5:C5 (14.7 µM)	Not known	No known effect on TRPC4:C4, TRPC6:C6 and kinases; suitable for in vivo use	[71]

Currently, the most promising TRPC1/4/5 activator for functional studies is (−)EA, which has unrivalled potency, efficacy and selectivity, making it a valuable probe of TRPC1/4/5 in cellular studies. However, its toxicity and instability in rodent serum and in the gastrointestinal (GI) tract limit its use for in vivo studies. BTD has the advantage that it activates (mouse) TRPC5 channels selectively with respect to TRPC4:C4 and TRPC1:C4 channels. It is selective against several other TRP channels, but potential off-targets have not been profiled comprehensively yet. The marketed drug riluzole can be used in vivo, but has relatively low potency and is thought to affect many ion channels [64].

The most promising TRPC1/4/5 inhibitors for functional studies are Pico145/HC-608 and HC-070. These compounds inhibit TRPC1/4/5 channels at (sub)nM concentrations, while at concentrations up to 1–2 µM, no significant effects on many other proteins have been found. Both compounds are orally bioavailable and are suitable for in vivo studies. AC1903 is an interesting compound because it can distinguish between TRPC5:C5 and TRPC4:C4 channels, while having no effect on TRPC6 or on a panel of kinases. In addition, its pharmacokinetic profile is compatible with in vivo use. However, its relatively low potency and unknown effects on different TRPC1/4/5 tetramers limit its current use as a chemical probe.

4. Using Small Molecules to Unravel (Patho)physiological Roles of TRPC1/4/5 Channels

Although observational clinical studies and changes detected in genetically- or pharmacologically-modified rodents and/or human tissue suggest multiple physiological roles of TRPC4/5 channels [1,73], disruption of the *Trpc4/5* genes [74] and global expression of a dominant-negative mutant TRPC5 [17] do not cause catastrophic phenotypes. However, TRPC1/4/5 channels have been implicated in various human diseases, including seizures (TRPC5 and TRPC1:C4) [75], fear-related behaviour (TRPC5) [76,77], severe pulmonary arterial hypertension (TRPC4) [78–80], heart failure (TRPC1/C4) [81], and chemotherapeutic resistance of cancers (TRPC5) [82,83]. This section contains a selection of recent studies on the roles of TRPC1/4/5 channels in health and disease to highlight examples of, and opportunities for, the use of small-molecule TRPC1/4/5 modulators to unravel TRPC1/4/5-mediated biological processes.

4.1. Roles of TRPC1/4/5 Channels in the Central Nervous System and Pain

4.1.1. Anxiety and Depression

One of the most researched areas of the role of TRPC1/4/5 channels is their potential involvement in the treatment of anxiety and depression. Evidence for these roles comes from studies utilising both transgenic mouse models and pharmacological modulators of these channels.

TRPC5 is expressed in brain regions associated with fear and anxiety, and *Trpc5*$^{−/−}$ mice show decreased fear behaviour compared to wild-type mice in behavioural tests [76], which was attributed to reduced potentiation of TRPC5 currents by G$_{q/11}$-coupled receptors, specifically those stimulated by glutamate and cholecystokinin 2 [76]. A similar anxiolytic phenotype was seen in mice lacking the TRPC4 subunit [84]. In addition, this study showed that TRPC4 protein knockdown limited to the lateral amygdala region—a region of the brain implicated in anxiety—showed the same phenotype as global *Trpc4*$^{−/−}$ mice. This suggests that both TRPC4 and TRPC5 channels in this specific area of the brain may be involved in the development of fear behaviours. It is not known if these TRPC4 and TRPC5 channels are homomers or heteromers, and whether TRPC1 is involved as well.

This proposed role of TRPC4/5 channels in fear behaviour has led to TRPC1/4/5 modulators being investigated as a possible treatment for anxiety. Indeed, the TRPC1/4/5 inhibitor M084 (see Section 3.2.2) [85] has anxiolytic and antidepressant effects in mice [77]. However, it is unknown whether this action of ML084 is due to its effects on homomeric or heteromeric channels, and whether the effect is specifically due to inhibition of TRPC4/5 channels located in the amygdala.

The xanthine HC-070, a highly potent and selective inhibitor of both homo- and heteromeric TRPC1/4/5 channels (see Section 3.2.1), reduces currents stimulated by CCK4 in basolateral amygdala in brain slices, and additionally shows anxiolytic and antidepressant effects in mouse behavioural studies, further confirming these channels as promising clinical targets in the treatment of anxiety and depression [67].

4.1.2. Epilepsy

TRPC1/4/5 channels have also been implicated in epilepsy. TRPC5 channels are highly expressed in rat hippocampal CA1 neurons, where they are thought to be involved in the formation of a prolonged depolarisation, the so-called plateau potential, following cholinergic innervation [86]. Thus far, inhibition of this process was only demonstrated with the non-specific compound 2-APB and with intracellular ATP. The effects of newer pharmacological modulators that show increased potency and selectivity are not known. Additionally, TRPC5 and TRPC1:4 channels are thought to be involved in epileptogenesis in mice, but via distinct expression patterns and mechanisms [75].

Evidence from human studies is limited, however both TRPC1 and TRPC4 proteins are upregulated in brain tissues of patients with focal cortical dysplasia, a common cause of refractory epilepsy [87,88]. Additionally, TRPC4 channel variants have also been implicated in generalised epilepsy [89]. Whether neuronal activity can be modulated by specific activators and inhibitors of TRPC1/4/5 remains to be elucidated.

4.1.3. Pain

TRPC1/4/5 channels have also been implicated in different types of pain. Westlund et al. investigated the role of TRPC4 channels in pain, using mice with a global knockout of the *Trpc4* gene [90]. The $Trpc4^{-/-}$ mice showed a resistance to mustard-oil induced visceral pain, as well as increased pain thresholds as compared to wild-type mice. In addition, animals treated with ML204 (0.5 and 1 mg/kg; orally administered) displayed reduced pain behaviours, similar to knockout mice. Wei et al. also investigated the role of TRPC4/5 channels in a spared nerve injury model of neuropathic pain with the TRPC4/5 inhibitor ML204 administered directly into the amygdala [91]. Administration of 5–10 µg ML204 decreased pain behaviour and showed an anti-hypersensitivity effect, which was not present when ML204 was injected into a control site.

4.1.4. Memory

Bröker-Lai et al. recently reported the presence of either TRPC1:C4:C5 channels or mixed populations of TRPC1:C4, TRPC1:C5 and TRPC4:C5 channels in mouse hippocampal cells (see Section 2.2) [18]. In this study, neurons and hippocampal slices from *Trpc1/Trpc4/Trpc5* triple knockout mice showed decreased (action potential-triggered) post-synaptic responses, while the animals displayed impaired cross-frequency coupling in hippocampal networks and deficits in spatial working memory and learning/adaptation. To date, the use of small-molecule TRPC1/4/5 modulators in studies of working memory and learning has not been reported, and it would be important to study whether TRPC1/4/5 inhibitors can have adverse effects on memory.

4.2. Roles of TRPC1/4/5 Channels in Kidney Disease

A role for TRPC1/4/5 has been postulated in the kidney, specifically in the development of kidney disease, however the literature provides conflicting findings in this field. TRPC5 channels are expressed in kidney podocytes, specialised cells that form the kidney filter. The channels form a molecular complex with the GTPase Rac1, and are involved in the regulation of cell migration and actin remodelling downstream of angiotensin stimulation [92]. *Trpc5* knockout protects mice from kidney filter barrier damage and resultant albuminuria caused by lipopolysaccharide (LPS), as well as protecting podocytes from barrier damage induced by protamine-sulfate. The same effects were seen in wild-type animals treated with the TRPC4/5 inhibitor ML204 [93]. This was also supported by in vitro data, showing an attenuation of cytoskeletal remodelling of podocytes, both after TRPC5 knockdown and pharmacological inhibition.

A role for TRPC5 in the development of focal segmental glomerusclerosis (FSGS), a leading cause of kidney failure, was also suggested by Zhou et al., who used a transgenic rat with a podocyte-specific overexpression of the angiotensin type 1 receptor (AT1R) [71]. These rats developed progressive kidney disease, and treatment of these rats with the TRPC4/5 inhibitor ML204 prevented podocyte death and attenuated the proteinuria caused by kidney damage. In addition, isolated cell studies showed increased riluzole-mediated single channel currents in rat glomeruli from AT1R animals, again inhibited by ML204. This study also introduced a novel TRPC5 inhibitor, named AC1903 (see Section 3.2.2), which showed similar effects to ML204 in suppressing proteinuria, in both AT1R transgenic animals and a model of hypertension-induced FSGS. However, a role of TRPC5 in progressive kidney disease was not supported by a study with transgenic mice overexpressing either wild-type TRPC5 or a dominant-negative TRPC5 mutant [94]. No difference in LPS-induced kidney damage was seen between the different animal groups, and treatment with the inhibitor ML204 (3×2 mg/kg) showed no effect on proteinuria in LPS-challenged animals. Treatment with the TRPC1/4/5 activator (−)EA (3 mg/kg, 24 h apart, i.p.) had no adverse effects on proteinuria in mice. However, as (−)EA displays poor stability in rodent plasma [51], it is debatable whether blood levels of (−)EA would reach levels sufficient to activate kidney TRPC5 channels and cause kidney damage. It is important to note, as stated by Van der Wijst and Bindels [95], that the two studies above used different doses of ML204 and different dosing regimens, which could account for the different effects seen. In addition, the exact identity of the TRPC1/4/5 channels expressed in the kidney is not known, and neither is the exact role of TRPC6 in FSGS. The channels may contain TRPC1, and although ML204 has recently been found to be a weak inhibitor of (−)EA-activated TRPC1:C5 channels, it is unknown how potent ML204 is against riluzole-activated channels. Overexpression of TRPC5 alone may not lead to formation of more channels linked to the studied phenotype, and knockout of *Trpc5* may lead to changes in formation of tetrameric ion channels by non-affected proteins such as TRPC1.

4.3. Roles of TRPC1/4/5 Channels in Cancer

It is well established that intracellular Ca^{2+} homeostasis is altered in cancer and that dysregulation of Ca^{2+} signalling is involved in tumour initiation, progression, metastasis, and angiogenesis. The roles of TRPC4 and TRPC5 in migration/proliferation of cancer cells, angiogenesis, cancer cell multi-drug resistance and (−)EA-induced renal cancer cell death have been reviewed in 2016 [96]. Here, we highlight the use of small-molecule TRPC1/4/5 modulators in the study of specific vulnerabilities of A498 renal carcinoma and SW982 synovial sarcoma cancer cells.

The discovery that the natural product (−)EA displays highly potent and selective cytotoxicity against eight renal cancer cell lines (GI_{50} values of under 1–87 nM; >1000-fold selectivity over other cell lines) led to target identification studies by several groups. PKCθ [56] and TRPC1:C4 channels (see Section 3.1.1) [14,15,51] have been proposed as the relevant target of (−)EA in renal cancer cells, and both proposals were based on extensive experimentation. A discussion of the evidence for these proposed mechanisms-of-action was included in a recent review on the englerins by Wu et al. [55]. It is possible that activation of TRPC1:C4 and effects on PKCθ-mediated gene regulation are linked in some cancer cells. However, in A498 cells and SW982 cells, both the potency of (−)EA in cell death assays (low nanomolar concentrations) and rapid onset of effects (minutes) are consistent with activation of TRPC1:C4 channels in these cells (low nanomolar EC_{50} values; similar to the potency in excised membrane patches from HEK293 cells containing TRPC1:C4 channels), but not with the proposed direct effects on PKCθ (majority of effects reported with 1–10 μM of (−)EA) and (much slower) downstream effects on gene transcription [14–16,51]. Furthermore, application of a PKCθ inhibitor has no effect on A498 cell proliferation and does not protect the cells from (−)EA-induced toxicity [51]. The analysis of >500 well characterized cancer cell lines revealed that TRPC4 mRNA abundance is the feature best correlated with sensitivity to (−)EA [51]. Knockdown of either TRPC1 or TRPC4 protects A498 and SW982 cells against (−)EA [14–16], while the Na^+/K^+ ATPase inhibitor ouabain increases the cytotoxic effect of (−)EA [15,16]. In addition, the well-characterised, highly potent and selective TRPC1/4/5 inhibitor Pico145 (see Section 3.2.1) strongly inhibits the cytotoxicity of (−)EA in SW982 cells [16], demonstrating the value of high-quality chemical probes in target validation studies. Overall, these studies suggest that (−)EA achieves its effect in A498 and SW982 cells through induction of sustained Na^+ entry through TRPC1:C4 channels, and that expression of functional TRPC1:C4 channels is necessary for potent and rapid (−)EA-induced cytotoxicity in these cell lines. In addition, Carson et al. demonstrated that overexpression of TRPC4 is sufficient to make HEK293 cells sensitive to growth inhibition by nanomolar concentrations of (−)EA (IC_{50} = 28 nM) [51].

A recent report by Wei et al. suggests that the expression of TRPC4-containing channels in medulloblastoma cells (which also express TRPC1 and TRPC5) promotes cell migration, contributing to invasion/metastasis [97]. However, the exact composition of these channels is not known, and inhibitory effects of (−)EA on migration of these cells are difficult to correlate with TRPC1/4/5 channel activity because the high concentration of (−)EA (10 μM) used in this study may affect additional mechanisms.

4.4. Roles of TRPC1/4/5 Channels in the Cardiovascular System

Several members of the TRP channel family have been implicated in the cardiovascular system, including TRPC1/4/5 (for reviews, see [98–101]). Here, we highlight a few recent examples. Based on studies in mice and rats, a role of TRPC5 channels as baroreceptor mechanosensors that regulate blood pressure has been suggested [73], although there was an error in the original published data and the findings have been challenged [102,103], indicating that further studies are needed.

Camacho Londoño et al. found that a background Ca^{2+} entry pathway that fine-tunes Ca^{2+} cycling in cardiomyocytes critically depends on TRPC1 and TRPC4 proteins. Suppression of this channel activity by *Trpc1/Trpc4* double knockout protects against pathological cardiac remodelling in mice, without affecting normal cardiac function [81].

TRPC4 channels have been studied in the development of pulmonary hypertension. Alzoubi et al. reported that *Trpc4* inactivation in rats confers a survival benefit in severe pulmonary arterial hypertension [78]. This was attributed to decreased occlusive remodelling of blood vessels in knockout animals. Recent reports suggest that TRPC4 channels are implicated in (bacterial toxin-induced/aggravated) pulmonary arterial hypertension/stenosis by increasing proliferation/permeability of endothelial and smooth muscle cells [79,80,104].

To date, no pharmacological modulators of TRPC1/4/5 have been reported in models of pathological cardiac remodelling or pulmonary hypertension.

4.5. Additional Roles and Opportunities

Trpc5 knockout animals have been used in the study of hepatic dyslipidaemia by Alawi et al. [105]. The authors compared cholestasis-induced liver injury in wild-type compared to *Trpc5* knockout mice, and found significantly reduced injury in knockout animals, as well as reduced dyslipidaemia and hypercholanemia, suggesting that TRPC5 channels could be involved in liver function.

TRPC5 channels have also been implicated in arthritis, although their role is unclear. Human fibroblast-like synoviocytes, the cells that secrete synovial fluid, express TRPC1 and TRPC5, and blocking their activity using antibodies or siRNA increases the secretion of matrix metalloproteases (MMPs), which is thought to lead to tissue remodelling and arthritis [34]. Additionally, TRPC5 channel expression is increased in the synovium in a mouse model of arthritis, and genetic deletion of TRPC5 as well as pharmacological inhibition with ML204 exacerbate arthritis induced by injection of complete Freud's adjuvant [106]. Whether pharmacological activation of TRPC5 is beneficial in arthritis is as yet unknown, but these results suggest a potentially protective role for TRPC5.

Mature adipocytes in murine and human perivascular fat express TRPC1 and TRPC5, and contain constitutively active channels with an I–V profile consistent with TRPC1:C5 channels [17]. These mature adipocytes also suppress excretion of adiponectin, an adipokine known to have anti-inflammatory, anti-atherosclerotic, and insulin-sensitising effects. Inhibition of TRPC1:C5 currents by genetic methods (RNAi or over-expression of a dominant-negative TRPC5 ion pore mutant) led to increased adiponectin secretion from adipocytes. The same effect was seen in vitro when TRPC1:C5 channels were blocked with a TRPC5 antibody or dietary fatty acids, revealing a potential mechanism for cardioprotection by these fatty acids.

TRPC channels have been implicated in diabetes-associated complications [107], and a recent study suggests that Ca^{2+}-permeable channels containing TRPC1 inhibit exercise-induced protection against high-fat diet-induced obesity and type II diabetes [108]. In addition, a recent study with $Trpc1/4/5/6^{-/-}$ mice suggests that TRPC channels contribute to the development of diabetic retinopathy. Knockout mice were protected from hyperglycaemia-evoked vasoregression and STZ-induced thinning of the retinal layer. These effects may be due to a role of TRPC channels in the regulation of expression/activity of glyoxalase 1 (GLO1), a key enzyme involved in the detoxification of the reactive metabolite methylglyoxal [109]. The exact nature of the channels involved in this phenotype is not known, and the effect of pharmacological TRPC1/4/5 modulators has not been reported yet.

5. Conclusions

Small-molecule modulators of TRPC1/4/5 channels can complement genetic approaches in dissecting the different roles of specific TRPC1/4/5 channels across species, tissues, and pathologies (see Section 4). Whereas genetic perturbation of TRPC proteins (overexpression, knockout/knockdown) can be performed with high precision, it may lead to secondary effects caused by alterations in native channel stoichiometries and protein–protein interactions, complicating data interpretation (and potentially masking the full potential of the channels as therapeutic targets) [110]. In contrast, chemical probes generally act quickly, acutely, reversibly, and can be used for experiments in cells, tissues and animals [111–113]. High-quality chemical probes are powerful tools in target validation studies, and can serve as useful starting points for drug development; however, their development is often costly in terms of time and resources. In addition, even high-quality chemical probes are likely to have off-targets, and potency and selectivity of a chemical probe may be dependent on cellular context (expression levels and localisation of targets, post-translational modifications, protein–protein interactions, presence of endogenous modulators, etc.). For these reasons, functional studies that carefully combine genetic and pharmacological approaches—and take limitations of both into account—are highly recommended for unravelling the biological roles of specific TRPC1/4/5 channels.

Traditionally, small-molecule modulation of TRPC1/4/5 channels has often relied on small-molecule modulators with low potency/selectivity. The emergence of highly potent and highly selective TRPC1/4/5 modulators such as (−)EA, Pico145 and HC-070 now offers unprecedented opportunities for TRPC1/4/5 research, and especially Pico145 and HC-070 are suitable for in vivo studies. The toxicity (depending on administration mode) [51,55,60] and instability of (−)EA in plasma and the digestive system [51,60] may limit its use for such studies though, and other activators such as BTD and riluzole have to be used at micromolar concentrations, increasing the chance of off-target effects. Therefore, additional potent and selective TRPC1/4/5 activators are needed.

The differentiation between different TRPC1/4/5 tetramers by compounds such as Pico145, ML204 and AC1903 suggests that development of tetramer-specific modulators is possible, and structural studies of TRPC1/4/5 channels may inform such developments. Such modulators could be used to reveal the composition of TRPC1/4/5 channels implicated in different (patho)physiological processes, which so far is often poorly understood (see Section 4). Studies of the roles of TRPC1/4/5 channels in anxiety, (−)EA-mediated cancer cell death and progressive kidney disease highlight the necessity and usefulness of small-molecule TRPC1/4/5 modulators for biological research. In addition, these studies show that it is essential to use carefully selected chemical probes and control compounds (with different selectivity profiles), at concentrations that are sufficient (and not much higher than that) to modulate the relevant TRPC1/4/5 channels under the tested conditions, and—where possible—to test dose-dependence of effects. When used appropriately, TRPC1/4/5 modulators can transform the understanding of TRPC1/4/5 channels in health and disease, and of the advantages and disadvantages of TRPC1/4/5 channels as drug targets.

Author Contributions: R.S.B. and D.J.B. planned the review. A.M., C.C.B., D.J.W., H.N.R. and R.S.B. performed literature searches. Drafts of sections were written by D.J.W. (Section 2), A.M. (Section 3), C.C.B. (Sections 4.1, 4.2, 4.4 and 4.5) and H.N.R. (Section 4.3). Data for Figure 2 were obtained by K.M. R.S.B. used these drafts to write the review with input from D.J.B. and K.M. All authors commented on the manuscript.

Funding: This work was supported by BBSRC research grant BB/P020208/1 (C.C.B., D.J.W., D.J.B. and R.S.B.) and a BBSRC studentship (A.M.). APC was sponsored by MDPI.

Conflicts of Interest: The authors declare no conflict of interest. A.M.'s PhD project is co-funded by AstraZeneca. The funders had no role in the design or preparation of this review, nor in the decision to publish it.

References

1. Bon, R.S.; Beech, D.J. In pursuit of small molecule chemistry for calcium-permeable non-selective TRPC channels—Mirage or pot of gold? *Br. J. Pharmacol.* **2013**, *170*, 459–474. [CrossRef] [PubMed]
2. Venkatachalam, K.; Montell, C. TRP channels. *Annu. Rev. Biochem.* **2007**, *76*, 387–417. [CrossRef] [PubMed]
3. Montell, C. The TRP superfamily of cation channels. *Sci. STKE* **2005**, *2005*, re3. [CrossRef] [PubMed]
4. Voets, T.; Talavera, K.; Owsianik, G.; Nilius, B. Sensing with TRP channels. *Nat. Chem. Biol.* **2005**, *1*, 85–92. [CrossRef] [PubMed]
5. Montell, C.; Birnbaumer, L.; Flockerzi, V.; Bindels, R.J.; Bruford, E.A.; Caterina, M.J.; Clapham, D.E.; Harteneck, C.; Heller, S.; Julius, D.; et al. A Unified Nomenclature for the Superfamily of TRP Cation Channels. *Mol. Cell* **2002**, *9*, 229–231. [CrossRef]
6. Abramowitz, J.; Birnbaumer, L. Physiology and pathophysiology of canonical transient receptor potential channels. *FASEB J.* **2009**, *23*, 297–328. [CrossRef] [PubMed]
7. Al-Shawaf, E.; Naylor, J.; Taylor, H.; Riches, K.; Milligan, C.J.; O'Regan, D.; Porter, K.E.; Li, J.; Beech, D.J. Short-term stimulation of calcium-permeable transient receptor potential canonical 5-containing channels by oxidized phospholipids. *Arterioscler. Thromb. Vasc. Biol.* **2010**, *30*, 1453–1459. [CrossRef] [PubMed]
8. Clapham, D.E. TRP channels as cellular sensors. *Nature* **2003**, *426*, 517–524. [CrossRef] [PubMed]
9. Vannier, B.; Peyton, M.; Boulay, G.; Brown, D.; Qin, N.; Jiang, M.; Zhu, X.; Birnbaumer, L. Mouse trp2, the homologue of the human trpc2 pseudogene, encodes mTrp2, a store depletion-activated capacitative Ca^{2+} entry channel. *Proc. Natl. Acad. Sci. USA* **1999**, *96*, 2060–2064. [CrossRef] [PubMed]
10. Plant, T.D.; Schaefer, M. TRPC4 and TRPC5: Receptor-operated Ca^{2+}-permeable nonselective cation channels. *Cell Calcium* **2003**, *33*, 441–450. [CrossRef]
11. Altschul, S.F.; Gish, W.; Miller, W.; Myers, E.W.; Lipman, D.J. Basic local alignment search tool. *J. Mol. Biol.* **1990**, *215*, 403–410. [CrossRef]
12. Bai, C.-X.; Giamarchi, A.; Rodat-Despoix, L.; Padilla, F.; Downs, T.; Tsiokas, L.; Delmas, P. Formation of a new receptor-operated channel by heteromeric assembly of TRPP2 and TRPC1 subunits. *EMBO Rep.* **2008**, *9*, 472–479. [CrossRef] [PubMed]
13. Ma, X.; Qiu, S.; Luo, J.; Ma, Y.; Ngai, C.-Y.; Shen, B.; Wong, C.; Huang, Y.; Yao, X. Functional role of vanilloid transient receptor potential 4-canonical transient receptor potential 1 complex in flow-induced Ca^{2+} influx. *Arterioscler. Thromb. Vasc. Biol.* **2010**, *30*, 851–858. [CrossRef] [PubMed]

14. Akbulut, Y.; Gaunt, H.J.; Muraki, K.; Ludlow, M.J.; Amer, M.S.; Bruns, A.; Vasudev, N.S.; Radtke, L.; Willot, M.; Hahn, S.; et al. (−)-Englerin A is a potent and selective activator of TRPC4 and TRPC5 calcium channels. *Angew. Chem. Int. Ed. Engl.* **2015**, *54*, 3787–3791. [CrossRef] [PubMed]

15. Ludlow, M.J.; Gaunt, H.J.; Rubaiy, H.N.; Musialowski, K.E.; Blythe, N.M.; Vasudev, N.S.; Muraki, K.; Beech, D.J. (−)-Englerin A-evoked Cytotoxicity Is Mediated by Na$^+$ Influx and Counteracted by Na$^+$/K$^+$-ATPase. *J. Biol. Chem.* **2017**, *292*, 723–731. [CrossRef] [PubMed]

16. Muraki, K.; Ohn, K.; Takezawa, A.; Su, H.; Hatano, N.; Muraki, Y.; Hamzah, N.; Foster, R.; Waldmann, H.; Christmann, M.; et al. Na$^+$ entry through heteromeric TRPC4/C1 channels mediates (−) Englerin A-induced cytotoxicity in synovial sarcoma cells. *Sci. Rep.* **2017**, *7*, 16988. [CrossRef] [PubMed]

17. Sukumar, P.; Sedo, A.; Li, J.; Wilson, L.A.; O'Regan, D.; Lippiat, J.D.; Porter, K.E.; Kearney, M.T.; Ainscough, J.F.X.; Beech, D.J. Constitutively active TRPC channels of adipocytes confer a mechanism for sensing dietary fatty acids and regulating adiponectin. *Circ. Res.* **2012**, *111*, 191–200. [CrossRef] [PubMed]

18. Bröker-Lai, J.; Kollewe, A.; Schindeldecker, B.; Pohle, J.; Chi, V.N.; Mathar, I.; Guzman, R.; Schwarz, Y.; Lai, A.; Weißgerber, P.; et al. Heteromeric channels formed by TRPC1, TRPC4 and TRPC5 define hippocampal synaptic transmission and working memory. *EMBO J.* **2017**, *36*, 2770–2789. [CrossRef] [PubMed]

19. Rubaiy, H.N.; Ludlow, M.J.; Henrot, M.; Gaunt, H.J.; Miteva, K.; Cheung, S.Y.; Tanahashi, Y.; Hamzah, N.; Musialowski, K.E.; Blythe, N.M.; et al. Picomolar, selective, and subtype-specific small-molecule inhibition of TRPC1/4/5 channels. *J. Biol. Chem.* **2017**, *292*, 8158–8173. [CrossRef] [PubMed]

20. Rubaiy, H.N.; Ludlow, M.J.; Bon, R.S.; Beech, D.J. Pico145—Powerful new tool for TRPC1/4/5 channels. *Channels* **2017**, *11*, 362–364. [CrossRef] [PubMed]

21. Chen, X.; Wang, Q.; Ni, F.; Ma, J. Structure of the full-length Shaker potassium channel Kv1.2 by normal-mode-based X-ray crystallographic refinement. *Proc. Natl. Acad. Sci. USA* **2010**, *107*, 11352–11357. [CrossRef] [PubMed]

22. Kühlbrandt, W. Biochemistry. The resolution revolution. *Science* **2014**, *343*, 1443–1444. [CrossRef] [PubMed]

23. Liao, M.; Cao, E.; Julius, D.; Cheng, Y. Structure of the TRPV1 ion channel determined by electron cryo-microscopy. *Nature* **2013**, *504*, 107–112. [CrossRef] [PubMed]

24. Winkler, P.A.; Huang, Y.; Sun, W.; Du, J.; Lü, W. Electron cryo-microscopy structure of a human TRPM4 channel. *Nature* **2017**, *552*, 200. [CrossRef] [PubMed]

25. Zhou, X.; Li, M.; Su, D.; Jia, Q.; Li, H.; Li, X.; Yang, J. Cryo-EM structures of the human endolysosomal TRPML3 channel in three distinct states. *Nat. Struct. Mol. Biol.* **2017**, *24*, 1146–1154. [CrossRef] [PubMed]

26. Grieben, M.; Pike, A.C.W.; Shintre, C.A.; Venturi, E.; El-Ajouz, S.; Tessitore, A.; Shrestha, L.; Mukhopadhyay, S.; Mahajan, P.; Chalk, R.; et al. Structure of the polycystic kidney disease TRP channel Polycystin-2 (PC2). *Nat. Struct. Mol. Biol.* **2017**, *24*, 114–122. [CrossRef] [PubMed]

27. Paulsen, C.E.; Armache, J.-P.; Gao, Y.; Cheng, Y.; Julius, D. Structure of the TRPA1 ion channel suggests regulatory mechanisms. *Nature* **2015**, *520*, 511–517. [CrossRef] [PubMed]

28. Fan, C.; Choi, W.; Sun, W.; Du, J.; Lu, W. Structure of the human lipid-gated cation channel TRPC3. *eLife* **2018**, *7*, e36852. [CrossRef] [PubMed]

29. Tang, Q.; Guo, W.; Zheng, L.; Wu, J.-X.; Liu, M.; Zhou, X.; Zhang, X.; Chen, L. Structure of the receptor-activated human TRPC6 and TRPC3 ion channels. *Cell Res.* **2018**. [CrossRef] [PubMed]

30. Duan, J.; Li, J.; Bo, Z.; Chen, G.-L.; Peng, X.; Zhang, Y.; Wang, J.; Clapham, D.E.; Li, Z.; Zhang, J. Structure of the mouse TRPC4 ion channel. *bioRxiv* **2018**, 282715. [CrossRef]

31. Vinayagam, D.; Mager, T.; Apelbaum, A.; Bothe, A.; Merino, F.; Hofnagel, O.; Gatsogiannis, C.; Raunser, S. Electron cryo-microscopy structure of the canonical TRPC4 ion channel. *eLife* **2018**, *7*, e36615. [CrossRef] [PubMed]

32. Cao, E.; Liao, M.; Cheng, Y.; Julius, D. TRPV1 structures in distinct conformations reveal activation mechanisms. *Nature* **2013**, *504*, 113–118. [CrossRef] [PubMed]

33. Gao, Y.; Cao, E.; Julius, D.; Cheng, Y. TRPV1 structures in nanodiscs reveal mechanisms of ligand and lipid action. *Nature* **2016**, *534*, 347. [CrossRef] [PubMed]

34. Xu, S.-Z.; Sukumar, P.; Zeng, F.; Li, J.; Jairaman, A.; English, A.; Naylor, J.; Ciurtin, C.; Majeed, Y.; Milligan, C.J.; et al. TRPC channel activation by extracellular thioredoxin. *Nature* **2008**, *451*, 69–72. [CrossRef] [PubMed]

35. Yoshida, T.; Inoue, R.; Morii, T.; Takahashi, N.; Yamamoto, S.; Hara, Y.; Tominaga, M.; Shimizu, S.; Sato, Y.; Mori, Y. Nitric oxide activates TRP channels by cysteine S-nitrosylation. *Nat. Chem. Biol.* **2006**, *2*, 596–607. [CrossRef] [PubMed]

36. Karakas, E.; Furukawa, H. Crystal structure of a heterotetrameric NMDA receptor ion channel. *Science* **2014**, *344*, 992–997. [CrossRef] [PubMed]

37. Lü, W.; Du, J.; Goehring, A.; Gouaux, E. Cryo-EM structures of the triheteromeric NMDA receptor and its allosteric modulation. *Science* **2017**, *355*, eaal3729. [CrossRef] [PubMed]

38. Morales-Perez, C.L.; Noviello, C.M.; Hibbs, R.E. X-ray structure of the human α4β2 nicotinic receptor. *Nature* **2016**, *538*, 411–415. [CrossRef] [PubMed]

39. Alfonso, S.; Benito, O.; Alicia, S.; Angélica, Z.; Patricia, G.; Diana, K.; Luis, V. Regulation of the cellular localization and function of human transient receptor potential channel 1 by other members of the TRPC family. *Cell Calcium* **2008**, *43*, 375–387. [CrossRef] [PubMed]

40. Liao, Y.; Erxleben, C.; Abramowitz, J.; Flockerzi, V.; Zhu, M.X.; Armstrong, D.L.; Birnbaumer, L. Functional interactions among Orai1, TRPCs, and STIM1 suggest a STIM-regulated heteromeric Orai/TRPC model for SOCE/Icrac channels. *Proc. Natl. Acad. Sci. USA* **2008**, *105*, 2895–2900. [CrossRef] [PubMed]

41. Storch, U.; Forst, A.-L.; Philipp, M.; Gudermann, T.; Mederos y Schnitzler, M. Transient receptor potential channel 1 (TRPC1) reduces calcium permeability in heteromeric channel complexes. *J. Biol. Chem.* **2012**, *287*, 3530–3540. [CrossRef] [PubMed]

42. Hofmann, T.; Schaefer, M.; Schultz, G.; Gudermann, T. Subunit composition of mammalian transient receptor potential channels in living cells. *Proc. Natl. Acad. Sci. USA* **2002**, *99*, 7461–7466. [CrossRef] [PubMed]

43. Barrera, N.P.; Shaifta, Y.; McFadzean, I.; Ward, J.P.T.; Henderson, R.M.; Edwardson, J.M. AFM imaging reveals the tetrameric structure of the TRPC1 channel. *Biochem. Biophys. Res. Commun.* **2007**, *358*, 1086–1090. [CrossRef] [PubMed]

44. Kunert-Keil, C.; Bisping, F.; Krüger, J.; Brinkmeier, H. Tissue-specific expression of TRP channel genes in the mouse and its variation in three different mouse strains. *BMC Genom.* **2006**, *7*, 159. [CrossRef] [PubMed]

45. Antoniotti, S.; Pla, A.F.; Barral, S.; Scalabrino, O.; Munaron, L.; Lovisolo, D. Interaction between TRPC Channel Subunits in Endothelial Cells. *J. Recept. Signal Transduct.* **2006**, *26*, 225–240. [CrossRef] [PubMed]

46. Zeng, B.; Yuan, C.; Yang, X.; Atkin, S.L.; Xu, S.-Z. TRPC Channels and Their Splice Variants are Essential for Promoting Human Ovarian Cancer Cell Proliferation and Tumorigenesis. *Curr. Cancer Drug Targets* **2012**, *13*, 103–116. [CrossRef]

47. Wes, P.D.; Chevesich, J.; Jeromin, A.; Rosenberg, C.; Stetten, G.; Montell, C. TRPC1, a human homolog of a Drosophila store-operated channel. *Proc. Natl. Acad. Sci. USA* **1995**, *92*, 9652–9656. [CrossRef] [PubMed]

48. Schaefer, M.; Plant, T.D.; Stresow, N.; Albrecht, N.; Schultz, G. Functional differences between TRPC4 splice variants. *J. Biol. Chem.* **2002**, *277*, 3752–3759. [CrossRef] [PubMed]

49. Mery, L.; Magnino, F.; Schmidt, K.; Krause, K.-H.; Dufour, J.-F. Alternative splice variants of hTrp4 differentially interact with the C-terminal portion of the inositol 1,4,5-trisphosphate receptors. *FEBS Lett.* **2001**, *487*, 377–383. [CrossRef]

50. Otsuguro, K.; Tang, J.; Tang, Y.; Xiao, R.; Freichel, M.; Tsvilovskyy, V.; Ito, S.; Flockerzi, V.; Zhu, M.X.; Zholos, A.V. Isoform-specific inhibition of TRPC4 channel by phosphatidylinositol 4,5-bisphosphate. *J. Biol. Chem.* **2008**, *283*, 10026–10036. [CrossRef] [PubMed]

51. Carson, C.; Raman, P.; Tullai, J.; Xu, L.; Henault, M.; Thomas, E.; Yeola, S.; Lao, J.; McPate, M.; Verkuyl, J.M.; et al. Englerin A Agonizes the TRPC4/C5 Cation Channels to Inhibit Tumor Cell Line Proliferation. *PLoS ONE* **2015**, *10*, e0127498. [CrossRef] [PubMed]

52. Gautier, M.; Dhennin-Duthille, I.; Ay, A.S.; Rybarczyk, P.; Korichneva, I.; Ouadid-Ahidouch, H. New insights into pharmacological tools to TR(i)P cancer up. *Br. J. Pharmacol.* **2014**, *171*, 2582–2592. [CrossRef] [PubMed]

53. Miller, M.; Shi, J.; Zhu, Y.; Kustov, M.; Tian, J.B.; Stevens, A.; Wu, M.; Xu, J.; Long, S.; Yang, P.; et al. Identification of ML204, a novel potent antagonist that selectively modulates native TRPC4/C5 ion channels. *J. Biol. Chem.* **2011**, *286*, 33436–33446. [CrossRef] [PubMed]

54. Ratnayake, R.; Covell, D.; Ransom, T.T.; Gustafson, K.R.; Beutler, J.A. Englerin A, a selective inhibitor of renal cancer cell growth, from *Phyllanthus engleri*. *Org. Lett.* **2009**, *11*, 57–60. [CrossRef] [PubMed]

55. Wu, Z.; Zhao, S.; Fash, D.M.; Li, Z.; Chain, W.J.; Beutler, J.A. Englerins: A Comprehensive Review. *J. Nat. Prod.* **2017**, *80*, 771–781. [CrossRef] [PubMed]

56. Sourbier, C.; Scroggins, B.T.; Ratnayake, R.; Prince, T.L.; Lee, S.; Lee, M.-J.; Nagy, P.L.; Lee, Y.H.; Trepel, J.B.; Beutler, J.A.; et al. Englerin A stimulates PKCθ to inhibit insulin signaling and to simultaneously activate HSF1: Pharmacologically induced synthetic lethality. *Cancer Cell* **2013**, *23*, 228–237. [CrossRef] [PubMed]

57. Rodrigues, T.; Sieglitz, F.; Somovilla, V.J.; Cal, P.M.S.D.; Galione, A.; Corzana, F.; Bernardes, G.J.L. Unveiling (−)-Englerin A as a Modulator of L-Type Calcium Channels. *Angew. Chem. Int. Ed.* **2016**, *55*, 11077–11081. [CrossRef] [PubMed]

58. Rubaiy, H.N.; Seitz, T.; Hahn, S.; Choidas, A.; Habenberger, P.; Klebl, B.; Dinkel, K.; Nussbaumer, P.; Waldmann, H.; Christmann, M.; et al. Identification of an (−)-englerin A analogue, which antagonizes (−)-englerin A at TRPC1/4/5 channels. *Br. J. Pharmacol.* **2018**, *175*, 830–839. [CrossRef] [PubMed]

59. Nicolaou, K.C.; Kang, Q.; Ng, S.Y.; Chen, D.Y.-K. Total synthesis of englerin A. *J. Am. Chem. Soc.* **2010**, *132*, 8219–8222. [CrossRef] [PubMed]

60. Fash, D.M.; Peer, C.J.; Li, Z.; Talisman, I.J.; Hayavi, S.; Sulzmaier, F.J.; Ramos, J.W.; Sourbier, C.; Neckers, L.; Figg, W.D.; et al. Synthesis of a Stable and Orally Bioavailable Englerin Analogue. *Bioorg. Med. Chem. Lett.* **2016**, *26*, 2641–2644. [CrossRef] [PubMed]

61. Beckmann, H.; Richter, J.; Hill, K.; Urban, N.; Lemoine, H.; Schaefer, M. A benzothiadiazine derivative and methylprednisolone are novel and selective activators of transient receptor potential canonical 5 (TRPC5) channels. *Cell Calcium* **2017**, *66*, 10–18. [CrossRef] [PubMed]

62. Schuster, J.E.; Fu, R.; Siddique, T.; Heckmann, C.J. Effect of prolongued riluzole exposure on cultured motoneurons in a mouse model of ALS. *J. Neurophysiol.* **2012**, *107*, 482–484. [CrossRef] [PubMed]

63. Grant, P.; Song, J.Y.; Swedo, S.E. Review of the Use of the Glutamate Antagonist Riluzole in Psychiatric Disorders and a Description of Recent Use in Childhood Obsessive-Compulsive Disorder. *J. Child Adolesc. Psychopharmacol.* **2010**, *20*, 309–315. [CrossRef] [PubMed]

64. Bellingham, M.C. A Review of the Neural Mechanisms of Action and Clinical Efficiency of Riluzole in Treating Amyotrophic Lateral Sclerosis: What have we Learned in the Last Decade? *CNS Neurosci. Ther.* **2011**, *17*, 4–31. [CrossRef] [PubMed]

65. Richter, J.M.; Schaefer, M.; Hill, K. Riluzole activates TRPC5 channels independently of PLC activity. *Br. J. Pharmacol.* **2014**, *171*, 158–170. [CrossRef] [PubMed]

66. Chenard, B.L.; Gallaschun, R.J. Substituted Xanthines and Methods of Use Thereof. WO/2014/143799, 18 September 2014.

67. Just, S.; Chenard, B.L.; Ceci, A.; Strassmaier, T.; Chong, A.; Blair, N.T.; Gallaschun, R.J.; Camino, D.; Cantin, S.; Amours, M.D.; et al. Treatment with HC-070, a potent inhibitor of TRPC4 and TRPC5, leads to anxiolytic and antidepressant effects in mice. *PLoS ONE* **2018**, *1*, 1–32. [CrossRef] [PubMed]

68. Einav, S.; Sobol, H.D.; Gehrig, E.; Glenn, J.S. The Hepatitis C virus (HCV) NS4B RNA binding inhibitor, clemizole, is highly synergistic with HCV protease inhibitors. *J. Infect. Dis.* **2010**, *202*, 65–74. [CrossRef] [PubMed]

69. Richter, J.M.; Schaefer, M.; Hill, K. Clemizole Hydrochloride is a Novel and Potent Inhibitor of Transient Receptor Potential Channel TRPC5. *Mol. Pharmacol.* **2014**, *86*, 514–521. [CrossRef] [PubMed]

70. Zhu, Y.; Lu, Y.; Qu, C.; Miller, M.; Tian, J.; Thakur, D.P.; Zhu, J.; Deng, Z.; Hu, X.; Wu, M.; et al. Identification and optimization of 2-aminobenzimidazole derivatives as novel inhibitors of TRPC4 and TRPC5 channels. *Br. J. Pharmacol.* **2015**, *172*, 3495–3509. [CrossRef] [PubMed]

71. Zhou, Y.; Castonguay, P.; Sidhom, E.H.; Clark, A.R.; Dvela-Levitt, M.; Kim, S.; Sieber, J.; Wieder, N.; Jung, J.Y.; Andreeva, S.; et al. A small-molecule inhibitor of TRPC5 ion channels suppresses progressive kidney disease in animal models. *Science* **2017**, *358*, 1332–1336. [CrossRef] [PubMed]

72. Naylor, J.; Minard, A.; Gaunt, H.J.; Amer, M.S.; Wilson, L.A.; Migliore, M.; Cheung, S.Y.; Rubaiy, H.N.; Blythe, N.M.; Musialowski, K.E.; et al. Natural and synthetic flavonoid modulation of TRPC5 channels. *Br. J. Pharmacol.* **2016**, *173*, 562–574. [CrossRef] [PubMed]

73. Lau, O.-C.; Shen, B.; Wong, C.-O.; Tjong, Y.-W.; Lo, C.-Y.; Wang, H.-C.; Huang, Y.; Yung, W.-H.; Chen, Y.-C.; Fung, M.-L.; et al. TRPC5 channels participate in pressure-sensing in aortic baroreceptors. *Nat. Commun.* **2016**, *7*, 11947. [CrossRef] [PubMed]

74. Babu, S.S.; Wojtowicz, A.; Freichel, M.; Birnbaumer, L.; Hecker, M.; Cattaruzza, M. Mechanism of Stretch-Induced Activation of the Mechanotransducer Zyxin in Vascular Cells. *Sci. Signal.* **2012**, *5*, ra91. [CrossRef]

75. Phelan, K.D.; Shwe, U.T.; Abramowitz, J.; Wu, H.; Rhee, S.W.; Howell, M.D.; Gottschall, P.E.; Freichel, M.; Flockerzi, V.; Birnbaumer, L.; et al. Canonical transient receptor channel 5 (TRPC5) and TRPC1/4 contribute to seizure and excitotoxicity by distinct cellular mechanisms. *Mol. Pharmacol.* **2013**, *83*, 429–438. [CrossRef] [PubMed]

76. Riccio, A.; Li, Y.; Moon, J.; Kim, K.-S.; Smith, K.S.; Rudolph, U.; Gapon, S.; Yao, G.L.; Tsvetkov, E.; Rodig, S.J.; et al. Essential role for TRPC5 in amygdala function and fear-related behavior. *Cell* **2009**, *137*, 761–772. [CrossRef] [PubMed]

77. Yang, L.-P.; Jiang, F.-J.; Wu, G.-S.; Deng, K.; Wen, M.; Zhou, X.; Hong, X.; Zhu, M.X.; Luo, H.-R. Acute Treatment with a Novel TRPC4/C5 Channel Inhibitor Produces Antidepressant and Anxiolytic-Like Effects in Mice. *PLoS ONE* **2015**, *10*, e0136255. [CrossRef] [PubMed]

78. Alzoubi, A.; Almalouf, P.; Toba, M.; O'Neill, K.; Qian, X.; Francis, M.; Taylor, M.S.; Alexeyev, M.; McMurtry, I.F.; Oka, M.; et al. TRPC4 Inactivation Confers a Survival Benefit in Severe Pulmonary Arterial Hypertension. *Am. J. Pathol.* **2013**, *183*, 1779–1788. [CrossRef] [PubMed]

79. Chen, G.-L.; Jiang, H.; Zou, F. Upregulation of Transient Receptor Potential Canonical Channels Contributes to Endotoxin-Induced Pulmonary Arterial Stenosis. *Med. Sci. Monit.* **2016**, *22*, 2679–2684. [CrossRef] [PubMed]

80. Francis, M.; Xu, N.; Zhou, C.; Stevens, T. Transient Receptor Potential Channel 4 Encodes a Vascular Permeability Defect and High-Frequency Ca^{2+} Transients in Severe Pulmonary Arterial Hypertension. *Am. J. Pathol.* **2016**, *186*, 1701–1709. [CrossRef] [PubMed]

81. Londoño, J.E.C.; Tian, Q.; Hammer, K.; Schröder, L.; Londoño, J.C.; Reil, J.C.; He, T.; Oberhofer, M.; Mannebach, S.; Mathar, I.; et al. A background Ca^{2+} entry pathway mediated by TRPC1/TRPC4 is critical for development of pathological cardiac remodelling. *Eur. Heart J.* **2015**, *36*, 2257–2266. [CrossRef] [PubMed]

82. Ma, X.; Chen, Z.; Hua, D.; He, D.; Wang, L.; Zhang, P.; Wang, J.; Cai, Y.; Gao, C.; Zhang, X.; et al. Essential role for TrpC5-containing extracellular vesicles in breast cancer with chemotherapeutic resistance. *Proc. Natl. Acad. Sci. USA* **2014**, *111*, 6389–6394. [CrossRef] [PubMed]

83. He, D.-X.; Ma, X. Transient receptor potential channel C5 in cancer chemoresistance. *Acta Pharmacol. Sin.* **2016**, *37*, 19–24. [CrossRef] [PubMed]

84. Riccio, A.; Li, Y.; Tsvetkov, E.; Gapon, S.; Yao, G.L.; Smith, K.S.; Engin, E.; Rudolph, U.; Bolshakov, V.Y.; Clapham, D.E. Decreased Anxiety-Like Behavior and G q/11-Dependent Responses in the Amygdala of Mice Lacking TRPC4 Channels. *J. Neurosci.* **2014**, *34*, 3653–3667. [CrossRef] [PubMed]

85. Chen, X.; Yang, D.; Ma, S.; He, H.; Luo, Z.; Feng, X.; Cao, T.; Ma, L.; Yan, Z.; Liu, D.; et al. Increased rhythmicity in hypertensive arterial smooth muscle is linked to transient receptor potential canonical channels. *J. Cell. Mol. Med.* **2010**, *14*, 2483–2494. [CrossRef] [PubMed]

86. Tai, C.; Hines, D.J.; Choi, H.B.; MacVicar, B.A. Plasma membrane insertion of TRPC5 channels contributes to the cholinergic plateau potential in hippocampal CA1 pyramidal neurons. *Hippocampus* **2011**, *21*, 958–967. [CrossRef] [PubMed]

87. Wang, L.-K.; Chen, X.; Zhang, C.-Q.; Liang, C.; Wei, Y.-J.; Yue, J.; Liu, S.-Y.; Yang, H. Elevated Expression of TRPC4 in Cortical Lesions of Focal Cortical Dysplasia II and Tuberous Sclerosis Complex. *J. Mol. Neurosci.* **2017**, *62*, 222–231. [CrossRef] [PubMed]

88. Zang, Z.; Li, S.; Zhang, W.; Chen, X.; Zheng, D.; Shu, H.; Guo, W.; Zhao, B.; Shen, K.; Wei, Y.J.; et al. Expression Patterns of TRPC1 in Cortical Lesions from Patients with Focal Cortical Dysplasia. *J. Mol. Neurosci.* **2015**, *57*, 265–272. [CrossRef] [PubMed]

89. Von Spiczak, S.; Muhle, H.; Helbig, I.; de Kovel, C.G.F.; Hampe, J.; Gaus, V.; Koeleman, B.P.C.; Lindhout, D.; Schreiber, S.; Sander, T.; et al. Association study of TRPC4 as a candidate gene for generalized epilepsy with photosensitivity. *Neuromol. Med.* **2010**, *12*, 292–299. [CrossRef] [PubMed]

90. Westlund, K.N.; Zhang, L.P.; Ma, F.; Nesemeier, R.; Ruiz, J.C.; Ostertag, E.M.; Crawford, J.S.; Babinski, K.; Marcinkiewicz, M.M. A rat knockout model implicates TRPC4 in visceral pain sensation. *Neuroscience* **2014**, *262*, 165–175. [CrossRef] [PubMed]

91. Wei, H.; Sagalajev, B.; Yüzer, M.A.; Koivisto, A.; Pertovaara, A. Regulation of neuropathic pain behavior by amygdaloid TRPC4/C5 channels. *Neurosci. Lett.* **2015**, *608*, 12–17. [CrossRef] [PubMed]

92. Tian, D.; Jacobo, S.M.P.; Billing, D.; Rozkalne, A.; Gage, S.D.; Anagnostou, T.; Pavenstädt, H.; Pavenstaedt, H.; Hsu, H.-H.; Schlondorff, J.; et al. Antagonistic regulation of actin dynamics and cell motility by TRPC5 and TRPC6 channels. *Sci. Signal.* **2010**, *3*, ra77. [CrossRef] [PubMed]

93. Schaldecker, T.; Kim, S.; Tarabanis, C.; Tian, D.; Hakroush, S.; Castonguay, P.; Ahn, W.; Wallentin, H.; Heid, H.; Hopkins, C.R.; et al. Inhibition of the TRPC5 ion channel protects the kidney filter. *J. Clin. Investig.* **2013**, *123*, 5298–5309. [CrossRef] [PubMed]

94. Wang, X.; Dande, R.R.; Yu, H.; Samelko, B.; Miller, R.E.; Altintas, M.M.; Reiser, J. TRPC5 Does Not Cause or Aggravate Glomerular Disease. *J. Am. Soc. Nephrol.* **2018**, *29*, 409–415. [CrossRef] [PubMed]

95. Van der Wijst, J.; Bindels, R.J.M. Renal physiology: TRPC5 inhibition to treat progressive kidney disease. *Nat. Rev. Nephrol.* **2018**, *14*, 145. [CrossRef] [PubMed]

96. Gaunt, H.J.; Vasudev, N.S.; Beech, D.J. Transient receptor potential canonical 4 and 5 proteins as targets in cancer therapeutics. *Eur. Biophys. J.* **2016**, *45*, 611–620. [CrossRef] [PubMed]

97. Wei, W.-C.; Huang, W.-C.; Lin, Y.-P.; Becker, E.B.E.; Ansorge, O.; Flockerzi, V.; Conti, D.; Cenacchi, G.; Glitsch, M.D. Functional expression of calcium-permeable canonical transient receptor potential 4-containing channels promotes migration of medulloblastoma cells. *J. Physiol.* **2017**, *595*, 5525–5544. [CrossRef] [PubMed]

98. Earley, S.; Brayden, J.E. Transient receptor potential channels in the vasculature. *Physiol. Rev.* **2015**, *95*, 645–690. [CrossRef] [PubMed]

99. Firth, A.L.; Remillard, C.V.; Yuan, J.X.-J. TRP channels in hypertension. *Biochim. Biophys. Acta Mol. Basis Dis.* **2007**, *1772*, 895–906. [CrossRef] [PubMed]

100. Yue, Z.; Xie, J.; Yu, A.S.; Stock, J.; Du, J.; Yue, L. Role of TRP channels in the cardiovascular system. *Am. J. Physiol. Circ. Physiol.* **2015**, *308*, H157–H182. [CrossRef] [PubMed]

101. Xiao, X.; Liu, H.-X.; Shen, K.; Cao, W.; Li, X.-Q. Canonical Transient Receptor Potential Channels and Their Link with Cardio/Cerebro-Vascular Diseases. *Biomol. Ther.* **2017**, *25*, 471–481. [CrossRef] [PubMed]

102. Thakore, P.; Brain, S.D.; Beech, D.J. Correspondence: Challenging a proposed role for TRPC5 in aortic baroreceptor pressure-sensing. *Nat. Commun.* **2018**, *9*, 1245. [CrossRef] [PubMed]

103. Lau, O.-C.; Shen, B.; Wong, C.-O.; Yao, X. Correspondence: Reply to 'Challenging a proposed role for TRPC5 in aortic baroreceptor pressure-sensing. *Nat. Commun.* **2018**, *9*, 1244. [CrossRef] [PubMed]

104. Jiang, H.-N.; Zeng, B.; Chen, G.-L.; Lai, B.; Lu, S.-H.; Qu, J.-M. Lipopolysaccharide potentiates endothelin-1-induced proliferation of pulmonary arterial smooth muscle cells by upregulating TRPC channels. *Biomed. Pharmacother.* **2016**, *82*, 20–27. [CrossRef] [PubMed]

105. Alawi, K.M.; Tandio, D.; Xu, J.; Thakore, P.; Papacleovoulou, G.; Fernandes, E.S.; Legido-Quigley, C.; Williamson, C.; Brain, S.D. Transient receptor potential canonical 5 channels plays an essential role in hepatic dyslipidemia associated with cholestasis. *Sci. Rep.* **2017**, *7*, 1–10. [CrossRef] [PubMed]

106. Alawi, K.M.; Russell, F.A.; Aubdool, A.A.; Srivastava, S.; Riffo-Vasquez, Y.; Baldissera, L.; Thakore, P.; Saleque, N.; Fernandes, E.S.; Walsh, D.A.; et al. Transient receptor potential canonical 5 (TRPC5) protects against pain and vascular inflammation in arthritis and joint inflammation. *Ann. Rheum. Dis.* **2017**, *76*, 252–260. [CrossRef] [PubMed]

107. Graham, S.; Yuan, J.P.; Ma, R. Canonical transient receptor potential channels in diabetes. *Exp. Biol. Med.* **2012**, *237*, 111–118. [CrossRef] [PubMed]

108. Krout, D.; Schaar, A.; Sun, Y.; Sukumaran, P.; Roemmich, J.N.; Singh, B.B.; Claycombe-Larson, K.J. The TRPC1 Ca^{2+}-permeable channel inhibits exercise-induced protection against high-fat diet-induced obesity and type II diabetes. *J. Biol. Chem.* **2017**, *292*, 20799–20807. [CrossRef] [PubMed]

109. Sachdeva, R.; Schlotterer, A.; Schumacher, D.; Matka, C.; Mathar, I.; Dietrich, N.; Medert, R.; Kriebs, U.; Lin, J.; Nawroth, P.; et al. TRPC proteins contribute to development of diabetic retinopathy and regulate glyoxalase 1 activity and methylglyoxal accumulation. *Mol. Metab.* **2018**, *9*, 1–12. [CrossRef] [PubMed]

110. Weiss, W.A.; Taylor, S.S.; Shokat, K.M. Recognizing and exploiting differences between RNAi and small-molecule inhibitors. *Nat. Chem. Biol.* **2007**, *3*, 739–744. [CrossRef] [PubMed]

111. Zamir, E.; Bastiaens, P.I.H. Reverse engineering intracellular biochemical networks. *Nat. Chem. Biol.* **2008**, *4*, 643–647. [CrossRef] [PubMed]

112. Frye, S.V. The art of the chemical probe. *Nat. Chem. Biol.* **2010**, *6*, 159–161. [CrossRef] [PubMed]

113. Arrowsmith, C.H.; Audia, J.E.; Austin, C.; Baell, J.; Bennett, J.; Blagg, J.; Bountra, C.; Brennan, P.E.; Brown, P.J.; Bunnage, M.E.; et al. The promise and peril of chemical probes. *Nat. Chem. Biol.* **2015**, *11*, 536–541. [CrossRef] [PubMed]

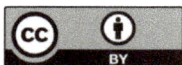

© 2018 by the authors. Licensee MDPI, Basel, Switzerland. This article is an open access article distributed under the terms and conditions of the Creative Commons Attribution (CC BY) license (http://creativecommons.org/licenses/by/4.0/).

cells

MDPI

Review

TRPC3 as a Target of Novel Therapeutic Interventions

Oleksandra Tiapko and Klaus Groschner *

Gottfried-Schatz-Research-Center—Biophysics, Medical University of Graz, Neue Stiftingtalstrasse 6/D04, 8010 Graz, Austria; oleksandra.tiapko@medunigraz.at
* Correspondence: klaus.groschner@medunigraz.at; Tel.: +43-316-385-71500

Received: 10 June 2018; Accepted: 20 July 2018; Published: 22 July 2018

Abstract: TRPC3 is one of the classical members of the mammalian transient receptor potential (TRP) superfamily of ion channels. TRPC3 is a molecule with intriguing sensory features including the direct recognition of and activation by diacylglycerols (DAG). Although TRPC3 channels are ubiquitously expressed, they appear to control functions of the cardiovascular system and the brain in a highly specific manner. Moreover, a role of TRPC3 in immunity, cancer, and tissue remodeling has been proposed, generating much interest in TRPC3 as a target for pharmacological intervention. Advances in the understanding of molecular architecture and structure-function relations of TRPC3 have been the foundations for novel therapeutic approaches, such as photopharmacology and optochemical genetics of TRPC3. This review provides an account of advances in therapeutic targeting of TRPC3 channels.

Keywords: transient receptor potential channels; TRPC3 pharmacology; channel structure; lipid mediators; photochromic ligands

1. Introduction to TRPC3

Mammalian transient receptor potential (TRP) channels of the classical subfamily (TRPC) are closely related to the founding member dTRP, which was discovered as a critical element in *Drosophila* visual transduction [1]. In human tissues, TRPCs typically serve signal transduction pathways downstream of G protein-coupled receptors [2]. All TRPCs are controlled by and able to sense membrane lipids [3,4], where TRPC3/6/7 channels display a direct mechanism of activation via diacylglycerols [5,6], which is generated in response to receptor-phospholipase C pathways. Like all other TRPC channels, TRPC3 features six transmembrane spanning segments with nitrogen (N) and carbon (C) termini residing in the cytoplasm. TRPC3 assembles into tetrameric complexes in which the cytoplasmic termini interact to form an inverted bell-shaped cytoplasmic layer, as revealed by single-particle cryo-electron microscopy (cryo-EM) [7,8]. The tetrameric assembly constitutes a cation permeation path with a selectivity filter harboring negatively charged residues (E630 in the 848aa variant; isoform 3/Q13507-3 in UniProt) to determine calcium ion (Ca^{2+}) transport within the pore domains, connecting transmembrane domains 5 and 6 (TM5 and TM6) [7,9]. Multiple cytoplasmic regulatory domains have been identified, including a highly conserved proline-rich and calmodulin/IP_3 receptor binding (CIRB) region in the C-terminus [10,11], which enable the channel to serve multimodal signaling functions. Initially, the channel was implicated in store-operated Ca^{2+} entry processes [12,13] but later on, a consent was reached among researchers that the prominent mechanism of TRPC3 activation and TRPC3-mediated Ca^{2+} signaling is based on a direct interaction with diacylglycerol. This was found to occur within a lateral gating fenestration of the pore domain [14]. Like its DAG-sensitive relatives TRPC6 and TRPC7, TRPC3 has been implicated in a wide array of pathologies and disorders ranging from tumors to cardiac arrhythmias [15]. Notably, expression of TRPC3 varies among tissues and their developmental state as well as cell phenotype. A prominent functional role of TRPC3 has been detected in both proliferating cells, such a vascular progenitors [16,17], but also in differentiated cell types [18,19]. Overall, pharmacological targeting of TRPC3 with high specificity and spatiotemporal precision has become feasible and emerged as an attractive perspective in TRPC pharmacology.

2. Potential Role of TRPC3 in Human Disease

Ca^{2+} influx is an essential determinant of cell function and fate, and TRPC3 serves to regulate Ca^{2+} entry via its nonselective permeation pathway by multiple mechanisms, including functional interaction with the sodium-calcium exchanger NCX1 [20–23]. TRPC3 mRNA was detected in both excitable and non-excitable cells, and changes in expression levels are reportedly correlated with pathological processes and organ disorders [24]. A gain in TRPC3 function was found to be associated with pathologies of the cardiovascular system and brain. In the heart, TRPC3 channels were confirmed as a major target of the angiotensin II- and noradrenaline-induced nuclear factor of activated T cells (NFAT) activation involved in maladaptive cardiac remodeling and arrhythmias [20,22,25,26]. TRPC3 overexpression and/or gain-of-function depolarizes myocytes, promotes the calcineurin/NFAT pathway, is involved in adverse mechanical stress responses, hypertrophy, and heart failure [25,26]. Importantly, NFAT signaling in myocytes has been linked to direct Ca^{2+} entry via TRPC3 channels [27]. Nonetheless, the pathophysiologicial role of TRPC3 in the heart appears, for a large part, to be based on its expression and function in cardiac fibroblasts. TRPC3 was identified as a crucial player in the proliferation and differentiation of fibroblasts in the myocardium and its activity was found to promote fibrosis, structural remodeling and arrhythmias, specifically atrial fibrillation [28–30].

TRPC3 channels are also expressed in other cardiovascular cells, including vascular smooth muscle and endothelial cells [31–33]. TRPC3 has been proposed to govern both the fate of endothelial progenitor cells and functions in the mature endothelium specifically vasodilatory responses [16]. TRPC3-mediated Ca^{2+} was reported to trigger NO-mediated [34] and NO-independent vasodilation [33]. For vascular smooth muscle, Dietrich et al. showed that up-regulated expression of TRPC3 channels, which features constitutive activity, is associated with high blood pressure in TRPC6-deficient mice [35]. Similar to cardiac muscle, a role of TRPC3 in phenotype transitions and vascular remodeling was suggested [36].

TRPC3 expression is detectable throughout the brain with prominent levels in cerebellar Purkinje cells in the adult mouse brain [37]. Notably, up-regulation of the neuronal TRPC3 conductance by the gain-of-function mutation T635A (moonwalker; *Mwk*) was shown to lead to Ca^{2+}-dependent degradation of Purkinje cells and, as a consequence, to impaired motor coordination [38,39]. In the hippocampus, TRPC3 activity was found to be negatively correlated with contextual fear memory [40].

A role in non-excitable cell signaling was proposed for the immune system. TRPC3 was reported to control Ca^{2+} waves and to facilitate the response to antigen stimulation [41]. Phillip et al. detected defects in the TRPC3 gene of immune cell lines with impaired Ca^{2+} signaling, which were initially described by Fanger et al. [42]. Phillip et al. were able to restore the Ca^{2+} influx and activation of T-cells by overexpression of functional TRPC3 channels [43]. Hence, TRPC3 was suggested to contribute to Ca^{2+} signaling in immune cells alongside the prominent players stromal interaction molecule (STIM) and Orai, which constitute the classical calcium release-activated Ca^{2+} channel (CRAC) conductance [44].

Growing consensus states that TRPC molecules impact on nearly all "cancer hallmarks" and drive cancer progression [45]. In particular, TRPC3 was found as an ion channel that governs proliferation and migration of a variety of tumor cells, including melanoma [46], lung [47], bladder [48], ovarian [49], and breast [50] cancers.

Current knowledge on the role of TRPC3 in most investigated pathologies suggests that channel blockers might be suitable for disease management. This has been suggested for cardiac fibrosis and hypertrophy [29,51], coronary stenosis [36], and melanoma [46]. Nonetheless, for certain disorders, selective block of TRPC3 channel functioning might not be a useful therapeutic strategy since the protein's cellular role is more complex, and TRPC3 function has also been assigned to beneficial effects, such as stabilization of cardiac contractility, and excitability and vasodilation or promotion of immune responses. Not only should the expression levels and overall channel activity be considered, but also the cell-type specific signaling signature of TRPC3 channels, which depends on factors like subcellular localization, composition of pore complex, and input signaling pattern, and are likely of relevance for disease etiology. The ability of TRPC proteins to assemble into specific heteromeric complexes, for which stoichiometry is likely to determine signaling features as well as sensitivity to pharmacological intervention, has long been recognized [52–54]. Moreover, native TRPC channels have been shown to operate in cell-specifically organized signalplexes, which enable efficient interactions with downstream signaling elements, such as CaN [27] or the electrogenic Ca^{2+} signaling partner NCX1 [22]. Dynamic organization of TRPC3 into such cell-type specific signalplexes, along with the TRPC channels cycling between activated, inactivated, and desensitized states, needs consideration as a basis of cell-type specific signaling and therapeutic targeting of TRPC3. In this context, more refined pharmacological interventions including also channel activators and modulators might be of value for therapeutic applications.

3. Pharmacological Inhibitors

Early attempts to identify and characterize TRPC3 channel function were based on non-specific channel blockers, such as the trivalent cations La^{3+} and Gd^{3+} [12,55,56], or commonly used nonselective inhibitors of receptor-mediated Ca^{2+} entry, verapamil or SKF96365 [55]. Due to their wide range of targets, these blockers were only of limited use for the characterization of TRPC3 in native tissues and not suitable for the development of therapeutic application. A first step toward the more specific targeting of TRPC3 function was achieved by He et al., showing that the 3,5-bis(trifluoromethyl)pyrazole (YM-58483 or BTP2), which was initially described as an inhibitor of T-lymphocytes store-operated Ca^{2+} entry (SOCE) [57,58], was inhibiting TRPC3 channel activity in different cell types including DT40 B-lymphocytes [59]. Based on the observation of BTP2 inhibition of TRPC3 conductance activated by carbachol (CCh) or oleoyl-acetyl glycerol (OAG; Figure 1) [59], these authors clearly identified the pyrazole derivative as an inhibitor of TRPC3. Since BTP2 still lacked appreciable selectivity among different Ca^{2+} entry pathways, Kiyonaka et al. synthesized and characterized a series of pyrazole derivatives to discriminate between SOCE, TRPC,3 and other TRPC isoforms. These authors reported a new pyrazole 3 (Pyr3) inhibitor of TRPC channels (Figure 1) with a striking preference for TRPC3. Notably, 3 μM of Pyr3, which effectively inhibited TRPC3, failed to suppress TRPC6, TRPM2, TRPM4, and TRPM7 channels overexpressed in HEK293 cells. Pyr3 was suggested to inhibit TRPC3 channels from the extracellular side and photoaffinity labeling of Pyr3 showed a strong incorporation of the inhibitor into TRPC3 but not into TRPC6 channels [60]. The exact site of molecular interaction has not been clearly defined, and even a principle blocking mechanism by occluding the permeation pathway has not been conclusively delineated. Pyr3 certainly advanced the field by enabling a pharmacological dissection of closely related TRPC channel subtypes. However, later investigations on the selectivity of pyrazole inhibitors demonstrated that Pyr3 inhibits STIM/Orai Ca^{2+} entry complexes [61]. The latter authors identified other pyrazole derivatives that are indeed able to discriminate between TRPC3 and Orai-mediated SOCE, including an acceptably selective TRPC3 blocker (Pyr10). This pyrazole blocked recombinant, homomeric TRPC3 channels were highly potent ($IC_{50} > 0.72$ μM) but affected SOCE only at concentrations more than one order of magnitude higher ($IC_{50} > 10$ μM) [61].

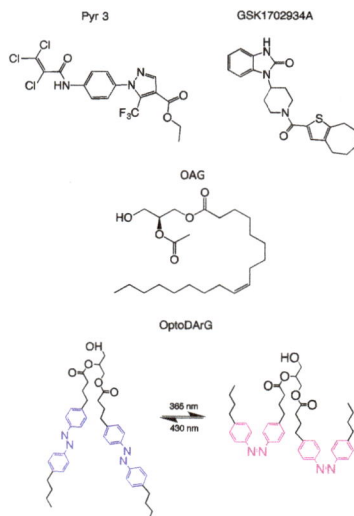

Figure 1. Chemical structures of prototypical antagonist and agonists of transient receptor potential channel 3/6 (TRPC3/6): Pyrazole 3 (Pyr3) as a most commonly used pore blocker; GSK1702934A and 2-Acetyl-1-oleoyl-sn-glycerol (OAG) represent channel agonists (a synthetic, non-lipid activator, and a diacylglycerol/lipid, respectively); OptoDArG as a photochromic agonist (photoswitchable lipid) and a powerful tool for precise control of TRP channels (TRPC) activity.

Another screening study by Washburn et al. identified two potent and selective thiazole inhibitors of TRPC channels. These compounds, assigned GSK2332255B (GSK255B) and GSK2833503A (GSK503A), are anilino-thiazoles and feature a nanomolar potency for blocking TRPC6 and TRPC3 and reportedly lack significant effects on many other calcium-permeable channels [62]. Since TRPC3/6 channels were implicated in the pathogenesis of hypertension and hypertrophy, GSK255B and GSK503A were tested in animal models of cardiac hypertrophy and remodeling. GSK255B and GSK503A, most likely by a combined suppression of TRPC3 and TRPC6 conductance, reduced hypertrophy and fibrosis induced by pressure overload in rodents [63].

Other TRPC3 blocking agents with ill-defined selectivity have been introduced, such as norgestamate [64], HC-C3A [40], 4-({(1R,2R)-2-[(3R)-3-aminopiperidin-1-yl]-2,3-dihydro-1H-inden-1-yl}oxy)-3-chlorobenzonitrile (SAR7334) [65], and 2-(benzo[d][1,3]dioxol-5-ylamino)thiazol-4-yl)((3S,5R)-3,5-dimethylpiperidin-1-yl)methanone (BTDM) [8]. The latter compound (BTDM), albeit incompletely characterized at the cellular and tissue level, was able to delineate TRPC6 and TRPC3 structure by cryo-EM [8]. Consequently, a BTDM binding site was localized within the TRPC6 tetrameric complex (Figure 1). Importantly, another study resolving the TRPC3 structure by cryo-EM [7] identified a highly charged extracellular cavity with close structural relation to the pore domain, therefore representing a potential interaction site for inhibitors and/or modulators of the channel. Thus, the first high-resolution structural information on the drug binding site in the TRPC3 complex has emerged, and this information will promote the development of therapeutic targeting of TRPC3 (Figure 1).

4. Endogenous and Synthetic Channel Activators

A hallmark of the cellular regulation of mammalian TRPC channels is the intimate linkage between channel activity and membrane lipid composition. TRPC3 is, for a large part, governed by its membrane lipid environment. Not only production of diacylglycerols (DAGs; Figure 1) in response to phospholipase C (PLC) activation activates the channel, but also phosphatidylinositol 4,5-bisphosphate PIP_2 as a precursor of DAG formation, has been identified as a determinant of TRPC3 activity [66]. Both PIP_2 and DAG appear to promote channel activity. Synthetic and photoswitchable DAGs have been introduced as activators that enable optical control of TRPC3 activity. As a highly active, unnatural lipid activator, a DAG with two arachidonyl-mimicking azobenzene moieties was introduced (OptoDArG; Figure 1) [14]. In addition to glycerol derivatives, membrane cholesterol was shown to initiate and enhance TRPC3 activity [67]. The effect of cholesterol was attributed in part by enhanced recruitment of the channel into the plasma membrane. Importantly, two distinct regulation mechanisms were reported for TRPC channels including TRPC3 in particular. This is, on the one hand, an increase in the open probability in membrane resident channels, as shown at the level of single TRPC3 channels for PLC-mediated activation, which is characterized by destabilized closed channel conformations [14]. On the other hand, the recruitment of a vesicular pool of TRPC channels into the plasma membrane was proposed. Through this mechanism, certain activating stimuli might enhance channel availability, and thereby TRPC3 currents and downstream signaling [68]. In this respect, TRPC3, in contrast to its close relative TRPC6, displays constitutive activity in resting cells, at essentially low PLC activity. Suppressed basal activity in TRPC6 was found to be related to the channel's glycosylation pattern. Dual glycosylation at two asparagine residues was found to be crucial for maintaining the basal activity of TRPC6 low compared to monoglycosylated TRPC3, which is marginally permeable for ions in a resting state [69]. Constitutive gating activity appears largely independent of basal levels of DAGs in the membrane, as a DAG-insensitive mutant (G652A) of TRPC3 retained constitutive activity [14]. The same mutation also retained sensitivity to activation by a synthetic activator GSK1702934A (GSK; Figure 1) that clearly acts in manner different from DAGs to enhance the open probability of TRPC3 [14]. Xu et al. introduced this small and apparently selective agonist of ligand-gated TRPC channels, which activated TRPC3/6 overexpressed in HEK293 cells and increased the perfusion pressure of isolated rat heart and transiently increased blood pressure in conscious Sprague Dawley rats [70]. Later, Qu et al. introduced a series of TRPC-selective agonists, which lacked effects on other members of the TRP family (TRPA, TRPM, and TRPV). These agonists were pyrazolopyrimidine-based and remarkably potent (EC_{50} in the nanomolar range) in the activation of recombinant TRPC3, TRPC6, and TRPC7 channels [71]. These synthetic small molecule agonists of TRPC channels (GSK-related and pyrazolopyrimidine-based structures) appear to bypass the PLC pathway and the TRPC lipid-gating machinery. Importantly, GSK has been found to exert little to no effect on membrane conductance of cardiomyocytes at an essentially low level of TRPC3 expression in the murine heart, but induced TRPC3 currents when the channel was overexpressed in a genetic mouse model [22]. This indicates a relatively high specificity of the GSK activator for TRPC3/6/7 channels, since none of the abundant voltage-gated cardiac conductances were affected [22]. For pyrazolopyrimidine-based agonists, Qu et al. confirmed the selectivity and efficiency in stimulating endogenous TRPC3/6 activity in rat primary glomerular mesangial cells by Ca^{2+} measurements [71]. Of note, limited therapeutic interest has been expressed as of yet for synthetic activators of TRPC3, since most TRPC3-associated pathologies are related to either an enhanced expression or a gain in function of phenotypes. Hence, drug development activities have focused primarily on selective antagonists or blockers of the channel. Nonetheless, TRPC3 has been identified as promoting proliferative cell phenotypes [16,29,36] and may be involved not only in maladaptive tissue remodeling but also in tissue regeneration. Therefore, unconventional approaches that provide high spatial precision of intervention, such as photopharmacology, may create the possibility of a therapeutic application for TRPC3 activators.

5. New Insights into the Ligand Binding Domains in TRPC3

The delineation of TRPC3 and TRPC6 structures by cryo-EM microscopy approaches succeeded in the localization of potential binding sites for blockers, modulators, as well as endogenous lipids. Tang et al. presented the structure of homotetrameric TRPC3 complexes at 4.4 Å [7]. A resolution along with the structure of TRPC6 (3.8 Å resolution), in which binding of the high affinity inhibitor BTDM was localized between the S1–S4 voltage sensor-like domain (VSLD) and the pore domain. This is a position in which an interaction is likely to hinder gating movements (Figure 1). The BTDM binding site is conserved between TRPC6 and TRPC3, and interaction of this potent inhibitor structure with the channel appears not to overlap with lipid regulation, as some mutations that prevent BTDM binding did not interfere with activation by DAGs. Tang et al. performed a structure analysis of TRPC3 reconstituted into nanodiscs in the presence of the diacylglycerol activator OAG, but obtained a closed channel conformation and could not discern the presence of the lipid activator [8]. Fan et al. reported the structure of tetrameric TRPC3 complexes in a lipid-occupied closed state at a 3.3 Å resolution and localized two lipid interaction sites without identifying the molecular nature of the lipid species [7]. One lipid molecule occupied a position between a pre-S1 elbow-like structure and the S4–S5 linker representing a pivotal element of TRPC gating. A second lipid-like density was found within a lateral fenestration in the pore domain (Figure 2). This second and potentially lipid-interaction site is close to the previously recognized critical LFW motif in the pore domain. It was identified by our laboratory as a structure essential for DAG recognition and lipid gating in the channel using homology modeling combined with structure-guided mutagenesis and a novel optical lipid-clamp approach [14]. Observation of a closed channel state may reflect either a desensitized or inactivated state of the channel or the presence of an inert, non-activating lipid species that occupies the channel in its resting state.

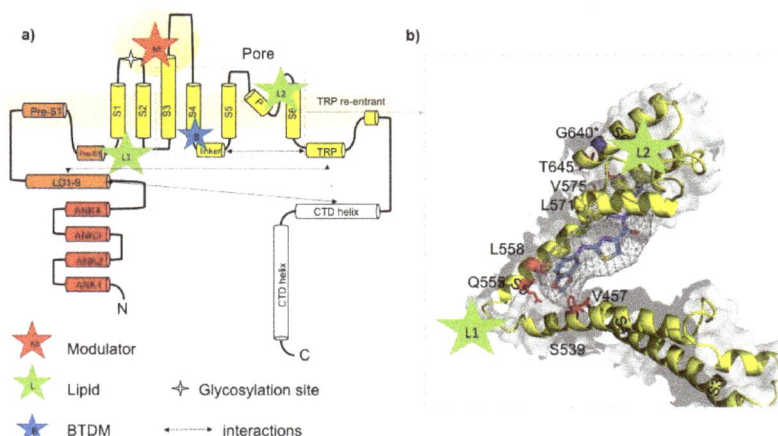

Figure 2. Ligand-channel interactions and potential drug binding sites in TRPC3. (**a**) Schematic illustration of the domain structure of one TRPC3 channel subunit according to information provided in Fan et al. [7]. Lipid binding sites (green stars) are indicated with L1 (formed by LD9, pre-S1, S1, S4, and S4–S5 linker) and L2 (between p-loop and S6 helix); potential modulator binding site (M) represented by a cavity (extracellular domain) formed by the extended S3 helix, S1–S2 and S3–S4 linkers as previously identified [7]. Proposed BTDM binding site formed by S3, S4–S5 linker, S4, S5, and S6 identified by Tang et al. [8]. (**b**) Detailed view on postulated 2-(benzo[d][1,3]dioxol-5-ylamino)thiazol-4-yl) ((3S,5R)-3,5-dimethylpiperidin-1-yl)methanone (BTDM) binding site in TRPC3: amino acids in the TRPC3 sequence, corresponding to the TRPC6 BTDM binding site are marked in red. The BTDM molecule is only schematically introduced into the TRPC structure and not adjusted in size. The glycine residue G652 (here G640, isoform 1/Q13507-1 in UniProt) identified as crucial for recognition and accommodation of lipid activators is highlighted in blue [14]. The BTDM molecule is schematically placed into the proposed binding site.

Both natural as well as synthetic modulators are likely to occupy distinct binding pockets to interfere with the gating machinery involving conformational changes in both the S1–S4 VSLD and the pore domains. Fan et al. identified a charged extracellular cavity formed by an extended S3 helix and the S3–S4 linker. This extracellular domain connects to the pore domain via hydrophobic interactions and represents a potential extracellular modulatory site for small molecules including pyrazole inhibitors [7].

Importantly, these advances in TRPC3 structural biology have created a basis for further advances with TRPC3 synthetic biology in terms of optogenetics and photopharmacology as outlined below. Availability of structural information at the atomic level will allow for tethered ligand approaches and optogating by crosslinking domains recognized as gating elements.

6. TRPC3 Photopharmacology—A Therapeutic Perspective

Therapeutic targeting of a multifunctional signaling molecule that is expressed in a wide range of tissues, as is the case for TRPC3 [23], typically requires refined pharmacological strategies to obtain sufficient tissue and/or cell-type specificity for clinically useful interventions. Of note, information on the viability in a genetic mouse model, which lacks expression of all TRPC species [72], indicated that the nonselective and simultaneous block of multiple TRPC conductances might not necessarily generate severe side effects in healthy tissues and organs. It is tempting to speculate that the impact of TRPC3 in organ dysfunction is based on either a certain expression profile of TRPC genes and/or a certain cell- or phenotype-dependent signaling signature of TRPC3, along with its closer relatives in diseased states. Hence, gaining understanding on the cell-type specific function of these channels in normal and pathological states is important. Cell-type specific interventions might be achievable by manipulating TRPC3 signaling in a spatiotemporally precise manner using photopharmacology.

Initial attempts adopted the caged ligand concept to gain optical control over TRPC channels [73]. This approach was based on the availability of caged lipid activators of TRPC3/6 channels. DAGs were fused to coumarin and nitroveratroyl molecules to prevent immediate interaction with their biological targets [74]. A significant increase in Ca^{2+} was generated in HeLa cells, which endogenously express TRPC3 and TRPC6 channels upon photorelease of the active lipid mediator with ultraviolet (UV)-A light. Notably, caged stearyl-arachinonyl-glycerol (SAG) was found to be the most potent agonist amongst different DAGs, consistent with the initial characterization of lipid sensitivity by Hofmann et al. [5]. Photoreleased SAG triggered the most sustained and largest increase in Ca^{2+} concentrations compared with other lipid activators, such as stearyl-linoenyl- and 1,2-dioctanoyl-glycerol. $NiCl_2$ and TRPC non-selective blocker SKF-96365 almost completely suppressed response in HeLa cells to lipid uncaging, suggesting a TRPC-dependent Ca^{2+} influx [74].

Disadvantages of the caged-lipid approach include the principle irreversibility of the chemical switch and the unavoidable generation of a second molecular structure represented by the released cage. Tiapko et al. clearly showed the undesirable off-target effect with the caged lipid strategy. Photorelease of caged 1,2-DOG was found to generate an artifact caused by UV light application in the presence of the generated free coumarin moiety, whereas the UV light itself did not affect membrane conductance. Hence, off-target effects, due to the phototoxicity of the caging structure, requires consideration and is expected to limit the therapeutic value of caged ligand strategies [75].

As an alternative approach, the photochromic ligand approach has been successfully adopted for TRPC photopharmacology [14,76]. Herein, the structure and activity of the ligand was reversibly controlled by light. As a conformation-flexible, light-sensing structure, azobenzene was introduced into the DAG structure. The biological activity of these photochromic activators is controlled by *cis-trans* photoisomerization of the azobenzene, which resides within the aliphatic side chains of the DAG. Azobenzene-modified DAGs successfully served as tools for studying TRPC cell-specific functions as well as ligand-protein interactions and channel activation-deactivation kinetics [14,76–78].

Initial characterization of different photochromic DAGs demonstrated precise and reversible control of Ca^{2+} signals in HeLa cells, with probes designated as PhoDAGs. PhoDAG-1 resembles

SAG with the arachidonyl side chain replaced by a corresponding structural element containing the azobenzene moiety. Two other structurally related lipids were predicted to functionally mimic 1,2-DOG (PhoDAG-2 and PhoDAG-3). Typically, the *trans*-conformation exerted little or no effect on intracellular Ca^{2+}, whereas *cis*-adopted molecules efficiently triggering Ca^{2+} influx through the plasma membrane. These actions were fully reversible and allowed for precise cyclic control of the signaling function [78].

With these new tools, Leinders-Zufall et al. demonstrated manipulation of mTRPC2 channels, endogenously expressed in neurons of murine sensory neurons from main olfactory and vomeronasal epithelium. As localization of these channels is confined to certain cell types and cellular structures, the spatial precision of the new technology provided important insight into DAG-sensitive TRPC2 function in the mouse olfactory system [76]. In another study, a photochromic DAG, containing two arachidonic acid-mimicking photochromic moieties, designated as OptoDArG, was introduced and successfully used to investigate the lipid sensing machinery [14]. This study used the intriguing temporal precision of the method and uncovered not only a structural element involved in lipid recognition by TRPC3, but also a cooperative slow gating processes, residing in a subunit interface within the pore domain. Such cooperative gating processes are potentially important determinants of frequency dependence of signaling, thereby generating specific signaling signatures dependent on complex composition, cellular localization of the complexes, or upstream signaling patterns. Detailed elucidation of cell- and phenotype-specific TRPC3 signaling features appears to be an essential next step toward the therapeutic targeting of this molecule.

7. Conclusions

Emerging technologies for precise spatiotemporal manipulation of the activity of TRPC channels by light, along with an increase in available structural information on drug interaction sites and gating processes in TRPC channels, are expected to promote the development of novel therapeutic concepts. TRPC photopharmacology will advance the field by enabling exact control over gating pattern, the option of spatially precise manipulation, as well as by providing a basis for efficient all-optical drug screening. As such, cell-type and tissue-specific targeting of TRPC3 and respective interventions of therapeutic value appear feasible and are awaited.

Funding: APC was sponsored by MDPI. Oleksandra Tiapko is member of the funded PhD program "Metabolic and Cardiovascular Disease" and was funded by the Austrian Science Fund (FWF W1226-B18).

Conflicts of Interest: The authors declare no competing interests.

References

1. Minke, B.; Cook, B. TRP channel proteins and signal transduction. *Physiol. Rev.* **2002**, *82*, 429–472. [CrossRef] [PubMed]
2. Zhu, X.; Jiang, M.; Peyton, M.; Boulay, G.; Hurst, R.; Stefani, E.; Birnbaumer, L. Trp, a novel mammalian gene family essential for agonist-activated capacitative Ca^{2+} entry. *Cell* **1996**, *85*, 661–671. [CrossRef]
3. Svobodova, B.; Groschner, K. Mechanisms of lipid regulation and lipid gating in TRPC channels. *Cell Calcium* **2016**, *59*, 271–279. [CrossRef] [PubMed]
4. Storch, U.; Forst, A.-L.; Pardatscher, F.; Erdogmus, S.; Philipp, M.; Gregoritza, M.; Mederos y Schnitzler, M.; Gudermann, T. Dynamic NHERF interaction with TRPC4/5 proteins is required for channel gating by diacylglycerol. *Proc. Natl. Acad. Sci. USA* **2017**, *114*, E37–E46. [CrossRef] [PubMed]
5. Hofmann, T.; Obukhov, A.G.; Schaefer, M.; Harteneck, C.; Gudermann, T.; Schultz, G. Direct activation of human TRPC6 and TRPC3 channels by diacylglycerol. *Nature* **1999**, *397*, 259–263. [CrossRef] [PubMed]
6. Beck, B.; Zholos, A.; Sydorenko, V.; Roudbaraki, M.; Lehen'kyi, V.; Bordat, P.; Prevarskaya, N.; Skryma, R. TRPC7 is a Receptor-Operated DAG-Activated Channel in Human Keratinocytes. *J. Investig. Dermatol.* **2006**, *126*, 1982–1993. [CrossRef] [PubMed]

7. Fan, C.; Choi, W.; Sun, W.; Du, J.; Lu, W. Structure of the human lipid-gated cation channel TRPC3. *eLife* **2018**, *7*, e36852. [CrossRef] [PubMed]
8. Tang, Q.; Guo, W.; Zheng, L.; Wu, J.-X.; Liu, M.; Zhou, X.; Zhang, X.; Chen, L. Structure of the receptor-activated human TRPC6 and TRPC3 ion channels. *Cell Res.* **2018**, *28*, 746–755. [CrossRef] [PubMed]
9. Lichtenegger, M.; Stockner, T.; Poteser, M.; Schleifer, H.; Platzer, D.; Romanin, C.; Groschner, K. A novel homology model of TRPC3 reveals allosteric coupling between gate and selectivity filter. *Cell Calcium* **2013**, *54*, 175–185. [CrossRef] [PubMed]
10. Vazquez, G.; Wedel, B.J.; Aziz, O.; Trebak, M.; Putney, J.W., Jr. The mammalian TRPC cation channels. *Biochim. Biophys. Acta (BBA) Mol. Cell Res.* **2004**, *1742*, 21–36. [CrossRef] [PubMed]
11. Wang, Y.; Bu, J.; Shen, H.; Li, H.; Wang, Z.; Chen, G. Targeting Transient Receptor Potential Canonical Channels for Diseases of the Nervous System. *Curr. Drug Targets* **2017**, *18*, 1460–1465. [CrossRef] [PubMed]
12. Vazquez, G.; Lievremont, J.P.; Bird, G.S.J.; Putney, J.W. Human Trp3 forms both inositol trisphosphate receptor-dependent and receptor-independent store-operated cation channels in DT40 avian B lymphocytes. *Proc. Natl. Acad. Sci. USA* **2001**, *98*, 11777–11782. [CrossRef] [PubMed]
13. Trebak, M.; Bird, G.S.J.; McKay, R.R.; Putney, J.W., Jr. Comparison of Human TRPC3 Channels in Receptor-activated and Store-operated Modes. *J. Biol. Chem.* **2002**, *277*, 21617–21623. [CrossRef] [PubMed]
14. Lichtenegger, M.; Tiapko, O.; Svobodova, B.; Stockner, T.; Glasnov, T.N.; Schreibmayer, W.; Platzer, D.; Cruz, G.G.; Krenn, S.; Schober, R. An optically controlled probe identifies lipid-gating fenestrations within the TRPC3 channel. *Nat. Chem. Biol.* **2018**, *14*, 1–9. [CrossRef] [PubMed]
15. Xiao, X.; Liu, H.-X.; Shen, K.; Cao, W.; Li, X.-Q. Canonical Transient Receptor Potential Channels and Their Link with Cardio/Cerebro-Vascular Diseases. *Biomol. Ther. (Seoul)* **2017**, *25*, 471–481. [CrossRef] [PubMed]
16. Poteser, M.; Graziani, A.; Eder, P.; Yates, A.; Mächler, H.; Romanin, C.; Groschner, K. Identification of a rare subset of adipose tissue-resident progenitor cells, which express CD133 and TRPC3 as a VEGF-regulated Ca^{2+} entry channel. *FEBS Lett.* **2008**, *582*, 2696–2702. [CrossRef] [PubMed]
17. Hao, H.B.; Webb, S.E.; Yue, J.; Moreau, M.; Leclerc, C.; Miller, A.L. TRPC3 is required for the survival, pluripotency and neural differentiation of mouse embryonic stem cells (mESCs). *Sci. China Life Sci.* **2018**, *61*, 253–265. [CrossRef] [PubMed]
18. Li, H.S.; Xu, X.Z.; Montell, C. Activation of a TRPC3-dependent cation current through the neurotrophin BDNF. *Neuron* **1999**, *24*, 261–273. [CrossRef]
19. Facemire, C.S.; Mohler, P.J.; Arendshorst, W.J. Expression and relative abundance of short transient receptor potential channels in the rat renal microcirculation. *Am. J. Physiol.-Ren. Physiol.* **2004**, *286*, F546–F551. [CrossRef] [PubMed]
20. Eder, P.; Probst, D.; Rosker, C.; Poteser, M.; Wolinski, H.; Kohlwein, S.D.; Romanin, C.; Groschner, K. Phospholipase C-dependent control of cardiac calcium homeostasis involves a TRPC3-NCX1 signaling complex. *Cardiovasc. Res.* **2007**, *73*, 111–119. [CrossRef] [PubMed]
21. Rosker, C.; Graziani, A.; Lukas, M.; Eder, P.; Zhu, M.X.; Romanin, C.; Groschner, K. Ca^{2+} signaling by TRPC3 involves Na$^+$ entry and local coupling to the Na$^+$/Ca^{2+} exchanger. *J. Biol. Chem.* **2004**, *279*, 13696–13704. [CrossRef] [PubMed]
22. Doleschal, B.; Primessnig, U.; Wolkart, G.; Wolf, S.; Schernthaner, M.; Lichtenegger, M.; Glasnov, T.N.; Kappe, C.O.; Mayer, B.; Antoons, G.; et al. TRPC3 contributes to regulation of cardiac contractility and arrhythmogenesis by dynamic interaction with NCX. *Cardiovasc. Res.* **2015**, *106*, 163–173. [CrossRef] [PubMed]
23. Lichtenegger, M.; Groschner, K. TRPC3: A multifunctional signaling molecule. *Handb. Exp. Pharmacol.* **2014**, *222*, 67–84. [PubMed]
24. Riccio, A.; Medhurst, A.D.; Mattei, C.; Kelsell, R.E.; Calver, A.R.; Randall, A.D.; Benham, C.D.; Pangalos, M.N. mRNA distribution analysis of human TRPC family in CNS and peripheral tissues. *Brain Res. Mol. Brain Res.* **2002**, *109*, 95–104. [CrossRef]
25. Bush, E.W.; Hood, D.B.; Papst, P.J.; Chapo, J.A.; Minobe, W.; Bristow, M.R.; Olson, E.N.; McKinsey, T.A. Canonical Transient Receptor Potential Channels Promote Cardiomyocyte Hypertrophy through Activation of Calcineurin Signaling. *J. Biol. Chem.* **2006**, *281*, 33487–33496. [CrossRef] [PubMed]

26. Onohara, N.; Nishida, M.; Inoue, R.; Kobayashi, H.; Sumimoto, H.; Sato, Y.; Mori, Y.; Nagao, T.; Kurose, H. TRPC3 and TRPC6 are essential for angiotensin II-induced cardiac hypertrophy. *EMBO J.* **2006**, *25*, 5305–5316. [CrossRef] [PubMed]

27. Poteser, M.; Schleifer, H.; Lichtenegger, M.; Schernthaner, M.; Stockner, T.; Kappe, C.O.; Glasnov, T.N.; Romanin, C.; Groschner, K. PKC-dependent coupling of calcium permeation through transient receptor potential canonical 3 (TRPC3) to calcineurin signaling in HL-1 myocytes. *Proc. Natl. Acad. Sci. USA* **2011**, *108*, 10556–10561. [CrossRef] [PubMed]

28. Harada, M.; Luo, X.; Qi, X.Y.; Tadevosyan, A.; Maguy, A.; Ordog, B.; Ledoux, J.; Kato, T.; Naud, P.; Voigt, N.; et al. Transient Receptor Potential Canonical-3 Channel-Dependent Fibroblast Regulation in Atrial Fibrillation. *Circulation* **2012**, *126*, 2051–2064. [CrossRef] [PubMed]

29. Numaga-Tomita, T.; Kitajima, N.; Kuroda, T.; Nishimura, A.; Miyano, K.; Yasuda, S.; Kuwahara, K.; Sato, Y.; Ide, T.; Birnbaumer, L.; et al. TRPC3-GEF-H1 axis mediates pressure overload-induced cardiac fibrosis. *Sci. Rep.* **2016**, *6*, 1–12. [CrossRef] [PubMed]

30. Thodeti, C.K.; Paruchuri, S.; Meszaros, J.G. A TRP to cardiac fibroblast differentiation. *Channels* **2014**, *7*, 211–214. [CrossRef] [PubMed]

31. Groschner, K.; Hingel, S.; Lintschinger, B.; Balzer, M.; Romanin, C.; Zhu, X.; Schreibmayer, W. Trp proteins form store-operated cation channels in human vascular endothelial cells. *FEBS Lett.* **1998**, *437*, 101–106. [CrossRef]

32. Yip, H.; Chan, W.-Y.; Leung, P.-C.; Kwan, H.-Y.; Liu, C.; Huang, Y.; Michel, V.; Yew, D.T.-W.; Yao, X. Expression of TRPC homologs in endothelial cells and smooth muscle layers of human arteries. *Histochem. Cell Biol.* **2004**, *122*, 553–561. [CrossRef] [PubMed]

33. Senadheera, S.; Kim, Y.; Grayson, T.H.; Toemoe, S.; Kochukov, M.Y.; Abramowitz, J.; Housley, G.D.; Bertrand, R.L.; Chadha, P.S.; Bertrand, P.P.; et al. Transient receptor potential canonical type 3 channels facilitate endothelium-derived hyperpolarization-mediated resistance artery vasodilator activity. *Cardiovasc. Res.* **2012**, *95*, 439–447. [CrossRef] [PubMed]

34. Huang, J.-H.; He, G.-W.; Xue, H.-M.; Yao, X.-Q.; Liu, X.-C.; Underwood, M.J.; Yang, Q. TRPC3 channel contributes to nitric oxide release: Significance during normoxia and hypoxia–reoxygenation. *Cardiovasc. Res.* **2011**, *91*, 472–482. [CrossRef] [PubMed]

35. Dietrich, A.; Mederos y Schnitzler, M.; Gollasch, M.; Gross, V.; Storch, U.; Dubrovska, G.; Obst, M.; Yildirim, E.; Salanova, B.; Kalwa, H.; et al. Increased vascular smooth muscle contractility in TRPC6-/- mice. *Mol. Cell. Biol.* **2005**, *25*, 6980–6989. [CrossRef] [PubMed]

36. Koenig, S.; Schernthaner, M.; Maechler, H.; Kappe, C.O.; Glasnov, T.N.; Hoefler, G.; Braune, M.; Wittchow, E.; Groschner, K. A TRPC3 blocker, ethyl-1-(4-(2,3,3-trichloroacrylamide) phenyl)-5-(trifluoromethyl)-1*H*-pyrazole-4-carboxylate (Pyr3), prevents stent-induced arterial remodeling. *J. Pharmacol. Exp. Ther.* **2013**, *344*, 33–40. [CrossRef] [PubMed]

37. Hartmann, J.; Konnerth, A. Mechanisms of metabotropic glutamate receptor-mediated synaptic signalling in cerebellar Purkinje cells. *Acta Physiol.* **2009**, *195*, 79–90. [CrossRef]

38. Becker, E.B.E.; Oliver, P.L.; Glitsch, M.D.; Banks, G.T.; Achilli, F.; Hardy, A.; Nolan, P.M.; Fisher, E.M.C.; Davies, K.E. A point mutation in TRPC3 causes abnormal Purkinje cell development and cerebellar ataxia in moonwalker mice. *Proc. Natl. Acad. Sci. USA* **2009**, *106*, 6706–6711. [CrossRef] [PubMed]

39. Fogel, B.L.; Hanson, S.M.; Becker, E.B.E. Do mutations in the murine ataxia gene TRPC3 cause cerebellar ataxia in humans? *Mov. Disord.* **2015**, *30*, 284–286. [CrossRef] [PubMed]

40. Neuner, S.M.; Wilmott, L.A.; Hope, K.A.; Hoffmann, B.; Chong, J.A.; Abramowitz, J.; Birnbaumer, L.; O'Connell, K.M.; Tryba, A.K.; Greene, A.S.; et al. TRPC3 channels critically regulate hippocampal excitability and contextual fear memory. *Behav. Brain Res.* **2015**, *281*, 69–77. [CrossRef] [PubMed]

41. Cohen, R.; Torres, A.; Ma, H.T.; Holowka, D.; Baird, B. Ca^{2+} Waves Initiate Antigen-Stimulated Ca^{2+} Responses in Mast Cells. *J. Immunol.* **2009**, *183*, 6478–6488. [CrossRef] [PubMed]

42. Fanger, C.M.; Hoth, M.; Crabtree, G.R.; Lewis, R.S. Characterization of T cell mutants with defects in capacitative calcium entry: Genetic evidence for the physiological roles of CRAC channels. *J. Cell Biol.* **1995**, *131*, 655–667. [CrossRef] [PubMed]

43. Philipp, S.; Strauss, B.; Hirnet, D.; Wissenbach, U.; Méry, L.; Flockerzi, V.; Hoth, M. TRPC3 Mediates T-cell Receptor-dependent Calcium Entry in Human T-lymphocytes. *J. Biol. Chem.* **2003**, *278*, 26629–26638. [CrossRef] [PubMed]

44. Wenning, A.S.; Neblung, K.; Strauss, B.; Wolfs, M.-J.; Sappok, A.; Hoth, M.; Schwarz, E.C. TRP expression pattern and the functional importance of TRPC3 in primary human T-cells. *Biochim. Biophys. Acta* **2011**, *1813*, 412–423. [CrossRef] [PubMed]

45. Bernardini, M.; Fiorio Pla, A.; Prevarskaya, N.; Gkika, D. Human transient receptor potential (TRP) channel expression profiling in carcinogenesis. *Int. J. Dev. Biol.* **2015**, *59*, 399–406. [CrossRef] [PubMed]

46. Oda, K.; Umemura, M.; Nakakaji, R.; Tanaka, R.; Sato, I.; Nagasako, A.; Oyamada, C.; Baljinnyam, E.; Katsumata, M.; Xie, L.-H.; et al. Transient receptor potential cation 3 channel regulates melanoma proliferation and migration. *J. Physiol. Sci.* **2017**, *67*, 497–505. [CrossRef] [PubMed]

47. Jiang, H.-N.; Zeng, B.; Zhang, Y.; Daskoulidou, N.; Fan, H.; Qu, J.-M.; Xu, S.-Z. Involvement of TRPC channels in lung cancer cell differentiation and the correlation analysis in human non-small cell lung cancer. *PLoS ONE* **2013**, *8*, e67637. [CrossRef] [PubMed]

48. Kim, J.-M.; Heo, K.; Choi, J.; Kim, K.; An, W. The histone variant MacroH2A regulates Ca^{2+} influx through TRPC3 and TRPC6 channels. *Oncogenesis* **2013**, *2*, e77. [CrossRef] [PubMed]

49. Yang, S.L.; Cao, Q.; Zhou, K.C.; Feng, Y.J.; Wang, Y.Z. Transient receptor potential channel C3 contributes to the progression of human ovarian cancer. *Oncogene* **2009**, *28*, 1320–1328. [CrossRef] [PubMed]

50. Aydar, E.; Yeo, S.; Djamgoz, M.; Palmer, C. Abnormal expression, localization and interaction of canonical transient receptor potential ion channels in human breast cancer cell lines and tissues: A potential target for breast cancer diagnosis and therapy. *Cancer Cell Int.* **2009**, *9*, 23. [CrossRef] [PubMed]

51. Seo, K.; Rainer, P.P.; Lee, D.I.; Hao, S.; Bedja, D.; Birnbaumer, L.; Cingolani, O.H.; Kass, D.A. Hyperactive Adverse Mechanical Stress Responses in Dystrophic Heart Are Coupled to Transient Receptor Potential Canonical 6 and Blocked by cGMP-Protein Kinase G Modulation. *Circ. Res.* **2014**, *114*, 823–832. [CrossRef] [PubMed]

52. Lintschinger, B.; Balzer-Geldsetzer, M.; Baskaran, T.; Graier, W.F.; Romanin, C.; Zhu, M.X.; Groschner, K. Coassembly of Trp1 and Trp3 proteins generates diacylglycerol- and Ca^{2+}-sensitive cation channels. *J. Biol. Chem.* **2000**, *275*, 27799–27805. [PubMed]

53. Strübing, C.; Krapivinsky, G.; Krapivinsky, L.; Clapham, D.E. Formation of Novel TRPC Channels by Complex Subunit Interactions in Embryonic Brain. *J. Biol. Chem.* **2003**, *278*, 39014–39019. [CrossRef] [PubMed]

54. Poteser, M.; Graziani, A.; Rosker, C.; Eder, P.; Derler, I.; Kahr, H.; Zhu, M.X.; Romanin, C.; Groschner, K. TRPC3 and TRPC4 associate to form a redox-sensitive cation channel. Evidence for expression of native TRPC3-TRPC4 heteromeric channels in endothelial cells. *J. Biol. Chem.* **2006**, *281*, 13588–13595. [CrossRef] [PubMed]

55. Zhu, X.; Jiang, M.; Birnbaumer, L. Receptor-activated Ca^{2+} influx via human Trp3 stably expressed in human embryonic kidney (HEK) 293 cells. Evidence for a non-capacitative Ca^{2+} entry. *J. Biol. Chem.* **1998**, *273*, 133–142. [CrossRef] [PubMed]

56. Kamouchi, M.; Philipp, S.; Flockerzi, V.; Wissenbach, U.; Mamin, A.; Raeymaekers, L.; Eggermont, J.; Droogmans, G.; Nilius, B. Properties of heterologously expressed hTRP3 channels in bovine pulmonary artery endothelial cells. *J. Physiol.* **1999**, *2*, 345–358. [CrossRef]

57. Ishikawa, J.; Ohga, K.; Yoshino, T.; Takezawa, R.; Ichikawa, A.; Kubota, H.; Yamada, T. A Pyrazole Derivative, YM-58483, Potently Inhibits Store-Operated Sustained Ca^{2+} Influx and IL-2 Production in T Lymphocytes. *J. Immunol.* **2003**, *170*, 4441–4449. [CrossRef] [PubMed]

58. Zitt, C.; Strauss, B.; Schwarz, E.C.; Spaeth, N.; Rast, G.; Hatzelmann, A.; Hoth, M. Potent Inhibition of Ca^{2+} Release-activated Ca^{2+} Channels and T-lymphocyte Activation by the Pyrazole Derivative BTPJ. *Biol. Chem.* **2004**, *279*, 12427–12437. [CrossRef] [PubMed]

59. He, L.-P.; Hewavitharana, T.; Soboloff, J.; Spassova, M.A.; Gill, D.L. A functional link between store-operated and TRPC channels revealed by the 3,5-bis(trifluoromethyl)pyrazole derivative, BTP. *J. Biol. Chem.* **2005**, *280*, 10997–11006. [CrossRef] [PubMed]

60. Kiyonaka, S.; Kato, K.; Nishida, M.; Mio, K.; Numaga, T.; Sawaguchi, Y.; Yoshida, T.; Wakamori, M.; Mori, E.; Numata, T.; et al. Selective and direct inhibition of TRPC3 channels underlies biological activities of a pyrazole compound. *Proc. Natl. Acad. Sci. USA* **2009**, *106*, 5400–5405. [CrossRef] [PubMed]

61. Schleifer, H.; Doleschal, B.; Lichtenegger, M.; Oppenrieder, R.; Derler, I.; Frischauf, I.; Glasnov, T.N.; Kappe, C.O.; Romanin, C.; Groschner, K. Novel pyrazole compounds for pharmacological discrimination between receptor-operated and store-operated Ca 2+entry pathways. *Br. J. Pharmacol.* **2012**, *167*, 1712–1722. [CrossRef] [PubMed]

62. Washburn, D.G.; Holt, D.A.; Dodson, J.; McAtee, J.J.; Terrell, L.R.; Barton, L.; Manns, S.; Waszkiewicz, A.; Pritchard, C.; Gillie, D.J.; et al. The discovery of potent blockers of the canonical transient receptor channels, TRPC3 and TRPC6, based on an anilino-thiazole pharmacophore. *Bioorganic Med. Chem. Lett.* **2013**, *23*, 4979–4984. [CrossRef] [PubMed]

63. Seo, K.; Rainer, P.P.; Shalkey Hahn, V.; Lee, D.I.; Jo, S.H.; Andersen, A.; Liu, T.; Xu, X.; Willette, R.N.; Lepore, J.J.; et al. Combined TRPC3 and TRPC6 blockade by selective small-molecule or genetic deletion inhibits pathological cardiac hypertrophy. *Proc. Natl. Acad. Sci. USA* **2014**, *111*, 1551–1556. [CrossRef] [PubMed]

64. Miehe, S.; Kleemann, H.-W.; Struebing, C. Use of Norgestimate as a Selective Inhibitor of Trpc3, Trpc6 and Trpc7 Ion Channels-European Patent Office-ep 2205247 B1use of Norgestimate as a Selective Inhibitor of Trpc3, Trpc6 and Trpc7 Ion Channels-European Patent Office-EP 2205247 B1 [Internet]. European Patent Office, 2013. Available online: https://patentimages.storage.googleapis.com/41/64/8c/b98422f55179fa/EP2205247B1.pdf (accessed on 21 July 2018).

65. Maier, T.; Follmann, M.; Hessler, G.; Kleemann, H.-W.; Hachtel, S.; Fuchs, B.; Weissmann, N.; Linz, W.; Schmidt, T.; Löhn, M.; et al. Discovery and pharmacological characterization of a novel potent inhibitor of diacylglycerol-sensitive TRPC cation channels. *Br. J. Pharmacol.* **2015**, *172*, 3650–3660. [CrossRef] [PubMed]

66. Lemonnier, L.; Trebak, M.; Putney, J.W., Jr. Complex regulation of the TRPC3, 6 and 7 channel subfamily by diacylglycerol and phosphatidylinositol-4,5-bisphosphate. *Cell Calcium* **2008**, *43*, 506–514. [CrossRef] [PubMed]

67. Graziani, A.; Rosker, C.; Kohlwein, S.D.; Zhu, M.X.; Romanin, C.; Sattler, W.; Groschner, K.; Poteser, M. Cellular cholesterol controls TRPC3 function: Evidence from a novel dominant-negative knockdown strategy. *Biochem. J.* **2006**, *396*, 147–155. [CrossRef] [PubMed]

68. Smyth, J.T.; Lemonnier, L.; Vazquez, G.; Bird, G.S.; Putney, J.W. Dissociation of regulated trafficking of TRPC3 channels to the plasma membrane from their activation by phospholipase C. *J. Biol. Chem.* **2006**, *281*, 11712–11720. [CrossRef] [PubMed]

69. Dietrich, A.; Mederos y Schnitzler, M.; Emmel, J.; Kalwa, H.; Hofmann, T.; Gudermann, T. N-Linked Protein Glycosylation Is a Major Determinant for Basal TRPC3 and TRPC6 Channel Activity. *J. Biol. Chem.* **2003**, *278*, 47842–47852. [CrossRef] [PubMed]

70. Xu, X.; Lozinskaya, I.; Costell, M.; Lin, Z.; Ball, J.A.; Bernard, R.; Behm, D.J.; Marino, J.P.; Schnackenberg, C.G. Characterization of Small Molecule TRPC3 and TRPC6 agonist and Antagonists. *Biophys. J.* **2013**, *104*, 454a. [CrossRef]

71. Qu, C.; Ding, M.; Zhu, Y.; Lu, Y.; Du, J.; Miller, M.; Tian, J.; Zhu, J.; Xu, J.; Wen, M.; et al. Pyrazolopyrimidines as Potent Stimulators for Transient Receptor Potential Canonical 3/6/7 Channels. *J. Med. Chem.* **2017**, *60*, 4680–4692. [CrossRef] [PubMed]

72. Lutas, A.; Birnbaumer, L.; Yellen, G. Metabolism Regulates the Spontaneous Firing of Substantia Nigra Pars Reticulata Neurons via K ATPand Nonselective Cation Channels. *J. Neurosci.* **2014**, *34*, 16336–16347. [CrossRef] [PubMed]

73. Fehrentz, T.; Schönberger, M.; Trauner, D. Optochemical genetics. *Angew. Chem. Int. Ed. Engl.* **2011**, *50*, 12156–12182. [CrossRef] [PubMed]

74. Nadler, A.; Reither, G.; Feng, S.; Stein, F.; Reither, S.; Müller, R.; Schultz, C. The fatty acid composition of diacylglycerols determines local signaling patterns. *Angew. Chem. Int. Ed. Engl.* **2013**, *52*, 6330–6334. [CrossRef] [PubMed]

75. Tiapko, O.; Bacsa, B.; la Cruz de, G.G.; Glasnov, T.; Groschner, K. Optopharmacological control of TRPC channels by coumarin-caged lipids is associated with a phototoxic membrane effect. *Sci. China Life Sci.* **2016**, *59*, 802–810. [CrossRef] [PubMed]

76. Leinders-Zufall, T.; Storch, U.; Bleymehl, K.; Schnitzler, M.M.Y.; Frank, J.A.; Konrad, D.B.; Trauner, D.; Gudermann, T.; Zufall, F. PhoDAGs Enable Optical Control of Diacylglycerol- Sensitive Transient Receptor Potential Channels. *Cell Chem. Biol.* **2018**, *25*, 215–223.e3. [CrossRef] [PubMed]

77. Frank, J.A.; Moroni, M.; Moshourab, R.; Sumser, M.; Lewin, G.R.; Trauner, D. Photoswitchable fatty acids enable optical control of TRPV. *Nat. Commun.* **2015**, *6*, 7118. [CrossRef] [PubMed]

78. Frank, J.A.; Yushchenko, D.A.; Hodson, D.J.; Lipstein, N.; Nagpal, J.; Rutter, G.A.; Rhee, J.-S.; Gottschalk, A.; Brose, N.; Schultz, C.; et al. Photoswitchable diacylglycerols enable optical control of protein kinase C. *Nat. Chem. Biol.* **2016**, *12*, 755–762. [CrossRef] [PubMed]

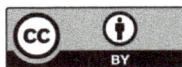

© 2018 by the authors. Licensee MDPI, Basel, Switzerland. This article is an open access article distributed under the terms and conditions of the Creative Commons Attribution (CC BY) license (http://creativecommons.org/licenses/by/4.0/).

![cells logo] *cells*

MDPI

Article

GABAB Receptors Augment TRPC3-Mediated Slow Excitatory Postsynaptic Current to Regulate Cerebellar Purkinje Neuron Response to Type-1 Metabotropic Glutamate Receptor Activation

Jinbin Tian and Michael X. Zhu *

Department of Integrative Biology and Pharmacology, McGovern Medical School, The University of Texas Health Science Center at Houston, Houston, TX 77030, USA; jin.bin.tian@uth.tmc.edu
* Correspondence: Michael.X.Zhu@uth.tmc.edu; Tel.: +1-713-500-7505

Received: 26 May 2018; Accepted: 27 July 2018; Published: 29 July 2018

Abstract: During strong parallel fiber stimulation, glutamate released at parallel fiber-Purkinje cell synapses activates type-1 metabotropic glutamate receptor (mGluR1) to trigger a slow excitatory postsynaptic current (sEPSC) in cerebellar Purkinje neurons. The sEPSC is mediated by transient receptor potential canonical 3 (TRPC3) channels. Often co-localized with mGluR1 in Purkinje neuron dendrites are type B γ-aminobutyric acid receptors (GABABRs) that respond to inhibitory synaptic inputs from interneurons located in the molecular layer of cerebellar cortex. It has been shown that activation of postsynaptic GABABRs potentiates mGluR1 activation-evoked sEPSC in Purkinje cells, but the underlying molecular mechanism remains elusive. Here we report that the augmentation of mGluR1-sEPSC by GABABR activation in Purkinje neurons is completely absent in TRPC3 knockout mice, but totally intact in TRPC1-, TRPC4-, and TRPC1,4,5,6-knockout mice, suggesting that TRPC3 is the only TRPC isoform that mediates the potentiation. Moreover, our results indicate that the potentiation reflects a postsynaptic mechanism that requires both GABABRs and mGluR1 because it is unaffected by blocking neurotransmission with tetrodotoxin but blocked by inhibiting either GABABRs or mGluR1. Furthermore, we show that the co-stimulation of GABABRs has an effect on shaping the response of Purkinje cell firing to mGluR1-sEPSC, revealing a new function of inhibitory input on excitatory neurotransmission. We conclude that postsynaptic GABABRs regulate Purkinje cell responses to strong glutamatergic stimulation through modulation of mGluR1-TRPC3 coupling. Since mGluR1-TRPC3 coupling is essential in cerebellar long-term depression, synapse elimination, and motor coordination, our findings may have implications in essential cerebellar functions, such as motor coordination and learning.

Keywords: transient receptor potential; TRPC3; mGluR1; GABAB; EPSC; Purkinje cell; cerebellum

---

1. Introduction

Purkinje cells in the cerebellum serve vital functions in motor coordination and motor learning. These neurons receive glutamatergic inputs at their extremely elaborated dendrites from parallel fibers at the molecular layer of cerebellar cortex and send outputs to deep cerebellar nuclei in the form of γ-aminobutyric acid (GABA) [1,2]. The excitatory postsynaptic potentials or currents (EPSPs or EPSCs) elicited by the glutamatergic inputs in Purkinje neurons include both fast and slow components, which have been referred to as fast EPSC (fEPSC) and slow EPSC (sEPSC) in the case of voltage-clamp recordings [3]. While fEPSC is mainly mediated by the ionotropic glutamate receptors, sEPSC is triggered by the activation of metabotropic glutamate receptors (mGluRs), mainly the type 1 mGluR (mGluR1) [4]. Importantly, sEPSC only develops when the Purkinje cell receives a strong glutamate input, which in experimental settings requires multiple pulses of high intensity and high frequency electrical stimulations of the parallel fibers [3,5]. This reflects high levels of glutamate release at the parallel fiber-Purkinje cell synapses, causing a spillover of the neurotransmitter from the synaptic clefts to activate mGluR1 abundantly present at the extra-postsynaptic sites of these synapses [6]. mGluR1 is highly expressed in the brain, particularly Purkinje cells [7,8]. The mGluR1-mediated signaling is essential for synaptic plasticity of Purkinje cells, such as cerebellar long-term depression (LTD), the long-lasting reduction of transmission efficiency at the parallel fiber-Purkinje cell synapses [9]. The activation of mGluR1 triggers sEPSC, which is exclusively mediated by channels made of the transient receptor potential canonical 3 (TRPC3) protein [3].

TRPC3 is a member of the TRPC subgroup of transient receptor potential (TRP) superfamily of cation channels. The seven members of the TRPC subgroup (TRPC1-7) function as receptor-operated, non-selective cation channels activated downstream from the stimulation of phospholipase C (PLC) [10,11]. Since mGluR1 is coupled to $G_{q/11}$ proteins which exert effects through PLCβ isoforms, it is natural for TRPC channels to be a part of signaling cascades associated with mGluR1 activation. Among all TRPCs, TRPC3 exhibits the highest expression in cerebellum, particularly Purkinje neurons [3,4], being most abundant in the somatodendritic compartment of these neurons [3]. Disruption of TRPC3 expression not only eliminated sEPSC in Purkinje neurons [3] but also impaired the normal cerebellar LTD induction [12]. Moreover, multiple motor deficits were observed in mice with an altered expression of TRPC3 or ablation of the *Trpc3* gene [4]. Therefore, by mediating sEPSC TRPC3 plays an important role in cerebellar function.

In addition to mGluR1, metabotropic $GABA_B$ receptors ($GABA_B$Rs) are also abundantly expressed at the extra-postsynaptic sites of the parallel fiber-Purkinje cell synapses [13–15]. It has been reported that in the continued activation of $GABA_B$Rs, mGluR1 agonist-evoked inward current, representing sEPSC, in cerebellar Purkinje cells is augmented [5]. However, it is not known whether the enhanced response to mGluR1 stimulation resulted from potentiation of the mGluR1-TRPC3 coupling or recruitment of a new channel(s); especially given that unlike mGluR1, $GABA_B$Rs are coupled to $G_{i/o}$ proteins. In the present study, we used whole-cell patch clamp recordings to examine the receptors and ion channels that underlie the potentiation of mGluR1-sEPSC by $GABA_B$Rs at the parallel fiber-Purkinje cell synapses. We found that $GABA_B$R activation still converges on mGluR1-TRPC3 coupling to augment sEPSC and this modulation helps shape the Purkinje cell firing response to mGluR1 activation.

2. Materials and Methods

2.1. Animals and Brain Slice Preparation

All animal procedures are approved by the Animal Welfare Committee of the University of Texas Health Science Center at Houston in accordance with NIH guidelines. TRPC3 knockout mice were generously provided by Dr. Oleh M. Pochynyuk at The University of Texas Health Science Center at Houston. TRPC1 knockout mice and TRPC1,4,5,6 quadruple knockout mice were generously offered by Dr. Lutz Birnbaumer at the National Institute of Environmental Health Sciences, USA. TRPC4 knockout mice were generously provide by Dr. Marc Freichel at Saarland University, Germany. The TRPC knockout mice are either in C57BL/6 background or mixed C57BL/6 × 129/Sv background. The wild-type (C57BL/6) and TRPC knockout mice used in this study were between postnatal days 17–22. Both male and female mice were used and no sex differences were found in the results. Mice were anesthetized by isoflurane before they were sacrificed. Whole cerebellum was excised quickly and immediately immersed into ice-cold, oxygenated artificial cerebrospinal fluid (aCSF, in mM): 125 NaCl, 26 $NaHCO_3$, 2.5 KCl, 1.25 NaH_2PO_4, 1 $MgCl_2$, 2 $CaCl_2$, and 10 glucose, bubbled with 5% CO_2 and 95% O_2 (pH 7.4). Sagittal cerebellar slices of 300 μm thickness were prepared from vermis of the cerebellum with a vibratome (VT1200S, Leica Biosystems, Wetzlar, Germany) in ice-cold, oxygenated aCSF. Slices were recovered at 35 °C for 1 h and then maintained at room temperature (22–24 °C) in aCSF until use.

2.2. Drug Delivery

Each cerebellar slice placed in the recording chamber was continuously perfused with the normal aCSF unless indicated otherwise. Drugs were diluted in aCSF and applied either through whole-chamber perfusion or by pressure ejection via a drug-delivery glass pipette positioned about 300 µm away from the targeted cell in the molecular layer of the cerebellar cortex (Figure 1A). The pressure ejections (puffs) were delivered by TooheySpritzer pressure system IIe (Toohey Company, Fairfield, NJ, USA) with the trigger controlled via stimulation protocols programmed using PatchMaster software (HEKA Instruments, Holliston, MA, USA). The puff duration was 100–200 ms and the air pressure ranged 5–20 psi. The recording chamber was continuously perfused with aCSF during the drug ejection.

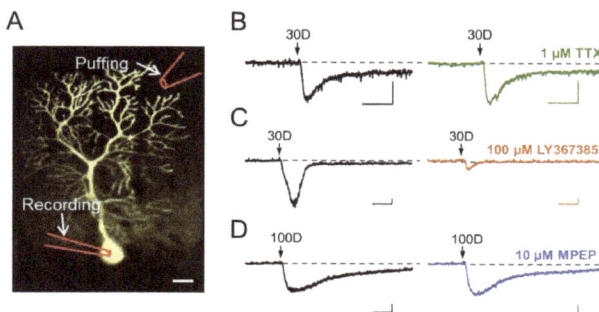

Figure 1. Activation of postsynaptic mGluR1 by a brief ejection of DHPG to dendrites triggers sEPSC in cerebellar Purkinje neurons. (**A**) Fluorescent image of a Purkinje cell loaded with Lucifer Yellow through the recording pipette placed at soma. The location of the puffing pipette for drug ejection is shown on the top. Scale bar: 50 µm. (**B–D**) Consecutive recordings of sEPSCs evoked by DHPG (30 or 100 µM, shown as 30D or 100D, respectively) from individual Purkinje cells before (left) and after (right) application of 1 µM TTX (B), 100 µM LY367385 (C), or 10 µM MPEP (D) through whole-chamber perfusion. Representative of 2–4 cells with similar results. Arrows point to the time when DHPG was ejected. Scale bars: 1 s, 100 pA.

2.3. Drugs

(S)-3,5-Dihydroxyphenylglycine (DHPG), LY367385, 2-methyl-6-(phenylethynyl)pyridine hydrochloride (MPEP), (R)-baclofen and CGP 55845 were purchased from Abcam Biochemicals (Cambridge, MA, USA). Tetrodotoxin (TTX) was purchased from Tocris Bioscience (Minneapolis, MN, USA). GSK2293017A was a kind gift from Prof. Xuechuan Hong (Wuhan University, China).

2.4. Electrophysiology

Glass pipettes (Sutter Instrument, Novato, CA, USA) were pulled using a Narishige PC-10 puller (Narishige International USA, Amityville, NY, USA). Whole-cell patch clamp recordings were made using pipettes with tip resistance of 3–6 MΩ when filled with internal solution containing (in mM): 130 K-methanesulfonate, 7 KCl, 0.05 EGTA, 1 Na_2-ATP, 3 Mg-ATP, 0.05 Na_2-GTP and 10 HEPES, with pH adjusted to 7.3 by KOH and osmolarity of 300 mOsm. Purkinje cells (lobules V-VII) were visualized using a 60x water objective lens and infrared-differential interference contrast videomicroscopy (Olympus BX51WI with OLY-150IR video camera, Olympus America, Center Valley, PA, USA). sEPSC was recorded in voltage-clamp mode when the cell was held at −70 mV. Membrane potential and action potential firing were recorded in current-clamp mode. Immediately before switching to current clamp, cells were held at −45 or −50 mV. After switching to current-clamp, a constant current based on the value in voltage-clamp mode was injected to maintain the membrane potential at the set level. Only Purkinje cells which showed tonic firing around −50 mV were included in the firing frequency analysis. The temperature of the recording chamber was maintained at approximately 32 °C by passing the perfusion solution (aCSF) through an in-line heater (Warner Instruments, Hamden, CT, USA) at 3 mL/min driven by a Rabbit™ peristaltic pump (Mettler-Toledo Rainin, Oakland, CA, USA).

2.5. Data Acquisition and Analysis

Data were acquired using an EPC10 amplifier operated by PatchMaster software (both from HEKA Instruments). Recordings were filtered at 2.9 kHz and digitized at 10 kHz. The amplitude of the sEPSC was measured at the time point when the inward current reached the maximum. All measurements were made off-line using the analysis function of the PatchMaster software. Data are presented as means ± SEM. Bar graphs were produced in GraphPad Prism 6 software (GraphPad software, Inc., San Diego, CA, USA). Differences are considered statistically significant when $P < 0.05$.

3. Results

3.1. Stimulation of Dendritic mGluR1 Evokes an sEPSC-Like Inward Current in Cerebellar Purkinje Neurons

Previous studies have shown the critical involvement of TRPC3 in mediating sEPSC of cerebellar Purkinje cells in response to stimulation of mGluR1 [3,4]. To confirm this in mouse brain slices, we used a pressure-driven drug ejection (puffing) system to eject varying concentrations of the mGluR1 agonist, (*S*)3,5-dihydroxyphenylglycine (DHPG), towards the molecular layer of cerebellum, which consists of dendritic trees of Purkinje cells. The response of individual Purkinje cells to DHPG stimulation was recorded by whole-cell patch clamp technique from the soma of each neuron (Figure 1A). As shown in Figure 1B–D (left panel), with the cells held at −70 mV under voltage clamp, the ejection of DHPG (30–100 μM, 100–200 ms) evoked inward currents that rose slowly and lasted for >1 s. These represent sEPSC because of the much slower kinetics of onset and longer lasting duration than fEPSCs typically mediated by ionotropic glutamate receptors [3]. The DHPG-elicited inward current (herein referred to as sEPSC) is independent of neurotransmission, as it was not affected by blocking neurotransmitter release with whole-chamber perfusion of 1 μM tetrodotoxin (TTX) (Figure 1B). Supporting the involvement of mGluR1, but not mGluR5, the DHPG-elicited sEPSC was abolished almost completely by LY367385 (100 μM), a specific mGluR1 antagonist (Figure 1C), but not MPEP (10 μM), a specific mGluR5 antagonist (Figure 1D), both applied through whole-chamber perfusion. These results suggest that postsynaptic mGluR1 expressed in the dendrites of cerebellar Purkinje neurons mediated DHPG-evoked sEPSCs.

3.2. TRPC3 Mediates the mGluR1 Activation-Evoked sEPSC in Cerebellar Purkinje Neurons

While the DHPG-evoked sEPSC in cerebellar Purkinje cells of adult mice has been shown to be mediated by TRPC3 [3], that in developing Purkinje neurons of young animals had been suggested to also depend on TRPC1 [16]. Given that the Purkinje cells also express other TRPC isoforms, albeit at lower levels than that of TRPC3 [4], we also evaluated the possible involvement of several TRPC isoforms in DHPG-evoked sEPSC under our experimental setting using transgenic mice with selective ablation of *Trpc* genes. With pressure ejection of 30 and 100 μM DHPG, we detected sEPSCs in cerebellar Purkinje neurons from brain slices prepared from *Trpc1* knockout (KO) mice, *Trpc4* KO mice, and *Trpc1,4,5,6* quadruple KO mice, but not that from *Trpc3* KO mice (Figure 2A,B), suggesting that among the 5 TRPC isoforms tested, only TRPC3 is involved in DHPG-elicited sEPSC response. For both DHPG concentrations, the mean amplitudes of the sEPSCs in all transgenic lines, except for the *Trpc3* KO mice, were not different from that of wild type mice (Figure 2B), confirming again the lack of contribution of TRPC1, C4, C5, and C6 to this response. Consistent with the absolute dependence on TRPC3, the strong sEPSC elicited by 100 µM DHPG in wild type Purkinje cells was abolished by whole-chamber perfusion of GSK2293017A (2 µM), a specific TRPC3/C6 antagonist [17] (Figure 2C). Taken together, these results confirm that TRPC3 is the sole TRPC isoform involved in mediating sEPSC in mouse cerebellar Purkinje neurons in response to DHPG stimulation of mGluR1 under our experimental conditions.

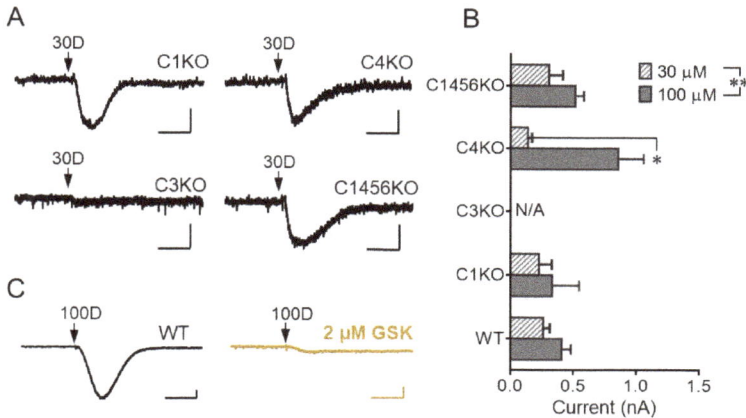

Figure 2. TRPC3 mediates DHPG-evoked sEPSC in mouse cerebellar Purkinje cells. (**A**) Representative current traces showing responses of cerebellar Purkinje cells in brain slices from different *Trpc* gene knockout mice to 30 µM DHPG (30D). C1KO, *Trpc1* knockout; C3KO, *Trpc3* knockout; C4KO, *Trpc4* knockout; C1456KO, *Trpc1,4,5,6* quadruple knockout. Note, only C3KO exhibited no response to DHPG. (**B**) Bar graph showing mean ± SEM of peak amplitudes of inward currents at −70 mV elicited by DHPG (30 and 100 µM) in Purkinje cells from wild type (WT) and *Trpc* knockout mice. $n = 3$–14 for each group. Two-way ANOVA analysis followed by Sidak post hoc test, * $P < 0.05$ between 30 and 100 µM in C4KO group, ** $P < 0.01$ for the factor of drug concentration, no significant difference for the factor of genotype. (**C**) Consecutive recordings of sEPSCs evoked by 100 µM DHPG before (left) and after (right) whole-chamber perfusion of 2 µM GSK2293017A in a Purkinje cell from wild type mouse. Representative of two cells with similar results. Arrows point to the time when DHPG was ejected. Scale bars: 1 s, 100 pA.

3.3. Stimulation of GABA$_B$R Potentiates mGluR1 Agonist-Evoked sEPSC in Cerebellar Purkinje Neurons via a Postsynaptic Mechanism

Previously, the mGluR1 agonist-activated currents in Purkinje neurons were shown to be enhanced following the activation of GABA$_B$Rs [5]. Different from mGluR1, which is coupled to G$_{q/11}$-PLCβ signaling, the GABA$_B$Rs are known to be preferentially coupled to pertussis-toxin sensitive G$_i$ and G$_o$ proteins [18]. Therefore, the co-stimulation of mGluR1 and GABA$_B$Rs represents co-incident G$_{q/11}$ and G$_{i/o}$ signaling. To test if GABA$_B$R signaling also affects the DHPG-evoked sEPSCs under our experimental setting, we used the GABA$_B$R agonist, baclofen. Pressure ejection of baclofen (10 µM) alone onto the molecular layer of cerebellum in brain slices from wild type mice evoked a small and slowly developing outward current (Figure 3A), consistent with the idea that GABA$_B$Rs are inhibitory because of their coupling to G$_{i/o}$ proteins [18]. The baclofen-evoked outward current lasted as long as the drug was present and persisted for seconds even after the drug had been washed out (data not shown, but see [13]). In the continued presence of baclofen (1–10 µM, applied through whole-chamber perfusion), the ejection of 30 µM DHPG evoked larger sEPSC than in the absence of baclofen (Figure 3A,B), indicating that instead of being inhibitory, the activation of GABA$_B$R actually enhances the excitatory response of mGluR1 activation by DHPG. On average, the whole-chamber perfusion of 1, 3, and 10 μM baclofen all potentiated sEPSC peak amplitude elicited by 30 μM DHPG by about double (Figure 3B), suggesting that either the potentiation only requires very weak GABA$_B$R activation or it is easily saturable. Thus, consistent with the previous study [5], the mGluR1 agonist-induced sEPSC in cerebellar Purkinje cells is potentiated by the co-activation of GABA$_B$Rs.

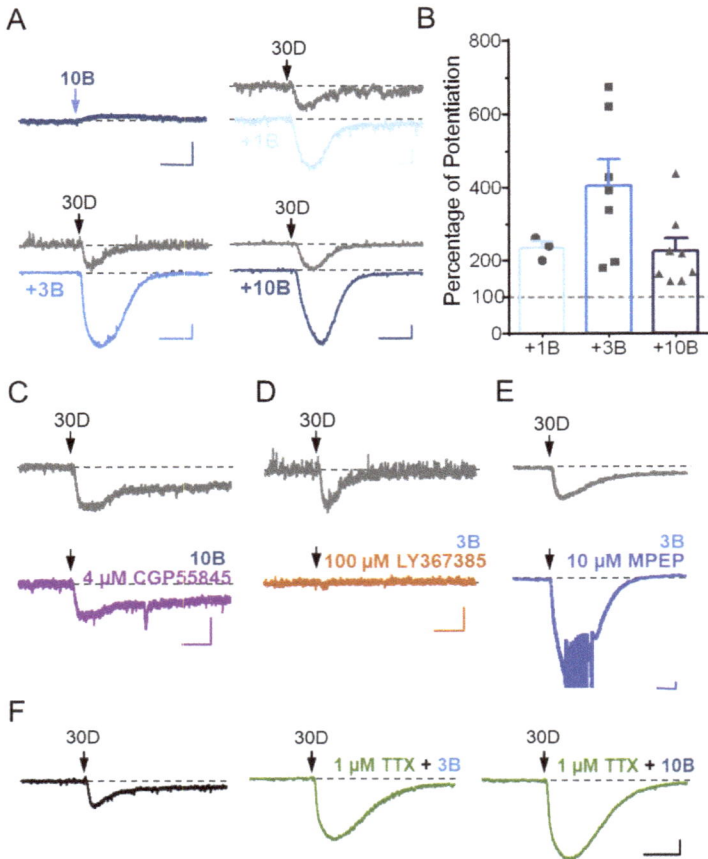

Figure 3. Stimulation of GABA$_B$Rs potentiates DHPG-evoked sEPSC in Purkinje neurons by a postsynaptic mechanism. (**A**) Representative current traces showing responses of Purkinje cells to pressure ejection of 10 μM baclofen (10B) or the ejection of 30 μM DHPG (30D) before (upper) and after (lower) the application of 1, 3, and 10 μM baclofen (+1B, +3B, and +10B, respectively) through whole-chamber perfusion. (**B**) Bar graph showing the potentiation of 30 μM DHPG-evoked sEPSC by 1, 3 and 10 μM baclofen. Peak sEPSC amplitudes were normalized to that before baclofen application (set as 100% and shown by the dotted line). Shown are individual data points and summary (mean ± SEM). One-way ANOVA analysis followed by Sidak post hoc test, no significant differences among three baclofen concentrations. (**C–F**) Receptor types and postsynaptic mechanism of GABA$_B$R action. Representative current traces showing responses of individual Purkinje cells to pressure ejection of 30 μM DHPG before and after application of 4 μM CPG55845 (**C**), 100 μM LY367385 (**D**), 10 μM MPEP (**E**), and 1 μM TTX (**F**) in combination with either 3 or 10 μM baclofen as indicated through whole-chamber perfusion. Representatives of 2–4 cells with similar results. For (**A,C–F**), arrows point to the time when baclofen or DHPG was ejected. Scale bars: 1 s, 100 pA.

To confirm that baclofen indeed acted at the GABA$_B$Rs to cause sEPSC potentiation in Purkinje neurons, we applied a specific GABA$_B$R antagonist, CGP55845, together with baclofen. In the presence of 4 µM CPG55845, baclofen (10 µM) failed to enhance the DHPG-evoked sEPSC (Figure 3C). On the other hand, the co-application of the mGluR1 antagonist LY367385 (100 µM), but not that of the mGluR5 antagonist MPEP (10 µM), completely abolished the generation of sEPSC in response to 30 µM DHPG even in the presence of 3 µM baclofen (Figure 3D–E), suggesting that baclofen did not recruit a separate mGluR subtype(s) or another DHPG-sensitive receptor type(s) to trigger a new form of sEPSC. Therefore, the co-activation of GABA$_B$Rs enhanced sEPSC triggered by the stimulation of mGluR1 in cerebellar Purkinje neurons.

Given that GABA$_B$Rs are present at both the presynaptic and postsynaptic sides of parallel fiber-Purkinje cell synapses [5,13–15,19,20], the potentiation action of GABA$_B$Rs on the DHPG-evoked sEPSC could arise either presynaptically or postsynaptically. To clarify these possibilities, we applied TTX (1 µM) to the brain slices through whole chamber perfusion. By blocking synaptic transmission, TTX should inhibit the presynaptic action of GABA$_B$Rs on postsynaptic currents. However, in the presence of TTX, baclofen (3 and 10 µM) still markedly enhanced the current evoked by pressure ejection of 30 µM DHPG (Figure 3F), suggesting a postsynaptic mechanism for the potentiation of DHPG-evoked sEPSC by GABA$_B$R activation in cerebellar Purkinje neurons.

3.4. TRPC3 Underlies the Potentiation of sEPSC by GABA$_B$R Stimulation

The potentiation of DHPG-evoked sEPSC by the postsynaptic GABA$_B$Rs could arise either from enhancing the activity of TRPC3, which underlies the DHPG-induced inward current in cerebellar Purkinje neurons, as shown earlier in Figure 2, or by recruiting other channels that respond specifically to mGluR1 and GABA$_B$R co-activation. To test these possibilities, we examined the effect of baclofen on DHPG-evoked currents in Purkinje cells of brain slices prepared from *Trpc* gene KO mice. We found that while neurons from *Trpc1* KO, *Trpc4* KO, and *Trpc1,4,5,6* quadruple KO mice showed similar responses as the wild type neurons to DHPG and the potentiation by baclofen, those from *Trpc3* KO animals failed to develop inward currents in response to DHPG (30 µM) either in the absence or presence of baclofen applied through whole-chamber perfusion (Figure 4A,B). Furthermore, in wild type Purkinje neurons, the TRPC3 blocker, GSK2293017A, not only inhibited the DHPG-elicited sEPSC in the absence of baclofen (Figure 2C) but also abolished it in the presence of the GABA$_B$R agonist (Figure 4C). Collectively, these results suggest an exclusive dependence on TRPC3 channels on not only the generation of sEPSC by mGluR1 agonist, but also its potentiation by postsynaptic GABA$_B$R activation in cerebellar Purkinje neurons.

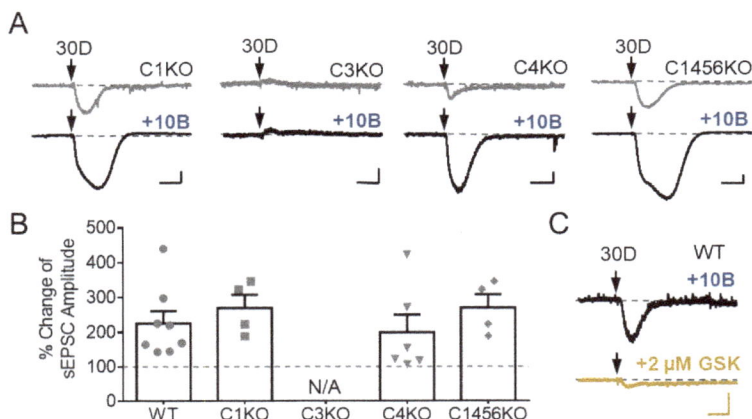

Figure 4. Baclofen potentiates TRPC3-mediated currents evoked by DHPG in cerebellar Purkinje neurons. (**A**) Representative current traces showing responses of cerebellar Purkinje cells in brain slices prepared from *Trpc1* KO (C1KO), *Trpc3* KO (C3KO), *Trpc4* KO (C4KO), and *Trpc1,4,5,6* quadruple KO (C1456KO), to pressure ejection of 30 μM DHPG (30D) in the absence (upper) and presence of 10 μM baclofen (10B) applied through whole-chamber perfusion. Only C3KO neurons failed to develop the inward current in response to DHPG no matter baclofen was applied or not. (**B**) Bar graph showing the effect of 10 μM baclofen on sEPSCs elicited by ejection of 30 μM DHPG in wild type (WT) and *Trpc* KO Purkinje neurons. Peak sEPSC amplitudes were normalized to that before baclofen application (set as 100% and shown by the dotted line). The values for C3KO ($n = 5$) could not be calculated because the sEPSC amplitudes are all 0. Shown are individual data points and summary (mean ± SEM). One-way ANOVA analysis followed by Sidak post hoc test did not show significant differences among different genotypes. (**C**) GSK2293017A strongly inhibited sEPSC evoked by ejection of DHPG (30 μM) in the presence of baclofen (10 μM) in wild type Purkinje neurons. Representative current trace for three neurons. For (A,C), arrows point to the time when DHPG was ejected. Scale bars: 1 s, 100 pA.

3.5. GABA$_B$R Co-Stimulation Reshapes mGluR1-mediated Increase of Purkinje Cell Firing

Like in most brain areas, GABA is commonly considered an inhibitory neurotransmitter in the cerebellar cortex. Upon parallel fiber stimulation, GABA is released from interneurons that make synaptic connections with Purkinje cells. This would suppress the excitatory action of glutamate released by the parallel fiber at the parallel fiber-Purkinje cell synapse through activation of both ionotropic GABA$_A$ receptors and metabotropic GABA$_B$Rs. The GABA$_B$R action can be both pre- and postsynaptic, as shown by the previous study [5]. Particularly, the presynaptic action of GABA$_B$Rs is purely inhibitory, resulting in reduced glutamate release and thereby inhibition of both fEPSC and sEPSC. By contrast, at the postsynaptic level, GABA$_B$R activation can assume both inhibitory or excitatory roles, with the latter being dependent on mGluR1 activation and the presence of TRPC3 channels. However, exactly how GABA$_B$R potentiation of the mGluR1 activation-induced TRPC3 inward cation currents might modulate Purkinje cell function remained mysterious, as the previous study did not attempt to separate the pre- and post-synaptic functions of GABA$_B$Rs by maintaining the constant stimulation levels of mGluR1 [5].

TRPC3 exerts a prominent effect on tonic firing frequency of Purkinje neurons [21]. Therefore, to address the functional significance of GABA$_B$R potentiation of TRPC3 activity, we used current clamp recording to examine how Purkinje neuron firing is altered by activating TRPC3 through stimulation of mGluR1 in the absence and presence of GABA$_B$R activation by baclofen. Purkinje cells in brain slices were initially held close to −50 mV, which produced spontaneous firing. When DHPG alone was applied by pressure ejection (100 ms), a significant increase of Purkinje cell firing was instantly initiated along with a small baseline membrane depolarization. It took about 1 s for the instant firing frequency to reach to a peak before the frequency winded down slowly with a time constant (Tau) of 2.5 s (Figure 5A,C). When DHPG was applied together with baclofen, increases in firing frequency were also observed. However, it took about 1.5 s for the instant firing frequency to achieve the maximum, which was less robust than that evoked by DHPG alone (Figure 5B,C). On the other hand, the decay of the firing frequency after reaching the peak was faster with the DHPG and baclofen co-stimulation, showing a time constant of 1.04 s. In appearance, such a negative impact of baclofen on mGluR1-TRPC3 mediated firing increase would be inconsistent with the strong potentiation of TRPC3 sEPSC by GABA$_B$R stimulation observed in voltage-clamp recordings. However, given that the action potentials were recorded under the current-clamp configuration, in which voltage-gated channels are allowed to be activated, it is reasonable to assume that the stronger activation of TRPC3 was also accompanied with greater activations of Ca^{2+}-activation and/or voltage-sensitive K$^+$ channels that could more quickly dampen the depolarizing effect of TRPC3. Thus, these results suggest that the activation of GABA$_B$Rs exerts a pronounced effect on shaping the TRPC3-mediated response of cerebellar Purkinje cells to mGluR1 activation.

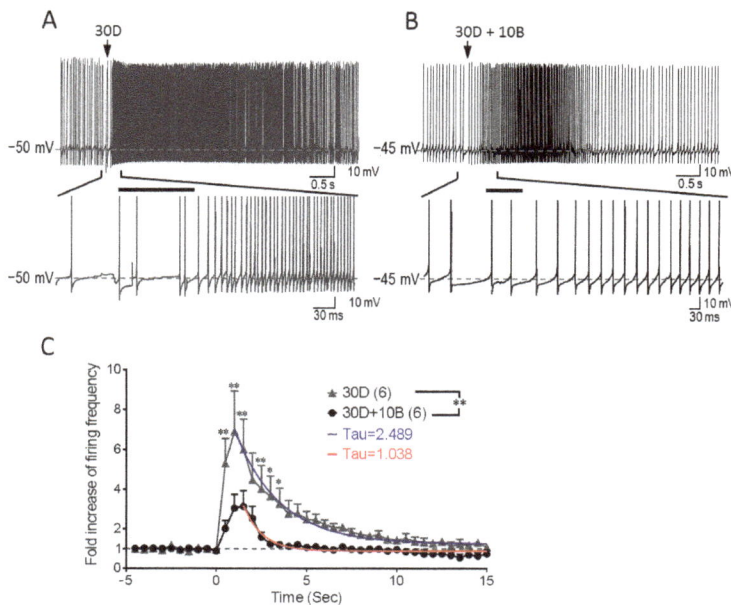

Figure 5. GABA$_B$Rs attenuate mGluR1-TRPC3-mediated firing increase and facilitate firing recovery in Purkinje cell. Current-clamp recordings of membrane depolarization and action potential generation (firing) in response to pressure ejection of 30 μM DHPG (30D) alone (**A**) or co-ejection of 30 μM DHPG and 10 μM baclofen (30D + 10B) (**B**). Lower traces are expanded regions indicated between the two short vertical lines from the top traces. The initial holding potentials were −50 mV (A) or −45 mV (B). Arrows in the top traces point to the time when drugs were ejected. Horizontal bars in the lower traces mark the time period when drugs were ejected. (**C**) Purkinje cell instant firing frequency changes before and after drug treatments. Co-ejection of 10 μM baclofen significantly attenuated firing increase evoked by 30 μM DHPG in Purkinje cells. It also significantly accelerated the recovery of the firing to the original frequency. $n = 6$ for each group. Two-way ANOVA analysis followed by Holm-Sidak post hoc test, ** $P < 0.01$ between the two drug treatments; ** $P < 0.01$, * $P < 0.05$ at individual time points between two drug groups.

4. Discussion

Increasing evidence has implicated the importance of TRPC3 in cerebellar Purkinje cell function by mediating sEPSCs in response to stimulation of mGluR1 [3,4,12]. The TRPC3 activity accelerates the firing rate of Purkinje neurons [21]. Given that TRPC channels are generally activated downstream from receptors that signal through PLC [4], the functional coupling between mGluR1 and the TRPC3 channel in Purkinje neurons is not surprising. However, it is not known that TRPC3 is also regulated by $G_{i/o}$ proteins although the $G_{i/o}$-dependence has been demonstrated for TRPC4/C5 [22–24]. The current study suggests that endogenous TRPC3 channels in cerebellar Purkinje cells are regulated by $G_{i/o}$ protein signaling, stimulated by postsynaptic GABA$_B$Rs in these neurons. Our data demonstrate that GABA$_B$R activation alone is insufficient to stimulate TRPC3, but when combined with mGluR1 activation, the GABA$_B$R-evoked signaling not only markedly enhances TRPC3 currents, but also alters the response of Purkinje cell firing to mGluR1 stimulation.

Previously, GABA$_B$R activation has been shown to enhance mGluR1 agonist-evoked inward currents in cerebellar Purkinje neurons [5]. The mGluR1 agonist-evoked inward currents were later determined to be exclusively dependent on TRPC3, but not other TRPC isoforms [3], a conclusion supported by our current study (Figure 2). We further demonstrate that the GABA$_B$R potentiation is also absolutely dependent on TRPC3 (Figure 4), ruling out the possibility that GABA$_B$Rs recruit additional channel types that only respond to the co-stimulation of both mGluR1 and GABA$_B$Rs. Thus, GABA$_B$Rs exert their potentiation effect on sEPSC through TRPC3, the same channel that responds to mGluR1 activation. The potentiation effect of GABA$_B$Rs was shown to be dependent on $G_{i/o}$ signaling with the use of *N*-ethylmaleimide (NEM) in the previous study [5]. Surprisingly, the same study also suggested that the $G_{i/o}$-dependent potentiation of the inward currents was specific for GABA$_B$Rs, as stimulation of other $G_{i/o}$-coupled receptors—such as acetylcholine, serotonin, and adenosine receptors—failed to mimic the effect of the GABA$_B$R agonist [5]. Therefore, $G_{i/o}$ protein signaling appears to be necessary but not sufficient for the potentiation of TRPC3-mediated sEPSC. It remains to be determined whether such specificity is a result of close colocalization between mGluR1 and GABA$_B$Rs at the peripheral of parallel fiber-Purkinje cell synapse [5] or unique signaling pathway(s) activated by GABA$_B$Rs but not other $G_{i/o}$-coupled receptors. In fact, it has been reported that in cerebellar Purkinje cells, GABA$_B$Rs constitutively enhance mGluR1 signaling in a manner that is dependent on the extracellular Ca^{2+} concentration, but independent of GABA$_B$R-mediated cell signaling. This presumably occurs through a direct binding of extracellular Ca^{2+} to GABA$_B$Rs, which alters the conformation of GABA$_B$Rs and further modifies the direct interaction between GABA$_B$Rs and mGluR1, leading to an enhanced function of mGluR1 [25]. Although co-immunoprecipitation experiments suggest that GABA$_B$Rs and mGluR1 form physical association at the dendritic synapses of Purkinje cells and both mGluRs and GABA$_B$Rs are atypical (Class C) G protein-coupled receptors that only work as dimers [26], to date, no evidence suggests that GABA$_B$Rs oligomerize with mGluR1. Even if they do oligomerize, the oligomerized receptor complex would unlikely be responsive to the GABA$_B$R agonist, as baclofen alone did not induce any inward current, meaning that without an mGluR1 agonist, the receptor complex could not trigger TRPC3 activation. It is possible that signaling pathway(s) downstream from GABA$_B$Rs is involved, which acts either at the level of mGluR1 or that of TRPC3 (Figure 6). Indeed, mGluR1 may be sensitized by shifting to a high affinity binding state [27] and TRPC3 can be activated via binding of β-arrestin, one of the signaling pathways associated with the activation of $G_{i/o}$-coupled receptors [28].

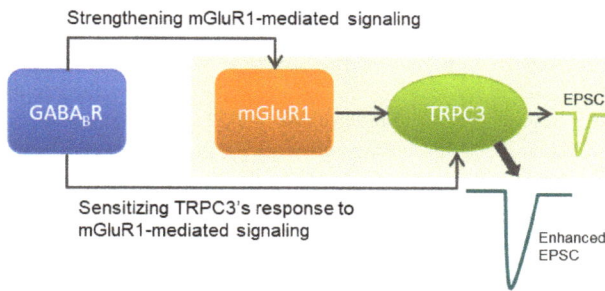

Figure 6. Diagram of GABA$_B$R-mediated potentiation of mGluR1-TRPC3 signaling pathway in cerebellar Purkinje cells. Stimulation of mGluR1 at the dendrites of Purkinje cells activates TRPC3 channels to evoke an excitatory postsynaptic current (EPSC). The EPSC is enhanced if GABA$_B$Rs expressed on the dendrites of the same Purkinje cell are activated at the same time. The enhanced EPSC is still mediated by mGluR1-TRPC3 coupling, presumably through enhancing mGluR1 function and/or increasing the sensitivity of TRPC3 to mGluR1 mediated signaling in Purkinje cells.

Our results indicate that TRPC3 expressed on Purkinje cell dendrites not only responds to postsynaptic mGluR1 activation with an inward cation current that induces membrane depolarization but also integrates the signals from G$_{i/o}$-coupled GABA$_B$Rs to shape the overall response of the Purkinje neuron to the co-transmission of the excitatory and inhibitory neurotransmitters, glutamate, and GABA, respectively. For the TRP channel, this appears to strengthen the channel activity, giving rise to potentiation of sEPSC; however, the net output of this integrated co-transmission is a better controlled time window of excitatory effect of mGluR1 activation on Purkinje neuron firing (Figure 5). The co-stimulation of GABA$_B$Rs helps shape the mGluR1-mediated firing changes in tonic firing Purkinje neurons, by slowing down and dampening the mGluR1-mediated firing increase and accelerating the recovery of the augmented firing (Figure 5). These results appear to be inconsistent with the voltage-clamp recording data showing that GABA$_B$Rs potentiate TRPC3 current (enhanced sEPSC). However, considering that membrane potentials are allowed to change freely under current-clamp but not voltage-clamp, the opposite net outcomes under the two recording modes are not unexpected. The voltage-gated K$^+$ channels and Ca^{2+}-activated and voltage-sensitive K$^+$ channels, such as the large conductance Ca^{2+}-activated K$^+$ channels, are likely activated subsequent to TRPC3 and voltage-gated Ca^{2+} channels during action potentials. The activation of K$^+$ channels counters the depolarization action of TRPC3. Depending on the types of K$^+$ channels involved and their voltage and Ca^{2+} sensitivities, the net effect of TRPC3 activation can be depolarizing or hyperpolarizing, but it is predictable that when TRPC3 is strongly activated, more K$^+$ channels will be recruited due to the very strong depolarization and Ca^{2+} influx, which will bring down the membrane potential. Therefore, TRPC3 plays a central role in mGluR1-mediated synaptic responses, which are further modulated by GABA input through GABA$_B$Rs to shape Purkinje cell firing in the cerebellum.

It is particularly worth noting that GABA$_B$R co-stimulation with mGluR1 accelerated the recovery of Purkinje cell firing to the original frequency (Figure 5). Such a modification may be functionally relevant. Because of the slow development of sEPSC, as opposed to fEPSC mediated by ionotropic glutamate receptors, the termination of sEPSC is also slow, leading to slow recovery of the tonic firing to the original rate. This may be undesirable for the neuron as the sluggish recovery interferes with subsequent neurotransmission. Thus, the co-activation of GABA$_B$Rs helps shut off the mGluR1 effect properly in Purkinje neurons. It remains to be clarified if this effect on termination is due to the hyperpolarization action of GABA$_B$Rs through stimulating K$^+$ channels or it is a result of TRPC3 channel potentiation. The outward current elicited by baclofen seen in the absence of mGluR1 activation represents K$^+$ conductance [5], but the identity of the K$^+$ channel(s) activated in response to GABA$_B$R agonist in Purkinje neurons remains undefined. Although Purkinje cells express G protein-activated inwardly rectifying K^+ (GIRK) channels, the $GABA_BR$ agonist-evoked outward current was unlikely mediated by GIRK, but instead might be attributable to Ca^{2+}-activated K^+ channels [5,18]. In such a case, the potentiated TRPC3 activity could have multiple ways to augment the activity of Ca^{2+}-activated K^+ channels. First, the enhanced Ca^{2+} influx through TRPC3 could increase the K^+ channel activity. Second, the enhanced Na^+ influx could induce stronger membrane depolarization, which could open more voltage-gated Ca^{2+} channels for more Ca^{2+} influx. Third, if the large conductance Ca^{2+}-activated K^+ channel, which is expressed in Purkinje cells, were involved, the membrane depolarization would also intensify its activity directly because of its voltage dependence. Finally, the rise of cytosolic Ca^{2+} also inhibits TRPC3 channel activity via a negative feedback mechanism [29,30]. Therefore, multiple mechanisms may act in concert to terminate the increase in Purkinje cell firing induced by mGluR1 activation in a timely manner.

Purkinje neurons represent the sole output of the cerebellar cortex. Their function is important for various motor functions, including movement control, learning, and coordination. Both mGluR1 and TRPC3 have been clearly shown to be critical for motor function. In mice, genetic deletion of mGluR1 leads to severe symptoms of ataxia [31]. The knockout of TRPC3 causes a less severe phenotype than that of mGluR1 but motor coordination deficit is clearly evident [3]. In humans, motor coordination is strongly impaired by autoantibodies against mGluR1 [32]. Patients with a point mutation of *TRPC3* gene (R762H) show late-onset unidentified ataxia [33,34]. It has also been postulated that TRPC3 signaling is disrupted in spinocerebellar ataxia 1 (SCA1) disease [4]. Interestingly, autoantibodies against $GABA_BRs$ have been found in an agrypnia patient showing ataxia [35]. Although no causal relationship has been established between the $GABA_BR$ antibodies and motor coordination impairment of this patient, the current finding that $GABA_BRs$ play an important role in shaping the response of Purkinje neuron firing to mGluR1 activation, a process mediated by the TRPC3 channel, brings an intriguing possibility that disrupting $GABA_BR$ function may interfere with motor coordination through deregulation of mGluR1/TRPC3 mediated activities in this cell type. In addition to regulating Purkinje cell firing frequency, sEPSC is closely associated to cerebellar LTD, a long term synaptic plasticity change that underlies motor learning [12]. It is therefore speculated that the potentiation of mGluR1/TRPC3 activity by $GABA_BRs$ can also impact motor learning. However, the more widespread expression of $GABA_BRs$ and TRPC3 in other cell types in the cerebellum rather than just Purkinje neurons plus the presence of both pre- and postsynaptic effects of the $GABA_BR$ function make the investigation of $GABA_BR$- and TRPC3-regulated processes in normal conditions and various diseases very challenging [4,18,19]. Nevertheless, the finding that $GABA_BRs$ and mGluR1 converge onto the TRPC3 channel in postsynaptic transmission in Purkinje neurons should open a new avenue to help improve cerebellar functions, such as motor coordination and learning, and combat cerebellar diseases, for instance the various types of ataxia.

5. Conclusions

We conclude that TRPC3 is responsible for the potentiation of mGluR1 activation-evoked sEPSC by $GABA_BRs$ at the parallel fiber-Purkinje cell synapses in the cerebellum and this regulation helps put a timed break on the sEPSC-induced increase in Purkinje cell firing.

Author Contributions: J.T. and M.X.Z. conceived and designed the experiments; J.T. performed the experiments; J.T. and M.X.Z. analyzed the data and wrote the paper.

Funding: This work was supported in part by NIH grant NS092377.

Acknowledgments: We thank Drs. Oleh M. Pochynyuk for kindly providing TRPC3 knockout mice; Lutz Birnbaumer for kindly providing TRPC1 and TRPC1,4,5,6 knockout mice; Marc Freichel for kindly providing TRPC4 knockout mice; Xuechuan Hong for kindly providing the TRPC3 antagonist. We thank members of Zhu laboratory for their suggestions and assistances in this study.

Conflicts of Interest: The authors declare no conflict of interest.

References

1. Apps, R.; Garwicz, M. Anatomical and physiological foundations of cerebellar information processing. *Nat. Rev. Neurosci.* **2005**, *6*, 297–311. [CrossRef] [PubMed]
2. Voogd, J.; Glickstein, M. The anatomy of the cerebellum. *Trends Neurosci.* **1998**, *21*, 370–375. [CrossRef]
3. Hartmann, J.; Dragicevic, E.; Adelsberger, H.; Henning, H.; Sumser, M.; Abramowitz, J.; Blum, R.; Dietrich, A.; Freichel, M.; Flockerzi, V.; et al. TRPC3 channels are required for synaptic transmission and motor coordination. *Neuron* **2008**, *59*, 392–398. [CrossRef] [PubMed]
4. Hartmann, J.; Konnerth, A. TRPC3-dependent synaptic transmission in central mammalian neurons. *J. Mol. Med. (Berl.)* **2015**, *93*, 983–989. [CrossRef] [PubMed]
5. Hirono, M.; Yoshioka, T.; Konishi, S. GABA_B receptor activation enhances mGluR-mediated responses at cerebellar excitatory synapses. *Nat. Neurosci.* **2001**, *4*, 1207–1216. [CrossRef] [PubMed]
6. Hartmann, J.; Henning, H.; Konnerth, A. mGluR1/TRPC3-mediated synaptic transmission and calcium signaling in mammalian central neurons. *Cold Spring Harb. Perspect. Biol.* **2011**, *3*, a006726. [CrossRef] [PubMed]
7. Lein, E.S.; Hawrylycz, M.J.; Ao, N.; Ayres, M.; Bensinger, A.; Bernard, A.; Boe, A.F.; Boguski, M.S.; Brockway, K.S.; Byrnes, E.J.; et al. Genome-wide atlas of gene expression in the adult mouse brain. *Nature* **2007**, *445*, 168–176. [CrossRef] [PubMed]
8. Shigemoto, R.; Nakanishi, S.; Mizuno, N. Distribution of the mRNA for a metabotropic glutamate receptor (mGluR1) in the central nervous system: An in situ hybridization study in adult and developing rat. *J. Comp. Neurol.* **1992**, *322*, 121–135. [CrossRef] [PubMed]
9. Ito, M.; Yamaguchi, K.; Nagao, S.; Yamazaki, T. Long-term depression as a model of cerebellar plasticity. *Prog. Brain Res.* **2014**, *210*, 1–30. [PubMed]
10. Abramowitz, J.; Birnbaumer, L. Physiology and pathophysiology of canonical transient receptor potential channels. *FASEB J.* **2009**, *23*, 297–328. [CrossRef] [PubMed]
11. Tian, J.B.; Thakur, D.; Lu, Y.; Zhu, M. TRPC Channels. In *Handbook of Ion Channels*; Zheng, J., Trudeau, M.C., Eds.; CRC Press: Boca Raton, FL, USA, 2015; pp. 411–426.
12. Chae, H.G.; Ahn, S.J.; Hong, Y.H.; Chang, W.S.; Kim, J.; Kim, S.J. Transient receptor potential canonical channels regulate the induction of cerebellar long-term depression. *J. Neurosci.* **2012**, *32*, 12909–12914. [CrossRef] [PubMed]
13. Kaupmann, K.; Malitschek, B.; Schuler, V.; Heid, J.; Froestl, W.; Beck, P.; Mosbacher, J.; Bischoff, S.; Kulik, A.; Shigemoto, R.; et al. GABA(B)-receptor subtypes assemble into functional heteromeric complexes. *Nature* **1998**, *396*, 683–687. [CrossRef] [PubMed]
14. Fritschy, J.M.; Meskenaite, V.; Weinmann, O.; Honer, M.; Benke, D.; Mohler, H. GABA_B-receptor splice variants GB1a and GB1b in rat brain: Developmental regulation, cellular distribution and extrasynaptic localization. *Eur. J. Neurosci.* **1999**, *11*, 761–768. [CrossRef] [PubMed]
15. Lujan, R.; Shigemoto, R. Localization of metabotropic GABA receptor subunits GABA_B1 and GABA_B2 relative to synaptic sites in the rat developing cerebellum. *Eur. J. Neurosci.* **2006**, *23*, 1479–1490. [CrossRef] [PubMed]
16. Kim, S.J.; Kim, Y.S.; Yuan, J.P.; Petralia, R.S.; Worley, P.F.; Linden, D.J. Activation of the TRPC1 cation channel by metabotropic glutamate receptor mGluR1. *Nature* **2003**, *426*, 285–291. [CrossRef] [PubMed]
17. Xu, X.; Lozinskaya, I.; Costell, M.; Lin, Z.A.; Ball, J.; Bernard, R.; Behm, D.P.; Marino, J.; Schnackenberg, C. Characterization of small molecule TRPC3 and TRPC6 agonist and antagonists. *Biophys. J.* **2013**, *104*, 454. [CrossRef]
18. Padgett, C.L.; Slesinger, P.A. GABA_B receptor coupling to G-proteins and ion channels. *Adv. Pharmacol.* **2010**, *58*, 123–147. [PubMed]
19. Hirano, T. GABA and synaptic transmission in the cerebellum. In *Handbook of the Cerebellum and Cerebellar Disorders*; Manto, M., Schmahmann, J., Rossi, F., Gruol, D., Koibuchi, N., Eds.; Springer: Berlin/Heidelberg, Germany, 2013; pp. 881–893.
20. Billinton, A.; Upton, N.; Bowery, N.G. GABA(B) receptor isoforms GBR1a and GBR1b, appear to be associated with pre- and post-synaptic elements respectively in rat and human cerebellum. *Br. J. Pharmacol.* **1999**, *126*, 1387–1392. [CrossRef] [PubMed]

21. Zhou, H.; Lin, Z.; Voges, K.; Ju, C.; Gao, Z.; Bosman, L.W.; Ruigrok, T.J.; Hoebeek, F.E.; De Zeeuw, C.I.; Schonewille, M. Cerebellar modules operate at different frequencies. *ELife* **2014**, *3*, e02536. [CrossRef] [PubMed]

22. Jeon, J.P.; Hong, C.; Park, E.J.; Jeon, J.H.; Cho, N.H.; Kim, I.G.; Choe, H.; Muallem, S.; Kim, H.J.; So, I. Selective Gαi subunits as novel direct activators of transient receptor potential canonical (TRPC)4 and TRPC5 channels. *J. Biol. Chem.* **2012**, *287*, 17029–17039. [CrossRef] [PubMed]

23. Otsuguro, K.-I.; Tang, J.; Tang, Y.; Xiao, R.; Freichel, M.; Tsvilovskyy, V.; Ito, S.; Flockerzi, V.; Zhu, M.; Zholos, A. Isoform-specific inhibition of TRPC4 channel by phosphatidylinositol 4,5-bisphosphate. *J. Biol. Chem.* **2008**, *283*, 10026–10036. [CrossRef] [PubMed]

24. Thakur, D.P.; Tian, J.B.; Jeon, J.; Xiong, J.; Huang, Y.; Flockerzi, V.; Zhu, M.X. Critical roles of $G_{i/o}$ proteins and phospholipase C-δ1 in the activation of receptor-operated TRPC4 channels. *Proc. Natl. Acad. Sci. USA* **2016**, *113*, 1092–1097. [CrossRef] [PubMed]

25. Tabata, T.; Araishi, K.; Hashimoto, K.; Hashimotodani, Y.; van der Putten, H.; Bettler, B.; Kano, M. Ca^{2+} activity at GABA_B receptors constitutively promotes metabotropic glutamate signaling in the absence of GABA. *Proc. Natl. Acad. Sci. USA* **2004**, *101*, 16952–16957. [CrossRef] [PubMed]

26. Pin, J.P.; Bettler, B. Organization and functions of mGlu and GABA_B receptor complexes. *Nature* **2016**, *540*, 60–68. [CrossRef] [PubMed]

27. Gerber, U.; Gee, C.; Benquet, P. Metabotropic glutamate receptors: Intracellular signaling pathways. *Curr. Opin. Pharmacol.* **2007**, *7*, 56–61. [CrossRef] [PubMed]

28. Liu, C.H.; Gong, Z.; Liang, Z.L.; Liu, Z.X.; Yang, F.; Sun, Y.J.; Ma, M.L.; Wang, Y.J.; Ji, C.R.; Wang, Y.H.; et al. Arrestin-biased AT1R agonism induces acute catecholamine secretion through TRPC3 coupling. *Nat. Commun.* **2017**, *8*, 14335. [CrossRef] [PubMed]

29. Ordaz, B.; Tang, J.; Xiao, R.; Salgado, A.; Sampieri, A.; Zhu, M.; Vaca, L. Calmodulin and calcium interplay in the modulation of TRPC5 channel activity. Identification of a novel C-terminal domain for calcium/calmodulin-mediated facilitation. *J. Biol. Chem.* **2005**, *280*, 30788–30796. [CrossRef] [PubMed]

30. Zhang, Z.; Tang, J.; Tikunova, S.; Johnson, J.; Chen, Z.; Qin, N.; Dietrich, A.; Stefani, E.; Birnbaumer, L.; Zhu, M. Activation of TRP3 by inositol 1,4,5-trisphosphate receptors through displacement of inhibitory calmodulin from a common binding domain. *Proc. Natl. Acad. Sci. USA* **2001**, *98*, 3168–3173. [CrossRef] [PubMed]

31. Aiba, A.; Kano, M.; Chen, C.; Stanton, M.E.; Fox, G.D.; Herrup, K.; Zwingman, T.A.; Tonegawa, S. Deficient cerebellar long-term depression and impaired motor learning in mGluR1 mutant mice. *Cell* **1994**, *79*, 377–388. [PubMed]

32. Coesmans, M.; Smitt, P.A.; Linden, D.J.; Shigemoto, R.; Hirano, T.; Yamakawa, Y.; van Alphen, A.M.; Luo, C.; van der Geest, J.N.; Kros, J.M.; et al. Mechanisms underlying cerebellar motor deficits due to mGluR1-autoantibodies. *Ann. Neurol.* **2003**, *53*, 325–336. [CrossRef] [PubMed]

33. Fogel, B.L.; Hanson, S.M.; Becker, E.B. Do mutations in the murine ataxia gene *trpc3* cause cerebellar ataxia in humans? *Mov. Disord.* **2015**, *30*, 284–286. [CrossRef] [PubMed]

34. Lichtenegger, M.; Groschner, K. TRPC3: A multifunctional signaling molecule. *Handb. Exp. Pharmacol.* **2014**, *222*, 67–84. [PubMed]

35. Frisullo, G.; Della Marca, G.; Mirabella, M.; Caggiula, M.; Broccolini, A.; Rubino, M.; Mennuni, G.; Tonali, P.A.; Batocchi, A.P. A human anti-neuronal autoantibody against GABA_B receptor induces experimental autoimmune agrypnia. *Exp. Neurol.* **2007**, *204*, 808–818. [CrossRef] [PubMed]

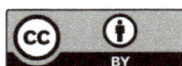

© 2018 by the authors. Licensee MDPI, Basel, Switzerland. This article is an open access article distributed under the terms and conditions of the Creative Commons Attribution (CC BY) license (http://creativecommons.org/licenses/by/4.0/).

cells

MDPI

Review

Emerging Roles of Diacylglycerol-Sensitive TRPC4/5 Channels

Michael Mederos y Schnitzler [1,2,*], Thomas Gudermann [1,2,3] and Ursula Storch [1,4,*]

[1] Walther Straub Institute of Pharmacology and Toxicology, Ludwig Maximilians University of Munich, 80336 Munich, Germany; thomas.gudermann@lrz.uni-muenchen.de
[2] DZHK (German Centre for Cardiovascular Research), Munich Heart Alliance, 80802 Munich, Germany
[3] Comprehensive Pneumology Center Munich (CPC-M), German Center for Lung Research, 81377 Munich, Germany
[4] Institute for Cardiovascular Prevention (IPEK), Ludwig Maximilians University of Munich, 80336 Munich, Germany
* Correspondence: mederos@lrz.uni-muenchen.de (M.M.y.S.); ursula.storch@lrz.uni-muenchen.de (U.S.); Tel.: +49-892-180-75744 (M.M.y.S.); +49-892-180-75745 (U.S.)

Received: 30 October 2018; Accepted: 16 November 2018; Published: 20 November 2018

Abstract: Transient receptor potential classical or canonical 4 (TRPC4) and TRPC5 channels are members of the classical or canonical transient receptor potential (TRPC) channel family of non-selective cation channels. TRPC4 and TRPC5 channels are widely accepted as receptor-operated cation channels that are activated in a phospholipase C-dependent manner, following the $G_{q/11}$ protein-coupled receptor activation. However, their precise activation mechanism has remained largely elusive for a long time, as the TRPC4 and TRPC5 channels were considered as being insensitive to the second messenger diacylglycerol (DAG) in contrast to the other TRPC channels. Recent findings indicate that the C-terminal interactions with the scaffolding proteins Na^+/H^+ exchanger regulatory factor 1 and 2 (NHERF1 and NHERF2) dynamically regulate the DAG sensitivity of the TRPC4 and TRPC5 channels. Interestingly, the C-terminal NHERF binding suppresses, while the dissociation of NHERF enables, the DAG sensitivity of the TRPC4 and TRPC5 channels. This leads to the assumption that all of the TRPC channels are DAG sensitive. The identification of the regulatory function of the NHERF proteins in the TRPC4/5-NHERF protein complex offers a new starting point to get deeper insights into the molecular basis of TRPC channel activation. Future studies will have to unravel the physiological and pathophysiological functions of this multi-protein channel complex.

Keywords: TRPC channels; diacylglycerol; TRPC4; TRPC5; NHERF

1. Introduction

Transient receptor potential classical or canonical 4 (TRPC4) and TRPC5 channels belong to the transient receptor potential classical or canonical (TRPC) cation channel subfamily, which comprises seven members. TRPC channels are regarded as non-selective, receptor-operated cation channels that are important for calcium homeostasis. They are activated via the $G_{q/11}$-signaling cascade as a function of phospholipase C (PLC) [1]. Moreover, the TRPC4 and TRPC5 channels can also be activated following the $G_{i/o}$-protein coupled receptor activation [2–4]. However, the mechanism of the $G_{i/o}$-mediated TRPC4/5 channel activation is still not completely understood and might involve either a direct $G_{i/o}$-protein interaction [3], or the activation of the PLC isoform, PLCδ1 [2]. Even a G_s-protein mediated activation mechanism was proposed for the TRPC5 channels [5]. Therefore, elevating the intracellular cyclic adenosine monophosphate (cAMP) levels might potentiate the TRPC5 currents by increasing the channel trafficking to the plasma membrane. Additionally, a store-operated activation mechanism for the TRPC4 [6–9] and TRPC5 channels [10–12] was proposed, and is still under discussion [13,14]. This article will only focus on the $G_{q/11}$-protein mediated signaling pathway leading to the TRPC4 and TRPC5 channel activation.

All of the TRPC channels are tetramers formed by four TRPC protein subunits, which was confirmed recently by structural analysis [15–18]. TRPC proteins can form not only homotetrameric but also heterotetrameric cation channels [19–22] with distinct channel properties, such as altered calcium permeability [21,23–25]. Because of their sequence homology, the TRPC channel family can be divided into the following subgroups: TRPC1, TRPC4/5, and TRPC3/6/7. TRPC2 has a special role as it represents a pseudogene in humans that is not functionally expressed because of several stop codons in the open reading frame [26,27]. However, in rodents, the TRPC2 channels are functionally expressed (e.g., in the olfactory cells of the vomeronasal organ, where they are important for pheromone sensing [28]).

Although the $G_{q/11}$-protein mediated TRPC channel activation is widely accepted, the precise signaling pathway resulting in the channel opening has remained elusive for quite some time. The activation of the $G_{q/11}$-protein coupled receptors leads to the activation of PLC, which cleaves phosphatidylinositol-4,5-bisphosphate (PIP$_2$) into the second messengers, inositol-1,4,5-trisphopshate (IP$_3$) and 1,2-diacyl-*sn*-glycerol (DAG), and to an oxonium ion [29,30]. There is broad agreement that the TRPC3/6/7 subfamily is directly activated by DAG, the cleavage product of PIP$_2$ [31]. However, IP$_3$ might also contribute to the activation of endogenously expressed TRPC7 channels [32]. Notably, a DAG binding site has not been identified until now, and it is not clear whether DAG directly activates the channel or whether it first interacts with an additional protein, which in turn causes the channel activation. Unfortunately, the recent structural analysis of the TRPC3, TRPC4, and TRPC6 channels only displays a closed channel conformation [15–18]. However, the structural model of TRPC3 reveals two lipid-binding sites, one being sandwiched between the pre-S1 elbow and the S4–S5 linker, and the other being close to the pore-forming domain, where the conserved "LWF" motif of the TRPC family is located [16]. Perhaps these lipid binding sites reflect potential DAG binding sites. Interestingly, it was recently reported that the exchange of a highly conserved amino acid located close to the pore-forming domain, affects the DAG recognition of the TRPC3 channels [33]. Thus, the second lipid binding site might indeed reflect a potential DAG binding site. TRPC2 channels are also regarded as being DAG sensitive [34,35]. In contrast to the TRPC2, TRPC3, TRPC6, and TRPC7 channels, the TRPC4 and TRPC5 channels were commonly considered as DAG insensitive [31], as DAG or the membrane permeable DAG analogue 1-oleoyl-2-acetyl-sn-glycerol (OAG) even inhibited the basal TRPC5 currents [36]. Interestingly, Venkatachalam and colleagues showed that the DAG-induced TRPC5 channel inhibition is related to the protein kinase C (PKC) activation [36]. Moreover, it was demonstrated that the homotetrameric TRPC4 and TRPC5 channels are activated by PIP$_2$ depletion [37,38]. In contrast, the heterotetrameric TRPC1/4 and TRPC1/5 [39] and homotetrameric TRPC6 and TRPC7 channels [40] are instead inhibited by the PIP$_2$ depletion. These contradictory findings suggest that the TRPC channel-lipid interaction is rather complex. Another unique structural feature of the TRPC4 and TRPC5 channels is their capability to interact with the PDZ I domain of the scaffolding proteins Na$^+$/H$^+$ exchanger regulatory factor 1 and 2 (NHERF1 and NHERF2) [41–43]. The NHERF1 and NHERF2 proteins are structurally related; can form homodimers [44]; and possess two PDZ binding domains as well as a C-terminal binding domain, which enables crosslinking with the actin cytoskeleton via ezrin, radixin, and moesin proteins [41,45]. Thus, NHERF1 and NHERF2 proteins are commonly regarded as adapter proteins that crosslink integral membrane proteins with the cytoskeleton, thereby increasing their membrane localization [46–48].

2. DAG-Mediated Activation Mechanism of TRPC4 and TRPC5 Channels

The first evidence that the TRPC5 channels might be DAG sensitive was presented by Lee and colleagues, who performed electrophysiological whole-cell measurements on murine gastric smooth muscle cells endogenously expressing TRPC5 channels, and found that the channels are activated by OAG [49]. However, the mechanistic insights into the DAG mediated TRPC5 channel activation were missing. A remarkable structural difference between TRPC4 and TRPC5, and the well characterized DAG sensitive TRPC3/6/7 channels, is the PDZ binding motif with the amino acid sequence "VTTRL" at the very end of the C-terminus [41,42,50]. This PDZ binding motif includes a potential PKC phosphorylation site, which was identified as being important for the TRPC5 current inactivation following the receptor activation [51]. The amino acid exchange from threonine to alanine at position 972 (T972A) in the murine TRPC5 channels resulted in a loss of current desensitization during the receptor activation with carbachol [51]. Thus, this was the first evidence that the PKC phosphorylation might regulate the TRPC5 channel function [36,51].

The C-terminal PDZ binding motif allows for interactions with the adapter proteins NHERF1 and NHERF2. This C-terminal TRPC4/5 interaction was demonstrated several times by performing co-immunoprecipitations and functional studies using the patch-clamp technique [41–43]. However, only a slight enhancement of the membrane expression was found to be similar to what was observed when analyzing the chloride channel cystic fibrosis transmembrane conductance regulator (CFTR) [52] and other integral membrane proteins. Thus, the functional implications of the TRPC4/5-NHERF interaction were missing. Interestingly, our recent findings indicate that the TRPC4 and TRPC5 channels are DAG-sensitive similar to other TRPC channels [53]. However, in contrast to TRPC3/6/7, their DAG-sensitivity is tightly regulated by the C-terminal NHERF1 and NHERF2 interaction. The $G_{q/11}$-protein coupled receptor activation causes a cleavage of PIP_2, resulting in a conformational change of the C-terminus, which in turn causes the dissociation of the NHERF proteins from the C-terminus of the channel. This dynamic dissociation was monitored employing the method of dynamic intermolecular fluorescence resonance energy transfer (FRET) between fluorescence tagged TRPC5 and NHERF proteins. The separation of the NHERF proteins from the C-terminus was a prerequisite for DAG sensitivity. Moreover, the C-terminal NHERF interaction strongly depended on the PKC phosphorylation status of the C-terminal PDZ binding motif "VTTRL" [53]. The PKC inhibition resulted in the DAG sensitivity, and the PKC phosphorylation mutant T972A of murine TRPC5 was sensitive to DAG, suggesting that PKC phosphorylation is a prerequisite for NHERF binding, thereby suppressing the DAG sensitivity. Thus, the NHERF proteins are dynamic regulators of the TRPC4 and TRPC5 channel activity. This signaling pathway was also observed in the primary cell lines (e.g., in proximal tubule cells and in hippocampal neurons, which endogenously express TRPC4 and TRPC5 channels, respectively) [53]. This activation model has the potential to integrate the contradictory findings of different research groups concerning the TRPC4 and TRPC5 channel activation. Therefore, the pieces of the puzzle like the PLC dependent receptor-mediated TRPC4/5 channel activation [1], the inhibitory effect of DAG or DAG analogues [31,36] on the native TRPC4/5-NHERF-channel complex [41–43], the activation by PIP_2 depletion [37,38], the inhibitory effect of PKC phosphorylation on DAG sensitivity [36], and the DAG sensitivity of the endogenous gastric TRPC5 channels [49] coalesce into a consistent picture. These findings lead to a new concept, that all of the TRPC channels are DAG-sensitive, and that classifying the TRPC channels as DAG-sensitive and -insensitive channels should be avoided. Consequently, a common DAG binding site for TRPC channels can be proposed. Perhaps the highly conserved amino acid near the TRPC pore domain that affects the DAG activation [33] participates in DAG binding.

Altogether, a new model of $G_{q/11}$-protein mediated TRPC4 and TRPC5 channel activation can be proposed. The agonist-induced $G_{q/11}$-protein coupled receptor activation causes the activation of PLC, which in turn cleaves PIP_2 into the two second messengers IP_3 and DAG. The PIP_2 cleavage causes a conformational change at the C-terminus of TRPC4 and TRPC5, which results in a dissociation of the NHERF proteins from the C-terminus, thereby evoking a DAG-sensitive channel conformation. Then, the PIP_2 cleavage product DAG can activate the channel. This model is illustrated in Figure 1.

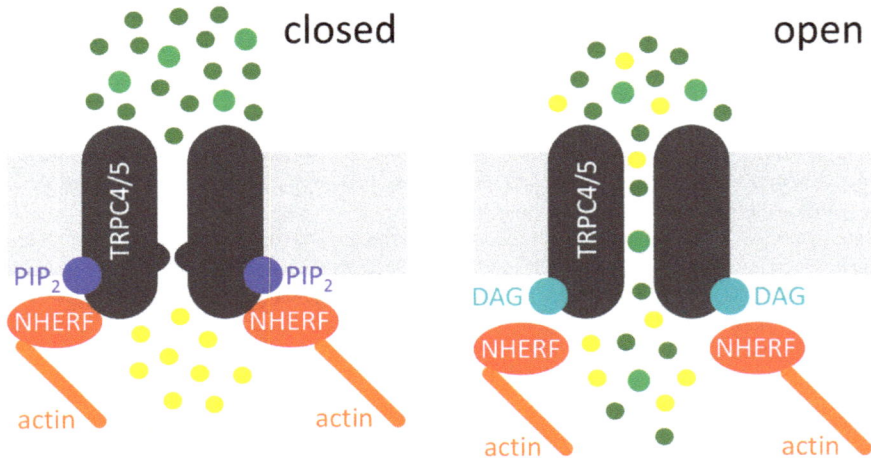

Figure 1. Diacylglycerol (DAG)-mediated activation of transient receptor potential classical or canonical 4/5 (TRPC4/5) channels. Left: Na^+/H^+ exchanger regulatory factor (NHERF) proteins and phosphatidylinositol-4,5-bisphosphate (PIP_2) interact with the C-termini of TRPC4/5, which depicts the closed state of the channel. Right: receptor activation (not displayed) leads to the cleavage of PIP_2, resulting in the dissociation of NHERF and in DAG binding, which represents the open state of the channel. Sodium cations (dark green circles), calcium cations (light green circles), and potassium cations (yellow circles) are displayed. The potassium efflux is mainly relevant in the excitable cells.

3. Physiological and Pathophysiological Roles of NHERF Proteins

NHERF1 and NHERF2 proteins belong to a family of scaffolding proteins that crosslink the integral membrane proteins with the cytoskeleton. It is commonly accepted that NHERF proteins increase the membrane localization of several membrane proteins, like transporters, receptors, and ion channels [46–48]. However, besides their anchoring function, the NHERF proteins are of the utmost importance for the maintenance of essential cellular functions (e.g., in the kidney or in the small intestine, where they interact with transporters, ion channels, signaling proteins, transcription factors, enzymes, G-protein coupled receptors, and tyrosine kinase receptors) [47,48,54–56]. Thus, NHERF proteins are involved in numerous physiological processes. For example, in proximal tubule cells, NHERF proteins regulate phosphate transport [57]. A mutation in the PDZ I domain of human NHERF1 was found in patients with impaired renal phosphate reabsorption due to a reduced expression of the renal phosphate transporter NPT2a [58]. In astrocytes, NHERF proteins regulate the activity of the glutamate transporter (GLAST) and of the metabotropic glutamate receptor (mGlu5) [59,60], and in the small intestine, they control ion transport via interactions with the Na^+/H^+ exchanger (NHE3) [61]. Moreover, the mice lacking NHERF1 and adult humans harboring NHERF1 mutations suffer from osteopenia [62,63], which might be due to abnormal osteoblast differentiation [64]. Furthermore, NHERF proteins influence proliferation [65,66], and they may be involved in carcinogenesis and in the progression of liver, breast, and colon cancer; small-cell lung carcinoma; and glioblastoma [67–70]. A mutation in the PDZ I domain of NHERF1 was identified in the patients with medullar breast carcinoma [71]. This mutation resulted in a reduced interaction of NHERF1 with the epidermal growth factor receptor, thereby promoting the progression of breast cancer. Another mutation in the PDZ II domain of human NHERF1 resulted in a nuclear translocation of NHERF1, thereby inducing carcinogenesis [72]. Recently, in the tumors from ovarian cancer patients, a mutation in the PDZ II domain of NHERF1 was identified, which might contribute to the disease progression [73]. These data suggest that wild-type NHERF1 may act as a tumor suppressor. The subcellular NHERF expression also plays a critical role in cancer cells. In breast cancer cells, the subcellular NHERF expression might even serve as a prognostic marker, as a high cytoplasmic expression of NHERF was associated with a high aggressiveness and poor prognosis [74]. Furthermore, aberrant nuclear NHERF1 expression might be important for the carcinogenesis and progression of colon [74] and breast cancer [72].

The specific role of NHERF proteins for channel function is poorly understood. Beside the regulatory role of NHERF proteins on TRPC4 and TRPC5 channel function [53], the interaction with NHERF was identified as playing an important role in the proper function of the CFTR chloride channel [52]. Mutations in the CFTR channel are known to cause cystic fibrosis [75], which is characterized by the accumulation of viscous mucus, because of impaired fluid transport. Furthermore, CFTR mutations can cause congenital absence of the vas deferens and male infertility [76]. Interestingly, the NHERF2 interaction with the lysophosphatidic acid receptor 2 (LPAR2) promotes the assembly of CFTR–NHERF2–LPAR2 protein complexes, which results in an impaired CFTR function [77,78]. The disruption of this protein complex might enhance the CFTR function of patients suffering from cystic fibrosis [52]. Altogether, the NHERF proteins or their protein complexes might be interesting novel targets for the treatment of diseases

4. Physiological and Pathophysiological Roles of TRPC4 and TRPC5 Channels

TRPC4 and TRPC5 channels are expressed in several cells and tissues (e.g., in the brain [79–83], kidney [80,84,85], and vascular system [7,8,86]). In particular, the TRPC4 and TRPC5 channel expression is very high in the central nervous system [7,79,82]. Here, the TRPC4 and TRPC5 channels are involved in the amygdala function and account for fear-related behavior against aversive stimuli [87,88]. In addition, the TRPC4 and TRPC5 channels are important for peripherally induced neuropathic pain behavior. Microinjections of the TRPC4 and TRPC5 channel blocker ML-204 into the amygdala of rats reduced the sensory and the affective pain sensitivity [89]. Thus, in the future, TRPC4/5 blockers that are able to cross the blood–brain barrier might be used as novel anxiolytics or even as innovative analgesics against peripheral neuropathies. Furthermore, the TRPC4 and TRPC5 channels are expressed in the dorsal root ganglia, where they contribute to axonal regeneration after nerve injury [90], to itching [91], and to cold detection [92].

Moreover, in the hippocampal CA1 pyramidal cells from rats, the calcium and sodium influx through the TRPC5 channels generated a plateau potential [93] that is also observed during epileptic seizures [94,95]. In accordance with this neurophysiological evidence, the TRPC5 gene-deficient mice exhibited significantly reduced seizures. Thus, future studies will have to show whether TRPC5 channels represent interesting novel target structures for the treatment of epileptic disorders.

Furthermore, the TRPC5 channels reduce the hippocampal neurite length and growth cone morphology by reducing the filopodia length growth, which leads to impaired axon guidance [96]. The TRPC5 channels also play a role in podocytes and in fibroblasts. Interestingly, in these cells, the TRPC5 and TRPC6 channels have opposite effects on the actin cytoskeleton [97]. The receptor-operated TRPC5 channel activation by angiotensin II decreased the number of parallel stress fibers via the activation of the small guanosine-5'-triphosphate (GTP)ase protein Rac1, leading to a motile and non-contractile phenotype in vitro, while the TRPC6 activation by angiotensin II increased the formation of parallel stress fibers via the activation of the small GTPase protein Rho A, resulting in a contractile but non-motile phenotype [97]. These differential channel functions might be due to a specific subcellular localization of TRPC5 and TRPC6 channels in podocytes, or be caused by a distinct signaling elicited by the podocyte-specific TRPC6 and slit membrane protein channel complex [98,99]. The reorganization of the actin cytoskeleton characterized by a reduction of the parallel stress fibers results in podocyte injury, leading to the loss of podocyte foot processes, which in the end results in the disruption of the slit diaphragm and in massive proteinuria [100–102]. Thus, the TRPC5 channel blockers might be useful for the treatment of podocyte diseases by preventing end-stage renal disease [103,104].

In addition, the TRPC4 and TRPC5 channels might play a pathophysiological role in cancer cells. The increased TRPC5 channel activity in breast cancer [105] and in colorectal cancer cells [106] caused an increased expression of the ABC transporter P-glycoprotein (MDR1). MDR1 is an important molecular correlate for drug-resistance against chemotherapeutic agents. For example, MDR1 eliminates the well-known and commonly used DNA intercalating drug doxorubicin, the tubulin-targeting drug paclitaxel, and the antimetabolite 5-fluorouracil. In breast cancer cells, the transcription factor NFATc3, and in colorectal cancer cells, the structural protein and transcription factor β-catenin, are thought to enhance the MDR1 expression [105,106]. In contrast, the potent TRPC4 and TRPC5 channel activator (-)-englerin A showed pronounced cytotoxic effects on diverse cancer cell lines, with an EC_{50} value of ~ 20 nM [107,108]. (-)-englerin A was even effective on triple-negative breast cancer cells [109], which do not express the drug targets of estrogen, progesterone, and human epithelial growth factor (HER2) receptor. Of all breast cancer patients, 15% have triple-negative breast cancer [110], which is regarded as very aggressive [111]. The main treatment is surgery, but specific targets for target-orientated chemotherapeutic agents are missing, and patients suffer from frequent relapses within the first three years [112]. A more targeted medical treatment would be of great benefit for these patients. Notably, although (-)-englerin A was selectively cytotoxic to cancer cell lines, adverse reactions were observed in mice and rats after (-)-englerin A injections [108], which were mediated by the TRPC4/5 channels [113]. Thus, the therapeutic application of (-)-englerin A might be limited.

There is evidence that the TRPC5 channel activity increases angiogenesis in cases of breast cancer by the activation of the transcription factor hypoxia-inducible factor 1 (HIF-1), leading to vascular endothelial growth factor (VEGF) formation [114], thereby promoting cancer growth. In contrast, it was reported that the TRPC4 channel activation reduces angiogenesis in cases of renal cell carcinoma cells by the secretion of the inhibitor of angiogenesis thrombospondin-1 [115]. Moreover, the TRPC4 and TRPC5 channel activation in the endothelial cells increases vasculogenesis [116,117], indicative of a pro-angiogenetic effect of these channels. Furthermore, the increased expression of TRPC1, TRPC3, TRPC4, and TRPC6 in ovarian cancer cells increased the migration and proliferation, and therefore had a tumorigenic effect [118]. Thus, other TRPC channels, like TRPC1, TRPC3, and TRPC6, might also function as targets for chemotherapeutic agents. However, at present, the majority of publications point to the TRPC4 and TRPC5 channels as potential new drug targets [119].

The novel role of the NHERF adapter proteins as dynamic regulators of the TRPC4 and TRPC5 channel activity [53,120] might also be important for several other physiological or pathophysiological processes. Interestingly, the NHERF1 protein/channel interaction is of the utmost importance for the proper function of CFTR channels. The NHERF1 proteins stabilized and enhanced the membrane expression of the misfolded CFTR mutant channels [121], which partially restored the channel activity after the NHERF binding.

The TRPC4 and TRPC5 channels, and the NHERF proteins are co-expressed in various excitable and non-excitable cells and tissues. Hence, it can be speculated that the inhibitory effect of the NHERF interaction on the TRPC4/5 channel function may contribute to several physiological or pathophysiological conditions. For example, in tumor cells, the TRPC4/5 channels and the NHERF proteins and NHERF mutations account for cancer progression. However, the effect of the TRPC4/5-NHERF protein complex on tumor growth has largely remained elusive until now. The NHERF interaction also inhibited the DAG mediated TRPC4/5 channel activation in murine hippocampal neurons and in proximal tubule cells [53], suggesting a regulatory role. Altogether, further studies will be needed to show whether the TRPC4/5-NHERF protein complexes have the potential to serve as novel target structures for therapeutics.

5. Conclusions

The new concept that all TRPC channels are DAG sensitive is not only a new starting point for deeper insights into the activation mechanism of TRPC channels on a molecular level, but it might also help to unravel the physiological and pathophysiological roles of these channels, which have not been fully understood until now. On the molecular level, the conformational changes and the kinetics of the conformational changes leading to the TRPC4 and TRPC5 channel activation are largely elusive, as a structure analysis only revealed the inactive channel states. Moreover, the role of the NHERF proteins as dynamic regulators of the TRPC4 and TRC5 channel activation sheds new light on the function of ion channels and adapter proteins in multi-protein complexes. In the TRPC4/5-NHERF protein complexes, the NHERF proteins suppress the DAG sensitivity. Thus, for screening purposes, wildtype TRPC5 channels as well as DAG sensitive PKC phosphorylation site mutant T972A, which cannot interact with NHERF, might be used. Without the inhibitory NHERF binding, it can be speculated that other hits will be identified. As the expression pattern of NHERF proteins and TRPC4/5 channels is altered in several cancer cell lines and might be linked to cancer progression, the TRPC4/5–NHERF channel complexes should also be reconsidered as potential novel targets for cancer therapeutics. Future studies will have to unravel the physiological and pathophysiological roles of these channel complexes. However, a thorough analysis of the TRPC channel functions on a molecular level is of the utmost importance to lay the foundation for a better understanding of the role of TRPC channels in health and disease.

Author Contributions: U.S. and M.M.y.S. planned the review; U.S. performed the literature searches; U.S., M.M.y.S., and T.G. wrote the review; M.M.y.S. created Figure 1.

Funding: This work was supported by the German Research Foundation (Deutsche Forschungsgemeinschaft) (project no. 406028471 and TRR-152).

Acknowledgments: We thank Anna-Lena Forst for her excellent work, and we thank Laura Danner for her brilliant technical support.

Conflicts of Interest: The authors declare no conflict of interest.

References

1. Rohacs, T. Regulation of transient receptor potential channels by the phospholipase c pathway. *Adv. Biol. Reg.* **2013**, *53*, 341–355. [CrossRef] [PubMed]
2. Thakur, D.P.; Tian, J.B.; Jeon, J.; Xiong, J.; Huang, Y.; Flockerzi, V.; Zhu, M.X. Critical roles of gi/o proteins and phospholipase c-delta1 in the activation of receptor-operated TRPC4 channels. *Proc. Natl. Acad. Sci. USA* **2016**, *113*, 1092–1097. [CrossRef] [PubMed]
3. Jeon, J.P.; Hong, C.; Park, E.J.; Jeon, J.H.; Cho, N.H.; Kim, I.G.; Choe, H.; Muallem, S.; Kim, H.J.; So, I. Selective Gαi subunits as novel direct activators of transient receptor potential canonical (TRPC)4 and TRPC5 channels. *J. Biol. Chem.* **2012**, *287*, 17029–17039. [CrossRef] [PubMed]
4. Jeon, J.P.; Lee, K.P.; Park, E.J.; Sung, T.S.; Kim, B.J.; Jeon, J.H.; So, I. The specific activation of TRPC4 by Gi protein subtype. *Biochem. Biophys. Res. Commun.* **2008**, *377*, 538–543. [CrossRef] [PubMed]
5. Hong, C.; Kim, J.; Jeon, J.P.; Wie, J.; Kwak, M.; Ha, K.; Kim, H.; Myeong, J.; Kim, S.Y.; Jeon, J.H.; et al. Gs cascade regulates canonical transient receptor potential 5 (TRPC5) through camp mediated intracellular Ca^{2+} release and ion channel trafficking. *Biochem. Biophys. Res. Commun.* **2012**, *421*, 105–111. [CrossRef] [PubMed]
6. Philipp, S.; Trost, C.; Warnat, J.; Rautmann, J.; Himmerkus, N.; Schroth, G.; Kretz, O.; Nastainczyk, W.; Cavalie, A.; Hoth, M.; et al. TRP4 (CCE1) protein is part of native calcium release-activated Ca^{2+}-like channels in adrenal cells. *J. Biol. Chem.* **2000**, *275*, 23965–23972. [CrossRef] [PubMed]
7. Freichel, M.; Suh, S.H.; Pfeifer, A.; Schweig, U.; Trost, C.; Weissgerber, P.; Biel, M.; Philipp, S.; Freise, D.; Droogmans, G.; et al. Lack of an endothelial store-operated Ca^{2+} current impairs agonist-dependent vasorelaxation in TRP4$^{-/-}$ mice. *Nat. Cell Biol.* **2001**, *3*, 121–127. [CrossRef] [PubMed]
8. Tiruppathi, C.; Freichel, M.; Vogel, S.M.; Paria, B.C.; Mehta, D.; Flockerzi, V.; Malik, A.B. Impairment of store-operated Ca^{2+} entry in TRPC4(-/-) mice interferes with increase in lung microvascular permeability. *Circ. Res.* **2002**, *91*, 70–76. [CrossRef] [PubMed]
9. Wang, X.; Pluznick, J.L.; Wei, P.; Padanilam, B.J.; Sansom, S.C. TRPC4 forms store-operated Ca2+ channels in mouse mesangial cells. *Am. J. Physiol. Cell Physiol.* **2004**, *287*, C357–C364. [CrossRef] [PubMed]
10. Xu, S.Z.; Boulay, G.; Flemming, R.; Beech, D.J. E3-targeted anti-TRPC5 antibody inhibits store-operated calcium entry in freshly isolated pial arterioles. *Am. J. Physiol. Heart Circ. Physiol.* **2006**, *291*, H2653–H2659. [CrossRef] [PubMed]

11. Liu, D.Y.; Thilo, F.; Scholze, A.; Wittstock, A.; Zhao, Z.G.; Harteneck, C.; Zidek, W.; Zhu, Z.M.; Tepel, M. Increased store-operated and 1-oleoyl-2-acetyl-sn-glycerol-induced calcium influx in monocytes is mediated by transient receptor potential canonical channels in human essential hypertension. *J. Hypertens.* **2007**, *25*, 799–808. [CrossRef] [PubMed]

12. Zeng, F.; Xu, S.Z.; Jackson, P.K.; McHugh, D.; Kumar, B.; Fountain, S.J.; Beech, D.J. Human TRPC5 channel activated by a multiplicity of signals in a single cell. *J. Physiol.* **2004**, *559*, 739–750. [CrossRef] [PubMed]

13. DeHaven, W.I.; Jones, B.F.; Petranka, J.G.; Smyth, J.T.; Tomita, T.; Bird, G.S.; Putney, J.W., Jr. TRPC channels function independently of STIM1 and Orai1. *J. Physiol.* **2009**, *587*, 2275–2298. [CrossRef] [PubMed]

14. Putney, J.W.; Steinckwich-Besancon, N.; Numaga-Tomita, T.; Davis, F.M.; Desai, P.N.; D'Agostin, D.M.; Wu, S.; Bird, G.S. The functions of store-operated calcium channels. *Biochim. Biophys. Acta Mol. Cell Res.* **2017**, *1864*, 900–906. [CrossRef] [PubMed]

15. Duan, J.; Li, J.; Zeng, B.; Chen, G.L.; Peng, X.; Zhang, Y.; Wang, J.; Clapham, D.E.; Li, Z.; Zhang, J. Structure of the mouse TRPC4 ion channel. *Nat. Commun.* **2018**, *9*. [CrossRef] [PubMed]

16. Fan, C.; Choi, W.; Sun, W.; Du, J.; Lu, W. Structure of the human lipid-gated cation channel TRPC3. *eLife* **2018**, *7*. [CrossRef] [PubMed]

17. Tang, Q.; Guo, W.; Zheng, L.; Wu, J.X.; Liu, M.; Zhou, X.; Zhang, X.; Chen, L. Structure of the receptor-activated human TRPC6 and TRPC3 ion channels. *Cell Res.* **2018**, *28*, 746–755. [CrossRef] [PubMed]

18. Vinayagam, D.; Mager, T.; Apelbaum, A.; Bothe, A.; Merino, F.; Hofnagel, O.; Gatsogiannis, C.; Raunser, S. Electron cryo-microscopy structure of the canonical TRPC4 ion channel. *eLife* **2018**, *7*. [CrossRef] [PubMed]

19. Strübing, C.; Krapivinsky, G.; Krapivinsky, L.; Clapham, D.E. TRPC1 and TRPC5 form a novel cation channel in mammalian brain. *Neuron* **2001**, *29*, 645–655. [CrossRef]

20. Strübing, C.; Krapivinsky, G.; Krapivinsky, L.; Clapham, D.E. Formation of novel TRPC channels by complex subunit interactions in embryonic brain. *J. Biol. Chem.* **2003**, *278*, 39014–39019. [CrossRef] [PubMed]

21. Storch, U.; Forst, A.L.; Philipp, M.; Gudermann, T.; Mederos y Schnitzler, M. Transient receptor potential channel 1 (TRPC1) reduces calcium permeability in heteromeric channel complexes. *J. Biol. Chem.* **2012**, *287*, 3530–3540. [CrossRef] [PubMed]

22. Hofmann, T.; Schaefer, M.; Schultz, G.; Gudermann, T. Subunit composition of mammalian transient receptor potential channels in living cells. *Proc. Natl. Acad. Sci. USA* **2002**, *99*, 7461–7466. [CrossRef] [PubMed]

23. Medic, N.; Desai, A.; Olivera, A.; Abramowitz, J.; Birnbaumer, L.; Beaven, M.A.; Gilfillan, A.M.; Metcalfe, D.D. Knockout of the Trpc1 gene reveals that TRPC1 can promote recovery from anaphylaxis by negatively regulating mast cell TNF-α production. *Cell Calcium* **2013**, *53*, 315–326. [CrossRef] [PubMed]

24. Kim, J.; Kwak, M.; Jeon, J.P.; Myeong, J.; Wie, J.; Hong, C.; Kim, S.Y.; Jeon, J.H.; Kim, H.J.; So, I. Isoform- and receptor-specific channel property of canonical transient receptor potential (TRPC)1/4 channels. *Pflugers Arch.* **2014**, *466*, 491–504. [CrossRef] [PubMed]

25. Erac, Y.; Selli, C.; Tosun, M. TRPC1 ion channel gene regulates store-operated calcium entry and proliferation in human aortic smooth muscle cells. *Turk. J. Biol.* **2016**, *40*, 1336–1344. [CrossRef]

26. Vannier, B.; Peyton, M.; Boulay, G.; Brown, D.; Qin, N.; Jiang, M.; Zhu, X.; Birnbaumer, L. Mouse trp2, the homologue of the human trpc2 pseudogene, encodes mtrp2, a store depletion-activated capacitative Ca^{2+} entry channel. *Proc. Natl. Acad. Sci. USA* **1999**, *96*, 2060–2064. [CrossRef] [PubMed]

27. Yildirim, E.; Dietrich, A.; Birnbaumer, L. The mouse c-type transient receptor potential 2 (TRPC2) channel: Alternative splicing and calmodulin binding to its n terminus. *Proc. Natl. Acad. Sci. USA* **2003**, *100*, 2220–2225. [CrossRef] [PubMed]

28. Liman, E.R.; Dulac, C. TRPC2 and the molecular biology of pheromone detection in mammals. In *TRP Ion Channel Function in Sensory Transduction and Cellular Signaling Cascades*; Liedtke, W.B., Heller, S., Eds.; Taylor and Francis: Boca Raton, FL, USA, 2007; ISBN 9781420005844.

29. Gudermann, T.; Mederos y Schnitzler, M. Phototransduction: Keep an eye out for acid-labile TRPs. *Curr. Biol.* **2010**, *20*, R149–R152. [CrossRef] [PubMed]

30. Huang, J.; Liu, C.H.; Hughes, S.A.; Postma, M.; Schwiening, C.J.; Hardie, R.C. Activation of TRP channels by protons and phosphoinositide depletion in drosophila photoreceptors. *Curr. Biol.* **2010**, *20*, 189–197. [CrossRef] [PubMed]

31. Hofmann, T.; Obukhov, A.G.; Schaefer, M.; Harteneck, C.; Gudermann, T.; Schultz, G. Direct activation of human TRPC6 and TRPC3 channels by diacylglycerol. *Nature* **1999**, *397*, 259–263. [CrossRef] [PubMed]

32. Vazquez, G.; Bird, G.S.; Mori, Y.; Putney, J.W., Jr. Native TRPC7 channel activation by an inositol trisphosphate receptor-dependent mechanism. *J. Biol. Chem.* **2006**, *281*, 25250–25258. [CrossRef] [PubMed]

33. Lichtenegger, M.; Tiapko, O.; Svobodova, B.; Stockner, T.; Glasnov, T.N.; Schreibmayer, W.; Platzer, D.; de la Cruz, G.G.; Krenn, S.; Schober, R.; et al. An optically controlled probe identifies lipid-gating fenestrations within the TRPC3 channel. *Nat. Chem. Biol.* **2018**, *14*, 396–404. [CrossRef] [PubMed]

34. Lucas, P.; Ukhanov, K.; Leinders-Zufall, T.; Zufall, F. A diacylglycerol-gated cation channel in vomeronasal neuron dendrites is impaired in TRPC2 mutant mice: Mechanism of pheromone transduction. *Neuron* **2003**, *40*, 551–561. [CrossRef]

35. Leinders-Zufall, T.; Storch, U.; Bleymehl, K.; Mederos, Y.S.M.; Frank, J.A.; Konrad, D.B.; Trauner, D.; Gudermann, T.; Zufall, F. PhoDAGs enable optical control of diacylglycerol-sensitive transient receptor potential channels. *Cell Chem. Biol.* **2018**, *25*, 215–223. [CrossRef] [PubMed]

36. Venkatachalam, K.; Zheng, F.; Gill, D.L. Regulation of canonical transient receptor potential (TRPC) channel function by diacylglycerol and protein kinase c. *J. Biol. Chem.* **2003**, *278*, 29031–29040. [CrossRef] [PubMed]

37. Otsuguro, K.; Tang, J.; Tang, Y.; Xiao, R.; Freichel, M.; Tsvilovskyy, V.; Ito, S.; Flockerzi, V.; Zhu, M.X.; Zholos, A.V. Isoform-specific inhibition of TRPC4 channel by phosphatidylinositol 4,5-bisphosphate. *J. Biol. Chem.* **2008**, *283*, 10026–10036. [CrossRef] [PubMed]

38. Trebak, M.; Lemonnier, L.; DeHaven, W.I.; Wedel, B.J.; Bird, G.S.; Putney, J.W., Jr. Complex functions of phosphatidylinositol 4,5-bisphosphate in regulation of TRPC5 cation channels. *Pflugers Arch.* **2009**, *457*, 757–769. [CrossRef] [PubMed]

39. Myeong, J.; Ko, J.; Kwak, M.; Kim, J.; Woo, J.; Ha, K.; Hong, C.; Yang, D.; Kim, H.J.; Jeon, J.H.; et al. Dual action of the $G\alpha_q$-PLCβ-PI(4,5)P$_2$ pathway on TRPC1/4 and TRPC1/5 heterotetramers. *Sci. Rep.* **2018**, *8*. [CrossRef] [PubMed]

40. Itsuki, K.; Imai, Y.; Hase, H.; Okamura, Y.; Inoue, R.; Mori, M.X. Plc-mediated PI(4,5)P2 hydrolysis regulates activation and inactivation of TRPC6/7 channels. *J. Gen. Physiol.* **2014**, *143*, 183–201. [CrossRef] [PubMed]

41. Tang, Y.; Tang, J.; Chen, Z.; Trost, C.; Flockerzi, V.; Li, M.; Ramesh, V.; Zhu, M.X. Association of mammalian trp4 and phospholipase c isozymes with a PDZ domain-containing protein, NHERF. *J. Biol. Chem.* **2000**, *275*, 37559–37564. [CrossRef] [PubMed]

42. Obukhov, A.G.; Nowycky, M.C. TRPC5 activation kinetics are modulated by the scaffolding protein ezrin/radixin/moesin-binding phosphoprotein-50 (ebp50). *J. Cell. Physiol.* **2004**, *201*, 227–235. [CrossRef] [PubMed]

43. Lee-Kwon, W.; Wade, J.B.; Zhang, Z.; Pallone, T.L.; Weinman, E.J. Expression of TRPC4 channel protein that interacts with NHERF-2 in rat descending vasa recta. *Am. J. Physiol. Cell Physiol.* **2005**, *288*, C942–C949. [CrossRef] [PubMed]

44. Shenolikar, S.; Minkoff, C.M.; Steplock, D.A.; Evangelista, C.; Liu, M.; Weinman, E.J. N-terminal pdz domain is required for NHERF dimerization. *FEBS Lett.* **2001**, *489*, 233–236. [CrossRef]

45. Mamonova, T.; Kurnikova, M.; Friedman, P.A. Structural basis for NHERF1 PDZ domain binding. *Biochemistry* **2012**, *51*, 3110–3120. [CrossRef] [PubMed]

46. Shenolikar, S.; Weinman, E.J. NHERF: Targeting and trafficking membrane proteins. *Am. J. Physiol. Renal. Physiol.* **2001**, *280*, F389–F395. [CrossRef] [PubMed]

47. Hall, R.A.; Ostedgaard, L.S.; Premont, R.T.; Blitzer, J.T.; Rahman, N.; Welsh, M.J.; Lefkowitz, R.J. A C-terminal motif found in the beta2-adrenergic receptor, P2Y1 receptor and cystic fibrosis transmembrane conductance regulator determines binding to the Na+/H+ exchanger regulatory factor family of PDZ proteins. *Proc. Natl. Acad. Sci. USA* **1998**, *95*, 8496–8501. [CrossRef] [PubMed]

48. Hall, R.A.; Premont, R.T.; Chow, C.W.; Blitzer, J.T.; Pitcher, J.A.; Claing, A.; Stoffel, R.H.; Barak, L.S.; Shenolikar, S.; Weinman, E.J.; et al. The beta2-adrenergic receptor interacts with the Na+/H+-exchanger regulatory factor to control Na+/H+ exchange. *Nature* **1998**, *392*, 626–630. [CrossRef] [PubMed]

49. Lee, Y.M.; Kim, B.J.; Kim, H.J.; Yang, D.K.; Zhu, M.H.; Lee, K.P.; So, I.; Kim, K.W. TRPC5 as a candidate for the nonselective cation channel activated by muscarinic stimulation in murine stomach. *Am. J. Physiol. Gastrointest. Liver Physiol.* **2003**, *284*, G604–G616. [CrossRef] [PubMed]

50. Mery, L.; Strauss, B.; Dufour, J.F.; Krause, K.H.; Hoth, M. The PDZ-interacting domain of TRPC4 controls its localization and surface expression in HEK293 cells. *J. Cell Sci.* **2002**, *115*, 3497–3508. [PubMed]

51. Zhu, M.H.; Chae, M.; Kim, H.J.; Lee, Y.M.; Kim, M.J.; Jin, N.G.; Yang, D.K.; So, I.; Kim, K.W. Desensitization of canonical transient receptor potential channel 5 by protein kinase c. *Am. J. Physiol. Cell Physiol.* **2005**, *289*, C591–C600. [CrossRef] [PubMed]

52. Holcomb, J.; Spellmon, N.; Trescott, L.; Sun, F.; Li, C.; Yang, Z. PDZ structure and implication in selective drug design against cystic fibrosis. *Curr. Drug Targets* **2015**, *16*, 945–950. [CrossRef] [PubMed]

53. Storch, U.; Forst, A.L.; Pardatscher, F.; Erdogmus, S.; Philipp, M.; Gregoritza, M.; Mederos y Schnitzler, M.; Gudermann, T. Dynamic NHERF interaction with TRPC4/5 proteins is required for channel gating by diacylglycerol. *Proc. Natl. Acad. Sci. USA* **2017**, *114*, E37–E46. [CrossRef] [PubMed]

54. Hall, R.A.; Spurney, R.F.; Premont, R.T.; Rahman, N.; Blitzer, J.T.; Pitcher, J.A.; Lefkowitz, R.J. G protein-coupled receptor kinase 6a phosphorylates the na(+)/h(+) exchanger regulatory factor via a pdz domain-mediated interaction. *J. Biol. Chem.* **1999**, *274*, 24328–24334. [CrossRef] [PubMed]

55. Maudsley, S.; Zamah, A.M.; Rahman, N.; Blitzer, J.T.; Luttrell, L.M.; Lefkowitz, R.J.; Hall, R.A. Platelet-derived growth factor receptor association with Na+/H+-exchanger regulatory factor potentiates receptor activity. *Mol. Cell Biol.* **2000**, *20*, 8352–8363. [CrossRef] [PubMed]

56. Weinman, E.J.; Hall, R.A.; Friedman, P.A.; Liu-Chen, L.Y.; Shenolikar, S. The association of NHERF adaptor proteins with g protein-coupled receptors and receptor tyrosine kinases. *Annu. Rev. Physiol.* **2006**, *68*, 491–505. [CrossRef] [PubMed]

57. Cunningham, R.; Biswas, R.; Steplock, D.; Shenolikar, S.; Weinman, E. Role of NHERF and scaffolding proteins in proximal tubule transport. *Urol. Res.* **2010**, *38*, 257–262. [CrossRef] [PubMed]

58. Courbebaisse, M.; Leroy, C.; Bakouh, N.; Salaun, C.; Beck, L.; Grandchamp, B.; Planelles, G.; Hall, R.A.; Friedlander, G.; Prie, D. A New Human NHERF1 Mutation Decreases Renal Phosphate Transporter NPT2a Expression by a PTH-Independent Mechanism. *PloS ONE* **2012**, *7*. [CrossRef] [PubMed]

59. Paquet, M.; Asay, M.J.; Fam, S.R.; Inuzuka, H.; Castleberry, A.M.; Oller, H.; Smith, Y.; Yun, C.C.; Traynelis, S.F.; Hall, R.A. The PDZ scaffold NHERF-2 interacts with mGluR5 and regulates receptor activity. *J. Biol. Chem.* **2006**, *281*, 29949–29961. [CrossRef] [PubMed]

60. Ritter, S.L.; Asay, M.J.; Paquet, M.; Paavola, K.J.; Reiff, R.E.; Yun, C.C.; Hall, R.A. GLAST stability and activity are enhanced by interaction with the PDZ scaffold NHERF-2. *Neurosci. Lett.* **2011**, *487*, 3–7. [CrossRef] [PubMed]

61. Ghishan, F.K.; Kiela, P.R. Small intestinal ion transport. *Curr. Opin. Gastroenterol.* **2012**, *28*, 130–134. [CrossRef] [PubMed]

62. Weinman, E.J.; Mohanlal, V.; Stoycheff, N.; Wang, F.; Steplock, D.; Shenolikar, S.; Cunningham, R. Longitudinal study of urinary excretion of phosphate, calcium, and uric acid in mutant NHERF-1 null mice. *Am. J. Physiol. Renal. Physiol.* **2006**, *290*, F838–F843. [CrossRef] [PubMed]

63. Karim, Z.; Gerard, B.; Bakouh, N.; Alili, R.; Leroy, C.; Beck, L.; Silve, C.; Planelles, G.; Urena-Torres, P.; Grandchamp, B.; et al. NHERF1 mutations and responsiveness of renal parathyroid hormone. *N. Engl. J. Med.* **2008**, *359*, 1128–1135. [CrossRef] [PubMed]

64. Liu, L.; Alonso, V.; Guo, L.; Tourkova, I.; Henderson, S.E.; Almarza, A.J.; Friedman, P.A.; Blair, H.C. Na+/H+ exchanger regulatory factor 1 (NHERF1) directly regulates osteogenesis. *J. Biol. Chem.* **2012**, *287*, 43312–43321. [CrossRef] [PubMed]

65. Bhattacharya, R.; Wang, E.; Dutta, S.K.; Vohra, P.K.; E, G.; Prakash, Y.S.; Mukhopadhyay, D. NHERF-2 maintains endothelial homeostasis. *Blood* **2012**, *119*, 4798–4806. [CrossRef] [PubMed]

66. Kruger, W.A.; Monteith, G.R.; Poronnik, P. NHERF-1 regulation of EGF and neurotensin signalling in HT-29 epithelial cells. *Biochem. Biophys. Res. Commun.* **2013**, *432*, 568–573. [CrossRef] [PubMed]

67. Voltz, J.W.; Weinman, E.J.; Shenolikar, S. Expanding the role of NHERF, a PDZ-domain containing protein adapter, to growth regulation. *Oncogene* **2001**, *20*, 6309–6314. [CrossRef] [PubMed]

68. Georgescu, M.M.; Morales, F.C.; Molina, J.R.; Hayashi, Y. Roles of NHERF1/EBP50 in cancer. *Curr. Mol. Med.* **2008**, *8*, 459–468. [CrossRef] [PubMed]

69. Lee, S.J.; Ritter, S.L.; Zhang, H.; Shim, H.; Hall, R.A.; Yun, C.C. MAGI-3 competes with NHERF-2 to negatively regulate LPA2 receptor signaling in colon cancer cells. *Gastroenterology* **2011**, *140*, 924–934. [CrossRef] [PubMed]

70. Mangia, A.; Partipilo, G.; Schirosi, L.; Saponaro, C.; Galetta, D.; Catino, A.; Scattone, A.; Simone, G. Fine needle aspiration cytology: A tool to study NHERF1 expression as a potential marker of aggressiveness in lung cancer. *Mol. Biotechnol.* **2015**, *57*, 549–557. [CrossRef] [PubMed]

71. Du, G.; Hao, C.; Gu, Y.; Wang, Z.; Jiang, W.G.; He, J.; Cheng, S. A novel NHERF1 mutation in human breast cancer inactivates inhibition by NHERF1 protein in EGFR signaling. *Anticancer Res.* **2016**, *36*, 1165–1173. [PubMed]

72. Yang, X.; Du, G.; Yu, Z.; Si, Y.; Martin, T.A.; He, J.; Cheng, S.; Jiang, W.G. A novel NHERF1 mutation in human breast cancer and effects on malignant progression. *Anticancer Res.* **2017**, *37*, 67–73. [CrossRef] [PubMed]

73. Kreimann, E.L.; Ratajska, M.; Kuzniacka, A.; Demacopulo, B.; Stukan, M.; Limon, J. A novel splicing mutation in the SLC9A3R1 gene in tumors from ovarian cancer patients. *Oncology Lett.* **2015**, *10*, 3722–3726. [CrossRef] [PubMed]

74. Saponaro, C.; Malfettone, A.; Dell'Endice, T.S.; Brunetti, A.E.; Achimas-Cadariu, P.; Paradiso, A.; Mangia, A. The prognostic value of the Na$^+$/H$^+$ exchanger regulatory factor 1 (NHERF1) protein in cancer. *Cancer Biomark.* **2014**, *14*, 177–184. [CrossRef] [PubMed]

75. Guggino, W.B.; Stanton, B.A. New insights into cystic fibrosis: Molecular switches that regulate cftr. *Nat. Rev. Mol. Cell Biol.* **2006**, *7*, 426–436. [CrossRef] [PubMed]

76. Cuppens, H.; Cassiman, J.J. CFTR mutations and polymorphisms in male infertility. *Int. J. Androl.* **2004**, *27*, 251–256. [CrossRef] [PubMed]

77. Holcomb, J.; Jiang, Y.; Lu, G.; Trescott, L.; Brunzelle, J.; Sirinupong, N.; Li, C.; Naren, A.P.; Yang, Z. Structural insights into PDZ-mediated interaction of NHERF2 and LPA(2), a cellular event implicated in CFTR channel regulation. *Biochem. Biophys. Res. Commun.* **2014**, *446*, 399–403. [CrossRef] [PubMed]

78. Zhang, W.; Penmatsa, H.; Ren, A.; Punchihewa, C.; Lemoff, A.; Yan, B.; Fujii, N.; Naren, A.P. Functional regulation of cystic fibrosis transmembrane conductance regulator-containing macromolecular complexes: A small-molecule inhibitor approach. *Biochem. J.* **2011**, *435*, 451–462. [CrossRef] [PubMed]

79. Sossey-Alaoui, K.; Lyon, J.A.; Jones, L.; Abidi, F.E.; Hartung, A.J.; Hane, B.; Schwartz, C.E.; Stevenson, R.E.; Srivastava, A.K. Molecular cloning and characterization of TRPC5 (HTRP5), the human homologue of a mouse brain receptor-activated capacitative Ca^{2+} entry channel. *Genomics* **1999**, *60*, 330–340. [CrossRef] [PubMed]

80. Philipp, S.; Hambrecht, J.; Braslavski, L.; Schroth, G.; Freichel, M.; Murakami, M.; Cavalie, A.; Flockerzi, V. A novel capacitative calcium entry channel expressed in excitable cells. *EMBO J.* **1998**, *17*, 4274–4282. [CrossRef] [PubMed]

81. Philipp, S.; Cavalie, A.; Freichel, M.; Wissenbach, U.; Zimmer, S.; Trost, C.; Marquart, A.; Murakami, M.; Flockerzi, V. A mammalian capacitative calcium entry channel homologous to drosophila TRP and TRPL. *EMBO J.* **1996**, *15*, 6166–6171. [CrossRef] [PubMed]

82. Mori, Y.; Takada, N.; Okada, T.; Wakamori, M.; Imoto, K.; Wanifuchi, H.; Oka, H.; Oba, A.; Ikenaka, K.; Kurosaki, T. Differential distribution of TRP Ca^{2+} channel isoforms in mouse brain. *Neuroreport* **1998**, *9*, 507–515. [PubMed]

83. Munsch, T.; Freichel, M.; Flockerzi, V.; Pape, H.C. Contribution of transient receptor potential channels to the control of GABA release from dendrites. *Proc. Natl. Acad. Sci. USA* **2003**, *100*, 16065–16070. [CrossRef] [PubMed]

84. Okada, T.; Shimizu, S.; Wakamori, M.; Maeda, A.; Kurosaki, T.; Takada, N.; Imoto, K.; Mori, Y. Molecular cloning and functional characterization of a novel receptor-activated TRP Ca^{2+} channel from mouse brain. *J. Biol. Chem.* **1998**, *273*, 10279–10287. [CrossRef] [PubMed]

85. Turvey, M.R.; Wang, Y.; Gu, Y. The effects of extracellular nucleotides on [Ca^{2+}]$_i$ signalling in a human-derived renal proximal tubular cell line (HKC-8). *J. Cell. Biochem.* **2010**, *109*, 132–139. [PubMed]

86. Yip, H.; Chan, W.Y.; Leung, P.C.; Kwan, H.Y.; Liu, C.; Huang, Y.; Michel, V.; Yew, D.T.; Yao, X. Expression of TRPC homologs in endothelial cells and smooth muscle layers of human arteries. *Histochem. Cell Biol.* **2004**, *122*, 553–561. [CrossRef] [PubMed]

87. Riccio, A.; Li, Y.; Moon, J.; Kim, K.S.; Smith, K.S.; Rudolph, U.; Gapon, S.; Yao, G.L.; Tsvetkov, E.; Rodig, S.J.; et al. Essential role for TRPC5 in amygdala function and fear-related behavior. *Cell* **2009**, *137*, 761–772. [CrossRef] [PubMed]

88. Riccio, A.; Li, Y.; Tsvetkov, E.; Gapon, S.; Yao, G.L.; Smith, K.S.; Engin, E.; Rudolph, U.; Bolshakov, V.Y.; Clapham, D.E. Decreased anxiety-like behavior and Gαq/11-dependent responses in the amygdala of mice lacking TRPC4 channels. *J. Neurosci.* **2014**, *34*, 3653–3667. [CrossRef] [PubMed]

89. Wei, H.; Sagalajev, B.; Yuzer, M.A.; Koivisto, A.; Pertovaara, A. Regulation of neuropathic pain behavior by amygdaloid TRPC4/C5 channels. *Neurosci. Lett.* **2015**, *608*, 12–17. [CrossRef] [PubMed]

90. Wu, D.; Huang, W.; Richardson, P.M.; Priestley, J.V.; Liu, M. TRPC4 in rat dorsal root ganglion neurons is increased after nerve injury and is necessary for neurite outgrowth. *J. Biol. Chem.* **2008**, *283*, 416–426. [CrossRef] [PubMed]

91. Lee, S.H.; Cho, P.S.; Tonello, R.; Lee, H.K.; Jang, J.H.; Park, G.Y.; Hwang, S.W.; Park, C.K.; Jung, S.J.; Berta, T. Peripheral serotonin receptor 2b and transient receptor potential channel 4 mediate pruritus to serotonergic antidepressants in mice. *J. Allergy Clin. Immunol.* **2018**, *142*, 1349–1352. [CrossRef] [PubMed]

92. Zimmermann, K.; Lennerz, J.K.; Hein, A.; Link, A.S.; Kaczmarek, J.S.; Delling, M.; Uysal, S.; Pfeifer, J.D.; Riccio, A.; Clapham, D.E. Transient receptor potential cation channel, subfamily c, member 5 (TRPC5) is a cold-transducer in the peripheral nervous system. *Proc. Natl. Acad. Sci. USA* **2011**, *108*, 18114–18119. [CrossRef] [PubMed]

93. Tai, C.; Hines, D.J.; Choi, H.B.; MacVicar, B.A. Plasma membrane insertion of TRPC5 channels contributes to the cholinergic plateau potential in hippocampal CA1 pyramidal neurons. *Hippocampus* **2011**, *21*, 958–967. [CrossRef] [PubMed]

94. Dichter, M.A.; Ayala, G.F. Cellular mechanisms of epilepsy: A status report. *Science* **1987**, *237*, 157–164. [CrossRef]

95. Fraser, D.D.; MacVicar, B.A. Cholinergic-dependent plateau potential in hippocampal CA1 pyramidal neurons. *J. Neurosci.* **1996**, *16*, 4113–4128. [CrossRef] [PubMed]

96. Greka, A.; Navarro, B.; Oancea, E.; Duggan, A.; Clapham, D.E. TRPC5 is a regulator of hippocampal neurite length and growth cone morphology. *Nat. Neurosci.* **2003**, *6*, 837–845. [CrossRef] [PubMed]

97. Tian, D.; Jacobo, S.M.; Billing, D.; Rozkalne, A.; Gage, S.D.; Anagnostou, T.; Pavenstadt, H.; Hsu, H.H.; Schlondorff, J.; Ramos, A.; et al. Antagonistic regulation of actin dynamics and cell motility by TRPC5 and TRPC6 channels. *Sci. Signal.* **2010**, *3*. [CrossRef] [PubMed]

98. Huber, T.B.; Schermer, B.; Benzing, T. Podocin organizes ion channel-lipid supercomplexes: Implications for mechanosensation at the slit diaphragm. *Nephron Exp. Nephrol.* **2007**, *106*, e27–e31. [CrossRef] [PubMed]

99. Huber, T.B.; Schermer, B.; Muller, R.U.; Hohne, M.; Bartram, M.; Calixto, A.; Hagmann, H.; Reinhardt, C.; Koos, F.; Kunzelmann, K.; et al. Podocin and MEC-2 bind cholesterol to regulate the activity of associated ion channels. *Proc. Natl. Acad. Sci. USA* **2006**, *103*, 17079–17086. [CrossRef] [PubMed]

100. Takeda, T.; McQuistan, T.; Orlando, R.A.; Farquhar, M.G. Loss of glomerular foot processes is associated with uncoupling of podocalyxin from the actin cytoskeleton. *J. Clin. Invest.* **2001**, *108*, 289–301. [CrossRef] [PubMed]

101. Asanuma, K.; Yanagida-Asanuma, E.; Faul, C.; Tomino, Y.; Kim, K.; Mundel, P. Synaptopodin orchestrates actin organization and cell motility via regulation of RhoA signalling. *Nat. Cell Biol.* **2006**, *8*, 485–491. [CrossRef] [PubMed]

102. Faul, C.; Asanuma, K.; Yanagida-Asanuma, E.; Kim, K.; Mundel, P. Actin up: Regulation of podocyte structure and function by components of the actin cytoskeleton. *Trends Cell Biol.* **2007**, *17*, 428–437. [CrossRef] [PubMed]

103. Zhou, Y.; Castonguay, P.; Sidhom, E.H.; Clark, A.R.; Dvela-Levitt, M.; Kim, S.; Sieber, J.; Wieder, N.; Jung, J.Y.; Andreeva, S.; et al. A small-molecule inhibitor of TRPC5 ion channels suppresses progressive kidney disease in animal models. *Science* **2017**, *358*, 1332–1336. [CrossRef] [PubMed]

104. Schaldecker, T.; Kim, S.; Tarabanis, C.; Tian, D.; Hakroush, S.; Castonguay, P.; Ahn, W.; Wallentin, H.; Heid, H.; Hopkins, C.R.; et al. Inhibition of the TRPC5 ion channel protects the kidney filter. *J. Clin. Invest.* **2013**, *123*, 5298–5309. [CrossRef] [PubMed]

105. Ma, X.; Cai, Y.; He, D.; Zou, C.; Zhang, P.; Lo, C.Y.; Xu, Z.; Chan, F.L.; Yu, S.; Chen, Y.; et al. Transient receptor potential channel TRPC5 is essential for p-glycoprotein induction in drug-resistant cancer cells. *Proc. Natl. Acad. Sci. USA* **2012**, *109*, 16282–16287. [CrossRef] [PubMed]

106. Wang, T.; Chen, Z.; Zhu, Y.; Pan, Q.; Liu, Y.; Qi, X.; Jin, L.; Jin, J.; Ma, X.; Hua, D. Inhibition of transient receptor potential channel 5 reverses 5-fluorouracil resistance in human colorectal cancer cells. *J. Biol. Chem.* **2015**, *290*, 448–456. [CrossRef] [PubMed]

107. Akbulut, Y.; Gaunt, H.J.; Muraki, K.; Ludlow, M.J.; Amer, M.S.; Bruns, A.; Vasudev, N.S.; Radtke, L.; Willot, M.; Hahn, S.; et al. (-)-Englerin a is a potent and selective activator of TRPC4 and TRPC5 calcium channels. *Angew Chem. Int. Ed. Engl.* **2015**, *54*, 3787–3791. [CrossRef] [PubMed]

108. Carson, C.; Raman, P.; Tullai, J.; Xu, L.; Henault, M.; Thomas, E.; Yeola, S.; Lao, J.M.; McPate, M.; Verkuyl, J.M.; et al. Englerin A agonizes the TRPC4/C5 cation channels to inhibit tumor cell line proliferation. *PloS ONE* **2015**, *10*. [CrossRef] [PubMed]

109. Ratnayake, R.; Covell, D.; Ransom, T.T.; Gustafson, K.R.; Beutler, J.A. Englerin A, a selective inhibitor of renal cancer cell growth, from Phyllanthus engleri. *Org. Lett.* **2009**, *11*, 57–60. [CrossRef] [PubMed]
110. Gluz, O.; Liedtke, C.; Gottschalk, N.; Pusztai, L.; Nitz, U.; Harbeck, N. Triple-negative breast cancer–current status and future directions. *Ann. Oncol.* **2009**, *20*, 1913–1927. [CrossRef] [PubMed]
111. Dent, R.; Trudeau, M.; Pritchard, K.I.; Hanna, W.M.; Kahn, H.K.; Sawka, C.A.; Lickley, L.A.; Rawlinson, E.; Sun, P.; Narod, S.A. Triple-negative breast cancer: Clinical features and patterns of recurrence. *Clin. Cancer Res.* **2007**, *13*, 4429–4434. [CrossRef] [PubMed]
112. Liedtke, C.; Mazouni, C.; Hess, K.R.; Andre, F.; Tordai, A.; Mejia, J.A.; Symmans, W.F.; Gonzalez-Angulo, A.M.; Hennessy, B.; Green, M.; et al. Response to neoadjuvant therapy and long-term survival in patients with triple-negative breast cancer. *J. Clin. Oncol.* **2008**, *26*, 1275–1281. [CrossRef] [PubMed]
113. Cheung, S.Y.; Henrot, M.; Al-Saad, M.; Baumann, M.; Muller, H.; Unger, A.; Rubaiy, H.N.; Mathar, I.; Dinkel, K.; Nussbaumer, P.; et al. TRPC4/TRPC5 channels mediate adverse reaction to the cancer cell cytotoxic agent (-)-Englerin A. *Oncotarget* **2018**, *9*, 29634–29643. [CrossRef] [PubMed]
114. Zhu, Y.; Pan, Q.; Meng, H.; Jiang, Y.; Mao, A.; Wang, T.; Hua, D.; Yao, X.; Jin, J.; Ma, X. Enhancement of vascular endothelial growth factor release in long-term drug-treated breast cancer via transient receptor potential channel 5-Ca(2+)-hypoxia-inducible factor 1α pathway. *Pharmacol. Res.* **2015**, *93*, 36–42. [CrossRef] [PubMed]
115. Veliceasa, D.; Ivanovic, M.; Hoepfner, F.T.; Thumbikat, P.; Volpert, O.V.; Smith, N.D. Transient potential receptor channel 4 controls thrombospondin-1 secretion and angiogenesis in renal cell carcinoma. *FEBS J.* **2007**, *274*, 6365–6377. [CrossRef] [PubMed]
116. Antigny, F.; Girardin, N.; Frieden, M. Transient receptor potential canonical channels are required for in vitro endothelial tube formation. *J. Biol. Chem.* **2012**, *287*, 5917–5927. [CrossRef] [PubMed]
117. Song, H.B.; Jun, H.O.; Kim, J.H.; Fruttiger, M.; Kim, J.H. Suppression of transient receptor potential canonical channel 4 inhibits vascular endothelial growth factor-induced retinal neovascularization. *Cell Calcium* **2015**, *57*, 101–108. [CrossRef] [PubMed]
118. Zeng, B.; Yuan, C.; Yang, X.; Atkin, S.L.; Xu, S.Z. TRPC channels and their splice variants are essential for promoting human ovarian cancer cell proliferation and tumorigenesis. *Curr. Cancer Drug Targets* **2013**, *13*, 103–116. [CrossRef] [PubMed]
119. Gaunt, H.J.; Vasudev, N.S.; Beech, D.J. Transient receptor potential canonical 4 and 5 proteins as targets in cancer therapeutics. *Eur. Biophys. J.* **2016**, *45*, 611–620. [CrossRef] [PubMed]
120. Gough, N.R. New connections: NHERF gates activity. *Sci. Signal.* **2017**, *10*. [CrossRef] [PubMed]
121. Loureiro, C.A.; Matos, A.M.; Dias-Alves, A.; Pereira, J.F.; Uliyakina, I.; Barros, P.; Amaral, M.D.; Matos, P. A molecular switch in the scaffold NHERF1 enables misfolded CFTR to evade the peripheral quality control checkpoint. *Sci. Signal.* **2015**, *8*. [CrossRef] [PubMed]

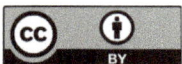

© 2018 by the authors. Licensee MDPI, Basel, Switzerland. This article is an open access article distributed under the terms and conditions of the Creative Commons Attribution (CC BY) license (http://creativecommons.org/licenses/by/4.0/).

Review

Ion Channels and Transporters in Inflammation: Special Focus on TRP Channels and TRPC6

Giuseppe A. Ramirez [1,2,3,*], **Lavinia A. Coletto** [1,2,3], **Clara Sciorati** [1,3], **Enrica P. Bozzolo** [1,2], **Paolo Manunta** [1,4], **Patrizia Rovere-Querini** [1,2,3] and **Angelo A. Manfredi** [1,2,3]

[1] Unit of Immunology, Rheumatology, Allergy and Rare Diseases, Università Vita-Salute San Raffaele, 20132 Milan, Italy; lavinia.coletto@gmail.com (L.A.C.); sciorati.clara@hsr.it (C.S.); bozzolo.enrica@hsr.it (E.P.B.); manunta.paolo@hsr.it (P.M.); rovere.patrizia@hsr.it (P.R.-Q.); manfredi.angelo@hsr.it (A.A.M.)

[2] Unit of Immunology, Rheumatology, Allergy and Rare Diseases, IRCCS Ospedale San Raffaele, 20132 Milan, Italy

[3] Division of Immunology, Transplantation and Infectious Immunity, IRCCS Ospedale San Raffaele, 20132 Milan, Italy

[4] Unit of Nephrology, IRCCS Ospedale San Raffaele, 20132 Milan, Italy

[*] Correspondence: ramirez.giuseppealvise@hsr.it; Tel.: +39-022-643-3950

Received: 11 June 2018; Accepted: 29 June 2018; Published: 4 July 2018

Abstract: Allergy and autoimmune diseases are characterised by a multifactorial pathogenic background. Several genes involved in the control of innate and adaptive immunity have been associated with diseases and variably combine with each other as well as with environmental factors and epigenetic processes to shape the characteristics of individual manifestations. Systemic or local perturbations in salt/water balance and in ion exchanges between the intra- and extracellular spaces or among tissues play a role. In this field, usually referred to as elementary immunology, novel evidence has been recently acquired on the role of members of the transient potential receptor (TRP) channel family in several cellular mechanisms of potential significance for the pathophysiology of the immune response. TRP canonical channel 6 (TRPC6) is emerging as a functional element for the control of calcium currents in immune-committed cells and target tissues. In fact, TRPC6 influences leukocytes' tasks such as transendothelial migration, chemotaxis, phagocytosis and cytokine release. TRPC6 also modulates the sensitivity of immune cells to apoptosis and influences tissue susceptibility to ischemia-reperfusion injury and excitotoxicity. Here, we provide a view of the interactions between ion exchanges and inflammation with a focus on the pathogenesis of immune-mediated diseases and potential future therapeutic implications.

Keywords: TRPC6; elementary immunology; inflammation; calcium; sodium; neutrophils; lymphocytes; endothelium; platelets

---

1. Introduction

Ion exchanges between the intra- and extracellular spaces constitute fundamental mechanisms for the control of cell metabolism and activation state. Changes in the rate of crucial cell reactions such as energy accumulation, protein synthesis and cytoskeleton assembly in response to environmental stimuli are required for the long-term maintenance of homeostasis in complex organisms. Accordingly, genes encoding proteins expressed on the cell membrane to regulate its permeability to ions are crucial for the most complex intra- and intercellular tasks. In particular, ion channels (which account for up to 1% of the human genome [1] and allow the communication among different cells in an organism [1]. The nervous system is important to coordinate the ability of multicellular organisms to sense, adapt, record and possibly predict external stimuli [2]. The role of ion channels in neuronal activation has been investigated leading to seminal discoveries on their role in physiology and disease.

The current set of human ion channels genes marks the pillars of adaptive immunity [2], suggesting a link between ion channel specialisation and novel biological functions committed to host defence. Consistently, growing evidence is accumulating on the ability of ions, ion channels and transporters and their pharmacological modulators to influence the behaviour of the immune system at the cellular and clinical level, a phenomenon also known as elementary immunology [3].

Transient receptor potential (TRP) channels comprise a wide family of membrane proteins behaving as sodium/calcium permeable molecules. Their role in the deployment of the innate and adaptive immune response has received growing attention [4]. In this setting, TRP canonical channel 6 (TRPC6) has emerged as a modulator of calcium homeostasis in leukocytes and tissues involved by the inflammatory response. Here, we will review the potential mechanisms related to TRPC6 function considering its similarities and interactions with the elements of the cellular machinery committed to ion balance control.

2. Elementary Immunology: An Expanding Landscape

Ion channels and transporters affect immune responses [5] mainly by trimming endosomal pH [6–9] and intracellular calcium concentrations [3,10,11] (Table 1, Figure 1). This latter mechanism involves the intrinsic biophysical properties of a given ion channels or transporter and its ability to allow or facilitate the passage of calcium through the cell membrane. Changes in permeability of calcium channels or transporters can be triggered by either engagement of specific ligands (receptor-operated calcium entry, ROCE), feedforward responses to the release of calcium from intracellular stores (store-operated calcium entry, SOCE) and/or changes in cell polarisation (voltage-operated calcium entry, VOCE) and in the strength of the sodium driving force.

In the majority of cells, the most significant contribution to the rise of intracellular calcium concentrations is due to SOCE events [12–15], which are primed by the release of intracellular calcium stores downstream cell-specific activation pathways. These latter include the B- and T-cell receptor (BcR and TcR) or the Fc receptors pathways [15,16]. The main player in this setting is constituted by a functional triad comprising (a) an inositol-1,4,5-triphosphate (IP$_3$) receptor channel expressed on the endoplasmic reticulum, which allows calcium to flow into the cytoplasm; (b) a set of cytoplasmic sensors called stromal interaction molecules (STIM); and (c) a membrane channel, bound to STIMs and composed of homo- or heteromers of members of the ORAI channel family [17,18]. The combination of ORAI and STIM protein is usually referred to as the calcium release-activated calcium channel (CRAC). The generation of IP$_3$ is due to the activity of several types of phospholipases and is paired with the production of diacylglycerol (DAG), which in turn constitutes a ligand for several receptor/channels [19,20]. Intracellular phospholipases are involved in the signal cascades downstream BcR or TcR and can be modulated by the activity of ancillary ion-pathways such as those involving magnesium or zinc interchanges between the intra and extracellular space [21–26]. Auto- or paracrine adenosine triphosphate (ATP), adenosine diphosphate ribose (ADPR), and multiple other chemical ligands or physical stimuli modulate ROCE [27–30].

Voltage-gated calcium channels (Ca$_V$) are required for leukocyte survival and are thought to be responsive to variations in cell polarisation [31]. Among the Ca$_V$ subtypes, those belonging to the α1 pore-forming subunit family have been identified in lymphocytes [32]. Indirect pharmacological evidence suggests a role of Ca$_V$ in myeloid-derived cells [31]. Sodium–calcium exchangers exploit gradients provided by the sodium-potassium ATPases to extrude calcium from the intracellular space. However, sodium depletion and prolonged cell depolarisation promote calcium entry through these transporters and favour cell activation [33,34].

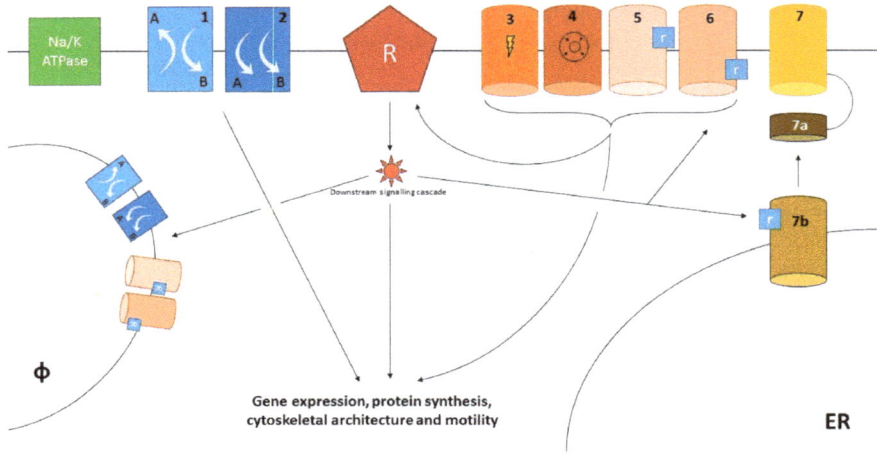

Figure 1. Ion channels and transporters. Ion channels and transporters may affect the behaviour of innate and adaptive immune cells at several levels. Under resting conditions, ion gradients between the intra- and extracellular space are actively generated through the Na/K ATPases. These gradients are exploited by transporters (1, 2) to trim the concentrations of other ions, including calcium. Cell activation after engagement of a cell-specific receptor (R), e.g., the BcR or TcR for lymphocytes or the FcR for myeloid cells, promotes the deployment of downstream signalling cascades that ultimately affect gene expression, protein synthesis and cause cytoskeletal remodelling, enabling cells to perform effector tasks such as chemotaxis, phagocytosis and release of antimicrobial moieties or cytokines. Activation of surface ion channels is integral to these events. A first set of ion channels are activated by physical or biochemical stimuli such as voltage (3), intracellular osmotic pressure (4) or engagement of extracellular (5) or intracellular (6) ligands, which in turn may be directly or indirectly induced by the activation of cell-specific receptors. Conversely, ion currents generated by voltage-operated or receptor-operated channels can exert feedback or feedforward effects on cell activating receptors. Specifically, raised calcium concentrations play a prominent role in mediating cell activation. However, to this regard store-operated calcium entry (SOCE, 7) generally provides a more significant contribution compared to voltage-operated or receptor-operated calcium entry (VOCE, ROCE). SOCE is propitiated by the activation of a inositol-1,4,5-triphosphate (IP$_3$) receptor channel on the surface of the endoplasmic reticulum (ER, 7b). Increased intracellular IP$_3$ concentrations are part of the changes induced by cell activation downstream cell-specific receptors (R). The release of calcium from ER stores is then sensed by adaptor proteins such as stromal interaction molecules (STIM; 7a), which in turn activate surface receptors (7), such as those of the ORAI family. Beside the cell surface, ion channels and transporters can also be expressed on intracellular compartments such as the phagolysosomes (φ). In this setting, they trim the endosomal pH, thus favouring the digestion of microbes and/or other dangerous moieties.

Gain of function mutations in the sodium–calcium exchanger 1 (*NCX1*) gene, highly expressed at the level of arterial smooth muscle cells, which show a constitutively slow recovery from depolarisation, associate with arterial hypertension, especially in the setting of sodium overload [35,36]. Enhanced activation and pro-inflammatory differentiation of macrophages and T-lymphocytes and enhanced formation of neutrophil extracellular traps occur in sodium-enriched extracellular environments [37–42]. *NCX1* risk alleles for salt-sensitive hypertension influences the course of nephritis in patients with systemic lupus erythematosus (SLE) [43]. While sodium overload can prompt NCX1 overactivity and enhanced cell activation, sodium-depleting conditions can also promote NCX1-mediated calcium responses and induce TNFalpha release from macrophages, mimicking lipopolysaccharide stimulation [44], and accelerate neutrophil recovery from an activation boost by increasing the speed of replenishment of intracellular calcium stores [11]. Voltage-gated potassium or sodium channels such as $K_v1.3$ and $Na_v1.5$, calcium-activated potassium channels such as $K_{Ca}3.1$ and chloride channels, all play significant roles in the modulation of membrane polarisation, respectively, favouring or limiting calcium currents [27,45–49]. Macrophages from patients with cystic fibrosis, who have dysfunctional chloride currents due to mutations in the Cystic Fibrosis Transmembrane Conductance Regulator (*CFTR*) gene, are characterised by persistent pro-inflammatory activation and defective phagocytosis, facilitating chronic infection [50,51]. Ion channels and transporters also selectively exert a specifying modulatory role on geographically distinct compartments within immune-committed cells [52].

Besides the modulation of calcium currents, ion channels and transporters involved in the modulation of protons, sodium and calcium influence the functionality of immune cells by regulating the generation of reactive oxygen species (ROS) and interfering with the signalling pathways involved in the processing of immune stimuli [53,54]. Sodium-based transporters are fundamental for the modulation of energy uptake, which ultimately affect the cell lifespan [55]. Immune cells alternatively exploit ion channels and transporters to regulate the unconventional release of cytokines such IL-1β [29,56,57] or modulate their expression by modifying ion balances within the cell nucleus [58,59].

The variety of biochemical effects of ion channels and transporters on cell homeostasis ultimately influences the processing of immune stimuli [15]. Persistent alterations in the control of ion exchanges at the cellular level might ultimately contribute to hypersensitivity and autoimmunity while altered function of ion channels and transporters might influence the ability of target tissues to cope with inflammation-induced damage.

Table 1. Functional impact of selected ion channels and transporters on inflammation.

			1. Modulation of Calcium Currents		
			1.1 Through Direct Involvement in Calcium Influx/Efflux		
			1.1.1 SOCE		
Channel	Permeability	Expression (immune cells)	Biological effects	Clinical correlates	Ref.
ORAI1	Ca^{2+}	Neutrophils, Lymphocytes	*Neutrophils*: proliferation, degranulation, cytokines production, cell polarization, migrational guidance with LFA1. *Lymphocytes*: B, T and NK cell proliferation, cytokine production and/or cytotoxicity in vitro; immunity to infection, T cell-mediated autoimmunity and inflammation, and allogeneic T cell responses in vivo; Treg cell development	CRAC channelopathy with immunodeficiency, autoimmunity, lymphoproliferation, muscular hypotonia and ectodermal dysplasia caused by mutations in STIM1 and ORAI1	[10,27,60,61]
ORAI2/3	Ca^{2+}	Neutrophils, Lymphocytes	Cell proliferation, Cytokines production	ND	
STIM1	NA	Neutrophils, Lymphocytes, DC, mast cells	*Neutrophils*: phagocytosis and ROS production *Lymphocytes*: cytokine production in T and B cells, Treg functionality *Mast cells*: FcεR-triggered SOCE	ND	[13,14,27,62–64]
STIM2	NA			Mice deficient of STIM1/2 develop a lymphoproliferative disorder because of dysfunction of Treg cells.	
IP3Rs	Ca^{2+}	All cells	Physiological development of B and T cells	ND	[16–19]
TRPC1	Ca^{2+}, Na^+	Endothelium	Enhanced vascular permeability after TNF/thrombin stimulation	ND	[65–67]
TRPC6	Ca^{2+}, Na^+	Platelets	Dense granules secretion after thrombin stimulation	ND	[68]
			1.1.2 ROCE		
Channel	Permeability	Expression (immune cells)	Biological effects	Clinical correlates	Ref.
TRPM2	Ca^{2+}, Na^+	Neutrophils, lymphocytes, macrophages and DC	*Neutrophils*: increased activation and endothelial adhesion *Lymphocytes*: T cell proliferation and cytokine secretion *Macrophages and dendritic cells*: regulation of ROS formation	Mice lacking TRPM2 have milder ischaemia-reperfusion injury after myocardial infarction and attenuated experimental brain inflammation	[54,69–75]
TRPC3	Ca^{2+}, Na^+	Lymphocytes, macrophages	*Lymphocytes*: T cell activation downstream the TCR *Macrophages*: enhanced pro-inflammatory activation	Mice: accelerated atherosclerosis	[76–78]
TRPC6	Ca^{2+}, Na^+	Lymphocytes, neutrophils, endothelium, platelets	*Lymphocytes*: T cell activation *Neutrophils*: chemotaxis, *Endothelium*: enhanced endothelial permeability and activation *Platelets*: TXA2-dependent expression of glycoproteins IIb-IIIa and P-selectin, release of platelet dense granules	Mice: TRPC6 ko associates with milder airway hypersensitivity in asthma models Humans: single study suggesting an association between a TRPC6 polymorphism and neuropsychiatric SLE	[79–85]

Table 1. Cont.

Channel	Permeability	Expression (immune cells)	Biological effects	Clinical correlates	Ref.
TRPV4	Ca^{2+}, Na^+	Macrophages	Cell activation after lung barotrauma.	Mice: exacerbated lung inflammation in acute lung injury and increased inflammatory hyperalgesia	[30]
P2X1R, P2X4R	Ca^{2+}, Na^+	Lymphocytes, neutrophils, eosinophils, monocytes/macrophages, mast cells, and DC	*Lymphocytes*: T cell proliferation; cytokine production; thymocyte apoptosis. *Macrophages*: PGE2 release, inflammasome activation	ND	[86,87]
P2X7R	Ca^{2+}, Na^+, other cations		*Lymphocytes*: T cell survival and cytokine production (downstream the TCR); T cell differentiation into Th17 vs. Treg. *Macrophages*: activation of the NLRP3 inflammasome. *Mast cells, eosinophils, DC*: inflammatory activation	Mice lacking P2X7R have attenuated allergic airway response, graft vs. host disease, allograft rejection	[88–90]

1.1.3 VOCE

Channel	Permeability	Expression (immune cells)	Biological effects	Clinical correlates	Ref.
Cav1.1-4	Ca^{2+}	Lymphocytes	T cell survival, differentiation and progression to effector function	ND	[31,32]

1.1.4 Direct calcium entry following upregulation

Channel	Permeability	Expression (immune cells)	Biological effects	Clinical correlates	Ref.
TRPC3	Ca^{2+}, Na^+	Macrophages/microglia	Regulation of cellular activation	Mice: reduced brain inflammation and post-ischaemic myocardial damage	[28,91,92]
TRPC5	Ca^{2+}, Na^+	Lymphocytes	Inhibition of Teff activation by Treg	Mice: protection from experimental arthritis	[93,94]
TRPV1	Ca^{2+}, Na^+	T lymphocytes	Cell activation (by associating to TCR)	ND	[95]
TRPV2	Ca^{2+}, Na^+	Macrophages	Phagocytosis, chemotaxis, following FCγR activation	Mice: TRPV2 deletion prompts accelerated mortality in bacterial infections. Humans: cystic Fibrosis macrophages exhibit a defect in TRPV2-mediated calcium influx	[51,96]
TRPV5,6	Ca^{2+}, Na^+	Lymphocytes	Cell activation and proliferation (the channels are constitutively active and regulated by endocytosis or at gene expression level).	ND	[97]

1.2 Through intracellular second messengers

Channel	Permeability	Expression (immune cells)	Biological effects	Clinical correlates	Ref.
TRPM7	Mg^{2+}, Ca^{2+}	Lymphocytes, macrophages, mast cells	Lymphocytes: activation downstream BCR and TCR; thymocyte development; production of thymocyte growth factor. Macrophages: survival and M2 polarisation. Mast cells: survival and activation	ND	[98–103]

Table 1. *Cont.*

MAGT1	Mg^{2+}	Lymphocytes	CD4+ T cell development and activation; immunity to EBV	XMEN syndrome (X-linked mutations in MAGT1)	[104]
ZIP6	Zn^{2+}	T cells, DC	*T cells*: sustained calcium currents enhancing TCR-related pathways and promoting T cell activation. *DC*: inhibition of maturation for antigen presentation	Genetically determined zinc deficit (mutated ZIP4 in the intestinal mucosa) causes acrodermatitis enteropathica with immunodeficiency	[26]
ZIP8		T cells	Sustained calcium currents enhancing TCR-related pathways and promoting T cell activation		

1.3 Through alterations of cell polarisation

Channel	*Permeability*	*Expression (immune cells)*	*Biological effects*	*Clinical correlates*	*Ref.*
NCX1	Ca^{2+}, Na^+	Neutrophils Macrophages	Neutrophils: recovery from activation. Macrophages: activation, cytokine (TNF) secretion	A single association study suggests potential links among NCX polymorphisms and SLE phenotypes (including severe nephritis)	[11,43,44]
NKCC2	Na^+, K^+, $2Cl^-$	Lymphocytes	Adaptation to extracellular hypertonicity, which eventually leads to the activation of the p38/MAPK $\rightarrow$ NFAT5 $\rightarrow$ SGK pathway, which favours Th17 differentiation	ND	[37]
ENaC	Na^+				
NHE1	Na^+, H^+				
TRPM4	Na^+, Ca^{2+}	Lymphocytes, macrophages and DC, mast cells	*Lymphocytes*: T helper motility and cytokine production (IL2, IL4, and IFNγ). *Macrophages*: phagocytosis and cytokine release. *DC*: motility. *Mast cells*: regulation of cell activation	Mice: lack of TRPM4 associates with reduced survival in sepsis and more intense anaphylaxis	[105–108]
GABA$_A$-R	Cl^-	Lymphocytes, macrophages and DC, neutrophils	Inhibition of cell activation	In preclinical models GABAergic drugs, protects against type 1 diabetes (T1D), experimental autoimmune encephalomyelitis (EAE), collagen-induced arthritis (CIA), contact dermatitis and allergic asthma. Treatment with gabapentin and pregabalin improved psoriasis (case report).	[49]
CFTR	Cl^-	Lymphocytes, macrophages	*Lymphocytes*: modulation of cytokine secretory profile (IL5, IL10) in T cells. *Macrophages*: cytokine release, phagocytosis	Cystic fibrosis	[51,109]
$K_V1.3$	K^+	Lymphocytes	Enhanced activation of the NLRP3 inflammasome and of IL1β production. Enhanced cell survival and prolonged activation.	A single phase Ib study on dalazatide (a specific $K_V1.3$ inhibitor) shows promise. Applications in SLE have been proposed.	[110–112]

Table 1. *Cont.*

Channel	Permeability	Expression (immune cells)	Biological effects	Clinical correlates	Ref.
KCa3.1	K$^+$	Lymphocytes, macrophages, endothelium	*Lymphocytes*: sustained TCR-induced calcium currents to support long-lasting effector functions. *Macrophages*: activation, chemotaxis, infiltration of atherosclerotic plaques *Endothelium*: proliferation	Encouraging evidence of efficacy of K$_{Ca}$3.1blockers in several models of inflammatory vasculopathy and autoimmunity.	[47,113–116]
Na$_V$1.5 (SCN5A)	Na$^+$	T cells	Positive selection of thymocytes	ND	[46]
P2X$_7$R	Ca^{2+}, Na$^+$ and other cations	Macrophages	Cell death for prolonged depolarisation in case of sustained receptor ligation.	ND	[117]

1.4 Through alterations in the geographical distribution of intracellular calcium

Channel	Permeability	Expression (immune cells)	Biological effects	Clinical correlates	Ref.
TRPC1	Ca^{2+}, Na$^+$	Neutrophils	Cell polarisation for chemotaxis	ND	[65–67]

2. Modulation of intracellular pH and production of reactive oxygen species

Channel	Permeability	Expression (immune cells)	Biological effects	Clinical correlates	Ref.
TRPM2	Ca^{2+}, Na$^+$	Macrophages and DC	*Macrophages and DC*: regulation of ROS formation, phagocytosis and bacterial killing	ND	[71,75]
H$_V$1/VSOP	H$^+$	lymphocytes, granulocytes, macrophages and DC	All cells: phagocytosis and ROS production B cells: BCR signalling	Mice: loss of the receptor prompts impaired killing of phagocytosed bacteria, ROS production and migration by leukocytes and impaired antibody responses.	[15,53]
NCX	Ca^{2+}, Na$^+$		Activation of NADPH oxidase and polarisation towards pro-inflammatory DC.		
ENac	Na$^+$	DC		ND	[42]
NHE	Na$^+$, H$^+$				

3. Modulation of endosomal pH

Channel	Permeability	Expression (immune cells)	Biological effects	Clinical correlates	Ref.
TRPC6	Ca^{2+}, Na$^+$	Macrophages	Phagocytosis and bacterial killing	ND	[8]
TRPM2	Ca^{2+}, Na$^+$	Macrophages and DC	Phagocytosis and bacterial killing	ND	[71,75]
Proton ATPases	H$^+$	Macrophages	Phagocytosis and bacterial killing	ND	[118]
Na$_V$1.5 (SCN5A)	Na$^+$	Macrophages	endosomal acidification and phagocytosis. Possible polarisation towards an antiinflammatory phenotype	Mice: enhanced recovery from EAE.	[45,119]
CLIC 1	Cl$^-$	Macrophages and DC	Phagocytosis, antigen processing and presentation.	ND	[9,120]

Table 1. *Cont.*

4. Modulation of other intracellular signalling pathways

Channel	Permeability	Expression (immune cells)	Biological effects	Clinical correlates	Ref.
TRPC1	Ca^{2+}, Na^+	Macrophages, Mast cells	*Macrophages*: inhibition of IL1β through other ion channels and transporters *Mast-cells*: inhibition of calcium-dependent release of TNF in the late phase of cell activation	Mice: delayed recovery from anaphylaxis	[77,121]

5. Other effects

Channel	Permeability	Expression (immune cells)	Biological effects	Clinical correlates	Ref.
SLC5A11	Na^+, glucose	Leukocytes (low)	Leukocytes: control of cell osmolarity under hypernatriemic environment, energy uptake, TNF-dependent apoptosis	Polymorphisms associated with susceptibility to SLE	[55,122]
CLIC 1	Cl^-		Modulation of cytokine gene expression and processing (conflicting results)	ND	[9,58,59]
CLIC 4	Cl^-	Macrophages			

Abbreviations. Ca_V: voltage-gated calcium channels; CFTR: cystic fibrosis transmembrane conductance regulator; CLIC: chloride intracellular channels; DC: dendritic cells; EAE: experimental allergic encephalomyelitis; ENaC: epithelial sodium channel; $GABA_A$-R: gamma-aminobutyric acid receptor type A; NADPH: nicotinamide adenine dinucleotide phosphate; NCX1: sodium-calcium exchanger 1; ND: not determined; NHE1: sodium-hydrogen exchanger 1; NKCC2: sodium-potassium-2 chloride exchanger; PGE2: prostaglandin E2; ROCE: receptor-operated calcium entry; SLC5A11: sodium glucose cotransporter; SOCE: store-operated calcium entry; STIM: stromal interaction molecule; TCR, T cell receptor; TRP: transient receptor potential channel; TXA2: thromboxane A2; VOCE: voltage-operated calcium entry; VSOP: voltage-sensing domain only protein; XMEN, X-linked immunodeficiency with Mg^{2+} defect and EBV infection and neoplasia; ZIP: zinc-regulated transporter (ZRT)/iron regulated transporter(IRT)-like protein.

3. Multiple Roles for Members of the TRP Channel Family in Inflammation

TRP channels are widely expressed and contribute to the control of cell homeostasis. Thus, variations in the functionality of TRP might influence the physiological deployment of the immune response [4,123,124] (Table 1). Six subgroups within the TRP family have been described in humans according to structural homology between members: canonical (i.e., more similar to the original set of channels isolated in *Drosophila* [125], TRPC), vanilloid (TRPV), analogues of melastatin-1 receptor (TRPM), mucolipins (TRPML), polycystins (TRPP), endowed with ankyrin repeats (TRPA). The TRPN subclass owes its name to the NO-mechano-potential C receptor of the worm *Caenorhabditis elegans*. No members of this subclass have been identified in humans, with fishes being the only vertebrates in which this TRP subclass appears to be expressed [123,126].

TRPC channels play a major role in the modulation of calcium currents. In this setting, the formation of heteromeric complexes between different TRPC monomers might extend the spectrum of potential effects of this subclass of TRP channels on calcium homeostasis. In particular, TRPC1, has been proposed as a prototypic biochemical regulator for other membrane receptors thanks to its supposed ability to form heteromers [127–130]. TRPC1 might thus affect the activity of the ORAI/STIM complex as well as of other TRPC, such as TRPC6, to regulate SOCE. However, the evidence supporting this hypothesis is controversial due to the lack of highly specific anti-TRPC1 antibodies and to the need of tissue-restricted models of ORAI/STIM knockout (complete ORAI/STIM deficit is lethal at the embryonic stage in mice) [127]. TRPC1 is highly expressed in the endothelium, where it enhances vascular permeability after TNF/thrombin stimulation [65–67]. The potential ability of TRPC1 to orchestrate the function of other calcium channels is crucial for the maintenance of an intracellular calcium gradient for neutrophil chemotaxis in experimental models [52]. Animal models also suggest that TRPC1 plays a role in the control of IL1β release from macrophages [57]. Similarly, TRPC1 might affect the late effects of anaphylaxis by controlling TNF release from mast cells [121].

TRP channels play an even more relevant role as receptor-operated channels. TRPM2 and TRPC3 are expressed in a wide range of immune cells, including macrophages and lymphocytes, and play a role in T-cell activation after TcR engagement [69,70,76]. TRPM2 is responsible for a significant fraction of calcium currents within endothelial cells and neutrophils [71]. Accordingly, mice lacking TRPM2 show reduced neutrophil infiltrate and less extensive damage following myocardial infarction [72,73]. The main ligand of TRPM2 is ADPR, which lies downstream an intracellular stress-response pathway to ROS. ADPR-mediated activation of TRPM2, in turn, promotes the final step of a regulatory feedback loop that leads to the inhibition of NADPH-oxidase. This process is crucial in macrophages to control the extent of oxidative stress generation during the inflammatory response [54,74]. In this setting, lysosomal expression of TRPM2 is also required for phagocytosis [71,75]. In contrast to the anti-inflammatory effects of TRPM2 on macrophage activity, the role of TRPC3 on macrophage-driven inflammation is less clear. TRPC3 can be activated by DAG and is thought to contribute to vascular inflammation [77,78]. On the other hand, upregulation of TRPC3 downstream the pathway of brain-derived neurotrophic factor might have a protective role against neuronal inflammation and myocardial injury [28,91,92].

TRPV1 contributes to T cell activation by associating to TCR and responding to its engagement with increased calcium flux towards the intracellular space [95], whereas TRPV2 is upregulated by FCγR activation in macrophages and is involved in the deployment of phagocytosis and chemotaxis [96]. A recent study suggests that clustering of TRPV2 in lipid rafts is crucial for bacterial phagocytosis and is defective in patients with cystic fibrosis [51]. TRPM7 has also a crucial role in macrophage activation and is required for the physiological development of functional B- and T cells. Similar to the role of MagT1 receptor in T cells, TRPM7 responds to variation in Mg^{2+} concentrations (itself being more permeable to Mg^{2+} than to Ca^{2+}) and enhances phospholipase activity downstream the BCR/TCR [98,99]. In addition, TRPM7 is crucial for mast cell survival and activation [100,101] as well as for macrophage survival and alternative activation [102]. TRPM7 might work by sensitising leukocytes to relatively low Mg^{2+} levels, rather than responding to acute variations in the concentration of the cation [103]. This is consistent with the evidence of lon8g-term, rather than sudden effects of TRPM7 deletion on leukocytes, with the partial compensatory role of exogenous Mg^{2+} [24] and with the clinical efficacy of $MgSO_4$ in acute allergic reactions.

TRPC5, TRPV5 and TRPV6 have also been proposed to mediate calcium-dependent activation of leukocytes, although their precise pathways of activation have been less clearly defined [93,94,97,131–133]. TRPM4 exerts an inhibitory effect on calcium currents by promoting membrane depolarisation through calcium-induced sodium entry in macrophages and mast cells [105,106]. In addition, thanks to differential expression levels, TRPM4 exhibits distinct regulatory effects in Th1 and Th2 lymphocytes [107].

4. TRPC6 and Immune Responses

TRPC6 is a member of a TRP subgroup with a probable dual role in SOCE and ROCE (Table 1) [20]. The fraction of calcium currents sustained by TRPC6 varies according to the inciting stimulus and to the cell type [134]. Evidence from neoplastic cell lines suggests that TRPC6-related calcium currents are crucial for the survival and activation of a multitude of histotypes [135–140]. The main physiological agonist of the receptor in the setting of ROCE is DAG. Conversely, endocytosis is the main mechanism for regulating TRPC6 function [141]. TRPC6 is expressed in a wide range of cell types, including neutrophils, lymphocytes, platelets and the endothelium (Table 1, Figure 2) [5]. During the acute phase response, TRPC6 plays a crucial role in neutrophil mobilisation as it enhances macrophage inflammatory protein 2 (MIP-2)- and CXCR2-related chemotactic responses by increasing Ca^{2+} concentration within the intracellular space and promoting actin-based cytoskeleton remodelling [79,80].

During trans-endothelial leukocyte migration TRPC6 acts on the endothelial side by mediating the downstream effects of platelet/endothelial cell adhesion molecule (PECAM/CD31) engagement, thus modulating endothelial permissibility [81]. TRPC6 contributes to loosen the endothelial junctions during acute inflammation, enhancing the effects of cellular and humoral immune mediators on target tissues [82,83]. Histamine-induced vascular leakage, which constitutes the core pathogenic mechanism in an acute hypersensitivity response, is also dependent on TRPC6, at least in animal models [142]. Finally, TRPC6 cooperates in lipopolysaccharide-induced endothelial activation after being itself activated by increasing intracellular concentrations of DAG, downstream the activation of Toll-like receptor 4 [143]. TRPC6 expressed on macrophage phagolysosomes is thought to promote their acidification and ultimately favour anti-microbial responses [8]. Chronically stimulated lung macrophages from patients with chronic obstructive pulmonary disease (COPD) express TRPC6 at high levels [144].

Calcium currents within T-lymphocytes are influenced by TRPC6 [145,146]. TRPC6 knockout dampens Th2-driven hypersensitivity responses in sensitised mice after airway allergen re-challenge [147] while sustained inward calcium currents due to TRPC6 may be indispensable for antimicrobial T cell responses during sepsis [148]. Notably, inhibitors of TRPC6 also have protective effects on the development of lymphocyte apoptosis [84]. This finding is in line with observations from others and us on the potential modulatory role of TRPC6 on cell death. TRPC6 influences endothelial apoptosis in an experimental model of atherosclerosis [148] and we observed that polymorphic gene variants of TRPC6 associate with susceptibility to apoptosis of peripheral blood mononuclear cells and diverging responses to the pharmacological inhibition of the channel in patients with SLE [84].

Enhanced apoptosis and unbalanced cell debris production to clearance ratios are fundamental, often calcium-dependent, events in autoimmunity, especially in the setting of SLE [149–152], a systemic autoimmune disease characterised by the production of autoantibodies against cell nuclear components and inflammatory manifestations involving multiple tissues and organs, such as skin and mucosal surfaces, joints, kidneys, serosae, central and peripheral nerves as well as circulating blood cells. TRPC6 gene variants might influence the secretory profile of SLE lymphocytes [84]. Retrospective clinical data from a well-characterised cohort of patients with SLE suggests the association between TRPC6 genetic polymorphisms and the risk of developing neuropsychiatric manifestations [85].

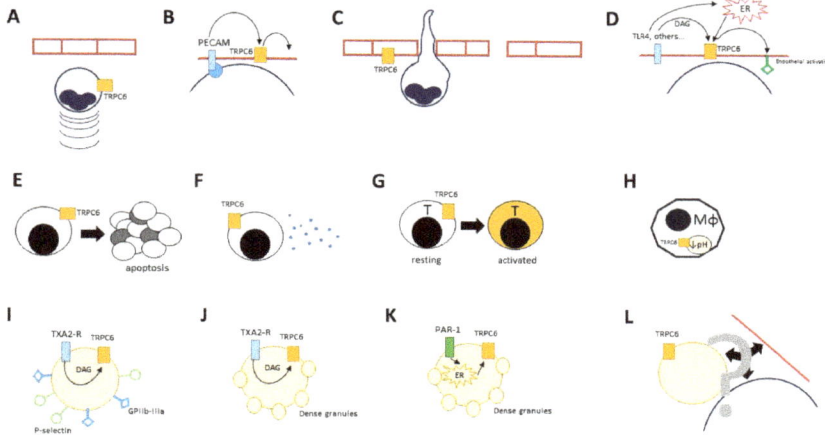

Figure 2. Effects of TRPC6 on immune cells. Activation of TRPC6 plays a critical role in the control of key cellular functions in several immune-committed cells, such as neutrophils (panel (**A–D**)), lymphocytes (panel (**E–G**)), macrophages (panel (**H**)), platelets (panel (**I–L**)) and the endothelium (panel (**A–D,L**)). TRPC6 contributes to neutrophil activation, adhesion to the vascular walls and extravasation by enhancing the stimulatory effects on chemo-attractants such as MIP-2 and CXCR2 (**A**); by promoting the downstream effects of endothelial cell adhesion molecules such as platelet/endothelial cell adhesion molecule (PECAM; (**B**)) or surface sensors of pro-inflammatory stimuli such as TLR-4 (**D**); by favouring the signal cascades that lead to looser transcellular junction between endothelial cells (**C**). Enhanced TRPC6 activation in lymphocytes might accelerate apoptosis, which could constitute a further trigger for inflammation in autoimmune disorders such as SLE (**E**). The expression of TRPC6 in T cells promotes cytokine release (**F**) and cell activation (**G**), which eventually translate in more aggressive inflammatory or allergic responses. In macrophages, TRPC6 is required for the acidification of endophagolysosomes (**H**). Platelets express high amounts of TRPC6 and might exploit its activation within ROCE (**I,J**) or SOCE (**K**) to undergo activation. Receptor-operated stimulation of TRPC6 downstream the thromboxane A2 (TXA2) pathway might be responsible for surface expression of crucial adhesion molecules such as GPIIb-IIIa or P-selectin (**J**) and for the release of platelet dense granules (**J**). This latter event might also occur as the result of TRPC6 activation after mobilisation of calcium from intracellular stores (**K**). Whether these events might impact on the interaction between platelets, leukocytes and the endothelium is still unknown (**L**).

Megakaryocytes and platelets abundantly express TRPC6 on the plasma membrane [153]. TRPC6 promotes calcium entry after being activated by intracellular ligands such as DAG. TRPC6-mediated ROCE in human platelets is restricted to the thromboxane pathway and might induce the expression of surface molecules such as glycoproteins IIb-IIIa or P-selectin and the release of platelet-dense granules. TRPC6 might also be involved in dense granules secretion downstream the thrombin receptors pathway through SOCE [68]. These events play a role in haemostasis and accordingly, prolonged bleeding time and delayed formation of clots have been observed after TRPC6 inhibition or genetic deletion in mice [154,155]. However, evidence from murine models is controversial, as other authors reported normal platelet function and haemostasis in TRPC6 knockout mice [153]. Platelets are part of an interactive network that involves the endothelium and circulating leukocytes and sustains acute and long-term inflammatory responses [156,157]. While evidence has been provided to support a potential place for TRPC6 as a target for anticoagulation [154], little is known about the impact of TRPC6 inhibition in modulating platelet–leukocyte interactions and related clinical phenotypes [158–161].

5. Effects of TRPC6 Activation and Function on Inflamed Tissues

TRPC6 is a modulator of tissue susceptibility to inflammatory injuries. The channel is expressed in the lungs and is involved in the pathogenesis of ischaemia-reperfusion lung injury [162], septic acute lung injury [143] and idiopathic pulmonary arterial hypertension [163,164]. These events reflect the prominent expression and homeostatic action of TRPC6 on the lung vasculature, in particular at the level of the endothelium and of pulmonary artery smooth muscle cells [163,165]. TRPC6 might also play a role in the biology of other lung-residing cells [136]. Hypoxia-induced elevation of DAG vascular smooth muscle cells promotes ROCE through TRPC6 and subsequent vasoconstriction, which eventually exacerbates ischaemia [166]. Similar vasomotor effects have been demonstrated in aortic smooth muscle cells [167,168] and in the medial layer of coronary arteries in porcine models [169]. In addition, TRPC6-dependent surges in intracellular calcium concentrations contribute to the susceptibility of cardiomyocytes to ischaemia-reperfusion injury [170,171] and to long-term maladaptive responses leading to cardiac remodelling [172,173].

Animal models in which TRPC6 expression had been silenced revealed that TRPC6-mediated cellular responses prevented necroptosis of renal tubular epithelial cells [174], suggesting that TRPC6 contributes to protect the kidney from ischemia-reperfusion injury. Downregulation of TRPC6 influences the ability of mesangial cells to contract following angiotensin II stimulation [175,176] while overactive TRPC6 in podocytes promotes cytoskeletal remodelling due to sustained increased intracellular calcium concentrations with podosome disassembly and eventual proteinuria. Gain of function mutations of TRPC6 have been associated with familial forms of focal segmental glomerular sclerosis [177,178]. TRPC6 inhibition improves protein retention in rat models of nephrosis, suggesting that aberrant TRPC6 function might also exacerbate the clinical picture of patients with acquired forms of glomerular injury [179,180]. Accordingly, higher levels of TRPC6 RNA were found in urines of patients with more aggressive forms of lupus nephritis in a pilot study [181]. More recently, TRPC6 has also been implicated in the pathogenesis of tubular interstitial fibrosis [182].

These latter observations are consistent with the wider role of TRPC6 in sustaining wound healing and tissue remodelling responses after injury. In particular, in line with its role as a promoter of vascular smooth muscle cell contraction, TRPC6 is required for myofibroblast trans-differentiation from resting fibroblasts [183]. Recent evidence suggests the implication of this phenomenon in pulmonary fibrosis [184] and in intestinal strictures in patients with Crohn's disease [185].

TRPC6 is expressed in neuronal tissues. TRPC6 activity in the nervous system seems to contrast the sequelae of brain ischaemia and reperfusion. Neurons are protected from post-ischaemic excitotoxicity by an indirect effect of TRPC6 on NMDA receptors [186,187] while under ischaemic conditions, TRPC6 degradation is enhanced in murine neurons by an IL17-dependent pathway. Inhibition of IL17 or of the downstream proteolytic enzyme calpain restores TRPC6 functions and reduces the area of post-ischemic necrosis [188]. A role for TRPC6 in modulating synaptic plasticity [189,190] and enhancing microglial activation [62] has been proposed.

6. Conclusions

The modulation of salt–water balance and electrolyte exchanges between the intra- and extra-cellular space has effects on the deployment of the immune response. Among the ion channels and transporters concurring to define the shape of the landscape of elementary immunology, TRPC6 seems to play a role in the regulation of several inflammatory events. More robust evidence from controlled human studies is required to pave the way to possible applications of TRPC6 as a target for diagnostic assessment or therapeutic intervention.

Acknowledgments: This work has been supported by grants from the Italian Association for Cancer Research (AIRC), the Cariplo Foundation and the Italian Ministry of Health (Ministero della Salute).

Conflicts of Interest: The authors declare that they have no conflict of interest in connection with this paper.

References

1. Venter, J.C.; Adams, M.D.; Myers, E.W.; Li, P.W.; Mural, R.J.; Sutton, G.G.; Smith, H.O.; Yandell, M.; Evans, C.A.; Holt, R.A.; et al. The sequence of the human genome. *Science* **2001**, *291*, 1304–1351. [CrossRef] [PubMed]

2. Chen, S.; He, F.F.; Wang, H.; Fang, Z.; Shao, N.; Tian, X.J.; Liu, J.S.; Zhu, Z.H.; Wang, Y.M.; Wang, S.; et al. Calcium entry via TRPC6 mediates albumin overload-induced endoplasmic reticulum stress and apoptosis in podocytes. *Cell Calcium* **2011**, *50*, 523–529. [CrossRef] [PubMed]

3. Schatz, V.; Neubert, P.; Schroder, A.; Binger, K.; Gebhard, M.; Muller, D.N.; Luft, F.C.; Titze, J.; Jantsch, J. Elementary immunology: Na(+) as a regulator of immunity. *Pediatr. Nephrol.* **2017**, *32*, 201–210. [CrossRef] [PubMed]

4. Parenti, A.; De Logu, F.; Geppetti, P.; Benemei, S. What is the evidence for the role of TRP channels in inflammatory and immune cells? *Br. J. Pharmacol.* **2016**, *173*, 953–969. [CrossRef] [PubMed]

5. European Bioinformatics Institute (EMBL-EBI); SIB Swiss Institute of Bioinformatics; (PIR), P.I.R. Universal Protein Resource (Uniprot). Available online: http://www.uniprot.org/ (accessed on 5 June 2018).

6. Sumoza-Toledo, A.; Lange, I.; Cortado, H.; Bhagat, H.; Mori, Y.; Fleig, A.; Penner, R.; Partida-Sanchez, S. Dendritic cell maturation and chemotaxis is regulated by TRPM2-mediated lysosomal Ca^{2+} release. *FASEB J. Off. Publ. Fed. Am. Soc. Exp. Biol.* **2011**, *25*, 3529–3542. [CrossRef] [PubMed]

7. Maxson, M.E.; Grinstein, S. *The Vacuolar-Type H^+-ATPase at a Glance—More Than a Proton Pump*; The Company of Biologists Ltd.: Cambridge, UK, 2014.

8. Riazanski, V.; Gabdoulkhakova, A.G.; Boynton, L.S.; Eguchi, R.R.; Deriy, L.V.; Hogarth, D.K.; Loaec, N.; Oumata, N.; Galons, H.; Brown, M.E.; et al. TRPC6 channel translocation into phagosomal membrane augments phagosomal function. *Proc. Natl. Acad. Sci. USA* **2015**, *112*, E6486–E6495. [CrossRef] [PubMed]

9. Salao, K.; Jiang, L.; Li, H.; Tsai, V.W.; Husaini, Y.; Curmi, P.M.; Brown, L.J.; Brown, D.A.; Breit, S.N. Clic1 regulates dendritic cell antigen processing and presentation by modulating phagosome acidification and proteolysis. *Biol. Open* **2016**, *5*, 620–630. [CrossRef] [PubMed]

10. Clemens, R.A.; Lowell, C.A. Store-operated calcium signaling in neutrophils. *J. Leukoc. Biol.* **2015**, *98*, 497–502. [CrossRef] [PubMed]

11. Tintinger, G.R.; Steel, H.C.; Theron, A.J.; Anderson, R. Pharmacological control of neutrophil-mediated inflammation: Strategies targeting calcium handling by activated polymorphonuclear leukocytes. *Drug Des. Dev. Ther.* **2009**, *2*, 95–104.

12. Vaeth, M.; Maus, M.; Klein-Hessling, S.; Freinkman, E.; Yang, J.; Eckstein, M.; Cameron, S.; Turvey, S.E.; Serfling, E.; Berberich-Siebelt, F. Store-operated Ca^{2+} entry controls clonal expansion of T cells through metabolic reprogramming. *Immunity* **2017**, *47*, 664–679. [CrossRef] [PubMed]

13. Clemens, R.A.; Chong, J.; Grimes, D.; Hu, Y.; Lowell, C.A. STIM1 and STIM2 cooperatively regulate mouse neutrophil store-operated calcium entry and cytokine production. *Blood* **2017**, *130*, 1565–1577. [CrossRef] [PubMed]

14. Vaeth, M.; Eckstein, M.; Shaw, P.J.; Kozhaya, L.; Yang, J.; Berberich-Siebelt, F.; Clancy, R.; Unutmaz, D.; Feske, S. Store-operated Ca(2+) entry in follicular T cells controls humoral immune responses and autoimmunity. *Immunity* **2016**, *44*, 1350–1364. [CrossRef] [PubMed]

15. Vaeth, M.; Feske, S. Ion channelopathies of the immune system. *Curr. Opin. Immunol.* **2018**, *52*, 39–50. [CrossRef] [PubMed]

16. Harr, M.W.; Rong, Y.; Bootman, M.D.; Roderick, H.L.; Distelhorst, C.W. Glucocorticoid-mediated inhibition of LCK modulates the pattern of T cell receptor-induced calcium signals by down-regulating inositol 1,4,5-trisphosphate receptors. *J. Biol. Chem.* **2009**, *284*, 31860–31871. [CrossRef] [PubMed]

17. Tang, H.; Wang, H.; Lin, Q.; Fan, F.; Zhang, F.; Peng, X.; Fang, X.; Liu, J.; Ouyang, K. Loss of IP3 receptor-mediated Ca(2+) release in mouse B cells results in abnormal B cell development and function. *J. Immunol.* **2017**, *199*, 570–580. [CrossRef] [PubMed]

18. Ouyang, K.; Leandro Gomez-Amaro, R.; Stachura, D.L.; Tang, H.; Peng, X.; Fang, X.; Traver, D.; Evans, S.M.; Chen, J. Loss of IP3R-dependent Ca^{2+} signalling in thymocytes leads to aberrant development and acute lymphoblastic leukemia. *Nat. Commun.* **2014**, *5*, 4814. [CrossRef] [PubMed]

19. Lichtenegger, M.; Tiapko, O.; Svobodova, B.; Stockner, T.; Glasnov, T.N.; Schreibmayer, W.; Platzer, D.; Cruz, G.G.; Krenn, S.; Schober, R. An optically controlled probe identifies lipid-gating fenestrations within the TRPC3 channel. *Nat. Chem. Biol.* **2018**, *14*, 396. [CrossRef] [PubMed]

20. Dietrich, A.; Gudermann, T. TRPC6: Physiological function and pathophysiological relevance. *Handb. Exp. Pharmacol.* **2014**, *222*, 157–188. [PubMed]

21. Li, F.-Y.; Chaigne-Delalande, B.; Kanellopoulou, C.; Davis, J.C.; Matthews, H.F.; Douek, D.C.; Cohen, J.I.; Uzel, G.; Su, H.C.; Lenardo, M.J. Signaling role for Mg^{2+} revealed by immunodeficiency due to loss of MAGT1. *Nature* **2011**, *475*, 471. [CrossRef] [PubMed]

22. Deason-Towne, F.; Perraud, A.-L.; Schmitz, C. Identification of SER/THR phosphorylation sites in the C2-domain of phospholipase c γ2 (plcγ2) using TRPM7-kinase. *Cell. Signal.* **2012**, *24*, 2070–2075. [CrossRef] [PubMed]

23. Cahalan, M.D.; Chandy, K.G. The functional network of ion channels in T lymphocytes. *Immunol. Rev.* **2009**, *231*, 59–87. [CrossRef] [PubMed]

24. Schmitz, C.; Perraud, A.-L.; Johnson, C.O.; Inabe, K.; Smith, M.K.; Penner, R.; Kurosaki, T.; Fleig, A.; Scharenberg, A.M. Regulation of vertebrate cellular Mg^{2+} homeostasis by TRPM7. *Cell* **2003**, *114*, 191–200. [CrossRef]

25. Gotru, S.K.; Gil-Pulido, J.; Beyersdorf, N.; Diefenbach, A.; Becker, I.C.; Vögtle, T.; Remer, K.; Chubanov, V.; Gudermann, T.; Hermanns, H.M. Cutting edge: Imbalanced cation homeostasis in MAGT1-deficient B cells dysregulates B cell development and signaling in mice. *J. Immunol.* **2018**, *200*, 2529–2534. [CrossRef] [PubMed]

26. Hojyo, S.; Fukada, T. Roles of zinc signaling in the immune system. *J. Immunol. Res.* **2016**, *2016*. [CrossRef] [PubMed]

27. Feske, S.; Wulff, H.; Skolnik, E.Y. Ion channels in innate and adaptive immunity. *Annu. Rev. Immunol.* **2015**, *33*, 291–353. [CrossRef] [PubMed]

28. Mizoguchi, Y.; Monji, A. TRPC channels and brain inflammation. In *Transient Receptor Potential Canonical Channels and Brain Diseases*; Springer: Berlin/Heidelberg, Germany, 2017; pp. 111–121.

29. Di Virgilio, F.; Dal Ben, D.; Sarti, A.C.; Giuliani, A.L.; Falzoni, S. The P2X7 receptor in infection and inflammation. *Immunity* **2017**, *47*, 15–31. [CrossRef] [PubMed]

30. Hamanaka, K.; Jian, M.Y.; Townsley, M.I.; King, J.A.; Liedtke, W.; Weber, D.S.; Eyal, F.G.; Clapp, M.M.; Parker, J.C. TRPV4 channels augment macrophage activation and ventilator-induced lung injury. *Am. J. Physiol. Lung Cell. Mol. Physiol.* **2010**, *299*, L353–L362. [CrossRef] [PubMed]

31. Davenport, B.; Li, Y.; Heizer, J.W.; Schmitz, C.; Perraud, A.L. Signature channels of excitability no more: L-type channels in immune cells. *Front. Immunol.* **2015**, *6*, 375. [CrossRef] [PubMed]

32. Badou, A.; Jha, M.K.; Matza, D.; Flavell, R.A. Emerging roles of L-type voltage-gated and other calcium channels in T lymphocytes. *Front. Immunol.* **2013**, *4*, 243. [CrossRef] [PubMed]

33. Blaustein, M.P.; Zhang, J.; Chen, L.; Song, H.; Raina, H.; Kinsey, S.P.; Izuka, M.; Iwamoto, T.; Kotlikoff, M.I.; Lingrel, J.B.; et al. The pump, the exchanger, and endogenous Ouabain: Signaling mechanisms that link salt retention to hypertension. *Hypertension* **2009**, *53*, 291–298. [CrossRef] [PubMed]

34. Boscia, F.; D'Avanzo, C.; Pannaccione, A.; Secondo, A.; Casamassa, A.; Formisano, L.; Guida, N.; Scorziello, A.; Di Renzo, G.; Annunziato, L. New roles of NCX in glial cells: Activation of microglia in ischemia and differentiation of oligodendrocytes. *Adv. Exp. Med. Biol.* **2013**, *961*, 307–316. [PubMed]

35. Iwamoto, T.; Kita, S.; Zhang, J.; Blaustein, M.P.; Arai, Y.; Yoshida, S.; Wakimoto, K.; Komuro, I.; Katsuragi, T. Salt-sensitive hypertension is triggered by Ca^{2+} entry via Na^+/Ca^{2+} exchanger type-1 in vascular smooth muscle. *Nat. Med.* **2004**, *10*, 1193. [CrossRef] [PubMed]

36. Citterio, L.; Simonini, M.; Zagato, L.; Salvi, E.; Delli Carpini, S.; Lanzani, C.; Messaggio, E.; Casamassima, N.; Frau, F.; D'Avila, F.; et al. Genes involved in vasoconstriction and vasodilation system affect salt-sensitive hypertension. *PLoS ONE* **2011**, *6*, e19620. [CrossRef] [PubMed]

37. Kleinewietfeld, M.; Manzel, A.; Titze, J.; Kvakan, H.; Yosef, N.; Linker, R.A.; Muller, D.N.; Hafler, D.A. Sodium chloride drives autoimmune disease by the induction of pathogenic TH17 cells. *Nature* **2013**, *496*, 518–522. [CrossRef] [PubMed]

38. Hernandez, A.L.; Kitz, A.; Wu, C.; Lowther, D.E.; Rodriguez, D.M.; Vudattu, N.; Deng, S.; Herold, K.C.; Kuchroo, V.K.; Kleinewietfeld, M.; et al. Sodium chloride inhibits the suppressive function of FOXP3+ regulatory T cells. *J. Clin. Investig.* **2015**, *125*, 4212–4222. [CrossRef] [PubMed]

39. Junger, W.G.; Liu, F.C.; Loomis, W.H.; Hoyt, D.B. Hypertonic saline enhances cellular immune function. *Circ. Shock* **1994**, *42*, 190–196. [PubMed]
40. Binger, K.J.; Gebhardt, M.; Heinig, M.; Rintisch, C.; Schroeder, A.; Neuhofer, W.; Hilgers, K.; Manzel, A.; Schwartz, C.; Kleinewietfeld, M.; et al. High salt reduces the activation of IL-4- and IL-13-stimulated macrophages. *J. Clin. Investig.* **2015**, *125*, 4223–4238. [CrossRef] [PubMed]
41. Shapiro, L.; Dinarello, C.A. Osmotic regulation of cytokine synthesis in vitro. *Proc. Natl. Acad. Sci. USA* **1995**, *92*, 12230–12234. [CrossRef] [PubMed]
42. Barbaro, N.R.; Foss, J.D.; Kryshtal, D.O.; Tsyba, N.; Kumaresan, S.; Xiao, L.; Mernaugh, R.L.; Itani, H.A.; Loperena, R.; Chen, W.; et al. Dendritic cell amiloride-sensitive channels mediate sodium-induced inflammation and hypertension. *Cell Rep.* **2017**, *21*, 1009–1020. [CrossRef] [PubMed]
43. Ramirez, G.A.; Lanzani, C.; Bozzolo, E.P.; Zagato, L.; Citterio, L.; Casamassima, N.; Canti, V.; Sabbadini, M.G.; Rovere-Querini, P.; Manunta, P.; et al. Beta-adducin and sodium-calcium exchanger 1 gene variants are associated with systemic lupus erythematosus and lupus nephritis. *Rheumatol. Int.* **2015**, *35*, 1975–1983. [CrossRef] [PubMed]
44. Staiano, R.I.; Granata, F.; Secondo, A.; Petraroli, A.; Loffredo, S.; Frattini, A.; Annunziato, L.; Marone, G.; Triggiani, M. Expression and function of Na$^+$/Ca^{2+} exchangers 1 and 3 in human macrophages and monocytes. *Eur. J. Immunol.* **2009**, *39*, 1405–1418. [CrossRef] [PubMed]
45. Carrithers, L.M.; Hulseberg, P.; Sandor, M.; Carrithers, M.D. The human macrophage sodium channel NAV1.5 regulates mycobacteria processing through organelle polarization and localized calcium oscillations. *FEMS Immunol. Med. Microbiol.* **2011**, *63*, 319–327. [CrossRef] [PubMed]
46. Lo, W.L.; Donermeyer, D.L.; Allen, P.M. A voltage-gated sodium channel is essential for the positive selection of Cd4(+) T cells. *Nat. Immunol.* **2012**, *13*, 880–887. [CrossRef] [PubMed]
47. Di, L.; Srivastava, S.; Zhdanova, O.; Ding, Y.; Li, Z.; Wulff, H.; Lafaille, M.; Skolnik, E.Y. Inhibition of the K$^+$ channel KCa3.1 ameliorates T cell-mediated colitis. *Proc. Natl. Acad. Sci. USA* **2010**, *107*, 1541–1546. [CrossRef] [PubMed]
48. Grimaldi, A.; D'Alessandro, G.; Golia, M.T.; Grossinger, E.M.; Di Angelantonio, S.; Ragozzino, D.; Santoro, A.; Esposito, V.; Wulff, H.; Catalano, M.; et al. KCa3.1 inhibition switches the phenotype of glioma-infiltrating microglia/macrophages. *Cell Death Dis.* **2016**, *7*, e2174. [CrossRef] [PubMed]
49. Prud'homme, G.J.; Glinka, Y.; Wang, Q. Immunological gabaergic interactions and therapeutic applications in autoimmune diseases. *Autoimmun. Rev.* **2015**, *14*, 1048–1056. [CrossRef] [PubMed]
50. Simonin-Le Jeune, K.; Le Jeune, A.; Jouneau, S.; Belleguic, C.; Roux, P.F.; Jaguin, M.; Dimanche-Boitre, M.T.; Lecureur, V.; Leclercq, C.; Desrues, B.; et al. Impaired functions of macrophage from cystic fibrosis patients: Cd11b, TLR-5 decrease and SCD14, inflammatory cytokines increase. *PLoS ONE* **2013**, *8*, e75667. [CrossRef] [PubMed]
51. Leveque, M.; Penna, A.; Le Trionnaire, S.; Belleguic, C.; Desrues, B.; Brinchault, G.; Jouneau, S.; Lagadic-Gossmann, D.; Martin-Chouly, C. Phagocytosis depends on TRPV2-mediated calcium influx and requires TRPV2 in lipids rafts: Alteration in macrophages from patients with cystic fibrosis. *Sci. Rep.* **2018**, *8*, 4310. [CrossRef] [PubMed]
52. Lindemann, O.; Strodthoff, C.; Horstmann, M.; Nielsen, N.; Jung, F.; Schimmelpfennig, S.; Heitzmann, M.; Schwab, A. TRPC1 regulates FMLP-stimulated migration and chemotaxis of neutrophil granulocytes. *Biochim. Biophys. Acta* **2015**, *1853*, 2122–2130. [CrossRef] [PubMed]
53. Capasso, M.; Bhamrah, M.K.; Henley, T.; Boyd, R.S.; Langlais, C.; Cain, K.; Dinsdale, D.; Pulford, K.; Khan, M.; Musset, B. HVCN1 modulates BCR signal strength via regulation of BCR-dependent generation of reactive oxygen species. *Nat. Immunol.* **2010**, *11*, 265. [CrossRef] [PubMed]
54. Di, A.; Gao, X.P.; Qian, F.; Kawamura, T.; Han, J.; Hecquet, C.; Ye, R.D.; Vogel, S.M.; Malik, A.B. The redox-sensitive cation channel TRPM2 modulates phagocyte ROS production and inflammation. *Nat. Immunol.* **2011**, *13*, 29–34. [CrossRef] [PubMed]
55. Tsai, L.J.; Hsiao, S.H.; Tsai, L.M.; Lin, C.Y.; Tsai, J.J.; Liou, D.M.; Lan, J.L. The sodium-dependent glucose cotransporter SLC5A11 as an autoimmune modifier gene in SLE. *Tissue Antigens* **2008**, *71*, 114–126. [CrossRef] [PubMed]
56. Lopez-Castejon, G.; Brough, D. Understanding the mechanism of IL-1β secretion. *Cytokine Growth Factor Rev.* **2011**, *22*, 189–195. [CrossRef] [PubMed]

57. Py, B.F.; Jin, M.; Desai, B.N.; Penumaka, A.; Zhu, H.; Kober, M.; Dietrich, A.; Lipinski, M.M.; Henry, T.; Clapham, D.E. Caspase-11 controls interleukin-1β release through degradation of TRPC1. *Cell Rep.* **2014**, *6*, 1122–1128. [CrossRef] [PubMed]

58. Malik, M.; Jividen, K.; Padmakumar, V.; Cataisson, C.; Li, L.; Lee, J.; Howard, O.Z.; Yuspa, S.H. Inducible NOS-induced chloride intracellular channel 4 (CLIC4) nuclear translocation regulates macrophage deactivation. *Proc. Natl. Acad. Sci. USA* **2012**, *109*, 6130–6135. [CrossRef] [PubMed]

59. Domingo-Fernández, R.; Coll, R.C.; Kearney, J.; Breit, S.; O'Neill, L.A. The intracellular chloride channel proteins CLIC1 and CLIC4 induce IL-1β transcription and activate the NLRP3 inflammasome. *J. Biol. Chem.* **2017**, *292*, 12077–12087. [CrossRef] [PubMed]

60. Hogan, P.G.; Lewis, R.S.; Rao, A. Molecular basis of calcium signaling in lymphocytes: STIM and ORAI. *Annu. Rev. Immunol.* **2010**, *28*, 491–533. [CrossRef] [PubMed]

61. Bogeski, I.; Kummerow, C.; Al-Ansary, D.; Schwarz, E.C.; Koehler, R.; Kozai, D.; Takahashi, N.; Peinelt, C.; Griesemer, D.; Bozem, M. Differential redox regulation of ORAI ion channels: A mechanism to tune cellular calcium signaling. *Sci. Signal.* **2010**, *3*, ra24. [CrossRef] [PubMed]

62. Liu, N.; Zhuang, Y.; Zhou, Z.; Zhao, J.; Chen, Q.; Zheng, J. Nf-kappab dependent up-regulation of TRPC6 by abeta in bv-2 microglia cells increases Cox-2 expression and contributes to hippocampus neuron damage. *Neurosci. Lett.* **2017**, *651*, 1–8. [CrossRef] [PubMed]

63. Desvignes, L.; Weidinger, C.; Shaw, P.; Vaeth, M.; Ribierre, T.; Liu, M.; Fergus, T.; Kozhaya, L.; McVoy, L.; Unutmaz, D.; et al. Stim1 controls T cell-mediated immune regulation and inflammation in chronic infection. *J. Clin. Investig.* **2015**, *125*, 2347–2362. [CrossRef] [PubMed]

64. Nunes-Hasler, P.; Maschalidi, S.; Lippens, C.; Castelbou, C.; Bouvet, S.; Guido, D.; Bermont, F.; Bassoy, E.Y.; Page, N.; Merkler, D.; et al. STIM1 promotes migration, phagosomal maturation and antigen cross-presentation in dendritic cells. *Nat. Commun.* **2017**, *8*, 1852. [CrossRef] [PubMed]

65. Paria, B.C.; Vogel, S.M.; Ahmmed, G.U.; Alamgir, S.; Shroff, J.; Malik, A.B.; Tiruppathi, C. Tumor necrosis factor-alpha-induced TRPC1 expression amplifies store-operated Ca^{2+} influx and endothelial permeability. *Am. J. Physiol. Lung Cell. Mol. Physiol.* **2004**, *287*, L1303–L1313. [CrossRef] [PubMed]

66. Tiruppathi, C.; Ahmmed, G.U.; Vogel, S.M.; Malik, A.B. Ca^{2+} signaling, TRP channels, and endothelial permeability. *Microcirculation* **2006**, *13*, 693–708. [CrossRef] [PubMed]

67. Qu, Y.Y.; Wang, L.M.; Zhong, H.; Liu, Y.M.; Tang, N.; Zhu, L.P.; He, F.; Hu, Q.H. TRPC1 stimulates calciumsensing receptorinduced storeoperated Ca^{2+} entry and nitric oxide production in endothelial cells. *Mol. Med. Rep.* **2017**, *16*, 4613–4619. [CrossRef] [PubMed]

68. Lopez, E.; Bermejo, N.; Berna-Erro, A.; Alonso, N.; Salido, G.M.; Redondo, P.C.; Rosado, J.A. Relationship between calcium mobilization and platelet alpha- and delta-granule secretion. A role for TRPC6 in thrombin-evoked delta-granule exocytosis. *Arch. Biochem. Biophys.* **2015**, *585*, 75–81. [CrossRef] [PubMed]

69. Melzer, N.; Hicking, G.; Gobel, K.; Wiendl, H. TRPM2 cation channels modulate T cell effector functions and contribute to autoimmune CNS inflammation. *PLoS ONE* **2012**, *7*, e47617. [CrossRef] [PubMed]

70. Wehrhahn, J.; Kraft, R.; Harteneck, C.; Hauschildt, S. Transient receptor potential melastatin 2 is required for lipopolysaccharide-induced cytokine production in human monocytes. *J. Immunol.* **2010**, *184*, 2386–2393. [CrossRef] [PubMed]

71. Syed Mortadza, S.A.; Wang, L.; Li, D.; Jiang, L.H. TRPM2 channel-mediated ROS-sensitive Ca(2+) signaling mechanisms in immune cells. *Front. Immunol.* **2015**, *6*, 407. [CrossRef] [PubMed]

72. Hiroi, T.; Wajima, T.; Negoro, T.; Ishii, M.; Nakano, Y.; Kiuchi, Y.; Mori, Y.; Shimizu, S. Neutrophil TRPM2 channels are implicated in the exacerbation of myocardial ischaemia/reperfusion injury. *Cardiovasc. Res.* **2013**, *97*, 271–281. [CrossRef] [PubMed]

73. Mittal, M.; Nepal, S.; Tsukasaki, Y.; Hecquet, C.M.; Soni, D.; Rehman, J.; Tiruppathi, C.; Malik, A.B. Neutrophil activation of endothelial cell-expressed TRPM2 mediates transendothelial neutrophil migration and vascular injury. *Circ. Res.* **2017**, *121*, 1081–1091. [CrossRef] [PubMed]

74. Yamamoto, S.; Shimizu, S.; Kiyonaka, S.; Takahashi, N.; Wajima, T.; Hara, Y.; Negoro, T.; Hiroi, T.; Kiuchi, Y.; Okada, T. TRPM2-mediated Ca2+ influx induces chemokine production in monocytes that aggravates inflammatory neutrophil infiltration. *Nat. Med.* **2008**, *14*, 738. [CrossRef] [PubMed]

75. Di, A.; Kiya, T.; Gong, H.; Gao, X.; Malik, A.B. Role of the phagosomal redox-sensitive TRP channel TRPM2 in regulating bactericidal activity of macrophages. *J. Cell Sci.* **2017**, *130*, 735–744. [CrossRef] [PubMed]

76. Philipp, S.; Strauss, B.; Hirnet, D.; Wissenbach, U.; Mery, L.; Flockerzi, V.; Hoth, M. TRPC3 mediates T-cell receptor-dependent calcium entry in human T-lymphocytes. *J. Biol. Chem.* **2003**, *278*, 26629–26638. [CrossRef] [PubMed]

77. Solanki, S.; Dube, P.R.; Birnbaumer, L.; Vazquez, G. Reduced necrosis and content of apoptotic m1 macrophages in advanced atherosclerotic plaques of mice with macrophage-specific loss of TRPC3. *Sci. Rep.* **2017**, *7*, 42526. [CrossRef] [PubMed]

78. Feng, M.; Xu, D.; Wang, L. miR-26a inhibits atherosclerosis progression by targeting TRPC3. *Cell Biosci.* **2018**, *8*, 4. [CrossRef] [PubMed]

79. Damann, N.; Owsianik, G.; Li, S.; Poll, C.; Nilius, B. The calcium-conducting ion channel transient receptor potential canonical 6 is involved in macrophage inflammatory protein-2-induced migration of mouse neutrophils. *Acta Physiol.* **2009**, *195*, 3–11. [CrossRef] [PubMed]

80. Lindemann, O.; Umlauf, D.; Frank, S.; Schimmelpfennig, S.; Bertrand, J.; Pap, T.; Hanley, P.J.; Fabian, A.; Dietrich, A.; Schwab, A. TRPC6 regulates CXCR2-mediated chemotaxis of murine neutrophils. *J. Immunol.* **2013**, *190*, 5496–5505. [CrossRef] [PubMed]

81. Weber, E.W.; Han, F.; Tauseef, M.; Birnbaumer, L.; Mehta, D.; Muller, W.A. TRPC6 is the endothelial calcium channel that regulates leukocyte transendothelial migration during the inflammatory response. *J. Exp. Med.* **2015**. [CrossRef] [PubMed]

82. Singh, I.; Knezevic, N.; Ahmmed, G.U.; Kini, V.; Malik, A.B.; Mehta, D. Gαq-TRPC6-mediated Ca^{2+} entry induces RHOA activation and resultant endothelial cell shape change in response to thrombin. *J. Biol. Chem.* **2007**, *282*, 7833–7843. [CrossRef] [PubMed]

83. Kini, V.; Chavez, A.; Mehta, D. A new role for pten in regulating transient receptor potential canonical channel 6-mediated Ca^{2+} entry, endothelial permeability, and angiogenesis. *J. Biol. Chem.* **2010**, *285*, 33082–33091. [CrossRef] [PubMed]

84. Ramirez, G.; Sciorati, C.; Bozzolo, E.; Zagato, L.; Citterio, L.; Coletto, L.; Lanzani, C.; Rovere-Querini, P.; Sabbadini, M.; Manunta, P. TRPC6 and Neuropsychiatric SLE: From bedside to bench. In *Clinical and Experimental Rheumatology*; Clinical & Exper Rheumatology: Pisa, Italy, 2016; p. S67.

85. Ramirez, G.A.; Lanzani, C.; Bozzolo, E.P.; Citterio, L.; Zagato, L.; Casamassima, N.; Canti, V.; Sabbadini, M.G.; Rovere-Querini, P.; Manunta, P.; et al. TRPC6 gene variants and neuropsychiatric lupus. *J. Neuroimmunol.* **2015**, *288*, 21–24. [CrossRef] [PubMed]

86. Ulmann, L.; Hirbec, H.; Rassendren, F. P2X4 receptors mediate PGE2 release by tissue-resident macrophages and initiate inflammatory pain. *EMBO J.* **2010**, *29*, 2290–2300. [CrossRef] [PubMed]

87. Burnstock, G. P2X ion channel receptors and inflammation. *Purinergic Signal.* **2016**, *12*, 59–67. [CrossRef] [PubMed]

88. Savio, L.E.B.; de Andrade Mello, P.; da Silva, C.G.; Coutinho-Silva, R. The P2X7 receptor in inflammatory diseases: Angel or demon? *Front. Pharmacol.* **2018**, *9*, 52. [CrossRef] [PubMed]

89. Muller, T.; Vieira, R.P.; Grimm, M.; Durk, T.; Cicko, S.; Zeiser, R.; Jakob, T.; Martin, S.F.; Blumenthal, B.; Sorichter, S.; et al. A potential role for P2X7R in allergic airway inflammation in mice and humans. *Am. J. Respir. Cell Mol. Biol.* **2011**, *44*, 456–464. [CrossRef] [PubMed]

90. Labasi, J.M.; Petrushova, N.; Donovan, C.; McCurdy, S.; Lira, P.; Payette, M.M.; Brissette, W.; Wicks, J.R.; Audoly, L.; Gabel, C.A. Absence of the P2X7 receptor alters leukocyte function and attenuates an inflammatory response. *J. Immunol.* **2002**, *168*, 6436–6445. [CrossRef] [PubMed]

91. Hang, P.; Zhao, J.; Cai, B.; Tian, S.; Huang, W.; Guo, J.; Sun, C.; Li, Y.; Du, Z. Brain-derived neurotrophic factor regulates TRPC3/6 channels and protects against myocardial infarction in rodents. *Int. J. Biol. Sci.* **2015**, *11*, 536–545. [CrossRef] [PubMed]

92. Mizoguchi, Y.; Kato, T.A.; Seki, Y.; Ohgidani, M.; Sagata, N.; Horikawa, H.; Yamauchi, Y.; Sato-Kasai, M.; Hayakawa, K.; Inoue, R.; et al. Brain-derived neurotrophic factor (BDNF) induces sustained intracellular Ca^{2+} elevation through the up-regulation of surface transient receptor potential 3 (TRPC3) channels in rodent microglia. *J. Biol. Chem.* **2014**, *289*, 18549–18555. [CrossRef] [PubMed]

93. Wang, J.; Lu, Z.H.; Gabius, H.J.; Rohowsky-Kochan, C.; Ledeen, R.W.; Wu, G. Cross-linking of GM1 ganglioside by galectin-1 mediates regulatory T cell activity involving TRPC5 channel activation: Possible role in suppressing experimental autoimmune encephalomyelitis. *J. Immunol.* **2009**, *182*, 4036–4045. [CrossRef] [PubMed]

94. Alawi, K.M.; Russell, F.A.; Aubdool, A.A.; Srivastava, S.; Riffo-Vasquez, Y.; Baldissera, L., Jr.; Thakore, P.; Saleque, N.; Fernandes, E.S.; Walsh, D.A.; et al. Transient receptor potential canonical 5 (TRPC5) protects against pain and vascular inflammation in arthritis and joint inflammation. *Ann. Rheum. Dis.* **2017**, *76*, 252–260. [CrossRef] [PubMed]

95. Bertin, S.; Aoki-Nonaka, Y.; de Jong, P.R.; Nohara, L.L.; Xu, H.; Stanwood, S.R.; Srikanth, S.; Lee, J.; To, K.; Abramson, L.; et al. The ion channel TRPV1 regulates the activation and proinflammatory properties of Cd4(+) T cells. *Nat. Immunol.* **2014**, *15*, 1055–1063. [CrossRef] [PubMed]

96. Link, T.M.; Park, U.; Vonakis, B.M.; Raben, D.M.; Soloski, M.J.; Caterina, M.J. TRPV2 has a pivotal role in macrophage particle binding and phagocytosis. *Nat. Immunol.* **2010**, *11*, 232–239. [CrossRef] [PubMed]

97. Tomilin, V.N.; Cherezova, A.L.; Negulyaev, Y.A.; Semenova, S.B. TRPV5/V6 channels mediate Ca(2+) influx in jurkat T cells under the control of extracellular pH. *J. Cell. Biochem.* **2016**, *117*, 197–206. [CrossRef] [PubMed]

98. Kim, J.K.; Ko, J.H.; Nam, J.H.; Woo, J.E.; Min, K.M.; Earm, Y.E.; Kim, S.J. Higher expression of TRPM7 channels in murine mature B lymphocytes than immature cells. *Korean J. Physiol. Pharmacol.* **2005**, *9*, 69–75.

99. Jin, J.; Desai, B.N.; Navarro, B.; Donovan, A.; Andrews, N.C.; Clapham, D.E. Deletion of TRPM7 disrupts embryonic development and thymopoiesis without altering Mg^{2+} homeostasis. *Science* **2008**, *322*, 756–760. [CrossRef] [PubMed]

100. Wykes, R.C.; Lee, M.; Duffy, S.M.; Yang, W.; Seward, E.P.; Bradding, P. Functional transient receptor potential melastatin 7 channels are critical for human mast cell survival. *J. Immunol.* **2007**, *179*, 4045–4052. [CrossRef] [PubMed]

101. Huang, L.; Ng, N.M.; Chen, M.; Lin, X.; Tang, T.; Cheng, H.; Yang, C.; Jiang, S. Inhibition of TRPM7 channels reduces degranulation and release of cytokines in rat bone marrow-derived mast cells. *Int. J. Mol. Sci.* **2014**, *15*, 11817–11831. [CrossRef] [PubMed]

102. Schilling, T.; Miralles, F.; Eder, C. TRPM7 regulates proliferation and polarisation of macrophages. *J. Cell Sci.* **2014**, *127*, 4561–4566. [CrossRef] [PubMed]

103. Ryazanova, L.V.; Hu, Z.; Suzuki, S.; Chubanov, V.; Fleig, A.; Ryazanov, A.G. Elucidating the role of the TRPM7 alpha-kinase: TRPM7 kinase inactivation leads to magnesium deprivation resistance phenotype in mice. *Sci. Rep.* **2014**, *4*, 7599. [CrossRef] [PubMed]

104. Ravell, J.; Chaigne-Delalande, B.; Lenardo, M. X-linked immunodeficiency with magnesium defect, epstein-barr virus infection, and neoplasia disease: A combined immune deficiency with magnesium defect. *Curr. Opin. Pediatr.* **2014**, *26*, 713–719. [CrossRef] [PubMed]

105. Serafini, N.; Dahdah, A.; Barbet, G.; Demion, M.; Attout, T.; Gautier, G.; Arcos-Fajardo, M.; Souchet, H.; Jouvin, M.H.; Vrtovsnik, F.; et al. The TRPM4 channel controls monocyte and macrophage, but not neutrophil, function for survival in sepsis. *J. Immunol.* **2012**, *189*, 3689–3699. [CrossRef] [PubMed]

106. Vennekens, R.; Olausson, J.; Meissner, M.; Bloch, W.; Mathar, I.; Philipp, S.E.; Schmitz, F.; Weissgerber, P.; Nilius, B.; Flockerzi, V.; et al. Increased IGE-dependent mast cell activation and anaphylactic responses in mice lacking the calcium-activated nonselective cation channel TRPM4. *Nat. Immunol.* **2007**, *8*, 312–320. [CrossRef] [PubMed]

107. Weber, K.S.; Hildner, K.; Murphy, K.M.; Allen, P.M. TRPM4 differentially regulates th1 and TH2 function by altering calcium signaling and NFAT localization. *J. Immunol.* **2010**, *185*, 2836–2846. [CrossRef] [PubMed]

108. Barbet, G.; Demion, M.; Moura, I.C.; Serafini, N.; Leger, T.; Vrtovsnik, F.; Monteiro, R.C.; Guinamard, R.; Kinet, J.P.; Launay, P. The calcium-activated nonselective cation channel TRPM4 is essential for the migration but not the maturation of dendritic cells. *Nat. Immunol.* **2008**, *9*, 1148–1156. [CrossRef] [PubMed]

109. Moss, R.B.; Bocian, R.C.; Hsu, Y.P.; Dong, Y.J.; Kemna, M.; Wei, T.; Gardner, P. Reduced IL-10 secretion by Cd4+ T lymphocytes expressing mutant cystic fibrosis transmembrane conductance regulator (CFTR). *Clin. Exp. Immunol.* **1996**, *106*, 374–388. [CrossRef] [PubMed]

110. Zhu, J.; Yang, Y.; Hu, S.G.; Zhang, Q.B.; Yu, J.; Zhang, Y.M. T-lymphocyte KV1.3 channel activation triggers the NLRP3 inflammasome signaling pathway in hypertensive patients. *Exp. Ther. Med.* **2017**, *14*, 147–154. [CrossRef] [PubMed]

111. Stevens, A.; Yuasa, M.; Peckham, D.; Olsen, C.; Iadonato, S.; Probst, P. *Thu0285 Dalazatide, an Inhibitor of the KV1.3 Channel on Activated Effector Memory T Cells, Has Immunotherapy Potential in Systemic Lupus Erythematosus*; BMJ Publishing Group Ltd.: London, UK, 2016.

112. Tarcha, E.J.; Olsen, C.M.; Probst, P.; Peckham, D.; Munoz-Elias, E.J.; Kruger, J.G.; Iadonato, S.P. Safety and pharmacodynamics of dalazatide, a KV1.3 channel inhibitor, in the treatment of plaque psoriasis: A randomized phase 1b trial. *PLoS ONE* **2017**, *12*, e0180762. [CrossRef] [PubMed]

113. Grgic, I.; Wulff, H.; Eichler, I.; Flothmann, C.; Kohler, R.; Hoyer, J. Blockade of T-lymphocyte KCa3.1 and KV1.3 channels as novel immunosuppression strategy to prevent kidney allograft rejection. *Transplant. Proc.* **2009**, *41*, 2601–2606. [CrossRef] [PubMed]

114. Grgic, I.; Eichler, I.; Heinau, P.; Si, H.; Brakemeier, S.; Hoyer, J.; Kohler, R. Selective blockade of the intermediate-conductance Ca^{2+}-activated K^+ channel suppresses proliferation of microvascular and macrovascular endothelial cells and angiogenesis in vivo. *Arterioscler. Thromb. Vasc. Biol.* **2005**, *25*, 704–709. [CrossRef] [PubMed]

115. Chou, C.C.; Lunn, C.A.; Murgolo, N.J. KCa3.1: Target and marker for cancer, autoimmune disorder and vascular inflammation? *Expert Rev. Mol. Diagn.* **2008**, *8*, 179–187. [CrossRef] [PubMed]

116. Toyama, K.; Wulff, H.; Chandy, K.G.; Azam, P.; Raman, G.; Saito, T.; Fujiwara, Y.; Mattson, D.L.; Das, S.; Melvin, J.E.; et al. The intermediate-conductance calcium-activated potassium channel KCa3.1 contributes to atherogenesis in mice and humans. *J. Clin. Investig.* **2008**, *118*, 3025–3037. [CrossRef] [PubMed]

117. Buisman, H.P.; Steinberg, T.H.; Fischbarg, J.; Silverstein, S.C.; Vogelzang, S.A.; Ince, C.; Ypey, D.L.; Leijh, P.C. Extracellular ATP induces a large nonselective conductance in macrophage plasma membranes. *Proc. Natl. Acad. Sci. USA* **1988**, *85*, 7988–7992. [CrossRef] [PubMed]

118. Singh, C.R.; Moulton, R.A.; Armitige, L.Y.; Bidani, A.; Snuggs, M.; Dhandayuthapani, S.; Hunter, R.L.; Jagannath, C. Processing and presentation of a mycobacterial antigen 85b epitope by murine macrophages is dependent on the phagosomal acquisition of vacuolar proton ATPase and in situ activation of cathepsin D. *J. Immunol.* **2006**, *177*, 3250–3259. [CrossRef] [PubMed]

119. Rahgozar, K.; Wright, E.; Carrithers, L.M.; Carrithers, M.D. Mediation of protection and recovery from experimental autoimmune encephalomyelitis by macrophages expressing the human voltage-gated sodium channel nav1.5. *J. Neuropathol. Exp. Neurol.* **2013**, *72*, 489–504. [CrossRef] [PubMed]

120. Jiang, L.; Salao, K.; Li, H.; Rybicka, J.M.; Yates, R.M.; Luo, X.W.; Shi, X.X.; Kuffner, T.; Tsai, V.W.; Husaini, Y.; et al. Intracellular chloride channel protein clic1 regulates macrophage function through modulation of phagosomal acidification. *J. Cell Sci.* **2012**, *125*, 5479–5488. [CrossRef] [PubMed]

121. Medic, N.; Desai, A.; Olivera, A.; Abramowitz, J.; Birnbaumer, L.; Beaven, M.A.; Gilfillan, A.M.; Metcalfe, D.D. Knockout of the TRPC1 gene reveals that TRPC1 can promote recovery from anaphylaxis by negatively regulating mast cell TNF-alpha production. *Cell Calcium* **2013**, *53*, 315–326. [CrossRef] [PubMed]

122. Chung, S.A.; Brown, E.E.; Williams, A.H.; Ramos, P.S.; Berthier, C.C.; Bhangale, T.; Alarcon-Riquelme, M.E.; Behrens, T.W.; Criswell, L.A.; Graham, D.C.; et al. Lupus nephritis susceptibility loci in women with systemic lupus erythematosus. *J. Am. Soc. Nephrol.* **2014**. [CrossRef] [PubMed]

123. Nilius, B.; Owsianik, G. The transient receptor potential family of ion channels. *Genome Biol.* **2011**, *12*, 218. [CrossRef] [PubMed]

124. Freichel, M.; Almering, J.; Tsvilovskyy, V. The role of TRP proteins in mast cells. *Front. Immunol.* **2012**, *3*, 150. [CrossRef] [PubMed]

125. Montell, C.; Rubin, G.M. Molecular characterization of the drosophila TRP locus: A putative integral membrane protein required for phototransduction. *Neuron* **1989**, *2*, 1313–1323. [CrossRef]

126. Dietrich, A.; Chubanov, V.; Kalwa, H.; Rost, B.R.; Gudermann, T. Cation channels of the transient receptor potential superfamily: Their role in physiological and pathophysiological processes of smooth muscle cells. *Pharmacol. Ther.* **2006**, *112*, 744–760. [CrossRef] [PubMed]

127. Dietrich, A.; Fahlbusch, M.; Gudermann, T. Classical transient receptor potential 1 (TRPC1): Channel or channel regulator? *Cells* **2014**, *3*, 939–962. [CrossRef] [PubMed]

128. Kim, M.S.; Zeng, W.; Yuan, J.P.; Shin, D.M.; Worley, P.F.; Muallem, S. Native store-operated Ca^{2+} influx requires the channel function of orai1 and TRPC1. *J. Biol. Chem.* **2009**, *284*, 9733–9741. [CrossRef] [PubMed]

129. Ambudkar, I.S.; Ong, H.L.; Liu, X.; Bandyopadhyay, B.; Cheng, K.T. TRPC1: The link between functionally distinct store-operated calcium channels. *Cell Calcium* **2007**, *42*, 213–223. [CrossRef] [PubMed]

130. Storch, U.; Forst, A.L.; Philipp, M.; Gudermann, T.; Mederos y Schnitzler, M. Transient receptor potential channel 1 (TRPC1) reduces calcium permeability in heteromeric channel complexes. *J. Biol. Chem.* **2012**, *287*, 3530–3540. [CrossRef] [PubMed]

131. Vassilieva, I.O.; Tomilin, V.N.; Marakhova, I.I.; Shatrova, A.N.; Negulyaev, Y.A.; Semenova, S.B. Expression of transient receptor potential vanilloid channels TRPV5 and TRPV6 in human blood lymphocytes and Jurkat leukemia T cells. *J. Membr. Biol.* **2013**, *246*, 131–140. [CrossRef] [PubMed]

132. Ma, H.T.; Peng, Z.; Hiragun, T.; Iwaki, S.; Gilfillan, A.M.; Beaven, M.A. Canonical transient receptor potential 5 channel in conjunction with orai1 and stim1 allows Sr^{2+} entry, optimal influx of Ca^{2+}, and degranulation in a rat mast cell line. *J. Immunol.* **2008**, *180*, 2233–2239. [CrossRef] [PubMed]

133. Van Abel, M.; Hoenderop, J.G.; Bindels, R.J. The epithelial calcium channels TRPV5 and TRPV6: Regulation and implications for disease. *Naunyn-Schmiedeberg's Arch. Pharmacol.* **2005**, *371*, 295–306. [CrossRef] [PubMed]

134. Soboloff, J.; Spassova, M.; Xu, W.; He, L.P.; Cuesta, N.; Gill, D.L. Role of endogenous TRPC6 channels in Ca^{2+} signal generation in A7R5 smooth muscle cells. *J. Biol. Chem.* **2005**, *280*, 39786–39794. [CrossRef] [PubMed]

135. Guilbert, A.; Dhennin-Duthille, I.; Hiani, Y.E.; Haren, N.; Khorsi, H.; Sevestre, H.; Ahidouch, A.; Ouadid-Ahidouch, H. Expression of TRPC6 channels in human epithelial breast cancer cells. *BMC Cancer* **2008**, *8*, 125. [CrossRef] [PubMed]

136. Yang, L.L.; Liu, B.C.; Lu, X.Y.; Yan, Y.; Zhai, Y.J.; Bao, Q.; Doetsch, P.W.; Deng, X.; Thai, T.L.; Alli, A.A.; et al. Inhibition of TRPC6 reduces non-small cell lung cancer cell proliferation and invasion. *Oncotarget* **2017**, *8*, 5123–5134. [CrossRef] [PubMed]

137. Wen, L.; Liang, C.; Chen, E.; Chen, W.; Liang, F.; Zhi, X.; Wei, T.; Xue, F.; Li, G.; Yang, Q.; et al. Regulation of multi-drug resistance in hepatocellular carcinoma cells is TRPC6/calcium dependent. *Sci. Rep.* **2016**, *6*, 23269. [CrossRef] [PubMed]

138. Wang, D.; Li, X.; Liu, J.; Li, J.; Li, L.J.; Qiu, M.X. Effects of TRPC6 on invasibility of low-differentiated prostate cancer cells. *Asian Pac. J. Trop. Med.* **2014**, *7*, 44–47. [CrossRef]

139. Zhang, S.S.; Wen, J.; Yang, F.; Cai, X.L.; Yang, H.; Luo, K.J.; Liu, Q.W.; Hu, R.G.; Xie, X.; Huang, Q.Y.; et al. High expression of transient potential receptor C6 correlated with poor prognosis in patients with esophageal squamous cell carcinoma. *Med. Oncol.* **2013**, *30*, 607. [CrossRef] [PubMed]

140. Song, J.; Wang, Y.; Li, X.; Shen, Y.; Yin, M.; Guo, Y.; Diao, L.; Liu, Y.; Yue, D. Critical role of TRPC6 channels in the development of human renal cell carcinoma. *Mol. Biol. Rep.* **2013**, *40*, 5115–5122. [CrossRef] [PubMed]

141. Amin, M.R.; Piplani, H.; Sharma, T.; Mehta, D. Switching off TRPC6 signaling: A new anti-edemagenic strategy. *FASEB J.* **2017**, *31*, 676.4.

142. Chen, W.; Oberwinkler, H.; Werner, F.; Gassner, B.; Nakagawa, H.; Feil, R.; Hofmann, F.; Schlossmann, J.; Dietrich, A.; Gudermann, T.; et al. Atrial natriuretic peptide-mediated inhibition of microcirculatory endothelial Ca^{2+} and permeability response to histamine involves CGMP-dependent protein kinase I and TRPC6 channels. *Arterioscler. Thromb. Vasc. Biol.* **2013**, *33*, 2121–2129. [CrossRef] [PubMed]

143. Tauseef, M.; Knezevic, N.; Chava, K.R.; Smith, M.; Sukriti, S.; Gianaris, N.; Obukhov, A.G.; Vogel, S.M.; Schraufnagel, D.E.; Dietrich, A.; et al. TLR4 activation of TRPC6-dependent calcium signaling mediates endotoxin-induced lung vascular permeability and inflammation. *J. Exp. Med.* **2012**, *209*, 1953–1968. [CrossRef] [PubMed]

144. Finney-Hayward, T.K.; Popa, M.O.; Bahra, P.; Li, S.; Poll, C.T.; Gosling, M.; Nicholson, A.G.; Russell, R.E.; Kon, O.M.; Jarai, G.; et al. Expression of transient receptor potential c6 channels in human lung macrophages. *Am. J. Respir. Cell Mol. Biol.* **2010**, *43*, 296–304. [CrossRef] [PubMed]

145. Carrillo, C.; Hichami, A.; Andreoletti, P.; Cherkaoui-Malki, M.; del Mar Cavia, M.; Abdoul-Azize, S.; Alonso-Torre, S.R.; Khan, N.A. Diacylglycerol-containing oleic acid induces increases in [Ca(2+)](i) via TRPC3/6 channels in human T-cells. *Biochim. Biophys. Acta* **2012**, *1821*, 618–626. [CrossRef] [PubMed]

146. Wu, Q.-Y.; Sun, M.-R.; Wu, C.-L.; Li, Y.; Du, J.-J.; Zeng, J.-Y.; Bi, H.-L.; Sun, Y.-H. Activation of calcium-sensing receptor increases TRPC3/6 expression in T lymphocyte in sepsis. *Mol. Immunol.* **2015**, *64*, 18–25. [CrossRef] [PubMed]

147. Sel, S.; Rost, B.R.; Yildirim, A.O.; Sel, B.; Kalwa, H.; Fehrenbach, H.; Renz, H.; Gudermann, T.; Dietrich, A. Loss of classical transient receptor potential 6 channel reduces allergic airway response. *Clin. Exp. Allergy* **2008**, *38*, 1548–1558. [CrossRef] [PubMed]

148. Zhang, Y.; Qin, W.; Zhang, L.; Wu, X.; Du, N.; Hu, Y.; Li, X.; Shen, N.; Xiao, D.; Zhang, H.; et al. Microrna-26a prevents endothelial cell apoptosis by directly targeting TRPC6 in the setting of atherosclerosis. *Sci. Rep.* **2015**, *5*, 9401. [CrossRef] [PubMed]

149. Bouts, Y.M.; Wolthuis, D.F.; Dirkx, M.F.; Pieterse, E.; Simons, E.M.; van Boekel, A.M.; Dieker, J.W.; van der Vlag, J. Apoptosis and net formation in the pathogenesis of SLE. *Autoimmunity* **2012**, *45*, 597–601. [CrossRef] [PubMed]

150. Dieker, J.; Tel, J.; Pieterse, E.; Thielen, A.; Rother, N.; Bakker, M.; Fransen, J.; Dijkman, H.B.; Berden, J.H.; de Vries, J.M.; et al. Circulating apoptotic microparticles in systemic lupus erythematosus patients drive the activation of dendritic cell subsets and prime neutrophils for netosis. *Arthritis Rheumatol.* **2016**, *68*, 462–472. [CrossRef] [PubMed]

151. Souliotis, V.L.; Sfikakis, P.P. Increased DNA double-strand breaks and enhanced apoptosis in patients with lupus nephritis. *Lupus* **2015**, *24*, 804–815. [CrossRef] [PubMed]

152. Lu, M.C.; Lai, N.S.; Yu, H.C.; Hsieh, S.C.; Tung, C.H.; Yu, C.L. Nifedipine suppresses TH1/TH2 cytokine production and increased apoptosis of anti-Cd3 + anti-Cd28-activated mononuclear cells from patients with systemic lupus erythematosus via calcineurin pathway. *Clin. Immunol.* **2008**, *129*, 462–470. [CrossRef] [PubMed]

153. Ramanathan, G.; Mannhalter, C. Increased expression of transient receptor potential canonical 6 (TRPC6) in differentiating human megakaryocytes. *Cell Biol. Int.* **2016**, *40*, 223–231. [CrossRef] [PubMed]

154. Vemana, H.P.; Karim, Z.A.; Conlon, C.; Khasawneh, F.T. A critical role for the transient receptor potential channel type 6 in human platelet activation. *PLoS ONE* **2015**, *10*, e0125764. [CrossRef] [PubMed]

155. Espinosa, E.V.P.; Murad, J.P.; Ting, H.J.; Khasawneh, F.T. Mouse transient receptor potential channel 6: Role in hemostasis and thrombogenesis. *Biochem. Biophys. Res. Commun.* **2012**, *417*, 853–856. [CrossRef] [PubMed]

156. Semple, J.W.; Italiano, J.E., Jr.; Freedman, J. Platelets and the immune continuum. *Nat. Rev. Immunol.* **2011**, *11*, 264–274. [CrossRef] [PubMed]

157. Nurden, A.T. Platelets, inflammation and tissue regeneration. *Thromb. Haemost.* **2011**, *105*, S13–S33. [CrossRef] [PubMed]

158. Maugeri, N.; Baldini, M.; Rovere-Querini, P.; Maseri, A.; Sabbadini, M.G.; Manfredi, A.A. Leukocyte and platelet activation in patients with giant cell arteritis and polymyalgia rheumatica: A clue to thromboembolic risks? *Autoimmunity* **2009**, *42*, 386–388. [CrossRef] [PubMed]

159. Ramirez, G.A.; Rovere-Querini, P.; Sabbadini, M.G.; Manfredi, A.A. Parietal and intravascular innate mechanisms of vascular inflammation. *Arthritis Res. Ther.* **2015**, *17*, 16. [CrossRef] [PubMed]

160. Mantovani, A.; Cassatella, M.A.; Costantini, C.; Jaillon, S. Neutrophils in the activation and regulation of innate and adaptive immunity. *Nat. Rev. Immunol.* **2011**, *11*, 519–531. [CrossRef] [PubMed]

161. Scherlinger, M.; Guillotin, V.; Truchetet, M.E.; Contin-Bordes, C.; Sisirak, V.; Duffau, P.; Lazaro, E.; Richez, C.; Blanco, P. Systemic lupus erythematosus and systemic sclerosis: All roads lead to platelets. *Autoimmun. Rev.* **2018**, *17*, 625–635. [CrossRef] [PubMed]

162. Weissmann, N.; Sydykov, A.; Kalwa, H.; Storch, U.; Fuchs, B.; Mederos y Schnitzler, M.; Brandes, R.P.; Grimminger, F.; Meissner, M.; Freichel, M.; et al. Activation of TRPC6 channels is essential for lung ischaemia-reperfusion induced oedema in mice. *Nat. Commun.* **2012**, *3*, 649. [CrossRef] [PubMed]

163. Malczyk, M.; Erb, A.; Veith, C.; Ghofrani, H.A.; Schermuly, R.T.; Gudermann, T.; Dietrich, A.; Weissmann, N.; Sydykov, A. The role of transient receptor potential channel 6 channels in the pulmonary vasculature. *Front. Immunol.* **2017**, *8*, 707. [CrossRef] [PubMed]

164. Urban, N.; Hill, K.; Wang, L.; Kuebler, W.M.; Schaefer, M. Novel pharmacological TRPC inhibitors block hypoxia-induced vasoconstriction. *Cell Calcium* **2012**, *51*, 194–206. [CrossRef] [PubMed]

165. Lu, W.; Wang, J.; Shimoda, L.A.; Sylvester, J.T. Differences in STIM1 and TRPC expression in proximal and distal pulmonary arterial smooth muscle are associated with differences in Ca^{2+} responses to hypoxia. *Am. J. Physiol. Lung Cell. Mol. Physiol.* **2008**, *295*, L104–L113. [CrossRef] [PubMed]

166. Wang, J.; Shimoda, L.A.; Weigand, L.; Wang, W.; Sun, D.; Sylvester, J.T. Acute hypoxia increases intracellular $[Ca^{2+}]$ in pulmonary arterial smooth muscle by enhancing capacitative Ca^{2+} entry. *Am. J. Physiol. Lung Cell. Mol. Physiol.* **2005**, *288*, L1059–L1069. [CrossRef] [PubMed]

167. Jung, S.; Strotmann, R.; Schultz, G.; Plant, T.D. TRPC6 is a candidate channel involved in receptor-stimulated cation currents in A7R5 smooth muscle cells. *Am. J. Physiol. Cell Physiol.* **2002**, *282*, C347–C359. [CrossRef] [PubMed]

168. Erac, Y.; Selli, C.; Kosova, B.; Akcali, K.C.; Tosun, M. Expression levels of TRPC1 and TRPC6 ion channels are reciprocally altered in aging rat aorta: Implications for age-related vasospastic disorders. *Age* **2010**, *32*, 223–230. [CrossRef] [PubMed]

169. Li, W.; Chen, X.; Riley, A.M.; Hiett, S.C.; Temm, C.J.; Beli, E.; Long, X.; Chakraborty, S.; Alloosh, M.; White, F.A.; et al. Long-term spironolactone treatment reduces coronary TRPC expression, vasoconstriction, and atherosclerosis in metabolic syndrome pigs. *Basic Res. Cardiol.* **2017**, *112*, 54. [CrossRef] [PubMed]

170. He, X.; Li, S.; Liu, B.; Susperreguy, S.; Formoso, K.; Yao, J.; Kang, J.; Shi, A.; Birnbaumer, L.; Liao, Y. Major contribution of the 3/6/7 class of TRPC channels to myocardial ischemia/reperfusion and cellular hypoxia/reoxygenation injuries. *Proc. Natl. Acad. Sci. USA* **2017**, *114*, E4582–E4591. [CrossRef] [PubMed]

171. Zhou, R.; Hang, P.; Zhu, W.; Su, Z.; Liang, H.; Du, Z. Whole genome network analysis of ion channels and connexins in myocardial infarction. *Cell. Physiol. Biochem. Int. J. Exp. Cell. Physiol. Biochem. Pharmacol.* **2011**, *27*, 299–304. [CrossRef] [PubMed]

172. Kuwahara, K.; Wang, Y.; McAnally, J.; Richardson, J.A.; Bassel-Duby, R.; Hill, J.A.; Olson, E.N. TRPC6 fulfills a calcineurin signaling circuit during pathologic cardiac remodeling. *J. Clin. Investig.* **2006**, *116*, 3114–3126. [CrossRef] [PubMed]

173. Eder, P. Cardiac remodeling and disease: SOCE and TRPC signaling in cardiac pathology. *Adv. Exp. Med. Biol.* **2017**, *993*, 505–521. [PubMed]

174. Shen, B.; He, Y.; Zhou, S.; Zhao, H.; Mei, M.; Wu, X. TRPC6 may protect renal ischemia-reperfusion injury through inhibiting necroptosis of renal tubular epithelial cells. *Med. Sci. Monit. Int. Med. J. Exp. Clin. Res.* **2016**, *22*, 633. [CrossRef]

175. Li, W.; Ding, Y.; Smedley, C.; Wang, Y.; Chaudhari, S.; Birnbaumer, L.; Ma, R. Increased glomerular filtration rate and impaired contractile function of mesangial cells in TRPC6 knockout mice. *Sci. Rep.* **2017**, *7*, 4145. [CrossRef] [PubMed]

176. Graham, S.; Gorin, Y.; Abboud, H.E.; Ding, M.; Lee, D.Y.; Shi, H.; Ding, Y.; Ma, R. Abundance of TRPC6 protein in glomerular mesangial cells is decreased by ROS and PKC in diabetes. *Am. J. Physiol. Cell Physiol.* **2011**, *301*, C304–C315. [CrossRef] [PubMed]

177. Santin, S.; Ars, E.; Rossetti, S.; Salido, E.; Silva, I.; Garcia-Maset, R.; Gimenez, I.; Ruiz, P.; Mendizabal, S.; Luciano Nieto, J.; et al. TRPC6 mutational analysis in a large cohort of patients with focal segmental glomerulosclerosis. *Nephrol. Dial. Transplant. Off. Publ. Eur. Dial. Transpl. Assoc. Eur. Ren. Assoc.* **2009**, *24*, 3089–3096. [CrossRef] [PubMed]

178. Winn, M.P.; Conlon, P.J.; Lynn, K.L.; Farrington, M.K.; Creazzo, T.; Hawkins, A.F.; Daskalakis, N.; Kwan, S.Y.; Ebersviller, S.; Burchette, J.L.; et al. A mutation in the TRPC6 cation channel causes familial focal segmental glomerulosclerosis. *Science* **2005**, *308*, 1801–1804. [CrossRef] [PubMed]

179. Kim, E.Y.; Yazdizadeh Shotorbani, P.; Dryer, S.E. TRPC6 inactivation confers protection in a model of severe nephrosis in rats. *J. Mol. Med.* **2018**, *96*, 631–644. [CrossRef] [PubMed]

180. Krall, P.; Canales, C.P.; Kairath, P.; Carmona-Mora, P.; Molina, J.; Carpio, J.D.; Ruiz, P.; Mezzano, S.A.; Li, J.; Wei, C.; et al. Podocyte-specific overexpression of wild type or mutant TRPC6 in mice is sufficient to cause glomerular disease. *PLoS ONE* **2010**, *5*, e12859. [CrossRef] [PubMed]

181. Dos Santos, M.; Bringhenti, R.N.; Rodrigues, P.G.; do Nascimento, J.F.; Pereira, S.V.; Zancan, R.; Monticielo, O.A.; Gasparin, A.A.; de Castro, W.P.; Veronese, F.V. Podocyte-associated mRNA profiles in kidney tissue and in urine of patients with active lupus nephritis. *Int. J. Clin. Exp. Pathol.* **2015**, *8*, 4600–4613. [PubMed]

182. Wu, Y.L.; Xie, J.; An, S.W.; Oliver, N.; Barrezueta, N.X.; Lin, M.H.; Birnbaumer, L.; Huang, C.L. Inhibition of TRPC6 channels ameliorates renal fibrosis and contributes to renal protection by soluble klotho. *Kidney Int.* **2017**, *91*, 830–841. [CrossRef] [PubMed]

183. Davis, J.; Burr, A.R.; Davis, G.F.; Birnbaumer, L.; Molkentin, J.D. A TRPC6-dependent pathway for myofibroblast transdifferentiation and wound healing in vivo. *Dev. Cell* **2012**, *23*, 705–715. [CrossRef] [PubMed]

184. Hofmann, K.; Fiedler, S.; Vierkotten, S.; Weber, J.; Klee, S.; Jia, J.; Zwickenpflug, W.; Flockerzi, V.; Storch, U.; Yildirim, A.O.; et al. Classical transient receptor potential 6 (TRPC6) channels support myofibroblast differentiation and development of experimental pulmonary fibrosis. *Biochim. Biophys. Acta* **2017**, *1863*, 560–568. [CrossRef] [PubMed]

185. Kurahara, L.H.; Sumiyoshi, M.; Aoyagi, K.; Hiraishi, K.; Nakajima, K.; Nakagawa, M.; Hu, Y.; Inoue, R. Intestinal myofibroblast TRPC6 channel may contribute to stenotic fibrosis in crohn's disease. *Inflamm. Bowel Dis.* **2015**, *21*, 496–506. [CrossRef] [PubMed]

186. Du, W.; Huang, J.; Yao, H.; Zhou, K.; Duan, B.; Wang, Y. Inhibition of TRPC6 degradation suppresses ischemic brain damage in rats. *J. Clin. Investig.* **2010**, *120*, 3480–3492. [CrossRef] [PubMed]

187. Li, H.; Huang, J.; Du, W.; Jia, C.; Yao, H.; Wang, Y. TRPC6 inhibited NMDA receptor activities and protected neurons from ischemic excitotoxicity. *J. Neurochem.* **2012**, *123*, 1010–1018. [CrossRef] [PubMed]

188. Zhang, J.; Mao, X.; Zhou, T.; Cheng, X.; Lin, Y. IL-17a contributes to brain ischemia reperfusion injury through calpain-TRPC6 pathway in mice. *Neuroscience* **2014**, *274*, 419–428. [CrossRef] [PubMed]

189. Griesi-Oliveira, K.; Acab, A.; Gupta, A.R.; Sunaga, D.Y.; Chailangkarn, T.; Nicol, X.; Nunez, Y.; Walker, M.F.; Murdoch, J.D.; Sanders, S.J.; et al. Modeling non-syndromic autism and the impact of TRPC6 disruption in human neurons. *Mol. Psychiatry* **2015**, *20*, 1350–1365. [CrossRef] [PubMed]

190. Zhang, H.; Sun, S.; Wu, L.; Pchitskaya, E.; Zakharova, O.; Fon Tacer, K.; Bezprozvanny, I. Store-operated calcium channel complex in postsynaptic spines: A new therapeutic target for Alzheimer's disease treatment. *J. Neurosci. Off. J. Soc. Neurosci.* **2016**, *36*, 11837–11850. [CrossRef] [PubMed]

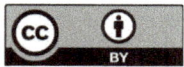

© 2018 by the authors. Licensee MDPI, Basel, Switzerland. This article is an open access article distributed under the terms and conditions of the Creative Commons Attribution (CC BY) license (http://creativecommons.org/licenses/by/4.0/).

cells

MDPI

Article

Transient Receptor Potential Channel A1 (TRPA1) Regulates Sulfur Mustard-Induced Expression of Heat Shock 70 kDa Protein 6 (*HSPA6*) In Vitro

Robin Lüling [1,2], Harald John [1], Thomas Gudermann [2], Horst Thiermann [1], Harald Mückter [2], Tanja Popp [1,2] and Dirk Steinritz [1,2,*]

[1] Bundeswehr Institute of Pharmacology and Toxicology, Ludwig-Maximilians-Universität Munich, 80937 Munich, Germany; robin1lueling@bundeswehr.org (R.L.); haraldjohn@bundeswehr.org (H.J.); horstthiermann@bundeswehr.org (H.T.); tanjapopp@bundeswehr.org (T.P.)
[2] Walther-Straub-Institute of Pharmacology and Toxicology, Ludwig-Maximilians-Universität Munich, 80336 Munich, Germany; thomas.gudermann@lrz.uni-muenchen.de (T.G.); Mueckter@lrz.uni-muenchen.de (H.M.)
* Correspondence: dirk.steinritz@lrz.uni-muenchen.de; Tel.: +49-89-992692-2304

Received: 26 July 2018; Accepted: 28 August 2018; Published: 31 August 2018

Abstract: The chemosensory transient receptor potential ankyrin 1 (TRPA1) ion channel perceives different sensory stimuli. It also interacts with reactive exogenous compounds including the chemical warfare agent sulfur mustard (SM). Activation of TRPA1 by SM results in elevation of intracellular calcium levels but the cellular consequences are not understood so far. In the present study we analyzed SM-induced and TRPA1-mediated effects in human TRPA1-overexpressing HEK cells (HEKA1) and human lung epithelial cells (A549) that endogenously exhibit TRPA1. The specific TRPA1 inhibitor AP18 was used to distinguish between SM-induced and TRPA1-mediated or TRPA1-independent effects. Cells were exposed to 600 μM SM and proteome changes were investigated 24 h afterwards by 2D gel electrophoresis. Protein spots with differential staining levels were analyzed by matrix-assisted laser desorption/ionization time-of-flight mass spectrometry and nano liquid chromatography electrospray ionization tandem mass spectrometry. Results were verified by RT-qPCR experiments in both HEKA1 or A549 cells. Heat shock 70 kDa protein 6 (*HSPA6*) was identified as an SM-induced and TRPA1-mediated protein. AP18 pre-treatment diminished the up-regulation. RT-qPCR measurements verified these results and further revealed a time-dependent regulation. Our results demonstrate that SM-mediated activation of TRPA1 influences the protein expression and confirm the important role of TRPA1 ion channels in the molecular toxicology of SM.

Keywords: 2D gel electrophoresis; AP18; HEK293; HSP70; MALDI-TOF MS(/MS); nanoHPLC-ESI MS/MS; proteomics; sulfur mustard; TRPA1

1. Introduction

The chemical warfare agent sulfur mustard (SM) causes severe damage to the skin, eyes, and the respiratory system [1,2]. Although SM and the associated injuries have been intensively investigated over decades, the molecular toxicology is still not understood in detail. In aqueous environments, SM forms a highly reactive sulfonium and subsequent carbenium ion [3]. A plethora of nucleophiles including the N7 atom of guanine bases in the DNA helix are targeted by SM. Monofunctional DNA alkylation and in particular DNA crosslinks were regarded as the exclusive mechanism of toxicity. However, Stenger et al. demonstrated that the alkylating substances CEES (2-chloroethyl-ethyl sulfide, a mono-functional SM analogue) and SM activate transient receptor potential ankyrin 1 cation channels (TRPA1) in vitro, thereby affecting cell viability [4].

TRPA1 channels belong to the TRP channel superfamily and are located in the plasma membrane of different human cell types, predominantly of neuronal cells [5].

They usually form homotetramers, but heterotetramers with TRPV1 have also been described [6,7]. TRP channels share the overall architecture of voltage-gated ion channels with six transmembrane domains (TMs). TM5 and TM6 form the pore region that is permeable for monovalent K^+, Na^+ and bivalent Ca^{2+} or Mg^{2+} cations [8]. The intracellular N-terminus of TRPA1 possesses multiple characteristic ankyrin repeat domains that contain free cysteine residues that are important for channel activity [9]. The physiological function of TRPA1 is the perception of sensory stimuli like pain and cold but also of certain reactive chemicals such as acrolein, a highly reactive substance present in tear gas or vehicle exhausts [10–12]. The activation of TRPA1 by reactive compounds is assumed to rely on covalent modification of cysteine residues in the ankyrin repeat sequence [9,10,12]. Reactive oxygen species (ROS), hypochlorite and protons were also identified as TRPA1 activators [13–18]. The latter seem to interact with an extracellular interaction site of TRPA1 and not via modification of intracellular cysteines [13].

The highly reactive SM and CEES were also identified as distinct TRPA1 activators with a not yet identified binding site [4,19]. Both chemicals provoked a TRPA1-dependent increase of intracellular calcium levels ($[Ca^{2+}]_i$) that could be efficiently prevented by pre-incubation with the TRPA1-specific blocker AP18 [4,19]. There is some evidence that TRPA1 activation is involved in the molecular toxicity of alkylating compounds [4,20,21]. However, the cellular consequences of an SM-induced and TRPA1-mediated elevation of $[Ca^{2+}]_i$ have not been investigated in detail so far. In the present study we analyzed TRPA1-dependent effects after SM exposure in human TRPA1-overexpressing HEK cells (HEKA1). Proteome changes were analyzed by 2D gel electrophoresis (2D-GE) with subsequent matrix-assisted laser desorption/ionization time-of-flight mass spectrometry (MALDI-TOF MS(/MS)) and nano high performance liquid chromatography electrospray ionization tandem mass spectrometry (nanoHPLC-ESI MS/MS). AP18 was used to distinguish between TRPA1-dependent and -independent effects on protein expression. Results were validated by RT-qPCR in HEKA1 cells and as well as in human A549 lung epithelial cells endogenously expressing TRPA1 channels [22–24].

2. Materials & Methods

2.1. Chemicals

SM was made available by the German Ministry of Defense and integrity as well as purity was proved by NMR in house. Allylisothiocyanat (AITC), iodoacetamid (IAA), ethanol (EtOH), glycerol, glycine, trifluoroacetic acid (TFA), acetonitrile (ACN), penicillin/streptomycin (P/S) and Trypsin Profile IGD Kit for proteolysis of protein spots were obtained from Sigma-Aldrich (Steinheim, Germany). 2D-Clean-UP Kit, Silver Staining Kit (protein), 2D-Quant-Kit and Coomassie Brilliant Blue Solution were obtained from GE Healthcare (Freiburg, Germany). Bromophenol blue and sodium dodecyl sulfate (SDS) were purchased from Bio-Rad (Munich, Germany). RT^2 First Strand Kit, RT^2 SYBR Green/ROX qPCR Mastermix, RNeasy Protect Mini Kit and RT^2 Custom Profiler PCR 96-well plates with specific customized primers were purchased from QIAGEN Sciences (Venlo, The Netherlands). Dulbecco's minimal Eagle medium (DMEM), fetal bovine serum (FBS), trypsin–EDTA (ethylenediaminetetraacetic acid) and phosphate-buffered saline (PBS) were obtained from Life Technologies (Gibco, Karlsruhe, Germany). AP18 was delivered by Bio-Techne (Wiesbaden-Nordenstadt, Germany). α-cyano-4-hydroxycinnamic acid (CHC) as matrix for MALDI-TOF measurements was obtained from Bruker Daltonics (Bremen, Germany).

2.2. Cell Culture

HEK293 wild-type cells (introduced as HEKwt) and HEK293-A1-E cells (introduced as HEKA1) with a stable expression of human TRPA1 (hTRPA1) were kindly donated by the Walther-Straub-Institute of Pharmacology and Toxicology (Ludwig-Maximilians-Universität, Munich).

Cells were grown in DMEM containing 4.5 g/L glucose, Earl's salts and L-glutamine. This medium was supplemented with 10% FBS (v/v) and 1% P/S (v/v). Cells were cultured in a humidified atmosphere at 5% (v/v) CO_2 and 37 °C (standard conditions). HEKwt cells were split every 2–3 days while HEKA1 cells were subcultivated every 3–4 days. Cells were detached using trypsin-EDTA for 3 min and resuspended in the respective medium. A549 cells were grown in DMEM (Biochrom, Berlin, Germany) supplemented with FBS (Biochrom, Berlin, Germany) and gentamycin (5 µg/mL). Cells were split every 2–3 days detached by trypsin-EDTA for 5 min.

2.3. Sample Preparation

HEKwt, HEKA1 or A549 cells were exposed to 600 µM SM according to Stenger et al. [4,19]. A concentration of 25 µM AITC was used to stimulate HEKwt and HEKA1 cells. Cell lysates of SM-exposed or AITC-treated cells were generated at 24 h for 2D-GE. Pre-incubation with the TRPA1-specific inhibitor AP18 (2 µM, application 5 min prior to SM or AITC exposure) was also performed according to Stenger et al. for all groups [4]. Controls were incubated without AITC or SM but with medium and, if applicable, with AP18. After the respective incubation time, cells were washed with PBS first and then harvested with trypsin-EDTA for 3 min and resuspended in 10 mL DMEM. Cell number was determined using a Neubauer counting chamber (NanoEnTek, Seoul, Korea). Cells were lysed in lysis buffer (7 M urea, 2 M thiourea, 4% w/v CHAPS, 2% v/v IPG buffer, 40 mM DTT) for 2D-GE. Samples were sonicated (4 cycles with 10 s) on ice. Supernatants were collected after centrifugation (30 min, 4 °C and 21,130 RCF) and subsequently cleaned up using the 2D Clean-Up Kit according to the manual of the provider. Protein concentration was determined using the 2D-Quant Kit. Samples were aliquoted and frozen at −80 °C.

For RT-qPCR, HEKA1 cells were investigated 1, 3, 5, or 24 h after exposure while HEKwt and A549 cells were analyzed after 24 h only. Approx. 10×10^6 cells were collected in 1 mL of RNA protection reagent from QIAGEN (Hilden, Germany) at the respective time points. RNA was extracted using the RNeasy Mini Protect Kit (QIAGEN, Hilden, Germany) according to the instructions given by the manufacturer. In brief, cell pellets were lysed in 600 µL RLT lysis buffer and homogenized using a QIA shredder (QIAGEN). RNA was precipitated in 600 µL 70% (v/v) EtOH and purified by washing several times in different buffers according to the manufacturer's protocol. The concentration of RNA was measured using the NanoDrop 8000 Spectrophotometer from Thermo Scientific (Schwerte, Germany).

2.4. 2D Gel Electrophoresis and Image Analysis

IPG strips (Immobiline Drystrips 7 cm, pH 4–7 or pH 6–11, linear, or pH 3-11 non-linear, GE ealthcare, Chicago, IL, USA) were rehydrated with 8 M urea, 2% (w/v) CHAPS, 0.5% (w/v) DTT, 0.5% (v/v) IPG buffer together with 60 µg for pH 4–7 strips, 150 µg for pH 6–11 strips or 6 µg for pH 3–11 strips of the protein lysates. Following rehydration loading for approx. 17 h in an Immobiline DryStrip IPGbox (GE Healthcare), first dimension isoelectric focusing (IEF) was performed using an Ettan IPGphor II (GE Healthcare) for 8 kVh at a maximum voltage of 5000 V and a limiting current of 50 µA/strip. Afterwards, gel strips were equilibrated in 10 mg/mL DTT equilibration buffer (6 M urea, 75 mM Tris-HCl pH 8.8, 29.3% v/v glycerol, 2% w/v SDS) for 15 min and afterwards in 25 mg/mL IAA equilibration buffer for further 15 min. Strips were transferred on 10% Bis-Tris gels (Thermofisher Scientific, Waltham, MA, USA), sealed with agarose sealing solution (25 mM Tris base, 192 mM glycine, 0.1% w/v SDS, 0.5% w/v agarose, 0.002% w/v bromophenol blue) and separated in a second dimension according to electrophoretic mobility with constant voltage of 180 V for 1 h (SDS-PAGE). Proteins separated by pH 4–7 strips or pH 6–11 strips were then stained with colloidal Coomassie Brilliant Blue (CBB, GE Healthcare) for 35 min and scanned on a Microtek Bio-5000 scanner (Serva, Heidelberg, Germany). Proteins separated on pH 3–11 strips were stained using the Silver Staining Kit (GE Healthcare). In short, gels were soaked in fixing solution (30% v/v EtOH, 10% v/v glacial acetic acid) for 60 min and then sensitized in sensitizing solution (30% v/v EtOH, 5% w/v sodium thiosulphate, 6.8% w/v sodium acetate) for a further 60 min. After washing with distilled water for four times, silver solution (2.5% w/v silver nitrate solution) was added for 60 min. A developing solution (2.5% w/v sodium carbonate, 37% w/v formaldehyde) was added until spots reached desired intensity. Then, gels were transferred to a stopping solution (1.5% w/v EDTA-Na$_2$) before a preserving solution (30% EtOH, 87% w/w glycerol) was added. Gels were scanned on a Microtek Bio-5000 scanner (Serva, Heidelberg, Germany).

Protein spots with significant different staining levels were identified using Progenesis SameSpots software v5.0.0.7 (Nonlinear Dynamics, Newcastle, UK). Threshold levels were defined with a fold change > 2.0 and an ANOVA p value < 0.05. Spots were filtered to identify only those which applied to both criteria. At least 3 biological replicates were investigated for each group. EtOH solvent control gels were chosen as reference.

2.5. MALDI-TOF MS(/MS) or NanoHPLC-ESI MS/MS Analysis

Relevant protein spots were excised and proteolyzed in-gel using the trypsin profile IGD kit (Sigma-Aldrich). In brief, the gel piece was covered with 200 µL destaining solution and incubated at 37 °C for 30 min. The gel piece was dried before 20 µL (0.4 µg of trypsin) of the prepared trypsin solution and 50 µL of the trypsin reaction buffer were added. It was incubated overnight at 37 °C. Following tryptic cleavage, peptides were desalted and concentrated using ZipTip-C18 pipette tips (Merck Millipore, Darmstadt, Germany). First, ZipTip was equilibrated using 10 µL methanol and 10 µL 0.1% (v/v) TFA. Afterwards, sample was loaded by pipetting the digested protein up and down for 10 times. ZipTip was washed with 10 µL 0.1% (v/v) TFA before sample was eluted with 10 µL of acetonitrile/0.1% (v/v) TFA (80/20 v/v). Using the dried-droplet technique, samples were spotted onto a polished steel target by mixing 1 µL each of sample and CHC (5 mg/mL in a 1:2 mixture of ACN and 0.1% v/v TFA).

MALDI-TOF MS(/MS) measurements were performed in the positive reflector ion mode using an Autoflex III smartbeam mass spectrometer (Bruker, Billerica, MA, USA) equipped with a modified pulsed all-solid-state laser 355 nm (Bruker Daltonics). A peptide mass fingerprint (PMF) was recorded in a mass range from m/z 900–3400 with the following settings: Ion source I, 19 kV; ion source II, 16.5 kV; lens, 8.3 kV; reflector I, 21 kV; reflector II, 9.75 kV. MS/MS experiments were executed in the LIFT mode with the following parameters: Ion source I, 6 kV; ion source II, 5.3 kV; lens, 3.0 kV; reflector I, 27 kV; reflector II, 11.6 kV; LIFT I, 19 kV; LIFT II, 4.2 kV.

The mass spectrometer was calibrated using the peptide standard mixture of bradykinin (1–7), angiotensin II, angiotensin I, substance P, bombesin, renin substrate, ACTH clip (1–17), ACTH clip (18–39) and somatostatin (peptide calibration standard II, Bruker Daltonics).

Mass spectra were recorded using the flex control software v.3.0 (Bruker, Billerica, MA, USA) and further processed by flex analysis v.3.0 and BioTools v.3.1.2.22 (both Bruker). Identification of proteins was achieved via the SwissProt protein database using MS ion search of the Mascot search engine (Matrix Science, London, England) with following search criteria: Taxonomy Homo sapiens (human), enzyme trypsin, fragment mass tolerance 0.1%, significance threshold $p < 0.05$, maximum number of hits 20.

Protein spots that could not be identified by MALDI-TOF MS(/MS) were analyzed by more sensitive nanoHPLC-ESI MS/MS (proteome factory AG, Berlin, Germany). The LC MS/MS system consisted of an Agilent 1100 nanoHPLC system (Agilent, Waldbronn, Germany), PicoTip electrospray emitter (New Objective, Woburn, MA, USA) and an Orbitrap XL mass spectrometer (ThermoFisher Scientific, Bremen, Germany). Peptides were first trapped and desalted on the enrichment column (Zorbax 300SB-C18, 0.3 × 0.5 mm, Agilent, Santa Clara, CA, USA) for five minutes (solvent: 2.5% ACN/0.5% formic acid). Then, they were separated on a Zorbax 300SB-C18, 75 µm × 150 mm column (Agilent) using a linear gradient from 15% to 40% B (solvent A: 0.1% formic acid in water, solvent B: 0.1% formic acid in ACN). Ions of interest were data-dependently subjected to MS/MS according to the expected charge state distribution of peptide ions. MS/MS data were matched against the SwissProt protein database using MS/MS ion search of the Mascot search engine (Matrix Science,

London, UK) with following parameters: Enzyme trypsin, fixed modifications carbamidomethyl (C), variable modifications deamidated (NQ) and oxidation (M), mass values monoisotopic, peptide mass tolerance 3 ppm, fragment mass tolerance 0.6 Da, significance threshold $p < 0.05$, taxonomy Homo sapiens (human).

2.6. Real-Time qPCR

Extracted RNA (500 ng) was transcribed into complementary DNA (cDNA) using the RT^2 First Strand Kit. Transcription was performed according to the manufacturer's protocol. In brief, 10 µL of a reverse transcriptase mixture was added to the RNA samples. The mixture was incubated for 15 min at 42 °C and then for another 5 min at 95 °C. From each resulting cDNA sample, 675 µL were mixed with 675 µL of RT^2 SYBR Green/ROX qPCR Mastermix. A volume of 25 µL from each sample was transferred into a specially designed RT^2 Custom Profiler PCR 96-well plate using a TECAN freedom evo (TECAN, Crailsheim, Germany). 96-well plates were pre-spotted with specific primers according to the results of 2D-GE. Plates were sealed with cap s–trips and placed into the Mastercycler 2S (Eppendorf, Hamburg, Germany). The qPCR was carried out with the following PCR program: 10 min at 95 °C followed by 40 cycles of 15 s at 95 °C, and 1 min at 60 °C. At the end of the PCR program, a melting profile of the DNA amplifications was measured with the following settings: 95 °C for 15 s, 60 °C for 15 s and a final temperature gradient from 60 °C to 95 °C over 20 min. PCR data were analyzed with the realplex software from Eppendorf and with an online software from QIAGEN [25].

3. Results

3.1. 2D Gel Electrophoresis and Mass Spectrometry

Analysis of HEKA1 cells exposed to SM and investigated after 24 h revealed differential detection of 22 protein spots compared to the control group (Figure 1A) in CBB-stained 2D gels. Three of these spots were identified with a threshold level of a fold change > 2.0 together with a p value < 0.05 and to be dependent on TRPA1 (Figure 1B–D). Dependency on TRPA1 was proven as pre-incubation with AP18 prevented SM-induced effects. Up-regulation of one (Figure 1B) and down-regulation of two protein spots (Figure 1C,D) were observed. The up-regulated protein was identified by MALDI-TOF MS peptide mass fingerprint (Figure 2A) and subsequent MS/MS analysis of characteristic protein-derived peptides as heat shock 70 kDa protein 6 (*HSPA6*, UniProtKB-P17066). Fragmenting of the ion at m/z 1487.5 is exemplarily shown in Figure 2B and documents the internal peptide (39–51). The overall sequence coverage was 35.5% (Figure 2C). The Mascot probability score was calculated to be 86.6. Identification of the two down-regulated protein spots was not successful by the MALDI-TOF technique. Therefore, spots were analyzed by the more sensitive nanoHPLC-ESI MS/MS which identified 4 proteins for each spot all with a high probability score. Table 1 gives an overview on the detected proteins. Values for the respective molecular weight were taken from UniProt database.

Silver-stained 2D gels identified 28 additional protein spots (12 up- and 16 down-regulated) that were affected after SM exposure (Figure S1). AP18 pre-incubation did not influence the SM-induced changes, thereby excluding the involvement of TRPA1 (data not shown).

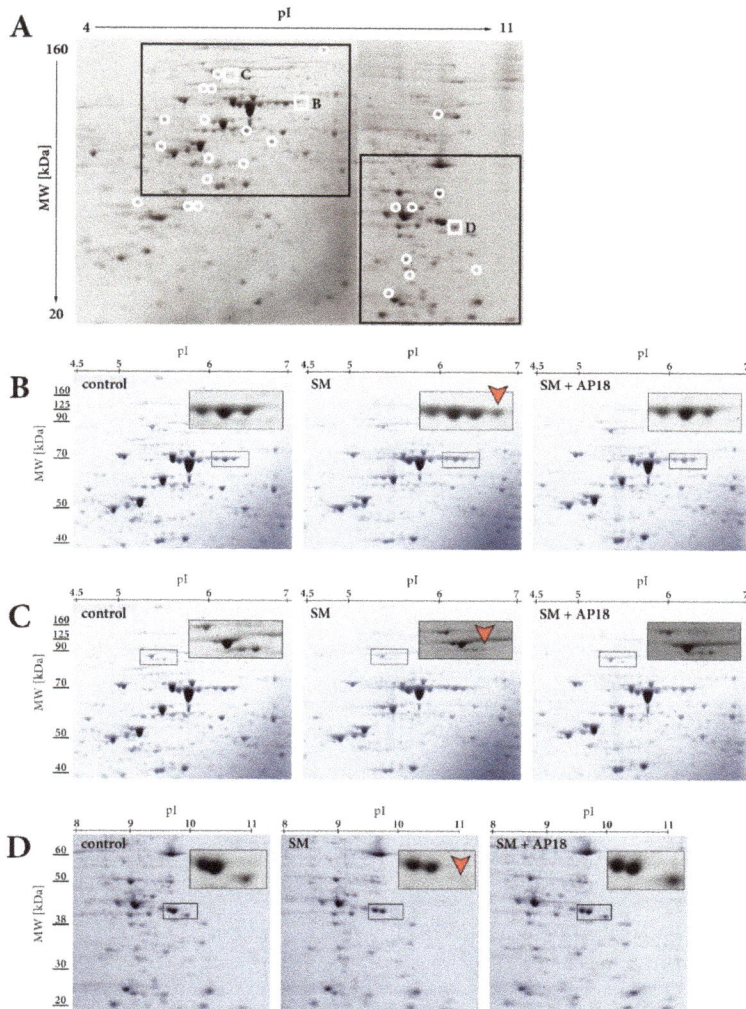

Figure 1. Representative 2D CBB-stained gel electrophoresis of HEKA1 cells. The proteome of HEKA1 control, 600 μM SM-exposed or 2 μM AP18-pre-incubated and SM-exposed cells was investigated. Isoelectric focusing of cell lysates was performed by 7 cm strips (pH 4–7 and pH 6–11, linear). Proteins were separated by 10% Bis-Tris gels. (**A**) Overview gel displaying 22 differential protein spots after SM exposure compared to controls (white open circles). White frames indicate three SM-induced and TRPA1-regulated proteins. (**B**) Zoom of the *HSPA6* spot and (**C,D**) zoom of the two protein spots which proteins are listed in Table 1. Experiments were carried out with *n* = 3 per group. Molecular weight is indicated on the left and the pI value on top of the gels.

A

B

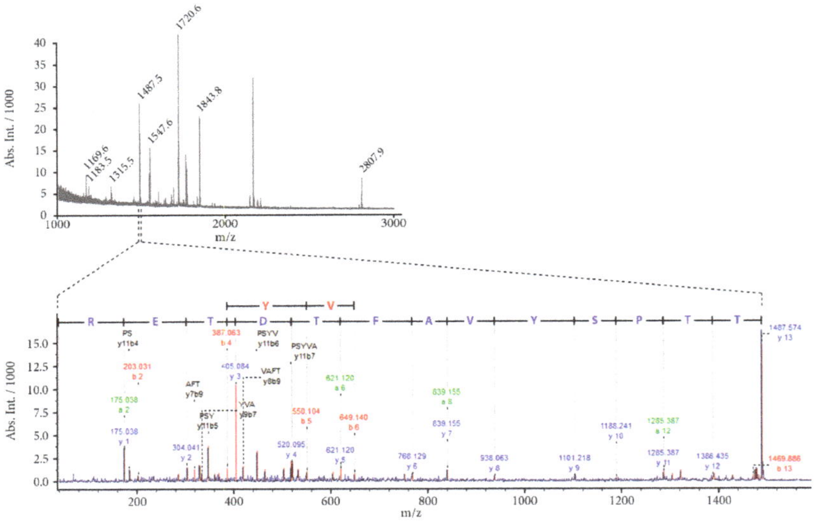

C

```
        10         20         30         40         50
MQAPRELAVG IDLGTTYSCV GVFQQGRVEI LANDQGNRTT PSYVAFTDTE
        60         70         80         90        100
RLVGDAAKSQ AALNPHNTVF DAKRLIGRKF ADTTVQSDMK HWPFRVVSEG
       110        120        130        140        150
GKPKVRVCYR GEDKTFYPEE ISSMVLSKMK ETAEAYLGQP VKHAVITVPA
       160        170        180        190        200
YFNDSQRQAT KDAGAIAGLN VLRIINEPTA AAIAYGLDRR GAGERNVLIF
       210        220        230        240        250
DLGGGTFDVS VLSIDAGVFE VKATAGDTHL GGEDFDNRLV NHFMEEFRRK
       260        270        280        290        300
HGKDLSGNKR ALRRLRTACE RAKRTLSSST QATLEIDSLF EGVDFYTSIT
       310        320        330        340        350
RARFEELCSD LFRSTLEPVE KALRDAKLDK AQIHDVVLVG GSTRIPKVQK
       360        370        380        390        400
LLQDFFNGKE LNKSINPDEA VAYGAAVQAA VLMGDKCEKV QDLLLLDVAP
       410        420        430        440        450
LSLGLETAGG VMTTLIQRNA TIPTKQTQTF TTYSDNQPGV FIQVYEGERA
       460        470        480        490        500
MTKDNNLLGR FELSGIPPAP RGVPQIEVTF DIDANGILSV TATDRSTGKA
       510        520        530        540        550
NKITITNDKG RLSKEEVERM VHEAEQYKAE DEAQRDRVAA KNSLEAHVFH
       560        570        580        590        600
VKGSLQEESL RDKIPEEDRR KMQDKCREVL AWLEHNQLAE KEEYEHQKRE
       610        620        630        640
LEQICRPIFS RLYGGPGVPG GSSCGTQARQ GDPSTGPIIE EVD
```

Figure 2. MALDI-TOF MS(/MS) measurements of a protein spot after tryptic cleavage identified HSP6A. (**A**) Peptide mass fingerprint of *HSPA6* identified by MASCOT database matching resulted in a score of 86.6. (**B**) MS/MS spectrum of the ion at m/z 1487.5 resulted in a sequence tag of 13 amino acids. The complete series of y-ions could be found. (**C**) A sequence coverage of 35.5% was found for *HSPA6* (UniProtKB-P17066). Assigned peptides are indicated with a yellow background. The sequence of the peptide subjected to MS/MS fragmentation depicted in (**B**) (amino acids 39–51) is highlighted with a red background.

Table 1. Protein assignment of differentially down-regulated protein spots. SM-induced and TRPA1-dependent down-regulated spots were analyzed by nanoHPLC-ESI MS/MS. Peptides were identified by NCBInr protein database search. Molecular weights (MW) were taken from UniProt database and theoretical pI values were calculated using isoelectric point calculators [26,27]. MS/MS scores represent sums over all MS/MS scores of every significant peptide.

	Gene Name	Protein Name	UniProt ID	MW [kDa]	pI [Calculated]	Number of Identified Peptides	MS/MS Score
Figure 1C	*CAPRIN1*	Caprin-1	Q14444	78.5	5.0	17	864
	STRN4	Striatin 4	Q9NRL3	81.3	5.1	13	787
	NCL	Nucleolin	P19338	76.6	4.5	10	443
	GPHN	Gephyrin	Q9NQX3	80.4	5.1	7	372
Figure 1D	*SFXN1*	Sideroflexin 1	Q9H9B4	35.9	9.4	10	689
	FHL1	Four and a half LIM domain protein 1	Q13642	38.0	9.2	9	592
	NOSIP	Nitric oxide synthase interacting protein	Q9Y314	33.7	9.1	11	554
	ELAVL1	ELAV like protein 1	Q15717	36.2	9.6	8	445

3.2. RT-qPCR

The results of 2D-GE analysis were confirmed by independent RT-qPCR experiments (Figure 3). Accordingly, genes for *HSPA6, CAPRIN1, ELAVL1, FHL1, GPHN, NOSIP, NCL, SFXN1* and *STRN4* were chosen as targets. Effects on transcription of these genes were assessed 24 h after SM exposure. In HEKA1 cells, SM significantly increased *HSPA6* mRNA ($16.0 \times [14.4 - 17.6, 95\%$ CI]) compared to controls (normalized to 1.0) (Figure 3A). AP18 attenuated this up-regulation significantly ($9.78 \times [8.9 - 10.66, 95\%$ CI]) (Figure 3A). As these results confirmed findings from the 2D-GE, additional time points (1, 3, 5 h and 24 h) were investigated. A minor increase of *HSPA6* mRNA levels was detectable already 1 h after SM exposure ($1.99 \times [1.75 - 2.23, 95\%$ CI]) (Figure 3A). After 3 h, a more pronounced increase ($9.5 \times [8.2 - 10.8, 95\%$ CI]) was observed, which further increased after 5 h ($11.7 \times [10.6 - 12.8, 95\%$ CI]) (Figure 3A). AP18 pre-incubation significantly decreased *HSPA6* mRNA levels after 3 h and beyond (1 h: $1.6 \times [1.5 - 1.9]$; 3 h: $6.7 \times [6.1 - 7.4]$; 5 h: $8.7 \times [7.0 - 10.4]$) (Figure 3A).

AITC treatment, also with AP18 pre-incubation, of HEKA1 was conducted to elucidate the role of TRPA1 activation in more detail (Figure S2). As expected, AITC resulted in a pronounced increase of *HSPA6* mRNA levels 24 h after treatment that was minimized to less than 50% by AP18. AP18 alone without AITC did not affect *HSPA6* mRNA. Also, no changes of *HSPA6* mRNA levels were observed in HEKwt cells after AP18 or SM exposure (Figure S2).

Human A549 cells, endogenously expressing TPRA1, responded with a distinct increase of *HSPA6* mRNA levels after SM exposure measured 24 h after exposure ($6.8 \times [6.5 - 7.2]$) that was significantly diminished by AP18 ($5.0 \times [4.7 - 5.3]$) (Figure 3B).

Levels of *FHL1, NOSIP* or *STRN4* mRNA showed some slight SM-induced changes, but levels were not in the range of ±1.5-fold compared to controls. *CAPRIN1, ELAVL1, GPHN, NCL* and *SFXN1* mRNA levels were down-regulated 24 h after SM exposure. However, AP18 was unable to increase these mRNA levels. A summary of the fold change values is given in Table S1.

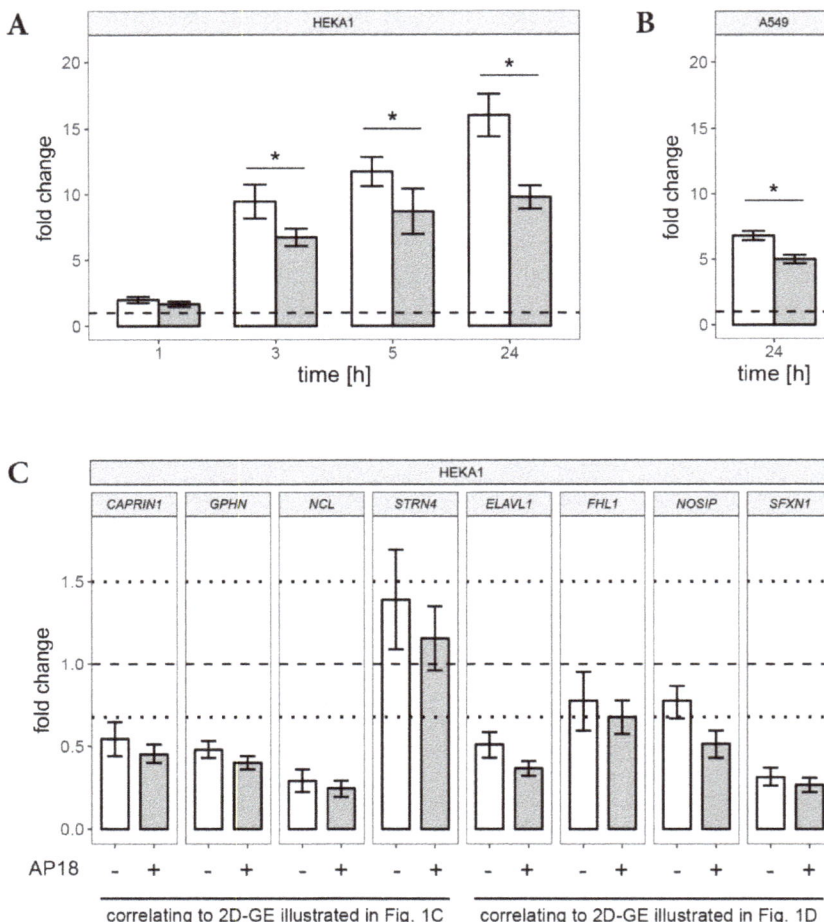

Figure 3. RT-qPCR measurements for potentially SM-affected and TRPA1-regulated genes. mRNA levels of (**A**) *HSPA6* in HEKA1 cells, (**B**) *HSPA6* in A549 cells and (**C**) *CAPRIN1*, *ELAVL1*, *FHL1*, *GPHN*, *NOSIP*, *NCL*, *SFXN1* and *STRN4* in HEKA1 cells were analyzed 24 h after 600 µM SM exposure by RT-qPCR. White bars indicate the fold change values after SM exposure while grey bars illustrate the effect of 2 µM AP18 pre-incubation on mRNA levels. The dashed lines represent normalized levels of the control samples and dotted lines indicate ±1.5-fold change ranges. Significant differences ($p < 0.05$) are displayed by asterisks (*). Error bars represent the 95% confidence intervals. Data are derived from independent biological experiments ($n = 3$). Gene names correspond to the following proteins: Caprin-1 (*CAPRIN1*), ELAV like protein 1 (*ELAVL1*), Four and a half LIM domain protein 1 (*FHL1*), Gephyrin (*GPHN*), Nitric oxide synthase interacting protein (*NOSIP*), Nucleolin (*NCL*), Sideroflexin 1 (*SFXN1*) and Striatin 4 (*STRN4*).

4. Discussion

Cell damage caused by alkylating compounds is assumed to rely on DNA mono-adducts and particularly on DNA crosslinks or the biological consequences thereof [28–30]. However, cytotoxic effects of alkylating agents are strongly attenuated by cellular DNA repair processes [29,31–33]. Therefore, additional complex mechanisms have been proposed including PARP signaling, nitric oxide and oxidative stress and activation of multiple cellular pathways that contribute to cytotoxicity [28,34–39]. In this context, chemosensing TRPA1 channels were described as targets of SM and related alkylating compounds [4,19]. A distinct increase of $[Ca^{2+}]_i$ occurred after the activation of TRPA1 by SM. Some biological effects thereof, e.g., influence on cell viability, have already been described [4]. Additional SM-induced and TRPA1-mediated effects have not been studied so far and were investigated in this study.

HEKA1 cells, overexpressing human TRPA1 channels, as well as human A549 lung epithelial cells, endogenously expressing TRPA1, were chosen as the in vitro model. Both cell types were used in several studies before and were found very well suited for the investigation of TRPA1-related effects [23,40,41]. Several genes and proteins have been reported to be specifically up-regulated in mouse skin and in human keratinocytes after exposure to SM [42,43]. Thus, we focused on proteome changes after SM exposure with special focus on the involvement of TRPA1.

2D-GE with subsequent protein identification by MS were used to detect changes of protein levels in HEKA1 cells. Cell lysates from controls, which were only treated with the solvent EtOH, were selected as control group. SM-treated or cells pre-incubated with the specific TRPA1 inhibitor AP18 [44], were examined to unambiguously identify SM-induced and TRPA1-regulated proteins.

Our results indicated 22 differentially expressed protein spots after SM exposure in HEKA1 cells compared to un-exposed controls (Figure 1A). It should be noted that we have chosen 7 cm first dimension gel strips covering pH-ranges between 4–7 or 6–11 and proteins were visualized after SDS-PAGE separation by CBB staining. CBB staining detects high-abundant proteins with a very good chance of success for the identification by MALDI-TOF MS(/MS) while changes in low-abundant proteins may be undiscovered. Additional silver staining experiments were conducted and identified 28 further protein spots. However, AP18 pre-incubation had no effect on these spots, thereby excluding a role of TRPA1. Nevertheless, we successfully identified three SM-induced and TRPA1-regulated protein spots 24 h after exposure with one up-regulated and two down-regulated proteins (Figure 1B–D). The up-regulated protein was unequivocally identified as heat shock 70 kDa protein 6 (*HSPA6*) by MALDI-TOF MS peptide mass fingerprint and further MS/MS fragmentation of prominent peptide ions (Figure 2A,B). Identification of the down-regulated protein spots by MALDI-TOF MS was not successful, most probably due to insufficient protein amounts. Therefore, nanoHPLC-ESI MS/MS was chosen as an alternative method. Using this highly sensitive MS/MS method, multiple proteins with high probability scores were unambiguously verified (Table 1). All proteins that were assigned to the respective spot revealed a similar MW and a pI, in line with the 2D-GE results. It is not uncommon in 2D-GE that protein spots, especially of high-abundant proteins, do not represent a single protein. Instead proteins with similar MW and pI can overlap which is also the case in our experiments. The identity of proteins was confirmed by RT-qPCR. SM exposure resulted in down-regulation of all investigated mRNA except *STRN4* (Figure 3C). Some effects were weak and failed to meet the criteria of a ±1.5-fold change (*STRN4, FHL1, NOSIP*) while *CAPRIN1, GPHN, NCL* and *ELAVL1* mRNA were down-regulated to some extend (Figure 3C). However, AP18 did not significantly influence mRNA levels in any case. Our results indicate that TRPA1 has no major effect on mRNA transcription of these genes. Effects on translation, post-translational modification or degradation of target proteins that could explain the obtained results in 2D-GE may be present but have not been elucidated so far.

SM-affected proteins identified in our study are involved in several steps of gene transcription or mRNA translation. Caprin-1 is discussed to mediate the transport and translation of mRNAs of proteins involved in cell proliferation and migration in multiple cell types [45]. Striatin-4 binds calmodulin in a calcium-dependent manner and may function as scaffolding or signaling protein [46]. Nucleolin is a nucleolar phosphoprotein involved in fundamental aspects of transcription regulation, cell proliferation and growth [47]. It is thought to play a role in pre-rRNA transcription and ribosome assembly and in the process of transcriptional elongation [48]. *GPHN* and *FHL1* are proteins involved in organization of the cytoskeleton and protein-cytoskeleton interactions [49,50]. In addition, *FHL1* is involved in nuclear gene regulation processes [50]. *ELAVL1* is an RNA-binding protein that binds to the 3′-UTR region of mRNAs and increases their stability [51,52]. Only for *SFXN1*, a protein that might be involved in the transport of a component required for iron utilization into or out of the mitochondria [53,54], and *NOSIP*, a ubiquitin-protein ligase that negatively regulates nitric oxide production by inducing NOS1 and NOS3 translocation to actin cytoskeleton and inhibiting their enzymatic activity [55], a direct function in protein biosynthesis has not been described yet. Whether the identified proteins are indeed involved in the molecular toxicology of SM or related compounds has to be proven but is not part of this study.

Exposure of human keratinocytes with CEES (a monofunctional analog of SM) increased *HSPA6* levels [56]. In addition, CEES was identified as an activator of TRPA1 [4]. Results obtained in our study suggest a link between the expression of *HSPA6* and TRPA1 activation by alkylating compounds: SM increased *HSPA6* mRNA levels beginning 3 h after exposure, which was significantly prevented by AP18 pre-treatment (Figure 3A) and induced *HSPA6* protein formation after 24 h (Figure 1B). HEKwt cells did not respond to SM while human A549 lung epithelial cells, endogenously expressing TRPA1, revealed similar results with regard to *HSPA6* mRNA levels compared to HEKA1 cells (Figure 3B).

HSPs are molecular chaperones that regulate the folding, degradation and assembly of proteins [57]. After cellular stress such as intense heat, heavy metal exposure, UVB light, oxidative stress or inflammation, HSPs are up-regulated to protect cell proteins against aggregation [58,59]. *HSPA6* is especially responsible for the correct folding and activation of many proteins [60].

It is well known that SM exposure results in the formation of reactive oxygen species (ROS) or reactive nitrogen species in vitro [34,35]. ROS can induce protein damage, instability, aggregation and can even provoke cell death but have also been shown to induce HSPs [61]. Therefore, it is reasonable to assume that HSP induction may also be the consequence of SM-induced oxidative stress in our experiments.

It was previously postulated that elevation of $[Ca^{2+}]_i$ through TRP channel activation (in particular TRPA1 and TRPV1) activates the mitochondrial tricarboxylic acid cycle, which generates ATP as well as ROS [62,63]. In a study by Gould et al., CEES was proven to affect mitochondrial function in lung cells resulting in ROS formation [64]. Ray et al. demonstrated that SM induced an increase of $[Ca^{2+}]_i$ localized to mitochondria [65]. However, TRP channels were not considered as potential mediators of the observed phenomena.

Our work suggests a distinct role of TRPA1 beyond an immediate effect of SM on mitochondria. Inhibition of TRPA1 by AP18 is suggested to attenuate the SM-induced increase of $[Ca^{2+}]_i$ and thus, the generation of ROS and *HSPA6* subsequently. However, AP18 was insufficient to completely prevent *HSPA6* induction in our experiments indicating that TRPA1 is not exclusively responsible for *HSPA6* up-regulation. In addition to TRPA1-mediated ROS formation, SM-induced depletion of antioxidants, lipid oxidation or direct effects on mitochondria can cause severe oxidative stress which is independent of TRPA1 and may also trigger *HSPA6* expression [66–68].

Other biological effects of SM-induced increase of $[Ca^{2+}]_i$ such as phospholipase A activation and subsequent arachidonate release, terminal differentiation of human keratinocytes, induction of cell death through caspases, in addition to the above discussed $Ca^{2+}/ROS/HSPA6$ cascade, were described [4,65,69–71]. A synopsis depicting the interaction of cellular events after SM-exposure with focus on TRPA1 and *HSPA6* is given in Figure 4.

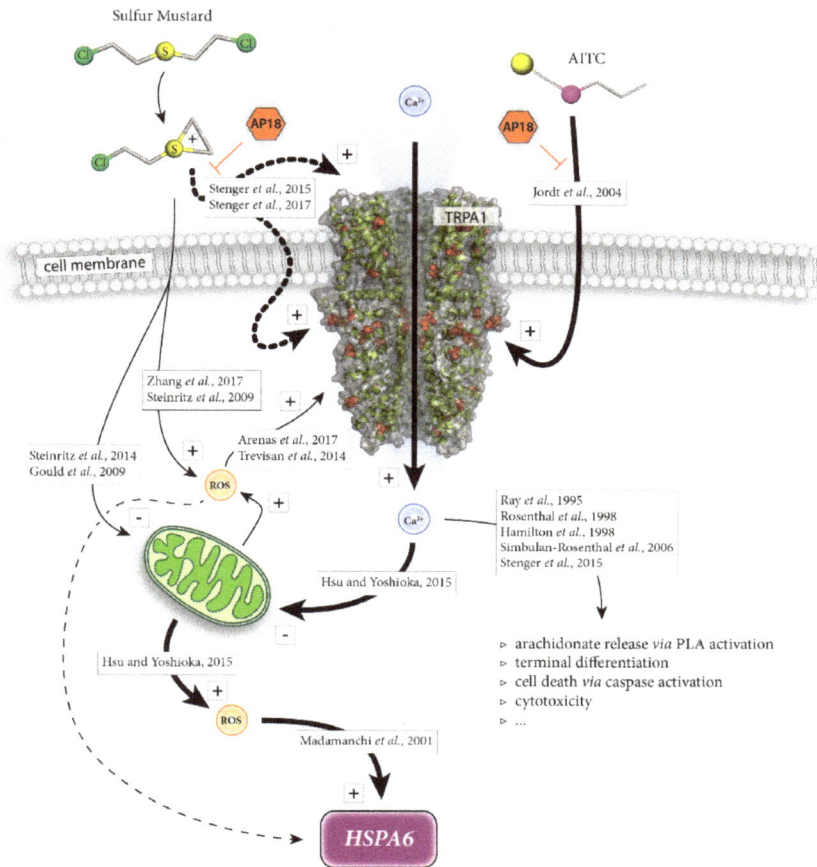

Figure 4. Schematic overview suggesting TRPA1-mediated induction of *HSPA6* after SM exposure. SM activates TRPA1 channels with a still unknown extra- or intracellular binding site (bold dotted lines). SM as well as AITC treatment increase intracellular Ca^{2+} ($[Ca^{2+}]_i$) levels. AP18 prevents both SM- and AITC-induced TRPA1 activation. $[Ca^{2+}]_i$ affects mitochondrial function thereby producing ROS which triggers *HSPA6* induction. SM may also cause ROS formation through disturbance of mitochondrial function or other yet not well-defined mechanisms thereby potentially contributing to *HSPA6* induction (dashed line) without involvement of TRPA1. Elevation of $[Ca^{2+}]_i$ also results in additional biological effects (open triangles). Text boxes list references describing the illustrated effects. Activation, increase or induction is marked with "+" while impairment of mitochondria is indicated with "−".

Our results suggest that SM causes an increase of $[Ca^{2+}]_i$ and subsequent induction of *HSPA6*, which is in part mediated by TRPA1 channels. Increase of ROS, presumably originating from mitochondrial stress, is a feasible cause for the observed *HSPA6* induction. An inhibition of TRPA1 in HEKA1 and A549 cells attenuated the SM-induced expression of *HSPA6* and thereby pointing to a distinct role of TRPA1 ion channels. Whether induction of *HSPA6* after SM exposure is a protective cellular defense mechanism as it may protect against stress-induced apoptosis [72] cannot be answered at this point and should be addressed in future research. Nevertheless, TRPA1 channels were proven to be part of the very complex molecular toxicology of SM and a step closer into the spotlight of SM research.

Supplementary Materials: The following are available online at http://www.mdpi.com/2073-4409/7/9/126/s1, Figure S1. Representative 2D silver-stained gel electrophoresis of 600 μM SM-exposed HEKA1 cells. Figure S2. RT-qPCR measurements of relative HSPA6 mRNA levels in HEKA1 and HEKwt cells. Table S1. Fold change values of RT-qPCR.

Author Contributions: Conceptualization D.S. and T.P.; Experiments R.L. and H.J.; Draft Preparation R.L. and T.P.; Writing & Editing, T.P., H.J. and D.S.; Visualization D.S.; Supervision, D.S., H.M. and T.G.

Funding: This research received no external funding

Conflicts of Interest: The authors declare no conflict of interest.

References

1. Steinritz, D.; Balszuweit, F.; Thiermann, H.; Kehe, K. Mustard: Pathophysiology and Therapeutic Approaches. In *Chemical Warfare Toxicology*; Worek, F., Jenner, J., Thiermann, H., Eds.; Royal Society of Chemistry: Cambridge, UK, 2016; pp. 120–156.

2. Kehe, K.; Steinritz, D.; Balszuweit, F.; Thiermann, H. Long-Term Effects of the Chemical Warfare Agent Sulfur Mustard. In *Chemical Warfare Toxicology*; Worek, F., Jenner, J., Thiermann, H., Eds.; Royal Society of Chemistry: Cambridge, UK, 2016; pp. 179–190.

3. Steinritz, D.; Thiermann, H. Sulfur Mustard. In *Critical Care Toxicology: Diagnosis and Management of the Critically Poisoned Patient*, 2nd ed.; Brent, J., Burkhart, K., Dargan, P.I., Hatten, B., Megarbane, B., Palmer, R., White, J., Eds.; Springer: Cham, Switzerland, 2017; pp. 2683–2712.

4. Stenger, B.; Zehfuss, F.; Mückter, H.; Schmidt, A.; Balszuweit, F.; Schäfer, E.; Büch, T.; Gudermann, T.; Thiermann, H.; Steinritz, D. Activation of the chemosensing transient receptor potential channel A1 (TRPA1) by alkylating agents. *Arch. Toxicol.* **2015**, *89*, 1631–1643. [CrossRef] [PubMed]

5. Ramsey, I.S.; Delling, M.; Clapham, D.E. An introduction to TRP channels. *Annu. Rev. Physiol.* **2006**, *68*, 619–647. [CrossRef] [PubMed]

6. Chen, J.; Hackos, D.H. TRPA1 as a drug target—Promise and challenges. *Naunyn-Schmiedeberg's Arch. Pharmacol.* **2015**, *388*, 451–463. [CrossRef] [PubMed]

7. Fischer, M.J.M.; Balasuriya, D.; Jeggle, P.; Goetze, T.A.; McNaughton, P.A.; Reeh, P.W.; Edwardson, J.M. Direct evidence for functional TRPV1/TRPA1 heteromers. *Pflug. Arch.-Eur. J. Physiol.* **2014**, *466*, 2229–2241. [CrossRef] [PubMed]

8. Madej, M.G.; Ziegler, C.M. Dawning of a new era in TRP channel structural biology by cryo-electron microscopy. *Pflug. Arch.-Eur. J. Physiol.* **2018**, *470*, 213–225. [CrossRef] [PubMed]

9. Macpherson, L.J.; Dubin, A.E.; Evans, M.J.; Marr, F.; Schultz, P.G.; Cravatt, B.F.; Patapoutian, A. Noxious compounds activate TRPA1 ion channels through covalent modification of cysteines. *Nature* **2007**, *445*, 541–545. [CrossRef] [PubMed]

10. Bessac, B.F.; Jordt, S.-E. Sensory detection and responses to toxic gases: Mechanisms, health effects, and countermeasures. *Proc. Am. Thorac. Soc.* **2010**, *7*, 269–277. [CrossRef] [PubMed]

11. Jordt, S.-E.; Bautista, D.M.; Chuang, H.-H.; McKemy, D.D.; Zygmunt, P.M.; Högestätt, E.D.; Meng, I.D.; Julius, D. Mustard oils and cannabinoids excite sensory nerve fibres through the TRP channel ANKTM1. *Nature* **2004**, *427*, 260–265. [CrossRef] [PubMed]

12. Achanta, S.; Jordt, S.-E. TRPA1: Acrolein meets its target. *Toxicol. Appl. Pharmacol.* **2017**, *324*, 45–50. [CrossRef] [PubMed]

13. De La Roche, J.; Eberhardt, M.J.; Klinger, A.B.; Stanslowsky, N.; Wegner, F.; Koppert, W.; Reeh, P.W.; Lampert, A.; Fischer, M.J.M.; Leffler, A. The molecular basis for species-specific activation of human TRPA1 protein by protons involves poorly conserved residues within transmembrane domains 5 and 6. *J. Biol. Chem.* **2013**, *288*, 20280–20292. [CrossRef] [PubMed]

14. Bessac, B.F.; Sivula, M.; Von Hehn, C.A.; Escalera, J.; Cohn, L.; Jordt, S.-E. TRPA1 is a major oxidant sensor in murine airway sensory neurons. *J. Clin. Investig.* **2008**, *118*, 1899–1910. [CrossRef] [PubMed]

15. Hox, V.; Vanoirbeek, J.A.; Alpizar, Y.A.; Voedisch, S.; Callebaut, I.; Bobic, S.; Sharify, A.; De Vooght, V.; Van Gerven, L.; Devos, F.; et al. Crucial role of transient receptor potential ankyrin 1 and mast cells in induction of nonallergic airway hyperreactivity in mice. *Am. J. Respir. Crit. Care Med.* **2013**, *187*, 486–493. [CrossRef] [PubMed]

16. Arenas, O.M.; Zaharieva, E.E.; Para, A.; Vásquez-Doorman, C.; Petersen, C.P.; Gallio, M. Activation of planarian TRPA1 by reactive oxygen species reveals a conserved mechanism for animal nociception. *Nat. Neurosci.* **2017**, *20*, 1686–1693. [CrossRef] [PubMed]

17. Lin, A.-H.; Liu, M.-H.; Ko, H.-K.; Perng, D.-W.; Lee, T.-S.; Kou, Y.R. Lung Epithelial TRPA1 Transduces the Extracellular ROS into Transcriptional Regulation of Lung Inflammation Induced by Cigarette Smoke: The Role of Influxed Ca^{2+}. *Mediat. Inflamm.* **2015**, *2015*. [CrossRef] [PubMed]

18. Trevisan, G.; Hoffmeister, C.; Rossato, M.F.; Oliveira, S.M.; Silva, M.A.; Silva, C.R.; Fusi, C.; Tonello, R.; Minocci, D.; Guerra, G.P.; et al. TRPA1 receptor stimulation by hydrogen peroxide is critical to trigger hyperalgesia and inflammation in a model of acute gout. *Free Radic. Biol. Med.* **2014**, *72*, 200–209. [CrossRef] [PubMed]

19. Stenger, B.; Popp, T.; John, H.; Siegert, M.; Tsoutsoulopoulos, A.; Schmidt, A.; Mückter, H.; Gudermann, T.; Thiermann, H.; Steinritz, D. *N*-Acetyl-L-cysteine inhibits sulfur mustard-induced and TRPA1-dependent calcium influx. *Arch. Toxicol.* **2017**, *91*, 2179–2189. [CrossRef] [PubMed]

20. Macpherson, L.J.; Xiao, B.; Kwan, K.Y.; Petrus, M.J.; Dubin, A.E.; Hwang, S.; Cravatt, B.; Corey, D.P.; Patapoutian, A. An ion channel essential for sensing chemical damage. *J. Neurosci.* **2007**, *27*, 11412–11415. [CrossRef] [PubMed]

21. Achanta, S.; Chintagari, N.R.; Brackmann, M.; Balakrishna, S.; Jordt, S.-E. TRPA1 and CGRP antagonists counteract vesicant-induced skin injury and inflammation. *Toxicol. Lett.* **2018**, *293*, 140–148. [CrossRef] [PubMed]

22. Nie, Y.; Huang, C.; Zhong, S.; Wortley, M.A.; Luo, Y.; Luo, W.; Xie, Y.; Lai, K.; Zhong, N. Cigarette smoke extract (CSE) induces transient receptor potential ankyrin 1(TRPA1) expression via activation of HIF1αin A549 cells. *Free Radic. Biol. Med.* **2016**, *99*, 498–507. [CrossRef] [PubMed]

23. Büch, T.R.H.; Schäfer, E.A.M.; Demmel, M.-T.; Boekhoff, I.; Thiermann, H.; Gudermann, T.; Steinritz, D.; Schmidt, A. Functional expression of the transient receptor potential channel TRPA1, a sensor for toxic lung inhalants, in pulmonary epithelial cells. *Chem.-Biol. Interact.* **2013**, *206*, 462–471. [CrossRef] [PubMed]

24. Mukhopadhyay, I.; Gomes, P.; Aranake, S.; Shetty, M.; Karnik, P.; Damle, M.; Kuruganti, S.; Thorat, S.; Khairatkar-Joshi, N. Expression of functional TRPA1 receptor on human lung fibroblast and epithelial cells. *J. Recept. Signal Transduct.* **2011**, *31*, 350–358. [CrossRef] [PubMed]

25. Qiagen. Data Analysis Center. 2018. Available online: https://www.qiagen.com/de/shop/genes-and-pathways/data-analysis-center-overview-page/?akamai-feo=off (accessed on 10 July 2018).

26. Protein Isoelectric Point Calculator. 2018. Available online: http://isoelectric.org/index.html (accessed on 23 August 2018).

27. Protein Isoelectric Point Calculator. 2018. Available online: http://www.bioinformatics.org/sms2/index.html (accessed on 23 August 2018).

28. Kehe, K.; Balszuweit, F.; Steinritz, D.; Thiermann, H. Molecular toxicology of sulfur mustard-induced cutaneous inflammation and blistering. *Toxicology* **2009**, *263*, 12–19. [CrossRef] [PubMed]

29. Fu, D.; Calvo, J.A.; Samson, L.D. Balancing repair and tolerance of DNA damage caused by alkylating agents. *Nat. Rev. Cancer* **2012**, *12*, 104–120. [CrossRef] [PubMed]

30. Dacre, J.C.; Goldman, M. Toxicology and pharmacology of the chemical warfare agent sulfur mustard. *Pharmacol. Rev.* **1996**, *48*, 289–326. [PubMed]

31. Deans, A.J.; West, S.C. DNA interstrand crosslink repair and cancer. *Nat. Rev. Cancer* **2011**, *11*, 467–480. [CrossRef] [PubMed]

32. Huang, Y.; Li, L. DNA crosslinking damage and cancer—A tale of friend and foe. *Transl. Cancer Res.* **2013**, *2*, 144–154. [PubMed]

33. Kondo, N.; Takahashi, A.; Ono, K.; Ohnishi, T. DNA damage induced by alkylating agents and repair pathways. *J. Nucleic Acids* **2010**, *2010*. [CrossRef] [PubMed]

34. Steinritz, D.; Elischer, A.; Balszuweit, F.; Gonder, S.; Heinrich, A.; Bloch, W.; Thiermann, H.; Kehe, K. Sulphur mustard induces time- and concentration-dependent regulation of NO-synthesizing enzymes. *Toxico. Lett.* **2009**, *188*, 263–269. [CrossRef] [PubMed]

35. O'Neill, H.C.; Orlicky, D.J.; Hendry-Hofer, T.B.; Loader, J.E.; Day, B.J.; White, C.W. Role of reactive oxygen and nitrogen species in olfactory epithelial injury by the sulfur mustard analogue 2-chloroethyl ethyl sulfide. *Am. J. Respir. Cell Mol. Biol.* **2011**, *45*, 323–331. [CrossRef] [PubMed]

36. Brent, J.; Burkhart, K.; Dargan, P.I.; Hatten, B.; Megarbane, B.; Palmer, R.; White, J. *Critical Care Toxicology. Diagnosis and Management of the Critically Poisoned Patient*, 2nd ed.; Springer: Cham, Switzerland, 2017.

37. Jain, A.K.; Tewari-Singh, N.; Gu, M.; Inturi, S.; White, C.W.; Agarwal, R. Sulfur mustard analog, 2-chloroethyl ethyl sulfide-induced skin injury involves DNA damage and induction of inflammatory mediators, in part via oxidative stress, in SKH-1 hairless mouse skin. *Toxicol. Lett.* **2011**, *205*, 293–301. [CrossRef] [PubMed]

38. Tewari-Singh, N.; Jain, A.K.; Inturi, S.; Agarwal, C.; White, C.W.; Agarwal, R. Silibinin attenuates sulfur mustard analog-induced skin injury by targeting multiple pathways connecting oxidative stress and inflammation. *PLoS ONE* **2012**, *7*, e46149. [CrossRef] [PubMed]

39. Steinritz, D.; Weber, J.; Balszuweit, F.; Thiermann, H.; Schmidt, A. Sulfur mustard induced nuclear translocation of glyceraldehyde-3-phosphate-dehydrogenase (GAPDH). *Chem.-Biol. Interact.* **2013**, *206*, 529–535. [CrossRef] [PubMed]

40. Steinritz, D.; Zehfuß, F.; Stenger, B.; Schmidt, A.; Popp, T.; Kehe, K.; Mückter, H.; Thiermann, H.; Gudermann, T. Zinc chloride-induced TRPA1 activation does not contribute to toxicity in vitro. *Toxicol. Lett.* **2018**, *293*, 133–139. [CrossRef] [PubMed]

41. Schaefer, E.A.M.; Stohr, S.; Meister, M.; Aigner, A.; Gudermann, T.; Buech, T.R.H. Stimulation of the chemosensory TRPA1 cation channel by volatile toxic substances promotes cell survival of small cell lung cancer cells. *Biochem. Pharmacol.* **2013**, *85*, 426–438. [CrossRef] [PubMed]

42. Everley, P.A.; Dillman, J.F. A large-scale quantitative proteomic approach to identifying sulfur mustard-induced protein phosphorylation cascades. *Chem. Res. Toxicol.* **2010**, *23*, 20–25. [CrossRef] [PubMed]

43. Rogers, J.V.; Choi, Y.W.; Kiser, R.C.; Babin, M.C.; Casillas, R.P.; Schlager, J.J.; Sabourin, C.L.K. Microarray analysis of gene expression in murine skin exposed to sulfur mustard. *J. Biochem. Mol. Toxicol.* **2004**, *18*, 289–299. [CrossRef] [PubMed]

44. Petrus, M.; Peier, A.M.; Bandell, M.; Hwang, S.W.; Huynh, T.; Olney, N.; Jegla, T.; Patapoutian, A. A role of TRPA1 in mechanical hyperalgesia is revealed by pharmacological inhibition. *Mol. Pain* **2007**, *3*, 40. [CrossRef] [PubMed]

45. Solomon, S.; Xu, Y.; Wang, B.; David, M.D.; Schubert, P.; Kennedy, D.; Schrader, J.W. Distinct structural features of caprin-1 mediate its interaction with G3BP-1 and its induction of phosphorylation of eukaryotic translation initiation factor 2α, entry to cytoplasmic stress granules, and selective interaction with a subset of mRNAs. *Mol. Cell. Biol.* **2007**, *27*, 2324–2342. [CrossRef] [PubMed]

46. Castets, F.; Rakitina, T.; Gaillard, S.; Moqrich, A.; Mattei, M.G.; Monneron, A. Zinedin, SG2NA, and striatin are calmodulin-binding, WD repeat proteins principally expressed in the brain. *J. Biol. Chem.* **2000**, *275*, 19970–19977. [CrossRef] [PubMed]

47. Losfeld, M.-E.; Khoury, D.E.; Mariot, P.; Carpentier, M.; Krust, B.; Briand, J.-P.; Mazurier, J.; Hovanessian, A.G.; Legrand, D. The cell surface expressed nucleolin is a glycoprotein that triggers calcium entry into mammalian cells. *Exp. Cell Res.* **2009**, *315*, 357–369. [CrossRef] [PubMed]

48. Cong, R.; Das, S.; Douet, J.; Wong, J.; Buschbeck, M.; Mongelard, F.; Bouvet, P. macroH2A1 histone variant represses rDNA transcription. *Nucleic Acids Res.* **2014**, *42*, 181–192. [CrossRef] [PubMed]

49. Reiss, J.; Lenz, U.; Aquaviva-Bourdain, C.; Joriot-Chekaf, S.; Mention-Mulliez, K.; Holder-Espinasse, M. A GPHN point mutation leading to molybdenum cofactor deficiency. *Clin. Genet.* **2011**, *80*, 598–599. [CrossRef] [PubMed]

50. Chu, P.-H.; Chen, J. The novel roles of four and a half LIM proteins 1 and 2 in the cardiovascular system. *Chang Gung Med. J.* **2011**, *34*, 127–134. [PubMed]

51. Doller, A.; Akool, E.-S.; Huwiler, A.; Müller, R.; Radeke, H.H.; Pfeilschifter, J.; Eberhardt, W. Posttranslational modification of the AU-rich element binding protein HuR by protein kinase Cdelta elicits angiotensin II-induced stabilization and nuclear export of cyclooxygenase 2 mRNA. *Mol. Cell. Biol.* **2008**, *28*, 2608–2625. [CrossRef] [PubMed]

52. Tran, H.; Maurer, F.; Nagamine, Y. Stabilization of Urokinase and Urokinase Receptor mRNAs by HuR Is Linked to Its Cytoplasmic Accumulation Induced by Activated Mitogen-Activated Protein Kinase-Activated Protein Kinase 2. *Mol. Cell. Biol.* **2003**, *23*, 7177–7188. [CrossRef] [PubMed]

53. Yoshikumi, Y.; Mashima, H.; Ueda, N.; Ohno, H.; Suzuki, J.; Tanaka, S.; Hayashi, M.; Sekine, N.; Ohnishi, H.; Yasuda, H.; et al. Roles of CTPL/Sfxn3 and Sfxn family members in pancreatic islet. *J. Cell. Biochem.* **2005**, *95*, 1157–1168. [CrossRef] [PubMed]

54. Xi, D.; He, Y.; Sun, Y.; Gou, X.; Yang, S.; Mao, H.; Deng, W. Molecular cloning, sequence identification and tissue expression profile of three novel genes Sfxn1, Snai2 and Cno from Black-boned sheep (Ovis aries). *Mol. Biol. Rep.* **2011**, *38*, 1883–1887. [CrossRef] [PubMed]

55. Dreyer, J.; Schleicher, M.; Tappe, A.; Schilling, K.; Kuner, T.; Kusumawidijaja, G.; Müller-Esterl, W.; Oess, S.; Kuner, R. Nitric oxide synthase (NOS)-interacting protein interacts with neuronal NOS and regulates its distribution and activity. *J. Neurosci.* **2004**, *24*, 10454–10465. [CrossRef] [PubMed]

56. Black, A.T.; Hayden, P.J.; Casillas, R.P.; Heck, D.E.; Gerecke, D.R.; Sinko, P.J.; Laskin, D.L.; Laskin, J.D. Regulation of Hsp27 and Hsp70 expression in human and mouse skin construct models by caveolae following exposure to the model sulfur mustard vesicant, 2-chloroethyl ethyl sulfide. *Toxicol. Appl. Pharmacol.* **2011**, *253*, 112–120. [CrossRef] [PubMed]

57. Liberek, K.; Lewandowska, A.; Zietkiewicz, S. Chaperones in control of protein disaggregation. *EMBO J.* **2008**, *27*, 328–335. [CrossRef] [PubMed]

58. Maytin, E.V. Heat Shock Proteins and Molecular Chaperones: Implication for Adaptive Responses in the Skin. *J. Investig. Dermatol.* **1995**, *104*, 448–455. [CrossRef] [PubMed]

59. Trautinger, F. Heat shock proteins in the photobiology of human skin. *J. Photochem. Photobiol. B Biol.* **2001**, *63*, 70–77. [CrossRef]

60. Macario, A.J.L. Molecular chaperones: Multiple functions, pathologies, and potential applications. *Front. Biosci.* **2007**, *12*, 2588–2600. [CrossRef] [PubMed]

61. Madamanchi, N.R.; Li, S.; Patterson, C.; Runge, M.S. Reactive Oxygen Species Regulate Heat-Shock Protein 70 via the JAK/STAT Pathway. *Arterioscler. Thromb. Vasc. Biol.* **2001**, *21*, 321–326. [CrossRef] [PubMed]

62. Brookes, P.S.; Yoon, Y.; Robotham, J.L.; Anders, M.W.; Sheu, S.-S. Calcium, ATP, and ROS: A mitochondrial love-hate triangle. *Am. J. Physiol.-Cell Physiol.* **2004**, *287*, C817–C833. [CrossRef] [PubMed]

63. Hsu, W.-L.; Yoshioka, T. Role of TRP channels in the induction of heat shock proteins (Hsps) by heating skin. *Biophysics* **2015**, *11*, 25–32. [CrossRef] [PubMed]

64. Gould, N.S.; White, C.W.; Day, B.J. A role for mitochondrial oxidative stress in sulfur mustard analog 2-chloroethyl ethyl sulfide-induced lung cell injury and antioxidant protection. *J. Pharmacol. Exp. Ther.* **2009**, *328*, 732–739. [CrossRef] [PubMed]

65. Ray, R.; Legere, R.H.; Majerus, B.J.; Petrali, J.P. Sulfur mustard-induced increase in intracellular free calcium level and arachidonic acid release from cell membrane. *Toxicol. Appl. Pharmacol.* **1995**, *131*, 44–52. [CrossRef] [PubMed]

66. Sawale, S.D.; Ambhore, P.D.; Pawar, P.P.; Pathak, U.; Deb, U.; Satpute, R.M. Ameliorating effect of S-2(ω-aminoalkylamino) alkylaryl sulfide (DRDE-07) on sulfur mustard analogue, 2-chloroethyl ethyl sulfide-induced oxidative stress and inflammation. *Toxicol. Mech. Methods* **2013**, *23*, 702–710. [CrossRef] [PubMed]

67. Zhang, X.; Mei, Y.; Wang, T.; Liu, F.; Jiang, N.; Zhou, W.; Zhang, Y. Early oxidative stress, DNA damage and inflammation resulting from subcutaneous injection of sulfur mustard into mice. *Environ. Toxicol. Pharmacol.* **2017**, *55*, 68–73. [CrossRef] [PubMed]

68. Steinritz, D.; Schmidt, A.; Simons, T.; Ibrahim, M.; Morguet, C.; Balszuweit, F.; Thiermann, H.; Kehe, K.; Bloch, W.; Bölck, B. Chlorambucil (nitrogen mustard) induced impairment of early vascular endothelial cell migration—Effects of α-linolenic acid and N-acetylcysteine. *Chem.-Biol. Interact.* **2014**, *219*, 143–150. [CrossRef] [PubMed]

69. Rosenthal, D.S.; Simbulan-Rosenthal, C.M.; Iyer, S.; Spoonde, A.; Smith, W.; Ray, R.; Smulson, M.E. Sulfur mustard induces markers of terminal differentiation and apoptosis in keratinocytes via a Ca^{2+}-calmodulin and caspase-dependent pathway. *J. Investig. Dermatol.* **1998**, *111*, 64–71. [CrossRef] [PubMed]

70. Simbulan-Rosenthal, C.M.; Ray, R.; Benton, B.; Soeda, E.; Daher, A.; Anderson, D.; Smith, W.J.; Rosenthal, D.S. Calmodulin mediates sulfur mustard toxicity in human keratinocytes. *Toxicology* **2006**, *227*, 21–35. [CrossRef] [PubMed]

71. Hamilton, M.G.; Dorandeu, F.M.; McCaffery, M.; Lundy, P.M.; Sawyer, T.W. Modification of cytosolic free calcium concentrations in human keratinocytes after sulfur mustard exposure. *Toxicol. In Vitro* **1998**, *12*, 365–372. [CrossRef]

72. Mosser, D.D.; Caron, A.W.; Bourget, L.; Meriin, A.B.; Sherman, M.Y.; Morimoto, R.I.; Massie, B. The Chaperone Function of hsp70 Is Required for Protection against Stress-Induced Apoptosis. *Mol. Cell. Biol.* **2000**, *20*, 7146–7159. [CrossRef] [PubMed]

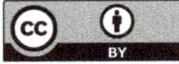

© 2018 by the authors. Licensee MDPI, Basel, Switzerland. This article is an open access article distributed under the terms and conditions of the Creative Commons Attribution (CC BY) license (http://creativecommons.org/licenses/by/4.0/).

Review

TRP Channel Involvement in Salivary Glands—Some Good, Some Bad

Xibao Liu, Hwei Ling Ong and Indu Ambudkar *

Secretory Physiology Section, National Institute of Dental Research, National Institutes of Health, Bethesda, MD 20892, USA; Xiliu@mail.nih.gov (X.L.); ongh@mail.nih.gov (H.L.O.)
* Correspondence: indu.ambudkar@nih.gov; Tel.: +1-301-496-5298

Received: 8 June 2018; Accepted: 8 July 2018; Published: 11 July 2018

Abstract: Salivary glands secrete saliva, a mixture of proteins and fluids, which plays an extremely important role in the maintenance of oral health. Loss of salivary secretion causes a dry mouth condition, xerostomia, which has numerous deleterious consequences including opportunistic infections within the oral cavity, difficulties in eating and swallowing food, and problems with speech. Secretion of fluid by salivary glands is stimulated by activation of specific receptors on acinar cell plasma membrane and is mediated by an increase in cytosolic $[Ca^{2+}]$ ($[Ca^{2+}]_i$). The increase in $[Ca^{2+}]_i$ regulates a number of ion channels and transporters that are required for establishing an osmotic gradient that drives water flow via aquaporin water channels in the apical membrane. The Store-Operated Ca^{2+} Entry (SOCE) mechanism, which is regulated in response to depletion of ER-Ca^{2+}, determines the sustained $[Ca^{2+}]_i$ increase required for prolonged fluid secretion. Core components of SOCE in salivary gland acinar cells are Orai1 and STIM1. In addition, TRPC1 is a major and non-redundant contributor to SOCE and fluid secretion in salivary gland acinar and ductal cells. Other TRP channels that contribute to salivary flow are TRPC3 and TRPV4, while presence of others, including TRPM8, TRPA1, TRPV1, and TRPV3, have been identified in the gland. Loss of salivary gland function leads to dry mouth conditions, or xerostomia, which is clinically seen in patients who have undergone radiation treatment for head-and-neck cancers, and those with the autoimmune exocrinopathy, Sjögren's syndrome (pSS). TRPM2 is a unique TRP channel that acts as a sensor for intracellular ROS. We will discuss recent studies reported by us that demonstrate a key role for TRPM2 in radiation-induced salivary gland dysfunction. Further, there is increasing evidence that TRPM2 might be involved in inflammatory processes. These interesting findings point to the possible involvement of TRPM2 in Sjögren's Syndrome, although further studies will be required to identify the exact role of TRPM2 in this disease.

Keywords: TRP channels; calcium signaling; salivary glands; xerostomia; radiation; inflammation

---

1. Introduction

Salivary glands secrete fluid composed of water and electrolytes in response to neurotransmitter stimulation of plasma membrane receptors that cause an elevation of cytosolic $[Ca^{2+}]$ ($[Ca^{2+}]_i$) in acinar cells, which are the primary site of fluid secretion [1–3] (Figure 1). The $[Ca^{2+}]_i$ increase is initiated by stimulation of the major receptors regulating fluid secretion, such as muscarinic cholinergic and α_1-adrenergic receptors, which triggers activation of phospholipase C (PLC), phosphatidylinositol 4,5-bisphosphate (PIP$_2$) hydrolysis, generation of inositol 1,4,5, trisphosphate (IP$_3$), and release of Ca^{2+} from the endoplasmic reticulum (ER) Ca^{2+} stores, mediated via the IP$_3$ receptors (IP$_3$R). In the absence of extracellular Ca^{2+}, release from the ER causes a transient increase in $[Ca^{2+}]_i$ that is not sufficient to maintain prolonged fluid secretion. The latter requires sustained increases in $[Ca^{2+}]_i$ that is supported by Ca^{2+} influx into the cells. The primary function of the $[Ca^{2+}]_i$ increase is to regulate the function of ion transporters and channels such as $Na^+/K^+/2Cl^-$ cotransporter 1 (NKCC1), Anoctamin 1 (ANO1), and Ca^{2+}-dependent K^+ (K_{Ca}), which cause vectorial transport of Cl^- from the basolateral to the luminal side of the cell, and the generation of an osmotic gradient across the luminal membrane of the cell. The latter provides the driving force for water secretion through the apical membrane via the water channel, Aquaporin 5 (AQP5).

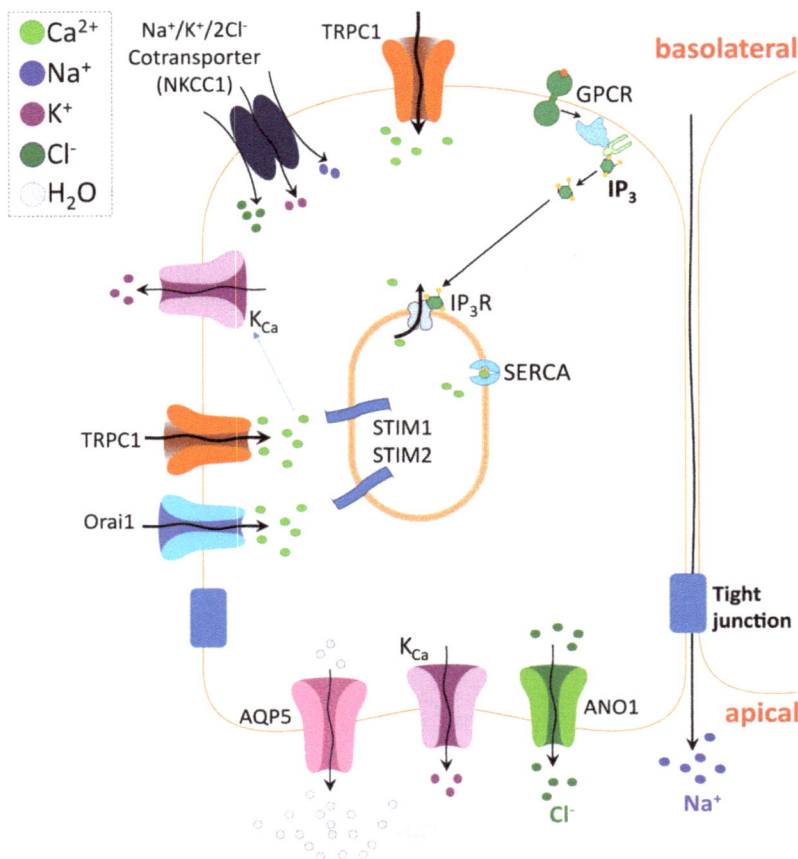

Figure 1. Ca^{2+} signaling and ion channel regulation underlying salivary gland fluid secretion. Salivary gland acinar cell (depicted in the figure) secretes fluid composed of water and electrolytes in response to neurotransmitter stimulation of plasma membrane receptors and consequent elevation of cytosolic $[Ca^{2+}]$ ($[Ca^{2+}]_i$) (see description in the text).

In salivary gland acinar cells, IP_3-mediated Ca^{2+} release occurs primarily via IP_3R2 and -3 [4,5]. Importantly, the resulting decrease in ER-$[Ca^{2+}]$ triggers the activation of Ca^{2+} influx. This type of Ca^{2+} entry, termed store-operated Ca^{2+} entry (SOCE), provides critical Ca^{2+} signals for regulation of salivary fluid secretion [6–8]. SOCE has two types of components; (i) plasma membrane Ca^{2+} channels and (ii) regulatory proteins that sense the change in ER-$[Ca^{2+}]$ and gate the channels. The main Ca^{2+} channels involved in SOCE in salivary gland cells are Orai1 and TRPC1. STIM1, an ER-Ca^{2+} binding protein, functions as the ER-$[Ca^{2+}]$ sensor and the gating component of both these channels [9–15]. In addition, STIM2 also contributes to SOCE by enhancing the sensitivity of SOCE activation under conditions when ER-Ca^{2+} stores are not substantially depleted [16]. Several different studies have demonstrated that TRPC1 is an essential channel for salivary gland function, where loss of the channel causes significant loss of fluid secretion and SOCE [17–19]. While Orai1 has been extensively studied, its exact role in salivary gland function has not yet been established. One possible function of Orai1 in the gland could be to regulate TRPC1 function, since studies with salivary gland cell lines have demonstrated that TRPC1 function is completely dependent on Orai1 [20–23].

While [Ca^{2+}]$_i$ increases are essential for the regulation of salivary gland function, disruption of Ca^{2+} homeostasis, either in resting or stimulated cells, results in salivary gland dysfunction. Two major conditions result in loss of salivary gland function and tissue damage: primary Sjögren's syndrome (pSS), a chronic autoimmune disease involving lymphocytic infiltration and loss of secretory function in salivary and lacrimal glands [24,25], and radiation-induced salivary gland dysfunction. Radiation-induced xerostomia, or dry mouth condition, occurs in patients who undergo radiation therapy for head-and-neck cancers, that results in irreversible damage of salivary glands. Loss of salivary fluid secretion leads to complications such as difficulty swallowing, rampant dental caries, oral mucosal lesions, and fungal infections that together severely affect the quality of life for patients [26,27]. This condition has been reproduced in several animal models, such as mouse, rats, mini-pigs, and non-human primates. Interestingly, irradiation (IR) induces considerable loss of saliva flow in the absence of extensive tissue damage or loss of acinar cells. While fibrosis and loss of tissue can occur, the onset and severity of this phase of cellular damage differs among the various species. Thus, the mechanism underlying IR-induced loss of salivary gland function is a subject of great interest in the field, with clinical studies being directed towards assessing therapies targeted to recovery of cell function, prevention of functional loss, or regrowth of salivary glands. In this review we will summarize the current knowledge regarding the role of TRP channels in salivary gland function and radiation-induced secretory dysfunction.

2. Historical Overview of Transient Receptor Potential (TRP) Channels

An extensive search for the molecular components of SOCE led to the identification of the transient receptor potential (TRP) superfamily of cation channels. These channels are expressed in a variety of organisms, including worms, flies, zebrafish, mice, and humans, and are broadly divided into two groups based on sequence and topological similarities. Group 1 TRPs consist of five subfamilies that bear strong homology to the founding member, *Drosophila* TRP [28]. Of these, the TRPC subfamily is most related to *Drosophila* TRP. Other subfamilies in the group include TRPV, TRPM, TRPA, and TRPN. The TRPN proteins are not found in mammals, although they are expressed in some vertebrates, such as zebrafish. The group 1 TRPs have six transmembrane segments, including a pore loop situated between the fifth and sixth transmembrane segments. TRPC, TRPM, and TRPN channels also contain a TRP domain, which follows the sixth transmembrane segment and is quite conserved between the channels. Apart from the TRPM channels, the other group 1 TRPs have multiple ankyrin repeats in the N-terminus. Three TRPM channel members, TRPM2, TRPM6, and TRPM7, are unique in that they have a pore as well as a catalytic functional domain and thus, are often referred to as chanzymes [29,30]. Group 2 TRPs consist of TRPP and TRPML channels, which share substantial sequence homology over the transmembrane segments and contain a large loop separating the first two transmembrane domains. The first TRPP and TRPML members were discovered as gene products mutated in autosomal dominant polycystic kidney disease (ADPKD) and mucolipidosis type IV (MLIV) respectively [31–34]. It should be noted that other TRP channels have also been associated with conditions of inflammation, cell damage, and disease. For example, TRPC5 and TRPC6 have been linked to the most common gastrointestinal obstruction disease in infants. TRPM2 have been suggested to underlie neurodegenerative disorders that cause movement disorders, whereas a mutation in TRPA1 was implicated in debilitating body pain. TRPV4 has been implicated to multiple channelopathies involving the musculo-skeletal system As such, it is not surprising that many members of the TRP superfamily are considered to be promising targets for the development of novel therapeutics [35–40].

TRPs are non-selective cation-channels which display variable calcium permeability. They, however, contribute to calcium signaling mechanisms and regulation of many physiological processes in a plethora of cell types. Almost all TRP channels, except TRPC subfamily members, have been reported to have sensory function. There is substantial evidence to show that regulation of TRP channels is polymodal and that they can mediate transduction of a wide variety of environmental stimuli including mechanical, thermal, or chemical stimuli [41]. A large group of TRP channels respond to thermal stimuli. While TRPV1 was the first heat-activated channel to be identified, to date, 10 thermoTRP channels with distinct range of thermoensitivity have been identified in mammals: TRPV (TRPV1, TRPV2, TRPV3, and TRPV4), TRPM (TRPM2, TRPM3, TRPM4, TRPM5, and TRPM8), and TRPA (TRPA1). In rodents, TRPV1, TRPV2, and TRPM3 are activated by noxious heat, while TRPV3, TRPV4, TRPM2, TRPM4, and TRPM5 are activated by warmth [42–44]. Channels such as TRPM8 [45–49] and TRPA1 [50] have been reported to be activated by cold stimuli. However, the thermal sensitivity of TRPA1 from both humans and rodents remains a subject of debate [51,52] due to contradictory observations. TRPA1 from mice was first reported to be activated by cold stimulation when heterologously expressed in cultured cells [50]. However, a later study contended that TRPA1 was not a temperature-sensitive channel [53]. Note that TRPA1 channel activity can be modulated by Ca^{2+}, receptor stimulation, pH, and osmotic pressure, which may explain the apparent contradictory observations by different studies [51,54–60]. A peculiar feature of thermoTRP channels is that they can also be activated by non-thermal stimulation. For example, TRPV4 is activated by hypotonic and mechanical stimulation [61,62], while TRPV1 is activated by capsaicin, contained in chili pepper, and also by extracellular acidic stimulation [46,63]. TRPA1 is activated by various irritating chemical compounds contained in plants, as well as environmental irritants such as acrolein contained in exhaust gas and cigarette smoke [64]. It is interesting that the sensitivity for thermal activation of TRP channels can be modified by other factors such as reduction of cellular PIP_2 levels [65–68]. The physiologic roles and activation mechanisms regulating thermoTRP channels have been summarized in several comprehensive reviews [69–71].

3. TRPC Channel Regulation and Function

The TRPC subfamily consists of seven members (TRPCs 1–7) that are divided into four subsets based on their amino acid homology: TRPC1, TRPC2, TRPC3/TRPC6/TRPC7, and TRPC4/TRPC5. All TRPC channels display channel activation in response to receptor-stimulated PIP_2 hydrolysis and have six transmembrane domains with a pore-forming domain located between the fifth and sixth domains. These channels contain N-terminal ankyrin repeats, and in the C-terminus, a highly conserved TRP domain, several calmodulin (CaM)-binding domains, and a putative IP_3R binding site [72–74]. TRPC channels show diverse tissue expression, physiological functions, and channel properties. Recent reviews have presented a general overview of the molecular components and mechanisms regulating SOCE [22,75], as well as overviews of the individual TRPC channels: TRPC1 [76], TRPC2 [77], TRPC3 [78], TRPC4 [79], TRPC5 [80], TRPC6 [81], and TRPC7 [82]. TRPC2 is a pseudogene in humans [83,84]. To date, almost all TRPC channels have been proposed as possible molecular components of channels mediating SOCE. However, data for some TRPCs are not very consistent. So far, the strongest evidence for the contribution of TRPC channels to SOCE has been provided for TRPC1 and TRPC4, whereas the contribution of TRPC3 to SOCE appears to be dependent on cell type and level of expression. TRPCs 5, 6, and 7 have been generally described to be store-independent, with a few exceptions. TRPC1 was the first mammalian TRPC channel to be cloned [83,84], and early studies established that it is activated by conditions resulting in store depletion and associated with the generation of a relatively Ca^{2+}-selective cation current that was termed I_{SOC} (store-operated Ca^{2+} current; [85]) to differentiate it from I_{CRAC}, the current generated by functional Orai1 [86]. TRPC1 has been reported to contribute to SOCE in a variety of cell types [87,88], although heterologous expression of the channel does not always result in enhancement of SOCE. Note that unlike with Orai1 or STIM1, TRPC channel contribution to SOCE is not seen in all cell types. Importantly, while TRPC1 clusters with and is activated by STIM1 following store-depletion, its function is also dependent on Orai1 channel activity [21]. It was shown that Orai1-mediated Ca^{2+} entry triggers recruitment of TRPC1 to the plasma membrane. Thus, TRPC1 and Orai1 form separate channels that are activated by STIM1 following neurotransmitter simulation of salivary gland cells and contribute to the $[Ca^{2+}]_i$ increase seen in stimulated cells. Orai1 is the first channel to be activated while recruitment and activation of TRPC1 leads to amplification and modulation of $[Ca^{2+}]_i$ increase that is induced by Orai1. However, since TRPC1 is activated by STIM1 following clustering of the two proteins within ER-PM-junctions, TRPC1 function is dependent on ER-Ca^{2+} depletion as well as Orai1 channel activity [21].

4. TRPC Channel Function in Exocrine Glands

As noted above, early studies established that Ca^{2+} influx is the primary determinant of sustained fluid secretion from salivary acinar cells [6]. It is now widely accepted that the primary mode of Ca^{2+} entry in acinar cells that is required for fluid secretion is mediated by SOCE. The main molecular components involved in SOCE in salivary gland acinar cells have now been identified as members of the transient receptor potential canonical (TRPC) family, TRPC1 and TRPC3. Both channels contribute to SOCE in dispersed acinar cell preparations, as well as cultured salivary gland cell lines [6,17,89]. Knockdown of endogenous TRPC1 significantly decreased SOCE in the human salivary gland (HSG) cell line, as well as primary cultures of mouse pancreatic and submandibular gland cells [17]. Further conclusive evidence was provided by studies with mice lacking TRPC1 (TRPC1$^{-/-}$), which showed reduced SOCE in salivary gland and pancreatic acinar cells as well as attenuation of Ca^{2+}-dependent physiological functions [17,18], despite having normal viability, development, and behavior [81]. SOCE is fundamentally important for fluid secretion in salivary glands and for protein secretion in the exocrine pancreas. TRPC1$^{-/-}$ mice displayed reduction in salivary gland fluid secretion that was associated with a decrease in SOCE and K_{Ca} activity in acinar cells from the mice [18,89]. Similarly defects in Ca^{2+}-activated Cl^- channel activity and protein secretion, as a consequence of reduced SOCE, were reported in pancreatic acinar cells [17]. Notably, while there is no change in Orai1 in salivary gland and pancreatic acinar cells from TRPC1$^{-/-}$ mice, the channel does not appear to compensate for the lack of TRPC1 or support cell function on its own. Hence, decreased secretory function in these exocrine glands is primarily due to the loss of TRPC1-mediated SOCE. The caveolae-residing protein, caveolin-1 (Cav-1), is an important modulator of TRPC1 activity and functions as a plasma membrane scaffold for the channel. In the absence of Cav-1, TRPC1 is mislocalized and unable to interact with STIM1 [90]. Consistent with this, localization of TRPC1, its interaction with STIM1, as well as SOCE were disrupted in salivary gland acinar cells from Cav-1$^{-/-}$ mice [91]. These cellular defects were associated with reduced fluid secretion in the mice. Together, these findings establish a vital role for TRPC1 in salivary gland fluid secretion.

TRPC3 is reported to contribute to both the store-operated and receptor-activated calcium entry pathways, and has been associated with the generation of a non-selective, Ca^{2+}-permeable channel in response to receptor-stimulated PIP_2 hydrolysis. While the channel can be directly activated by application of diacylglycerol to cells, it also contributes to SOCE under some conditions. Mice lacking TRPC3 show reduced SOCE and fluid secretion [92]. Interestingly, the contribution of TRPC3 to SOCE is dependent on the presence of TRPC1, as TRPC1$^{-/-}$ mice do not display TRPC3-dependent SOCE [93]. Thus, it has been proposed that either the channels are assembled as a store-operated heteromeric channel, or that TRPC1 is required for store-dependent regulation of TRPC3. Indeed, TRPC3–TRPC1 interaction is necessary for STIM1 regulation of the channels in salivary gland ductal cells. The two TRPC channels coimmunoprecipitate following cell stimulation together with STIM1. Loss of TRPC1 eliminates the association of STIM1 with TRPC3 [93,94]. TRPC3-mediated Ca^{2+} entry can also contribute to exocrine gland pathology and tissue damage. Pancreatic acini from TRPC3$^{-/-}$ mice showed significant protection from acute pancreatitis induced by hyper-activation of SOCE.

Similar effects were seen by blocking channel function in TRPC3$^{+/+}$ mice by treatment with pyrazole 3, a TRPC3 channel inhibitor [92,95].

Orai1 is a critical and essential component of SOCE [10,12]. Although the role of Orai1 in salivary gland function is yet to be determined, it has been examined in two other exocrine glands, lacrimal and pancreatic. Orai1$^{-/-}$ mice display loss of lacrimal gland function and reduced SOCE in lacrimal gland acinar cells [96]. Further, knockdown of Orai1 in isolated pancreatic ductal cells also resulted in loss of SOCE and Ca^{2+}-activated ion channel activity that was similar to that seen in TRPC1$^{-/-}$ cells [17]. Targeted knockout of Orai1 in pancreatic acinar cells of adult mice led to loss of SOCE and severely compromised pancreatic secretion. Antimicrobials secreted by pancreatic acini play an important role in shaping the gut microbiome, as well as maintaining the innate immunity and barrier function in the intestines [97]. Mice lacking acinar Orai1 exhibited intestinal bacterial outgrowth and dysbiosis, ultimately causing systemic translocation, inflammation, and death.

5. TRPV4 and Other TRP Channel Function in Salivary Glands

Regulation of cell volume in response to changes in osmolarity is critical in salivary gland fluid secretion. In response to carbachol (CCh) stimulation, cells undergo a decrease in cell volume, which then recovers via a regulatory volume increase (RVI). Conversely, hypotonic conditions lead to cell swelling and volume recovery via regulatory volume decrease (RVD). Both these processes depend on the water permeability of the cells, which in salivary gland cells is determined by the level of AQP5 in the membrane. A role for TRPV4 in RVD was previously reported by an earlier study reported by us [98]. TRPV4 was activated by cell swelling under hypoosmotic conditions and that Ca^{2+} entry via TRPV4 was important for regulating the ion fluxes involved in driving RVD. This study demonstrated a novel association between osmosensing TRPV4 and AQP5. Acinar cells from mice lacking either TRPV4 or AQP5 displayed greatly reduced Ca^{2+} entry and loss of RVD in response to hypotonicity, although the extent of cell swelling was similar. Recent studies have shown a more direct role for TRPV4 in fluid secretion. TRPV4 is activated by endogenous arachidonic acid metabolites, 4α-phorbol-12,13 didecanoate, GSK1016790A, moderate heat, and mechanical stress. Pharmacological TRPV4 activation using the selective agonist GSK1016790A caused Ca^{2+} influx in isolated acinar cells in a basal-to-apical wave. Consistent with these observations, GSK1016790A elicited salivation in the perfused submandibular gland that was dependent on extracellular Ca^{2+} [99]. Another study reported a functional interaction between TRPV4 and the Ca^{2+}-activated chloride channel, ANO1, in acinar cells isolated from mouse salivary and lacrimal glands [100]. Activation of TRPV4 induced an increase in fluid secretion, ANO1 activation and a volume decrease in acinar cells by increasing [Ca^{2+}]$_i$. Muscarinic stimulation of saliva and tear secretion was downregulated in both TRPV4-deficient mice and in acinar cells treated with a TRPV4-specific antagonist (HC-067047). Furthermore, the temperature dependence of muscarinic salivation was shown to depend mainly on TRPV4. This study also showed a novel association between TRPV4, IP$_3$Rs, and ANO1 that collectively contributes to the regulation of salivation and lacrimation.

Additional TRP channels have also been identified in salivary glands. Immunohistochemistry has revealed the presence of TRPM8, TRPA1, TRPV1, TRPV3, and TRPV4 in myoepithelial, acinar, and ductal cells of the sublingual, submandibular, and parotid glands. Interestingly, perfusion of the entire submandibular gland with the TRPV1 agonist capsaicin (1 μM) via the submandibular artery significantly increased CCh-induced salivation, whereas perfusion with TRPM8 and TRPA1 agonists (0.5 μM WS12 and 100 μM allyl isothiocyanate) decreased it. Application of agonists for each of the thermosensitive TRP channels increased [Ca^{2+}]$_i$ in a cultured submandibular epithelial cell line. These results indicate that temperature-sensitive TRP channels are localized and distributed in acinar, ductal and myoepithelial cells of salivary glands, and that they might have a functional role in regulating and/or modulating saliva secretion. Further studies will be needed to characterize the exact role of temperature-dependent regulation of salivary gland function and the involvement of TRP channels in this mechanism.

6. Role of TRPM2 in Salivary Gland Dysfunction

6.1. Regulation and Activation of TRPM2

TRPM2 is the second member of the TRPM subfamily, which includes eight functionally diverse members, namely TRPM 1–8. TRPM2 (previously known as LTRPC2 or TRPC7) is a Ca^{2+} permeable, non-selective cation channel. It is predominantly expressed in the brain and has also been detected in bone marrow, spleen, heart, liver, lung and immunocytes, salivary gland [101–103]. TRPM2 is unique in that its structure contains a Ca^{2+}-permeable non-selective cationic pore fused to an enzyme of the Nudix family of pyrophosphatases. Adenosine diphosphate ribose (ADPR) is considered the primary gating molecule of TRPM2 [104]. The channel displays a linear current-voltage (I–V) relationship, and substantial permeation to cations such as Na^+, K^+, Ca^{2+}, Mg^{2+}, and Zn^{2+}, with relative permeabilities of $P_K/P_{Na} \sim 1.1$, $P_{Ca}/P_{Na} \sim 0.9$, and $P_{Mg}/P_{Na} \sim 0.5$. Most importantly, TRPM2 serves as a sensor for reactive oxygen species (ROS) in cells, since increase in cellular ROS or nitrogen species, cause formation ADPR. Intracellular Ca^{2+} also facilitates TRPM2 activation by enhancing the channel sensitivity to ADPR [101].

Under oxidative stress, ADPR formation is mediated through activation of the PARP/PARG (Poly(ADP-ribose) polymerase/glycohydrolase) pathway in the nucleus. ADPR is also synthesized in the mitochondria, which contain the largest pool of intracellular nicotinamide adenosine diphosphate (NAD+), and is released into the cytosol [105,106]. Convincing evidence has been presented to show that ROS-induced TRPM2 activation is also triggered via the production of ADPR from mitochondria [107,108]. It is now clearly established that TRPM2 channel serves as an important pathway for oxidative stress-induced increases in $[Ca^{2+}]_i$, which regulate Ca^{2+} signaling mechanisms that include regulation of ion channel activities, gene expression, secretion, apoptosis, and inflammasome assembly. TRPM2 also responds to warm temperatures that act synergistically with ADPR, NAD^+, and cADPR at concentrations that otherwise cannot activate the channel [101,102,105,106,109]. In normal physiological states, a major function of TRPM2 is to modulate the immune system by controlling cytokine release in human monocytes, including tumor necrosis factor-alpha (TNFα), interleukin 6 (IL-6), IL-8, and IL-10, and the maturation and chemotaxis of dendritic cells. Non-physiological stimulation of TRPM2 is suggested to lead to pathology and dysfunction.

6.2. TRPM2 and Radiation-Induced Loss of Salivary Flow

A debilitating side effect of radiation treatment in patients with head and neck cancers is xerostomia, or dry mouth, as a result of severe decrease in saliva secretion. While acute effects of IR could be induced by membrane/protein damage, the more delayed and long-term effects have been proposed to be caused by damage of progenitor cells within the adult salivary gland [110–112]. However, the decrease in saliva secretion cannot be strictly correlated with a decrease in acinar cells or damage of the gland. In fact, in mouse models of radiation, glandular loss, and fibrosis are not seen for about four-to six months after radiation while loss of function is almost immediate and persists even after the radiation-induced ROS in the tissue has been cleared [113,114]. Our recent studies demonstrate a critical role for TRPM2 in radiation-induced persistent loss of salivary gland fluid secretion (Figure 2). TRPM2 is present in salivary gland acinar cells and is activated under conditions which increase ROS, such as by treatment with H_2O_2 or following radiation treatment of the salivary glands in mice [103]. Importantly, while TRPM2$^{+/+}$ mice display persistent loss of salivary gland fluid secretion that is detected within 10 days after radiation, mice lacking TRPM2 (TRPM2$^{-/-}$) demonstrate transient loss of function with >80% recovery of function by 30 days after IR. Activation of TRPM2 by radiation has been supported by data showing that Ca^{2+} influx is constitutively activated in acinar cells isolated from TRPM2$^{+/+}$ mice 24 h after radiation. This increase in plasma membrane Ca^{2+} permeability is not seen in acini from irradiated TRPM2$^{-/-}$ mice. Treatment of mice with the PARP1 inhibitor, 3-AB, prior to radiation suppresses TRPM2 activation and exerts protection of salivary gland function. Further, TEMPOL, a redox-cycling nitroxide and ROS scavenger that has been reported to protect several organs, including the heart and brain, from ischemia/reperfusion damage [115], also protects salivary gland function in irradiated mice [103,114]. Thus, the presence of TRPM2 in acinar cells converts an inherently reversible loss of salivary gland function, following radiation treatment to an irreversible one.

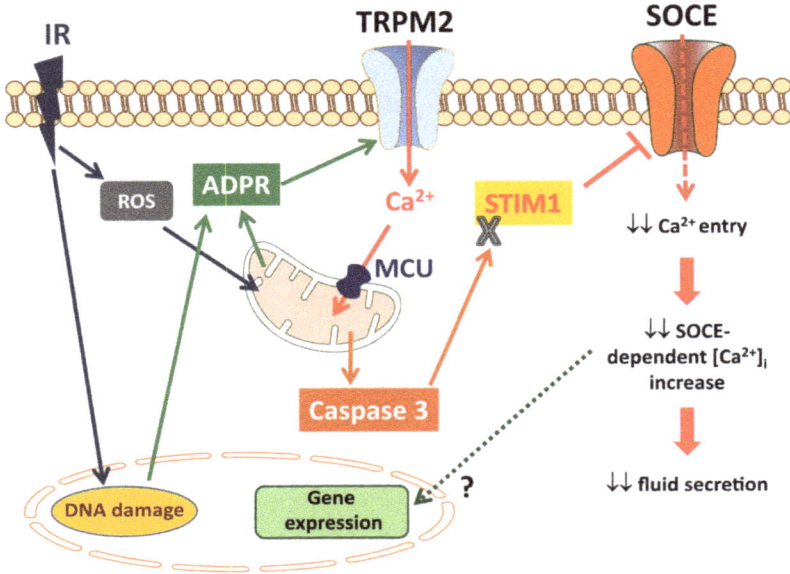

Figure 2. Role of TRPM2 in radiation -induced salivary gland dysfunction. See text for description.

In searching for the mechanism(s) linking early activation of TRPM2 by radiation to the persistent loss of salivary fluid secretion, we have now demonstrated that persistent reduction in STIM1 protein, and SOCE, underlies radiation-induced loss of salivary gland function. Furthermore, the decrease in STIM1 protein levels is linked to activation of TRPM2 [113]. A major finding of this study was that TRPM2-mediated increase in $[Ca^{2+}]_i$ in response to radiation causes an increase in mitochondrial $[Ca^{2+}]$ and ROS_{mt} but a decrease in mitochondrial membrane potential. This is accompanied by a relatively slower appearance of activated caspase-3 which persists for about a month after the treatment. In irradiated $TRPM2^{-/-}$ mice, the increases in $[Ca^{2+}]_{mt}$, ROS_{mt} and activated caspase-3 are substantially attenuated. Importantly, TRPM2-dependent activation of caspase-3 is correlated with loss of STIM1. These interesting findings reveal that radiation-induced loss of salivary gland fluid secretion is mediated via a TRPM2-dependent pathway that impacts mitochondrial function and leads to irreversible loss of SOCE. Notably, cleavage of STIM1 by calpain and γ-secretase has been associated with stress and Alzheimer's disease, respectively [116,117]. Further, proteasome inhibition reduces SOCE by promoting autophagy-mediated degradation of STIM1/2 [118]. Future studies will need to clarify exactly how the long-term suppression of STIM1 expression is controlled. Most likely, remodeling of gene expression or other epigenetic changes occurring in irradiated salivary glands might be involved. Ca^{2+} entry mediated by SOCE, via Orai1 channels, is critical for the regulation and activation of transcription factors such as NFAT and cFos, as well as other channels that regulate NFκB (e.g., TRPC1). Attenuation of these signaling mechanisms due to loss of channel activation could impact the expression of STIM1 or other cellular proteins, further depressing the occurrence of downstream events that are triggered by these signaling events. It is also important to consider that loss of STIM1 and SOCE can potentially affect other cellular processes, including regeneration of salivary gland cells [119]. In a salivary gland cell line, silencing the mitochondrial Ca^{2+} uniporter or caspase-3, or treatment with inhibitors of TRPM2 or caspase-3 prevented irradiation-induced loss of STIM1 and SOCE. Importantly, expression of exogenous STIM1 in the salivary glands of irradiated mice increases SOCE and fluid secretion. Thus, targeting the mechanisms underlying the loss of STIM1 would be a potentially useful approach for preserving salivary gland function after radiation therapy [113].

6.3. TRPM2 in Inflammatory Disorders

Oxidative stress plays a critical role in various pathophysiological processes, including cancer, acute and chronic neurodegenerative disorders (Alzheimer's and Parkinson's diseases); diabetes mellitus, atherosclerosis, ischemia/reperfusion injury, and autoimmune disease; and in normal cellular functions [120]. Main pro-inflammatory molecules present in chronic inflammatory responses are ROS, reactive nitrogen species (RNS), IL-2, IL-4, IL-5, IL-7, IL-13, IL-9, IL-10, IL-12, IL-17, IL-21, interferon (IFN)-γ, transforming growth factor (TGF)-β, and tumor necrosis factor (TNF)-α. Salivary gland epithelial cells themselves synthesize and secrete cytokines to maintain barrier protection and regulate anti-inflammatory processes. Furthermore, immune cells produce ADPR via CD38 and CD157 signaling or by activating the PARP pathway, both of which can facilitate activation of TRPM2. Although there are no data available presently that demonstrate a role for TRPM2 in inflammatory disorders of the salivary gland, the available information suggests that the channel could be activated in response to inflammatory conditions and contribute to the pathogenesis.

There is increasing evidence for the involvement of TRPM2 in innate immunity, inflammation, regulation of cytokine production, cellular migration and ROS production [105]. NADPH oxidase-dependent ROS production in phagocytic cells is triggered in response to infection and plays a key role in inflammation. Activation, migration as well as regulation of the effector mechanisms of immune cells critically depend on Ca^{2+}-entry into the cell. While Orai1 channels also mediate this type of calcium influx to regulate the function of T cells and B cells, TRPM2 can also contribute to the elevation of $[Ca^{2+}]_i$ as it is expressed in the plasma membrane of neutrophils, T and B lymphocytes, and dendritic cells. In T cells, cross-linking of cell surface receptors induces a rise of ADPR endogenously generated from NAD^+ which can activate TRPM2 [121]. Importantly, inhibition of NAADP signaling in T cells [122] reduces antigen-induced proliferation and cytokine production and ameliorates clinical symptoms of experimental autoimmune encephalomyelitis (EAE, [122]). The role for TRPM2 in lymphocyte function is now been widely accepted. It has been shown that TRPM2-mediated Ca^{2+} influx regulates T cell proliferation and proinflammatory cytokine secretion following polyclonal T cell receptor stimulation. TRPM2-deficiency or treatment with TRPM2 channel blockers significantly modulate effector T cell function [123,124]. Moreover, TRPM2 channels impact the maturation and chemokine-activated directional migration of dendritic cells, which function as antigen-presenting cells [125]. TRPM2 can also be activated by triggering of toll-like receptors by LPS and cytokine receptors (TNFα) as well as by intracellular ADPR. It is suggested that inhibition of TRPM2 channels in autoimmune inflammatory disorders will likely dampen the adaptive T cell-mediated immune response without favoring prolonged T cell survival and inflammatory tissue damage.

On the other hand, it has been reported that TRPM2-mediated Ca^{2+} influx controls the ROS-induced signaling cascade responsible for chemokine production, which aggravates inflammation [126]. TRPM2 expressed in macrophages and microglia aggravates peripheral and spinal pro-nociceptive inflammatory responses, and contributes to the pathogenesis of inflammatory and neuropathic pain [127]. TRPM2 critically influences T cell proliferation and proinflammatory cytokine secretion following polyclonal T cell receptor stimulation. Consistently, TRPM2-deficient mice exhibit an attenuated clinical phenotype of EAE with reduced inflammatory and demyelinating spinal cord lesions [128]. In addition, TRPM2 regulates macrophage polarization and gastric inflammation during *Helicobacter pylori* infection [129]. TRPM2 channels mediate bleomycin-induced lung inflammation in alveolar epithelial cells [130], and contributes to antigen-stimulated Ca^{2+} influx in mucosal mast cells [131].

Numerous proinflammatory cytokines are produced during the innate immune response to infection and inflammation, several of which have been linked with activation of TRPM2. Knockdown of TRPM2 attenuates LPS-induced production of IL-6, IL-8, IL-10, and TNF-α in THP1 monocytic cells. The corresponding decrease in LPS-induced Ca^{2+} influx under these conditions supports the suggestion that TRPM2-mediated Ca^{2+} influx has a significant role in generating these cytokines. Zymosan-induced production of granulocyte colony-stimulating factor (G-CSF) and IL-1α was also strongly attenuated in macrophages from the TRPM2$^{-/-}$ mice. Sulfur mustard (SM), an alkylating agent used in chemical warfare, causes tissue damage and induces inflammatory responses. SM-induced production of IL-6, IL-8, and TNF-α by human neutrophils requires TRPM2-mediated Ca^{2+} influx to activate the p38 mitogen-activated protein kinase (p38 MAPK) signaling pathway [132]. The production of IL-6 and TNF-α was however enhanced in LPS-treated macrophages from the TRPM2$^{-/-}$ mice and in response to LPS-induced infection in these mice [133]. Evidently, further studies are required to clarify the noticeable discrepancies from these studies that used different infection stimuli and cell preparations. The production of IL-12 and IFN-γ after dextran sulfate sodium-induced colon inflammation is significantly decreased in the TRPM2$^{-/-}$ mice [126]. Further analysis suggests that the TRPM2 channel function is required for the production of IL-12, the early inflammatory cytokine produced by dendritic cells and possibly other immune cells as well, which elicits IFN-γ-mediated innate immune responses. The deficient production of IL-12 and IFN-γ in the TRPM2$^{-/-}$ mice led to a significantly lower survival rate after *Listeria monocytogenes* infection, supporting a vital role for the TRPM2 channel in the innate immune response to this infection [134]. A recent study shows that LPS/IFN-γ-induced increase in the $[Ca^{2+}]_i$ and subsequent release of nitric oxide in microglia also depends on the TRPM2 channel function [135]. Immune cells such as macrophages and microglia also produce IL-1β, a key proinflammatory cytokine in innate immunity [136]. The priming signal stimulates a Toll-like receptor (TLR) such as TLR4 by LPS or other receptors to initiate signaling pathways leading to synthesis of pro-IL-1β. TRPM2 channels mediate Ca^{2+} influx as the major ROS-induced Ca^{2+} signaling mechanism in macrophages [137], which regulates NLRP3 inflammasome activation in macrophages by particulates such as charged lipids, silica, and alum. This process is impaired in macrophages from the TRPM2$^{-/-}$ mice [138]. Thus, TRPM2-mediated Ca^{2+} influx is a critical step in coupling ROS generation to NLRP3 inflammasome activation and IL-1β maturation.

Notably, Sjøgren's Syndrome (SS) has been associated with overexpression of proinflammatory cytokines, including TNF-α, IL-7, IL-1β, IL-6, IL-10, IL-17, IL-18 and gamma-interferon (γ-IFN) [139–141]. Moreover, one of these cytokines, IL-6, was correlated with poor quality of life in SS patients [140]. Based on a body of evidence related to different pathological conditions, TNF-α and its interactors are recognized to be involved in a pro-inflammatory/pro-oxidant condition, implicating the relevance of redox imbalances in SS pathogenesis [142,143]. Related to excess expression of proinflammatory cytokines, a pro-oxidant state could be postulated in SS based on the established evidence for a mechanistic association of a pro-inflammatory condition and oxidative stress in a number of disorders including, e.g., cancer, cardiovascular, neurological and pulmonary diseases, and diabetes [143–146]. Furthermore, it should be noted that ROS is also produced by activated granulocytes during inflammation both in SS pathogenesis and in other systemic disorders with autoimmune features (e.g., systemic sclerosis). Cejková et al. has reported that *Trpm2* knockout mice showed attenuation of inflammatory indicators such as production of CXCL2, neutrophil infiltration and ulceration [147]. Thus, ROS-evoked Ca^{2+} influx via TRPM2 could represent a key inflammatory mediator in monocytes and in the epithelium of both salivary and lacrimal glands of SS patients. It will be very important to investigate the role for this channel in SS-induced salivary gland pathology. Establishing this will provide new strategies for treatment of the disease.

7. Conclusions

Studies done over the past 30 years have provided a tremendous amount of information about the key molecular components that regulate salivary gland fluid secretion, including those involved in Ca^{2+} signaling, ion transport, and water transport. Future studies should be focused on establishing the mechanisms underlying salivary gland dysfunction. Such studies should provide novel targets and strategies for treatment. On such target in salivary glands is TRPM2, which appears to be critically involved in radiation-induced irreversible loss of salivary gland fluid secretion. Based on data reported by us and others, potential therapeutic strategies could include manipulating channel activity, developing specific inhibitors of the channel or TRPM2-dependent signal transduction cascade. In the case of radiation-induced salivary gland dysfunction, we propose that inhibitors of TRPM2 or caspase-3, scavengers of ROS in the cytosol or mitochondria, as well as inhibitors of PARP1 could be used to protect against loss of function. Additionally, its ability to respond to ROS has made TRPM2 a potential therapeutic target for chronic inflammation and neurodegenerative diseases. TRPM2 ion channel and its gating molecule ADPR are previously unsuspected players necessary for robust cytokine production and innate cell activation during intracellular bacterial infection. These findings highlight the potential of the metabolic manipulation of ADPR levels or modulating TRPM2 activation modalities to exert immunomodulation. However, currently, direct evidence for TRPM2 involvement in Sjøgren's Syndrome (SS) is lacking. Based on currently available data highlighting the role of TRPM2 in inflammatory process, it will be very important to assess whether TRPM2 contributes to Sjøgren's Syndrome (SS). Identification of the role of other, including sensory, TRP channels in salivary gland function will also provide additional targets for modulating water secretion from the gland. Future studies should focus on these potentially novel and important roles of these TRP channels.

Funding: Funding for this work was provided by NIDCR-DIR, NIH (Z01-DE00438-31).

Conflicts of Interest: The authors declare no conflicts of interest.

References

1. Ambudkar, I.S. Dissection of calcium signaling events in exocrine secretion. *Neurochem. Res.* **2011**, *36*, 1212–1221. [CrossRef] [PubMed]
2. Ambudkar, I.S. Polarization of calcium signaling and fluid secretion in salivary gland cells. *Curr. Med. Chem.* **2012**, *19*, 5774–5781. [CrossRef] [PubMed]
3. Melvin, J.E.; Yule, D.; Shuttleworth, T.; Begenisich, T. Regulation of fluid and electrolyte secretion in salivary gland acinar cells. *Annu. Rev. Physiol.* **2005**, *67*, 445–469. [CrossRef] [PubMed]
4. Futatsugi, A.; Nakamura, T.; Yamada, M.K.; Ebisui, E.; Nakamura, K.; Uchida, K.; Kitaguchi, T.; Takahashi-Iwanaga, H.; Noda, T.; Aruga, J.; et al. IP3 receptor types 2 and 3 mediate exocrine secretion underlying energy metabolism. *Science* **2005**, *309*, 2232–2234. [CrossRef] [PubMed]
5. Yule, D.I. Subtype-specific regulation of inositol 1,4,5-trisphosphate receptors: Controlling calcium signals in time and space. *J. Gen. Physiol.* **2001**, *117*, 431–434. [CrossRef] [PubMed]
6. Ambudkar, I.S. Ca^{2+} signaling and regulation of fluid secretion in salivary gland acinar cells. *Cell Calcium* **2014**, *55*, 297–305. [CrossRef] [PubMed]
7. Ambudkar, I.S. Calcium signalling in salivary gland physiology and dysfunction. *J. Physiol.* **2016**, *594*, 2813–2824. [CrossRef] [PubMed]
8. Putney, J.W., Jr. Capacitative calcium entry revisited. *Cell Calcium* **1990**, *11*, 611–624. [CrossRef]
9. Cheng, K.T.; Ong, H.L.; Liu, X.; Ambudkar, I.S. Contribution and regulation of TRPC channels in store-operated Ca^{2+} Entry. In *Store-Operated Calcium Channels*; Prakriya, M., Ed.; Elsevier: Amsterdam, The Netherlands, 2013; Volume 71, pp. 149–179.
10. Hogan, P.G.; Lewis, R.S.; Rao, A. Molecular basis of calcium signaling in lymphocytes: Stim and Orai. *Ann. Rev. Immunol.* **2010**, *28*, 491–533. [CrossRef] [PubMed]
11. Liou, J.; Kim, M.L.; Heo, W.D.; Jones, J.T.; Myers, J.W.; Ferrell, J.E., Jr.; Meyer, T. STIM is a Ca^{2+} sensor essential for Ca^{2+}-store-depletion-triggered Ca^{2+} influx. *Curr. Biol.* **2005**, *15*, 1235–1241. [CrossRef] [PubMed]

12. Prakriya, M. Store-operated Orai channels: Structure and function. *Curr. Top. Membr.* **2013**, *71*, 1–32. [PubMed]

13. Yuan, J.P.; Zeng, W.; Dorwart, M.R.; Choi, Y.J.; Worley, P.F.; Muallem, S. SOAR and the polybasic STIM1 domains gate and regulate Orai channels. *Nat. Cell Biol.* **2009**, *11*, 337–343. [CrossRef] [PubMed]

14. Zeng, W.; Yuan, J.P.; Kim, M.S.; Choi, Y.J.; Huang, G.N.; Worley, P.F.; Muallem, S. STIM1 gates TRPC channels, but not Orai1, by electrostatic interaction. *Mol. Cell* **2008**, *32*, 439–448. [CrossRef] [PubMed]

15. Zhang, S.L.; Yu, Y.; Roos, J.; Kozak, J.A.; Deerinck, T.J.; Ellisman, M.H.; Stauderman, K.A.; Cahalan, M.D. STIM1 is a Ca^{2+} sensor that activates CRAC channels and migrates from the Ca^{2+} store to the plasma membrane. *Nature* **2005**, *437*, 902–905. [CrossRef] [PubMed]

16. Ong, H.L.; de Souza, L.B.; Zheng, C.; Cheng, K.T.; Liu, X.; Goldsmith, C.M.; Feske, S.; Ambudkar, I.S. STIM2 enhances receptor-stimulated Ca^{2+} signaling by promoting recruitment of STIM1 to the endoplasmic reticulum-plasma membrane junctions. *Sci. Signal.* **2015**, *8*, ra3. [CrossRef] [PubMed]

17. Hong, J.H.; Li, Q.; Kim, M.S.; Shin, D.M.; Feske, S.; Birnbaumer, L.; Cheng, K.T.; Ambudkar, I.S.; Muallem, S. Polarized but differential localization and recruitment of STIM1, Orai1 and TRPC channels in secretory cells. *Traffic* **2011**, *12*, 232–245. [CrossRef] [PubMed]

18. Liu, X.; Cheng, K.T.; Bandyopadhyay, B.C.; Pani, B.; Dietrich, A.; Paria, B.C.; Swaim, W.D.; Beech, D.; Yildrim, E.; Singh, B.B.; et al. Attenuation of store-operated Ca^{2+} current impairs salivary gland fluid secretion in $TRPC1^{-/-}$ mice. *Proc. Natl. Acad. Sci. USA* **2007**, *104*, 17542–17547. [CrossRef] [PubMed]

19. Liu, X.; Wang, W.; Singh, B.B.; Lockwich, T.; Jadlowiec, J.; O'Connell, B.; Wellner, R.; Zhu, M.X.; Ambudkar, I.S. Trp1, a candidate protein for the store-operated Ca^{2+} influx mechanism in salivary gland cells. *J. Biol. Chem.* **2000**, *275*, 3403–3411. [CrossRef] [PubMed]

20. Cheng, K.T.; Liu, X.; Ong, H.L.; Ambudkar, I.S. Functional requirement for Orai1 in store-operated TRPC1-STIM1 channels. *J. Biol. Chem.* **2008**, *283*, 12935–12940. [CrossRef] [PubMed]

21. Cheng, K.T.; Liu, X.; Ong, H.L.; Swaim, W.; Ambudkar, I.S. Local Ca^{2+} entry via Orai1 regulates plasma membrane recruitment of TRPC1 and controls cytosolic Ca^{2+} signals required for specific cell functions. *PLoS Biol.* **2011**, *9*, e1001025. [CrossRef] [PubMed]

22. Choi, S.; Maleth, J.; Jha, A.; Lee, K.P.; Kim, M.S.; So, I.; Ahuja, M.; Muallem, S. The TRPCs-STIM1-Orai interaction. *Handbook Exp. Pharmacol.* **2014**, *223*, 1035–1054.

23. Lee, K.P.; Yuan, J.P.; Hong, J.H.; So, I.; Worley, P.F.; Muallem, S. An endoplasmic reticulum/plasma membrane junction: STIM1/Orai1/TRPCs. *FEBS Lett.* **2010**, *584*, 2022–2027. [CrossRef] [PubMed]

24. Delaleu, N.; Jonsson, R.; Koller, M.M. Sjögren's syndrome. *Eur. J. Oral. Sci.* **2005**, *113*, 101–113. [CrossRef] [PubMed]

25. Mavragani, C.P.; Moutsopoulos, H.M. Sjögren's syndrome. *Ann. Rev. Path.* **2014**, *9*, 273–285. [CrossRef] [PubMed]

26. Delli, K.; Spijkervet, F.K.; Kroese, F.G.; Bootsma, H.; Vissink, A. Xerostomia. *Monogr. Oral. Sci.* **2014**, *24*, 109–125. [PubMed]

27. Vissink, A.; Jansma, J.; Spijkervet, F.K.; Burlage, F.R.; Coppes, R.P. Oral sequelae of head and neck radiotherapy. *Crit. Rev. Oral. Biol. Med.* **2003**, *14*, 199–212. [CrossRef] [PubMed]

28. Montell, C.; Rubin, G.M. Molecular characterization of the Drosophila trp locus: A putative integral membrane protein required for phototransduction. *Neuron* **1989**, *2*, 1313–1323. [CrossRef]

29. Montell, C.; Birnbaumer, L.; Flockerzi, V. The TRP channels, a remarkably functional family. *Cell* **2002**, *108*, 595–598. [CrossRef]

30. Schlingmann, K.P.; Gudermann, T. A critical role of TRPM channel-kinase for human magnesium transport. *J. Physiol.* **2005**, *566*, 301–308. [CrossRef] [PubMed]

31. Bargal, R.; Avidan, N.; Ben-Asher, E.; Olender, Z.; Zeigler, M.; Frumkin, A.; Raas-Rothschild, A.; Glusman, G.; Lancet, D.; Bach, G. Identification of the gene causing mucolipidosis type IV. *Nat. Genet.* **2000**, *26*, 118–123. [PubMed]

32. Bassi, M.T.; Manzoni, M.; Monti, E.; Pizzo, M.T.; Ballabio, A.; Borsani, G. Cloning of the gene encoding a novel integral membrane protein, mucolipidin-and identification of the two major founder mutations causing mucolipidosis type IV. *Am. J. Hum. Genet.* **2000**, *67*, 1110–1120. [CrossRef]

33. Mochizuki, T.; Wu, G.; Hayashi, T.; Xenophontos, S.L.; Veldhuisen, B.; Saris, J.J.; Reynolds, D.M.; Cai, Y.; Gabow, P.A.; Pierides, A.; et al. Pkd2, a gene for polycystic kidney disease that encodes an integral membrane protein. *Science* **1996**, *272*, 1339–1342. [CrossRef] [PubMed]

34. Sun, M.; Goldin, E.; Stahl, S.; Falardeau, J.L.; Kennedy, J.C.; Acierno, J.S., Jr.; Bove, C.; Kaneski, C.R.; Nagle, J.; Bromley, M.C.; et al. Mucolipidosis type IV is caused by mutations in a gene encoding a novel transient receptor potential channel. *Hum. Mol. Genet.* **2000**, *9*, 2471–2478. [CrossRef] [PubMed]

35. Kaneko, Y.; Szallasi, A. TRP channels as therapeutic targets. *Curr. Top. Med. Chem.* **2013**, *13*, 241–243. [CrossRef] [PubMed]

36. Nilius, B.; Owsianik, G. Transient receptor potential channelopathies. *Pflugers Arch.* **2010**, *460*, 437–450. [CrossRef] [PubMed]

37. Nilius, B.; Szallasi, A. Transient receptor potential channels as drug targets: From the science of basic research to the art of medicine. *Pharmacol. Rev.* **2014**, *66*, 676–814. [CrossRef] [PubMed]

38. Tóth, B.I.; Nilius, B. Transient receptor potential dysfunctions in hereditary diseases. In *TRP Channels as Therapeutic Targets*; Szallasi, A., Ed.; Academic Press: Amsterdam, The Netherlands, 2015; pp. 13–33.

39. Kaneko, Y.; Szallasi, A. Transient receptor potential (TRP) channels: A clinical perspective. *Br. J. Pharmacol.* **2014**, *171*, 2474–2507. [CrossRef] [PubMed]

40. Smani, T.; Shapovalov, G.; Skryma, R.; Prevarskaya, N.; Rosado, J.A. Functional and physiopathological implications of TRP channels. *Biochim. Biophys. Acta* **2015**, *1853*, 1772–1782. [CrossRef] [PubMed]

41. Nilius, B.; Owsianik, G. The transient receptor potential family of ion channels. *Genome Biol.* **2011**, *12*, 218. [CrossRef] [PubMed]

42. Bandell, M.; Macpherson, L.J.; Patapoutian, A. From chills to chilis: Mechanisms for thermosensation and chemesthesis via thermotrps. *Curr. Opin. Neurobiol.* **2007**, *17*, 490–497. [CrossRef] [PubMed]

43. Patapoutian, A.; Peier, A.M.; Story, G.M.; Viswanath, V. ThermoTRP channels and beyond: Mechanisms of temperature sensation. *Nat. Rev. Neurosci.* **2003**, *4*, 529–539. [CrossRef] [PubMed]

44. Tominaga, M. The role of TRP channels in thermosensation. In *TRP Ion Channel Function in Sensory Transduction and Cellular Signaling Cascades*; Liedtke, W.B., Heller, S., Eds.; CRC Press: Boca Raton, FL, USA, 2007.

45. Caterina, M.J.; Rosen, T.A.; Tominaga, M.; Brake, A.J.; Julius, D. A capsaicin-receptor homologue with a high threshold for noxious heat. *Nature* **1999**, *398*, 436–441. [CrossRef] [PubMed]

46. Caterina, M.J.; Schumacher, M.A.; Tominaga, M.; Rosen, T.A.; Levine, J.D.; Julius, D. The capsaicin receptor: A heat-activated ion channel in the pain pathway. *Nature* **1997**, *389*, 816–824. [PubMed]

47. McKemy, D.D.; Neuhausser, W.M.; Julius, D. Identification of a cold receptor reveals a general role for TRP channels in thermosensation. *Nature* **2002**, *416*, 52–58. [CrossRef] [PubMed]

48. Peier, A.M.; Moqrich, A.; Hargarden, A.C.; Reeve, A.J.; Andersson, D.A.; Story, G.M.; Earley, T.J.; Dragoni, I.; MaIntyre, P.; Bevan, S.; et al. A TRP channel that senses cold stimuli and menthol. *Cell* **2002**, *108*, 705–715. [CrossRef]

49. Vriens, J.; Owsianik, G.; Hofmann, T.; Philipp, S.E.; Stab, J.; Chen, X.; Benoit, M.; Xue, F.; Janssens, A.; Kerselaers, S.; et al. TRPM3 is a nociceptor channel involved in the detection of noxious heat. *Neuron* **2011**, *70*, 482–494. [CrossRef] [PubMed]

50. Story, G.M.; Peier, A.M.; Reeve, A.J.; Eid, S.R.; Mosbacher, J.; Hricik, T.R.; Earley, T.J.; Hergarden, A.C.; Andersson, D.A.; Hwang, S.W.; et al. ANKTM1, a trp-like channel expressed in nociceptive neurons, is activated by cold temperatures. *Cell* **2003**, *112*, 819–829. [CrossRef]

51. Bandell, M.; Story, G.M.; Hwang, S.W.; Viswanath, V.; Eid, S.R.; Petrus, M.J.; Earley, T.J.; Patapoutian, A. Noxious cold ion channel TRPA1 is activated by pungent compounds and bradykinin. *Neuron* **2004**, *41*, 849–857. [CrossRef]

52. Chen, J.; Kang, D.; Xu, J.; Lake, M.; Hogan, J.O.; Sun, C.; Walter, K.; Yao, B.; Kim, D. Species differences and molecular determinant of TRPA1 cold sensitivity. *Nat. Commun.* **2013**, *4*, 2501. [CrossRef] [PubMed]

53. Jordt, S.E.; Bautista, D.M.; Chuang, H.H.; McKemy, D.D.; Zygmunt, P.M.; Hogestatt, E.D.; Meng, I.D.; Julius, D. Mustard oils and cannabinoids excite sensory nerve fibres through the TRP channel ANKTM1. *Nature* **2004**, *427*, 260–265. [CrossRef] [PubMed]

54. Bautista, D.M.; Pellegrino, M.; Tsunozaki, M. TRPA1: A gatekeeper for inflammation. *Annu. Rev. Physiol.* **2013**, *75*, 181–200. [CrossRef] [PubMed]

55. Caspani, O.; Heppenstall, P.A. TRPA1 and cold transduction: An unresolved issue? *J. Gen. Physiol.* **2009**, *133*, 245–249. [CrossRef] [PubMed]

56. Doerner, J.F.; Gisselmann, G.; Hatt, H.; Wetzel, C.H. Transient receptor potential channel A1 is directly gated by calcium ions. *J. Biol. Chem.* **2007**, *282*, 13180–13189. [CrossRef] [PubMed]

57. Fujita, F.; Uchida, K.; Moriyama, T.; Shima, A.; Shibasaki, K.; Inada, H.; Sokabe, T.; Tominaga, M. Intracellular alkalization causes pain sensation through activation of TRPA1 in mice. *J. Clin. Investig.* **2008**, *118*, 4049–4057. [CrossRef] [PubMed]
58. Nilius, B.; Appendino, G.; Owsianik, G. The transient receptor potential channel TRPA1: From gene to pathophysiology. *Pflugers Arch.* **2012**, *464*, 425–458. [CrossRef] [PubMed]
59. Nilius, B.; Prenen, J.; Owsianik, G. Irritating channels: The case of TRPA1. *J. Physiol.* **2011**, *589*, 1543–1549. [CrossRef] [PubMed]
60. Zhang, X.F.; Chen, J.; Faltynek, C.R.; Moreland, R.B.; Neelands, T.R. Transient receptor potential A1 mediates an osmotically activated ion channel. *Eur. J. Neurosci.* **2008**, *27*, 605–611. [CrossRef] [PubMed]
61. Liedtke, W.; Choe, Y.; Marti-Renom, M.A.; Bell, A.M.; Denis, C.S.; Sali, A.; Hudspeth, A.J.; Friendman, J.M.; Heller, S. Vanilloid receptor-related osmotically activated channel (VR-OAC), a candidate vertebrate osmoreceptor. *Cell* **2000**, *103*, 525–535. [CrossRef]
62. Strotmann, R.; Harteneck, C.; Nennenmacher, K.; Schultz, G.; Plant, T.D. OTRPC4, a nonselective cation channel that confers sensitivity to extracellular osmolarity. *Nat. Cell Biol.* **2000**, *2*, 695–702. [CrossRef] [PubMed]
63. Tominaga, M.; Caterina, M.J.; Malmberg, A.B.; Rosen, T.A.; Gilbert, H.; Skinner, K.; Raumann, B.E.; Basbaum, A.I.; Julius, D. The cloned capsaicin receptor integrates multiple pain-producing stimuli. *Neuron* **1998**, *21*, 531–543. [CrossRef]
64. Bautista, D.M.; Jordt, S.E.; Nikai, T.; Tsuruda, P.R.; Read, A.J.; Poblete, J.; Yamoah, E.N.; Basbaum, A.I.; Julius, D. TRPA1 mediates the inflammatory actions of environmental irritants and proalgesic agents. *Cell* **2006**, *124*, 1269–1282. [CrossRef] [PubMed]
65. Chuang, H.H.; Prescott, E.D.; Kong, H.; Shields, S.; Jordt, S.E.; Basbaum, A.I.; Chao, M.V.; Julius, D. Bradykinin and nerve growth factor release the capsaicin receptor from Ptdins(4,5)p2-mediated inhibition. *Nature* **2001**, *411*, 957–962. [CrossRef] [PubMed]
66. Liu, B.; Qin, F. Functional control of cold- and menthol-sensitive TRPM8 ion channels by phosphatidylinositol 4,5-bisphosphate. *J. Neurosci.* **2005**, *25*, 1674–1681. [CrossRef] [PubMed]
67. Prescott, E.D.; Julius, D. A modular PIP2 binding site as a determinant of capsaicin receptor sensitivity. *Science* **2003**, *300*, 1284–1288. [CrossRef] [PubMed]
68. Rohacs, T.; Lopes, C.M.; Michailidis, I.; Logothetis, D.E. PI(4,5)P2 regulates the activation and desensitization of TRPM8 channels through the TRP domain. *Nat. Neurosci.* **2005**, *8*, 626–634. [CrossRef] [PubMed]
69. Romanovsky, A.A.; Almeida, M.C.; Garami, A.; Steiner, A.A.; Norman, M.H.; Morrison, S.F.; Nakamura, K.; Burmeister, J.J.; Nucci, T.B. The transient receptor potential vanilloid-1 channel in thermoregulation: A thermosensor it is not. *Pharmacol. Rev.* **2009**, *61*, 228–261. [CrossRef] [PubMed]
70. Szolcsanyi, J. Effect of capsaicin on thermoregulation: An update with new aspects. *Temperature (Austin)* **2015**, *2*, 277–296. [CrossRef] [PubMed]
71. Wang, H.; Siemens, J. TRP ion channels in thermosensation, thermoregulation and metabolism. *Temperature (Austin)* **2015**, *2*, 178–187. [CrossRef] [PubMed]
72. Minke, H.; Cook, B. TRP channel proteins and signal transduction. *Physiol. Rev.* **2002**, *82*, 429–472. [CrossRef] [PubMed]
73. Montell, C. The TRP superfamily of cation channels. *Sci. STKE* **2005**, *272*, re3. [CrossRef] [PubMed]
74. Venkatachalam, K.; Montell, C. TRp channels. *Annu. Rev. Biochem.* **2007**, *76*, 387–417. [CrossRef] [PubMed]
75. Ong, H.L.; de Souza, L.B.; Cheng, K.T.; Ambudkar, I.S. Physiological functions and regulation of TRPC channels. *Handbook Exp. Pharmacol.* **2014**, *223*, 1005–1034.
76. Nesin, V.; Tsiokas, L. TRPC1. *Handbook Exp. Pharmacol.* **2014**, *222*, 15–51.
77. Miller, B.A. TRPC2. *Handbook Exp. Pharmacol.* **2014**, *222*, 53–65.
78. Lichtenegger, M.; Groschner, K. TRPC3: A multifunctional signaling molecule. *Handbook Exp. Pharmacol.* **2014**, *222*, 67–84.
79. Freichel, M.; Tsvilovskyy, V.; Camacho-Londono, J.E. TRPC4- and TRPC4-containing channels. *Handbook Exp. Pharmacol.* **2014**, *222*, 85–128.
80. Zholos, A.V. TRPC5. *Handbook Exp. Pharmacol.* **2014**, *222*, 129–156.
81. Dietrich, A.; Gudermann, T. TRPC6: Physiological function and pathophysiological relevance. *Handbook Exp. Pharmacol.* **2014**, *222*, 157–188.

82. Zhang, X.; Trebak, M. Transient receptor potential canonical 7: A diacylglycerol-activated non-selective cation channel. *Handbook Exp. Pharmacol.* **2014**, *222*, 189–204.

83. Wes, P.D.; Chevesich, J.; Jeromin, A.; Rosenberg, C.; Stetten, S.; Montell, C. TRPC1, a human homolog of a drosophila store-operated channel. *Proc. Natl. Acad. Sci. USA* **1995**, *92*, 9652–9656. [CrossRef] [PubMed]

84. Zhu, X.; Chu, P.B.; Peyton, M.; Birnbaumer, L. Molecular cloning of a widely expressed human homologue for the drosophila trp gene. *FEBS Lett.* **1995**, *373*, 193–198. [CrossRef]

85. Liu, X.; Singh, B.B.; Ambudkar, I.S. TRPC1 is required for functional store-operated Ca^{2+} channels. Role of acidic amino acid residues in the s5-s6 region. *J. Biol. Chem.* **2003**, *278*, 11337–11343. [CrossRef] [PubMed]

86. Hoth, M. Depletion of intracellular calcium stores activates an outward potassium current in mast and RBL-1 cells that is correlated with CRAC channel activation. *FEBS Lett.* **1996**, *390*, 285–288. [CrossRef]

87. Ambudkar, I.S. TRPC1: A core component of store-operated calcium channels. *Biochem. Soc. Trans.* **2007**, *35*, 96–100. [CrossRef] [PubMed]

88. Beech, D.J. TRPC1: Store-operated channel and more. *Pflugers Arch.* **2005**, *451*, 53–60. [CrossRef] [PubMed]

89. Sun, Y.; Birnbaumer, L.; Singh, B.B. TRPC1 regulates calcium-activated chloride channels in salivary gland cells. *J. Cell. Physiol.* **2015**, *230*, 2848–2856. [CrossRef] [PubMed]

90. Pani, B.; Ong, H.L.; Brazer, S.C.; Liu, X.; Rauser, K.; Singh, B.B.; Ambudkar, I.S. Activation of TRPC1 by STIM1 in ER-PM microdomains involves release of the channel from its scaffold caveolin-1. *Proc. Natl. Acad. Sci. USA* **2009**, *106*, 20087–20092. [CrossRef] [PubMed]

91. Pani, B.; Liu, X.; Bollimuntha, S.; Cheng, K.T.; Niesman, I.R.; Zheng, C.; Achen, V.R.; Patel, H.H.; Ambudkar, I.S.; Singh, B.B. Impairment of TRPC1-STIM1 channel assembly and aqp5 translocation compromise agonist-stimulated fluid secretion in mice lacking caveolin1. *J. Cell. Sci.* **2013**, *126*, 667–675. [CrossRef] [PubMed]

92. Kim, M.S.; Hong, J.H.; Li, Q.; Shin, D.M.; Abramowitz, J.; Birnbaumer, L.; Muallem, S. Deletion of TRPC3 in mice reduces store-operated Ca^{2+} influx and the severity of acute pancreatitis. *Gastroenterology* **2009**, *137*, 1509–1517. [CrossRef] [PubMed]

93. Lee, K.P.; Choi, S.; Hong, J.H.; Ahuja, M.; Graham, S.; Ma, R.; So, I.; Shin, D.M.; Muallem, S.; Yuan, J.P. Molecular determinants mediating gating of transient receptor potential canonical (TRPC) channels by stromal interaction molecule 1 (STIM1). *J. Biol. Chem.* **2014**, *289*, 6372–6382. [CrossRef] [PubMed]

94. Yuan, J.P.; Zeng, W.; Huang, G.N.; Worley, P.F.; Muallem, S. STIM1 heteromultimerizes TRPC channels to determine their function as store-operated channels. *Nat. Cell Biol.* **2007**, *9*, 636–645. [CrossRef] [PubMed]

95. Kim, M.S.; Lee, K.P.; Yang, D.; Shin, D.M.; Abramowitz, J.; Kiyonaka, S.; Birnbaumer, L.; Mori, Y.; Muallem, S. Genetic and pharmacologic inhibition of the Ca^{2+} influx channel TRPC3 protects secretory epithelia from Ca^{2+}-dependent toxicity. *Gastroenterology* **2011**, *140*, 2107–2115. [CrossRef] [PubMed]

96. Xing, J.; Petranka, J.G.; Davis, F.M.; Desai, P.N.; Putney, J.W.; Bird, G.S. Role of Orai1 and store-operated calcium entry in mouse lacrimal gland signalling and function. *J. Physiol.* **2014**, *592*, 927–939. [CrossRef] [PubMed]

97. Ahuja, M.; Jha, A.; Maleth, J.; Park, S.; Muallem, S. cAMP and Ca^{2+} signaling in secretory epithelia: Crosstalk and synergism. *Cell Calcium* **2014**, *55*, 385–393. [CrossRef] [PubMed]

98. Liu, X.; Bandyopadhyay, B.; Nakamoto, T.; Singh, B.; Liedtke, W.; Melvin, J.E.; Ambudkar, I. A role for AQP5 in activation of trpv4 by hypotonicity: Concerted involvement of AQP5 and TRPC4 in regulation of cell volume recovery. *J. Biol. Chem.* **2006**, *281*, 15485–15495. [CrossRef] [PubMed]

99. Zhang, Y.; Catalan, M.A.; Melvin, J.E. TRPV4 activation in mouse submandibular gland modulates Ca^{2+} influx and salivation. *Am. J. Physiol. Gastrointest. Liver Physiol.* **2012**, *303*, G1365–G1372. [CrossRef] [PubMed]

100. Derouiche, S.; Takayama, Y.; Murakami, M.; Tominaga, M. TRPV4 heats up ANO1-dependent exocrine gland fluid secretion. *FASEB J.* **2018**, *32*, 1841–1854. [CrossRef] [PubMed]

101. Sumoza-Toledo, A.; Penner, R. TRPM2: A multifunctional ion channel for calcium signalling. *J. Physiol.* **2011**, *589*, 1515–1525. [CrossRef] [PubMed]

102. Jiang, L.H.; Yang, W.; Zou, J.; Beech, D.J. TRPM2 channel properties, functions and therapeutic potentials. *Expert Opin. Ther. Targets* **2010**, *14*, 973–988. [CrossRef] [PubMed]

103. Liu, X.; Cotrim, A.; Teos, L.; Zheng, C.; Swaim, W.; Mitchell, J.; Mori, Y.; Ambudkar, I. Loss of TRPM2 function protects against irradiation-induced salivary gland dysfunction. *Nat. Commun.* **2013**, *4*, 1515. [CrossRef] [PubMed]

104. Perraud, A.L.; Shen, B.; Dunn, C.A.; Rippe, K.; Smith, M.K.; Bessman, M.J.; Stoddard, B.L.; Scharenberg, A.M. NUDT9, a member of the nudix hydrolase family, is an evolutionarily conserved mitochondrial ADP-ribose pyrophosphatase. *J. Biol. Chem.* **2003**, *278*, 1794–1801. [CrossRef] [PubMed]

105. Knowles, H.; Li, Y.; Perraud, A.L. The TRPM2 ion channel, an oxidative stress and metabolic sensor regulating innate immunity and inflammation. *Immunol. Res.* **2013**, *55*, 241–248. [CrossRef] [PubMed]

106. Li, J.; Gao, Y.; Bao, X.; Li, F.; Yao, W.; Feng, Z.; Yin, Y. TRPM2: A potential drug target to retard oxidative stress. *Front. Biosci. (Landmark Ed.)* **2017**, *22*, 1427–1438. [PubMed]

107. Perraud, A.L.; Takanishi, C.L.; Shen, B.; Kang, S.; Smith, M.K.; Schmitz, C.; Knowles, H.M.; Ferraris, D.; Li, W.; Zhang, J.; et al. Accumulation of free ADP-ribose from mitochondria mediates oxidative stress-induced gating of TRPM2 cation channels. *J. Biol. Chem.* **2005**, *280*, 6138–6148. [CrossRef] [PubMed]

108. Toth, B.; Iordanov, I.; Csanady, L. Ruling out pyridine dinucleotides as true TRPM2 channel activators reveals novel direct agonist ADP-ribose-2'-Phosphate. *J. Gen. Physiol.* **2015**, *145*, 419–430. [CrossRef] [PubMed]

109. Faouzi, M.; Penner, R. TRPM2. *Handbook Exp. Pharmacol.* **2014**, *222*, 403–426.

110. Konings, A.W.; Coppes, R.P.; Vissink, A. On the mechanism of salivary gland radiosensitivity. *Int. J. Rad. Oncol. Biol. Phys.* **2005**, *62*, 1187–1194. [CrossRef] [PubMed]

111. Stephens, L.C.; Schultheiss, T.E.; Price, R.E.; Ang, K.K.; Peters, L.J. Radiation apoptosis of serous acinar cells of salivary and lacrimal glands. *Cancer* **1991**, *67*, 1539–1543. [CrossRef]

112. Zeilstra, L.J.; Vissink, A.; Konings, A.W.; Coppes, R.P. Radiation induced cell loss in rat submandibular gland and its relation to gland function. *Int. J. Rad. Oncol. Biol. Phys.* **2000**, *76*, 419–429.

113. Liu, X.; Gong, B.; de Souza, L.B.; Ong, H.L.; Subedi, K.P.; Cheng, K.T.; Swaim, W.; Zheng, C.; Mori, Y.; Ambudkar, I.S. Radiation inhibits salivary gland function by promoting STIM1 cleavage by caspase-3 and loss of SOCE through a TRPM2-dependent pathway. *Sci. Signal.* **2017**, *10*, eaal4064. [CrossRef] [PubMed]

114. Teos, L.Y.; Zheng, C.Y.; Liu, X.; Swaim, W.D.; Goldsmith, C.M.; Cotrim, A.P.; Baum, B.J.; Ambudkar, I.S. Adenovirus-mediated hAQP1 expression in irradiated mouse salivary glands causes recovery of saliva secretion by enhancing acinar cell volume decrease. *Gene Ther.* **2016**, *23*, 572–579. [CrossRef] [PubMed]

115. Citrin, D.; Cotrim, A.P.; Hyodo, F.; Baum, B.J.; Krishna, M.C.; Mitchell, J.B. Radioprotectors and mitigators of radiation-induced normal tissue injury. *Oncologist* **2010**, *15*, 360–371. [CrossRef] [PubMed]

116. Prins, D.; Groenendyk, J.; Touret, N.; Michalak, M. Modulation of STIM1 and capacitative Ca^{2+} entry by the endoplasmic reticulum luminal oxidoreductase ERP57. *EMBO Rep.* **2011**, *12*, 1182–1188. [CrossRef] [PubMed]

117. Tong, B.C.; Lee, C.S.; Cheng, W.H.; Lai, K.O.; Foskett, J.K.; Cheung, K.H. Familial Alzheimer's disease-associated presenilin 1 mutants promote γ-secretase cleavage of STIM1 to impair store-operated Ca^{2+} entry. *Sci. Signal.* **2016**, *9*, ra89. [CrossRef] [PubMed]

118. Keil, J.M.; Shen, Z.; Briggs, S.P.; Patrick, G.N. Regulation of STIM1 and SOCE by the ubiquitin-proteasome system (UPS). *PLoS ONE* **2010**, *5*, e13465. [CrossRef] [PubMed]

119. Jang, S.I.; Ong, H.L.; Liu, X.; Alevizos, I.; Ambudkar, I.S. Up-regulation of store-operated Ca^{2+} entry and nuclear factor of activated T cells promote the acinar phenotype of the primary human salivary gland cells. *J. Biol. Chem.* **2016**, *291*, 8709–8720. [CrossRef] [PubMed]

120. Takahashi, N.; Kozai, D.; Kobayashi, R.; Ebert, M.; Mori, Y. Roles of TRPM2 in oxidative stress. *Cell Calcium* **2011**, *50*, 279–287. [CrossRef] [PubMed]

121. Gasser, A.; Glassmeier, G.; Fliegert, R.; Langhorst, M.F.; Meinke, S.; Hein, D.; Kruger, S.; Weber, K.; Heiner, I.; Oppenheimer, N.; et al. Activation of T cell calcium influx by the second messenger ADP-ribose. *J. Biol. Chem.* **2006**, *281*, 2489–2496. [CrossRef] [PubMed]

122. Dammermann, W.; Zhang, B.; Nebel, M.; Cordiglieri, C.; Odoardi, F.; Kirchberger, T.; Kawakami, N.; Dowden, J.; Schmid, F.; Dornmair, K.; et al. NAADP-mediated Ca^{2+} signaling via type 1 ryanodine receptor in T cells revealed by a synthetic NAADP antagonist. *Proc. Natl. Acad. Sci. USA* **2009**, *106*, 10678–10683. [CrossRef] [PubMed]

123. Bari, M.R.; Akbar, S.; Eweida, M.; Kuhn, F.J.; Gustafsson, A.J.; Luckhoff, A.; Islam, M.S. H_2O_2-induced Ca^{2+} influx and its inhibition by n-(p-amylcinnamoyl) anthranilic acid in the β-cells: Involvement of TRPM2 channels. *J. Cell. Mol. Med.* **2009**, *13*, 3260–3267. [CrossRef] [PubMed]

124. Kraft, R.; Grimm, C.; Frenzel, H.; Harteneck, C. Inhibition of TRPM2 cation channels by n-(p-amylcinnamoyl)anthranilic acid. *Br. J. Pharmacol.* **2006**, *148*, 264–273. [CrossRef] [PubMed]

125. Sumoza-Toledo, A.; Lange, I.; Cortado, H.; Bhagat, H.; Mori, Y.; Fleig, A.; Penner, R.; Partida-Sanchez, S. Dendritic cell maturation and chemotaxis is regulated by TRPM2-mediated lysosomal Ca^{2+} release. *FASEB J.* **2011**, *25*, 3529–3542. [CrossRef] [PubMed]

126. Yamamoto, S.; Shimizu, S.; Kiyonaka, S.; Takahashi, N.; Wajima, T.; Hara, Y.; Negoro, T.; Hiroi, T.; Kiuchi, Y.; Okada, T.; et al. TRPM2-mediated Ca^{2+}influx induces chemokine production in monocytes that aggravates inflammatory neutrophil infiltration. *Nat. Med.* **2008**, *14*, 738–747. [CrossRef] [PubMed]

127. Haraguchi, K.; Kawamoto, A.; Isami, K.; Maeda, S.; Kusano, A.; Asakura, K.; Shirakawa, H.; Mori, Y.; Nakagawa, T.; Kaneko, S. TRPM2 contributes to inflammatory and neuropathic pain through the aggravation of pronociceptive inflammatory responses in mice. *J. Neurosci.* **2012**, *32*, 3931–3941. [CrossRef] [PubMed]

128. Melzer, N.; Hicking, G.; Gobel, K.; Wiendl, H. TRPM2 cation channels modulate T cell effector functions and contribute to autoimmune CNS inflammation. *PLoS ONE* **2012**, *7*, e47617. [CrossRef] [PubMed]

129. Beceiro, S.; Radin, J.N.; Chatuvedi, R.; Piazuelo, M.B.; Horvarth, D.J.; Cortado, H.; Gu, Y.; Dixon, B.; Gu, C.; Lange, I.; et al. TRPM2 ion channels regulate macrophage polarization and gastric inflammation during helicobacter pylori infection. *Mucosal Immunol.* **2017**, *10*, 493–507. [CrossRef] [PubMed]

130. Yonezawa, R.; Yamamoto, S.; Takenaka, M.; Kage, Y.; Negoro, T.; Toda, T.; Ohbayashi, M.; Numata, T.; Nakano, Y.; Yamamoto, T.; et al. TRPM2 channels in alveolar epithelial cells mediate bleomycin-induced lung inflammation. *Free Radic. Biol. Med.* **2016**, *90*, 101–113. [CrossRef] [PubMed]

131. Oda, S.; Uchida, K.; Wang, X.; Lee, J.; Shimada, Y.; Tominaga, M.; Kadowaki, M. TRPM2 contributes to antigen-stimulated Ca^{2+} influx in mucosal mast cells. *Pflugers Arch.* **2013**, *465*, 1023–1030. [CrossRef] [PubMed]

132. Ham, H.Y.; Hong, C.W.; Lee, S.N.; Kwon, M.S.; Kim, Y.J.; Song, D.K. Sulfur mustard primes human neutrophils for increased degranulation and stimulates cytokine release via TRPM2/p38 MAPK signaling. *Toxicol. Appl. Pharmacol.* **2012**, *258*, 82–88. [CrossRef] [PubMed]

133. Di, A.; Gao, X.P.; Qian, F.; Kawamura, T.; Han, J.; Hecquet, C.; Ye, R.D.; Vogel, S.M.; Malik, A.B. The redox-sensitive cation channel TRPM2 modulates phagocyte ROS production and inflammation. *Nat. Immunol.* **2011**, *13*, 29–34. [CrossRef] [PubMed]

134. Knowles, H.; Heizer, J.W.; Li, Y.; Chapman, K.; Ogden, C.A.; Andreasen, K.; Shapland, E.; Kucera, G.; Mogan, J.; Humann, J.; et al. Transient receptor potential melastatin 2 (TRPM2) ion channel is required for innate immunity against listeria monocytogenes. *Proc. Natl. Acad. Sci. USA* **2011**, *108*, 11578–11583. [CrossRef] [PubMed]

135. Miyake, T.; Shirakawa, H.; Kusano, A.; Sakimoto, S.; Konno, M.; Nakagawa, T.; Mori, Y.; Kaneko, S. TRPM2 contributes to lPS/IFNγ-induced production of nitric oxide via the p38/JNK pathway in microglia. *Biochem. Biophys. Res. Commun.* **2014**, *444*, 212–217. [CrossRef] [PubMed]

136. Martinon, F.; Mayor, A.; Tschopp, J. The inflammasomes: Guardians of the body. *Annu. Rev. Immunol.* **2009**, *27*, 229–265. [CrossRef] [PubMed]

137. Zou, J.; Ainscough, J.F.; Yang, W.; Sedo, A.; Yu, S.P.; Mei, Z.Z.; Sivaprasadarao, A.; Beech, D.J.; Jiang, L.H. A differential role of macrophage TRPM2 channels in Ca^{2+} signaling and cell death in early responses to H$_2$O$_2$. *Am. J. Physiol. Cell. Physiol.* **2013**, *305*, C61–C69. [CrossRef] [PubMed]

138. Zhong, Z.Y.; Zhai, Y.G.; Liang, S.; Mori, Y.S.; Han, R.Z.; Sutterwala, F.S.; Qiao, L. TRPM2 links oxidative stress to NLRP3 inflammasome activation. *Nat. Commun.* **2013**, *4*, 1611. [CrossRef] [PubMed]

139. Bikker, A.; van Woerkom, J.M.; Kruize, A.A.; Wenting-van Wijk, M.; de Jager, W.; Bijlsma, J.W.; Lafeber, F.P.; van Roon, J.A. Increased expression of interleukin-7 in labial salivary glands of patients with primary Sjögren's Syndrome correlates with increased inflammation. *Arthritis Rheum.* **2010**, *62*, 969–977. [CrossRef] [PubMed]

140. Baturone, R.; Soto, M.J.; Marquez, M.; Macias, I.; de Oca, M.M.; Medina, F.; Chozas, N.; Garcia-Perez, S.; Giron-Gonzalez, J.A. Health-related quality of life in patients with primary Sjögren's Syndrome: Relationship with serum levels of proinflammatory cytokines. *Scand. J. Rheumatol.* **2009**, *38*, 386–389. [CrossRef] [PubMed]

141. Sakai, A.; Sugawara, Y.; Kuroishi, T.; Sasano, T.; Sugawara, S. Identification of il-18 and th17 cells in salivary glands of patients with sjogren's syndrome, and amplification of il-17-mediated secretion of inflammatory cytokines from salivary gland cells by il-18. *J. Immunol.* **2008**, *181*, 2898–2906. [CrossRef] [PubMed]

142. Lindholm, C.; Acheva, A.; Salomaa, S. Clastogenic plasma factors: A short overview. *Radiat. Environ. Biophys.* **2010**, *49*, 133–138. [CrossRef] [PubMed]

143. Obrador, E.; Navarro, J.; Mompo, J.; Asensi, M.; Pellicer, J.A.; Estrela, J.M. Regulation of tumour cell sensitivity to TNF-induced oxidative stress and cytotoxicity: Role of glutathione. *Biofactors* **1998**, *8*, 23–26. [CrossRef] [PubMed]

144. Chung, H.Y.; Lee, E.K.; Choi, Y.J.; Kim, J.M.; Kim, D.H.; Zou, Y.; Kim, C.H.; Lee, J.; Kim, H.S.; Kim, N.D.; et al. Molecular inflammation as an underlying mechanism of the aging process and age-related diseases. *J. Dent. Res.* **2011**, *90*, 830–840. [CrossRef] [PubMed]

145. Reuter, S.; Gupta, S.C.; Chaturvedi, M.M.; Aggarwal, B.B. Oxidative stress, inflammation, and cancer: How are they linked? *Free Radic. Biol. Med.* **2010**, *49*, 1603–1616. [CrossRef] [PubMed]

146. Elmarakby, A.A.; Sullivan, J.C. Relationship between oxidative stress and inflammatory cytokines in diabetic nephropathy. *Cardiovasc. Ther.* **2012**, *30*, 49–59. [CrossRef] [PubMed]

147. Cejkova, J.; Ardan, T.; Simonova, Z.; Cejka, C.; Malec, J.; Dotrelova, D.; Brunova, B. Decreased expression of antioxidant enzymes in the conjunctival epithelium of dry eye (Sjögren's Syndrome) and its possible contribution to the development of ocular surface oxidative injuries. *Histol. Histopathol.* **2008**, *23*, 1477–1483. [PubMed]

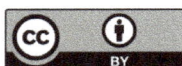

© 2018 by the authors. Licensee MDPI, Basel, Switzerland. This article is an open access article distributed under the terms and conditions of the Creative Commons Attribution (CC BY) license (http://creativecommons.org/licenses/by/4.0/).

Review

Role of the TRPM4 Channel in Cardiovascular Physiology and Pathophysiology

Chen Wang, Keiji Naruse and Ken Takahashi *

Department of Cardiovascular Physiology, Graduate School of Medicine, Dentistry and Pharmaceutical Sciences, Okayama University, Okayama 700-8558, Japan; wangchen11228@gmail.com (C.W.); knaruse@md.okayama-u.ac.jp (K.N.)
* Correspondence: takah-k2@okayama-u.ac.jp; Tel.: +81-86-235-7119

Received: 11 May 2018; Accepted: 14 June 2018; Published: 15 June 2018

Abstract: The transient receptor potential cation channel subfamily M member 4 (TRPM4) channel influences calcium homeostasis during many physiological activities such as insulin secretion, immune response, respiratory reaction, and cerebral vasoconstriction. This calcium-activated, monovalent, selective cation channel also plays a key role in cardiovascular pathophysiology; for example, a mutation in the TRPM4 channel leads to cardiac conduction disease. Recently, it has been suggested that the TRPM4 channel is also involved in the development of cardiac ischemia-reperfusion injury, which causes myocardial infarction. In the present review, we discuss the physiological function of the TRPM4 channel, and assess its role in cardiovascular pathophysiology.

Keywords: TRPM4 channel; cardiovascular system; physiology; pathophysiology

1. Introduction

The transient receptor potential (TRP) melastatin-like subfamily member 4 (TRPM4) is a 1214-amino-acid-long transmembrane protein encoded by *TRPM4*, which is located on human chromosome 19 [1,2]. As a member of the TRP family, it participates in mediating the flux of Na^+ and K^+ across the plasma membrane into the cytoplasm [3]. In contrast to most of the functionally characterized TRP channels, which are nonselective Ca^{2+}-permeable cation channels, TRPM4 and TRPM5 are permeable only to monovalent cations, and not to Ca^{2+} or Mg^{2+}. The Ca^{2+} impermeability of the TRPM4 channel plays a role in the accumulation of intracellular Ca^{2+}, which leads to the depolarization of the plasma membrane [2–5]. Although it is impermeable to Ca^{2+}, TRPM4 is a Ca^{2+}- and voltage-activated channel, and its activation is regulated via a variety of methods. Phosphatidylinositol 4,5-bisphosphate (PIP_2) is an effective modulator of TRPM4 as the channel can be rapidly desensitized to intracellular Ca^{2+} [6,7]. In addition, adenosine triphosphate (ATP), protein kinase C (PKC)-dependent phosphorylation, and calmodulin (CaM) also play a role in TRPM4 activation [8–11], which will be discussed later on in the review.

Like other TRP channels, TRPM4 also comprises six transmembrane domains. The NH_2 and COOH terminal regions of TRPM4 contain binding sites that are related to the channel's activation [1,10]. TRPM4 is highly expressed in a number of tissues and organs and involved in complicated physiological and pathological mechanisms, especially in calcium-dependent mechanisms, such as insulin secretion, immune response, respiratory reaction, tumor development, and cardiovascular diseases [12–15]. Cardiovascular risks have a detrimental impact on human health, and some research has implicated TRPM4 in cardiac hypertrophy, myocardial ischemia-reperfusion injury (IRI), and hereditary arrhythmia [16–24]. In the present review, we focus on the physiological role of TRPM4, and discuss its involvement in cardiovascular pathophysiology.

2. Physiological Characteristics of TRPM4

2.1. TRP Overview

TRP cation channels were first reported in *Drosophila* spp. In 1975, and over 50 family members have been characterized to date [1,25]. In general, they can be divided into seven subfamilies in accordance with the amino acid sequence homology: TRPC, TRPV, TRPM, TRPP, TRPML, TRPA, and TRPN. At present, 28 genes of the TRP family have been found to be expressed in mammalians in succession, but only 27 different members are in humans [1,3,26]. The biophysical properties of TRP family members have been described previously according to the reviews of Clapham et al., Watanabe et al., and Zheng et al. [11,15,26,27]. As mentioned earlier, all the TRPs contain six transmembrane domains and are tetramerized to form functional channels. Therefore, the classical structure of multiple cation channels is mimicked, such as voltage-dependent ion channels. It is well known that Ca^{2+} is involved in many important cellular response mechanisms as a major intracellular messenger [27–29]. The changes in intracellular Ca^{2+} concentration are closely related to the physiological and pathological mechanisms in important tissue systems; for example, alteration in calcium concentration in culture medium affects epidermal cell proliferation and differentiation [30].

It is widely acknowledged that the dynamic stability of extracellular and intracellular Ca^{2+} is beneficial to bone health and in maintaining the endocrine balance [31–33]. In recent years, intracellular Ca^{2+} overload has been regarded as key in a series of cardiovascular risks such as coronary artery diseases, arrhythmia, and cardiac failure; and clinically, calcium antagonists have been used effectively in treating angina, hypertension, and supraventricular tachyarrhythmias, which illustrates that maintenance of Ca^{2+} homeostasis confers cardioprotective benefits [34–40]. a majority of TRP channels are permeable to Ca^{2+} and play a unique role as cell sensors [41]. They are involved in various cellular functions mediated by Ca^{2+}, such as contraction, proliferation, and apoptosis [42–44]. In other words, TRP channels act as gatekeepers in homeostasis [14,45–48]; for example, it has been reported that the TRP channels maintain the dynamic equilibrium between Mg^{2+} and Ca^{2+} in epithelial tissues [49].

The multiple functions played by the TRP channels and their activated multimodality characteristics imply that correct channel gating or infiltration may facilitate the study of complex pathophysiological mechanisms [1,14,16,50]. In the last ten years, several studies from Nilius et al., Watanabe et al., and Kaneko et al. have successively shown that TRP channels are highly expressed in the gastrointestinal tract, genitourinary system, immune system, endocrine system, respiratory system, nervous system, and cardiovascular system, which are involved in complicated physiological and pathological processes [12–14].

In contrast to other TRP family members, TRPM4 can be activated by an intracellular accumulation of Ca^{2+} [8,51]. In addition, TRPM4 is permeable to the monovalent cations with the following ionic selectivity: $Na^+ > K^+ > Cs^+ > Li^+$ [52]. However, TRPM4 shows no Ca^{2+} permeability, which induces intracellular Ca^{2+} accumulation and overload to cause depolarization of the cell membrane, which further leads to cell damage or death [2,15]. Therefore, we will systematically analyze the physiological and pathological role of TRPM4 in the cardiovascular system as far as the specificity of TRPM4 for the non-permeability of Ca^{2+} is concerned.

2.2. Comparison between TRPM4 and TRPM5

Additionally, TRPM is a multifunctional group of TRP channels. As well as other TRPs, the majority of TRPM members are cation channels with Ca^{2+}-permeability, except for TRPM4 and TRPM5. It has been described that there is 50% amino acid sequence homology between the two channels [1,4]. The activity of TRPM5 is also initiated by a rise in the intracellular Ca^{2+}, which is quite similar to TRPM4, also being involved in numerous physiological and pathological mechanisms by modulating Ca^{2+} homeostasis. For example, according to Banik et al., TRPM4 and TRPM5 are both essential in transduction of taste stimuli [53]. Additionally, TRPM4 and TRPM5 are regulated by voltage and PIP2. TRPM5 has been regarded as a heat-activated channel, which shows temperature sensitivity in the range of 15–35 °C. As a close homolog of TRPM5, the temperature sensitivity of TRPM4 may be similar to that of TRPM5; studies have shown that its voltage-dependent activation curve may turn toward a more negative potential with an increasing temperature [9,54–56].

In contrast to the similarities described above, there are several differences between TRPM4 and TRPM5. For example, the tissue distributions of TRPM4 and TRPM5 are widely divergent. In research by Fonfria and colleagues, compared to TRPM4 expression, TRPM5 expression was observed only in a limited number of tissues including the intestine, pancreas, prostate, kidney, and pituitary. On the other hand, TRPM4 is highly expressed in the heart, lung, brain, bone, and stomach [57]. TRPM4 is involved in action potential generation in mouse atrial cardiomyocytes [58]. In 2014, Demir et al. found that the TRPM4 gene expression was increased slightly after exposure to myocardial ischemia-reperfusion. In contrast, TRPM5 was not detected in the heart [59].

2.3. TRPM4 Structure

As a member of the TRP channel family, TRPM4 contains various transmembrane and cytosolic domains that form a three-decker structure [60,61]. There is a wide selectivity filter of TRPM4 that is permeable to the monovalent cations owing to the pore-forming area between the transmembrane domains S5 and S6 [4,52,62]. As reported previously, the N-terminal nucleotide-binding domain and the C-terminal coiled coil in the NH_2 and COOH terminal regions influence the tetrameric composition of TRPM4, and two ATP-binding cassette transporter-like motifs at the N-terminal nucleotide-binding domain are involved in the inhibition of TRPM4 activity [60].

Moreover, there are several PKC phosphorylation sites, five CaM-binding sites, four Walker B motifs (which are putative ATP-binding sites), a putative PIP_2-binding site, and a coiled-coil domain, all of which participate in the modulation of TRPM4 function [1,10,60].

2.4. Activation of TRPM4

As a Ca^{2+}- and voltage-activated channel, there are diverse ways in which TRPM4 is activated, and we will discuss the mechanisms underlying TRPM4 activation in terms of the following modulators: PIP_2, ATP, PKC-dependent phosphorylation, and CaM.

2.4.1. PIP_2

PIP_2 is a minor phospholipid component of the cell membrane, where it is a substrate for a number of important signaling proteins [63,64]. As a substrate of phospholipase C (PLC), PIP_2 regulates all types of ion channels and transporters, including the voltage-gated K^+ and Ca^{2+} channels [65,66]. In 2005–2006, the studies of Zhang et al. and Nilius et al. showed that PIP_2 is a powerful enhancer of TRPM4, which may lead to a desensitization effect on TRPM4 activity through PLC-mediated PIP_2 decomposition [6,7]. With the hydrolysis of PIP_2 in the plasma membrane due to Ca^{2+}-mediated PLC activation, TRPM4 gradually becomes insensitive to Ca^{2+}, which leads to a move toward the state of negative potential [6,9]. Under a Ca^{2+}-desensitized condition, TRPM4 shows voltage-dependent gating with increased open-state probability at a depolarizing membrane potential [51,60]. It has been demonstrated that poly-L-lysine, which is a type of PIP_2 scavenger, can trigger a sharp desensitization [7].

Previous studies have additionally shown that loss of PIP_2 results in a rapid attenuation of the TRPM4 current, in accordance with Nilius et al., which has been detected by adding PIP_2 or inhibiting PIP_2 extracellularly of HEK293 cells, both of which can reverse the depletion of the TRPM4 current [6]. Furthermore, depression of PLC activity with U73122, an inhibitor of PLC [67], is also able to preserve the level of PIP_2 [6,9,68].

In summary, PIP_2 is a critical auxiliary factor in the activation of TRPM4. PIP_2 cannot activate TRPM4 on its own, but can rectify desensitization, increase the sensitivity of TRPM4 to Ca^{2+}, and restrict the voltage dependence of TRPM4 [6,7,10,69,70]. To date, two PIP_2-binding sites have been discovered at the C-terminal of TRPM4, which implies that the alteration of these binding sites may affect the sensitivity of TRPM4 to PIP$_2$ and Ca^{2+} [6,71].

2.4.2. ATP

Owing to the structure of TRPM4, Ca^{2+} sensitivity of TRPM4 can be modulated by ATP, PKC phosphorylation, and binding of CaM to the C-terminus [8–11]. ATP can restore the Ca^{2+} sensitivity of TRPM4 after desensitization has been clarified previously [8]. In the absence of Ca^{2+}, TRPM4 can revert from desensitization when the cytoplasmic side of the membrane is exposed to Mg^{2+}-chelated ATP [8,9]. However, TRPM4 currents would attenuate in the case of ATP deficiency after recovery. Therefore, addition or depletion of ATP has become vital in regulating the activation of TRPM4. As mentioned earlier, the ATP-binding sites, which include two Walker B motifs in the N-terminus and ABC transporter signature motifs, can be predicted from the amino acid sequence of TRPM4 [8,72,73]. It was also reported that TRPM4 currents are eliminated sharply when all the sites predicted to affect the ATP-binding of the channel carry mutations, which suggests that ATP is involved in the preservation of TRPM4's Ca^{2+} sensitivity [8].

2.4.3. PKC Phosphorylation

PKC-mediated TRPM4 phosphorylation can increase the Ca^{2+} sensitivity of TRPM4. A PKC activator, phorbol 12-myristate 13-acetate (PMA), can reduce the Half maximal effective concentration (EC$_{50}$) level of Ca^{2+} in TRPM4 from 15 to 4 μM [8,74], which suggests that the increased activity of PKC helps improve the Ca^{2+} sensitivity of TRPM4 and resist its desensitization. This effect of PMA disappears when both the readily-phosphorylated amino acid residues, S1145A and S1152A, at the C-terminus of TRPM4 carry mutations [8].

2.4.4. CaM

A previous study by Nilius et al. found that dominant-negative mutants of CaM reduce the activation of TRPM4. CaM partially counters the reduction of Ca^{2+} sensitivity of endogenous TRPM4. Mutations in the C-terminal binding site of CaM can significantly reduce TRPM4 current amplitude and promote faster current decay. This suggests that the C-terminal binding site of CaM is vital for the Ca^{2+} sensitivity of TRPM4 [8,75].

The following sections discuss why it is important to understand TRPM4's role in diseases by exploring the activated mechanism of the channel.

2.5. Inhibitors of TRPM4

Flufenamic acid is one of the inhibitors of TRPM4 and widely used in research [1]. Originally, according to Winder et al., flufenamic acid was identified in the 1960s as a member of the anthranilic acid-derivative class of nonsteroidal anti-inflammatory drugs (NSAID) due to its anti-inflammatory property, which is able to inhibit the production of prostaglandins. Subsequently, it has been found that flufenamic acid could act as an ion channel regulator that mainly impacts the nonselective cation channels. The TRPM4 channel can be significantly inhibited by flufenamic acid in the range of 4–12 μM. However, it affects sodium, potassium, calcium, and chloride channels as well [76].

Glibenclamide is another TRPM4 inhibitor, which can block TRPM4-like currents in sinoatrial node cells completely at a concentration of 100 μM [77]. The inhibiting effect of glibenclamide on TRPM4 channel is weaker than that on ATP-dependent K$^+$ channels, which are vital therapeutic targets of type II diabetes [78]. Compared to the chemicals above, 9-phenanthrol, which is a tricyclic aromatic compound, inhibits TRPM4 activity specifically [79,80].

3. TRPM4 and Cardiovascular Disease

3.1. TRPM4 and Arrhythmia

Arrhythmia is a group of conditions with abnormal frequency of cardiac pulsation and/or rhythm, caused in the origin of heart activity and/or conduction disturbances, such as atrial sinus node dysregulation, excitement outside the sinoatrial node, agitation, slow conduction, and blocked or abnormal channel conduction [81–84]. Arrhythmia is an important class of diseases with respect to cardiovascular risk. The reverse transport of the sodium–calcium exchanger (NCX) on cardiomyocytes is one of the major pathways that leads to intracellular Ca^{2+} overload [85–89]. The research of Voigt et al. In 2011 demonstrated that increased NCX expression and activity can delay afterdepolarization, which triggers and promotes chronic atrial fibrillation [86,90–92]. Interestingly, the coupling of TRP channels with NCX proteins (TRP–NCX-mediated Ca^{2+} signaling) is able to disrupt intracellular Na^+ and Ca^{2+} concentration, which produces a sudden accumulation of intracellular Ca^{2+}, especially in the case of TRPC3 [93–95].

It is clear that TRPM4 is highly expressed in atrial cardiomyocytes [1,77]. Being a member of the TRP channel family, it is worth considering whether a coupling between TRPM4 and reverse mode-NCX may induce atrial arrhythmias [12]. In 2009, a *TRPM4* mutation was detected in a patient with hereditary heart disease: the glutamate at position 7 was replaced with lysine, which induced progressive cardiac bundle-branch block [96]. This is the first case to closely link *TRPM4* mutation to the pathophysiology of human cardiovascular disease [1,96]. The researchers subsequently demonstrated that although these mutations did not change the physiological characteristics of TRPM4, the SUMOylation—a post-translational modification to regulate the protein function by combining a member of the small ubiquitin-like modifier (SUMO) family and the target protein—of the mutant protein caused the alternation of TRPM4 protein expression and its current level at the plasma membrane [16–18,97].

However, the link between the function of TRPM4 and cardiac conduction block remains unclear. Perhaps the dysfunction of the voltage-dependent Na^+ channel takes place, considering that TRPM4 switches on the depolarization of the cell membrane potential, which subsequently injures the cardiac conduction system [52,98,99]. Recently, other studies have also illustrated that *TRPM4* mutations are associated with isolated cardiac conduction disease, right bundle-branch block, tachycardia, and Brugada syndrome [17–21].

In summary, the fluctuation of Na^+ and Ca^{2+} is involved in the regulation of the cardiac conduction system and is closely linked to the development of arrhythmia. As a result, TRPM4, which is an important Ca^{2+} regulator, may also be involved in cardiac conduction system diseases.

3.2. TRPM4 and Cardiac Hypertrophy

Cardiac hypertrophy is one of powerful adaptive mechanisms of the cardiovascular system, which is mainly manifested by an increase in cell volume and weight [100–102]. Adaptive alteration, which is so-called physiological hypertrophy, occurs to meet the increased demand of blood circulation. Under the physiological condition, the cardiac function can be performed in an orderly manner [93]. However, if it exceeds the range of compensation owing to cardiac pressure or volume overload, such as high levels of angiotensin II (AII), chronic hypertension, valvular dysfunction, myocardial infarction, and even excessive training, the hypertrophy shifts to an irreversible pathology, which induces severe arrhythmia or cardiac failure [22,103–106].

Calcium is indispensable in the excitation–contraction coupling and heart contractility under normal physiological conditions [87,88]. In the opinion of Lopea et al. In 1997, intracellular Ca^{2+} levels in the cardiomyocytes of humans with myocardial hypertrophy were sustained at high levels [107], which might be due to the following two methods: First, the activation of the phosphoinositide-specific PLC pathway leads to the generation of inositol 1,4,5-trisphosphate and diacylglycerol (DAG) via the hydrolysis of PIP_2, both of which function as secondary messengers mediating the release of Ca^{2+}

from the smooth endoplasmic reticulum and sarcoplasmic reticulum [22,108–110]. Second, the nuclear factor of activated T cells (NFAT), one of the transcription factors regulated by calcium signaling, also takes part in the regulation of decompensated cardiac hypertrophy. CaM activates serine/threonine phosphatase calcineurin (CN), and activated CN rapidly dephosphorylates the serine-rich region and serine-proline (SP)-repeats in the amino termini of NFAT, resulting in its translocation from the cytoplasm to the nucleus and producing pathological cardiac hypertrophy [111–114]. There is no doubt that Ca^{2+} plays a significant role in inducing cardiac hypertrophy. Therefore, if the mechanisms that maintain intracellular Ca^{2+} homeostasis are perturbed, the evolution of the hypertrophic alteration at the stage of compensation and decompensation in the myocardium is affected. Thus, calcium-regulated ion channels act as typical mediators.

TRP channels are important targets in myocardial remodeling because they are capable of transmitting long-term calcium signals [115–117]. Studies have shown that TRPM4 seems to be involved in the occurrence and development of cardiac hypertrophy, in accordance with Demion et al., Kecskés et al., and Guefer et al. [104,118,119]. Indeed, TRPM4 has been shown to play a role in cardiac hypertrophy by the construction of a typical model that mimics the ventricular hypertrophic alteration in spontaneously hypertensive rats (SHRs) [120]. Changes in TRPM4 current and mRNA levels are detectable in SHRs. Compared with WKY rats (control group), the expression levels of TRPM4 mRNA in SHRs were almost 50-fold.

Although a significant level of TRPM4 current exists in SHRs, it is quite challenging to find it in WKY rats even by facilitating the TRPM4 current with application of PKC. TRPM4 properties can be monitored by the Patch-Clamp measurement to illustrate the existence of a nonselective cation channel in ventricular cardiomyocytes isolated from SHRs. Thus, TRPM4 is crucial during the process of ventricular remodeling [22,120].

TRPM4 is a negative regulator of cardiac hypertrophy induced by angiotensin II (AII) stimulation [104]. In this previous study, the researchers selectively removed the exons 15 and 16 from *TRPM4* for establishing a cardiac-specific TRPM4-knockout mouse line (TRPM4^{cKO}). They intended to compare cardiac hypertrophic changes between TRPM4^{cKO} mice and wild-type mice (littermate controls; TRPM4$^{+/+}$) under AII stimulation. Their results showed significantly higher cardiac hypertrophy at the morphological level in TRPM4^{cKO} mice compared with the wild-type mice, including increased heart size and weight. In addition, high levels of hypertrophy-related genes such as atrial natriuretic peptide (*ANP*), α-actin, and *Rcan1* were detected in the TRPM4^{cKO} mice.

TRPM4 deficiency increases the hypertrophic response to chronic AII in cultured neonatal myocytes. Increased intracellular Ca^{2+} concentration in isolated ventricular cardiomyocytes of TRPM4^{cKO} mice after AII stimulation reconfirmed that TRPM4 is a key regulator of intracellular Ca^{2+}. There was also a significant rise in CN phosphatase activity in the hearts of TRPM4^{cKO} mice following AII treatment. In these mice, Rcan1 mRNA, which is a reporter of the calcineurin–NFAT activation typical in cardiac hypertrophy, is overexpressed. Additionally, store-operated calcium entry (SOCE), which is helpful in promoting intracellular Ca^{2+} collection from the extracellular environment, has been regarded as having an important role in mediating cardiac hypertrophy [104,117,121]. The study of Kecskés et al. showed that AngII-mediated SOCE was increased in Trpm4$^{-/-}$ myocytes [104]. It means that TRPM4 is related to modulation of the Ca^{2+} influx through SOCE to induce pathological hypertrophy [104,117,121]

TRPM4 is important for the beneficial cardiac remodeling induced by endurance training, and the role of TRPM4 in physiological and pathological cardiac hypertrophy has also been studied [118]. In TRPM4$^{+/+}$ mice, enhanced cardiac function in response to endurance training was observed. In contrast, a high number of apoptotic DNA fragments are detectable in TRPM4$^{-/-}$ mice after endurance training. This illustrates that TRPM4 can obstruct the progress from adaptive hypertrophy to irreversible cardiac remodeling. In the pathological cardiac hypertrophy, Ca^{2+} entry via SOCs causes activation of the calcineurin–NFAT pathway. The TRPM4 channel inhibits the SOCs and thus prevents pathological remodeling [118].

The link between TRPM4 and arrhythmia, wherein 9-phenanthrol can inhibit TRPM4 and can shorten the duration of action potentials (APs), has been confirmed previously, which implies that TRPM4 can delay AP repolarization [119]. It has been hypothesized that TRPM4 is implicated in the prolongation of AP duration, which may be present in the hypertrophied heart, but has not been verified to date [122–124].

Thus, TRPM4 is an essential regulator of the hypertrophic alteration and is likely to supply a novel direction for the treatment of cardiovascular diseases caused by cardiac hypertrophy [22,122].

3.3. TRPM4 and Myocardial IRI

Ischemic heart diseases (IHDs) have become the most frequently reported threat to human health [125,126]. Myocardial ischemia originates owing to a reduction in coronary blood flow, which may result in an imbalance between myocardial supply and demand of oxygen. Typical symptoms include chest pain, chest discomfort, weakness or dyspnea after exercise, and mental stimulation or overeating, which are detrimental to the quality of life. Restoring the blood flow is an effective therapeutic strategy to treat ischemia, as achieved through thrombolysis, coronary artery bypass graft, and percutaneous coronary intervention. However, secondary injuries after recanalization are risk factors to IHD patients, such as contractile dysfunction, arrhythmia, and sudden death, which are also known as myocardial IRI [127–129].

The mechanism underlying myocardial ischemia-reperfusion injury (IRI) is complex [130–132]. At the onset of ischemia, ATP decreases progressively, which subsequently causes a dysfunction of ion pumps, leading to the accumulation of intracellular Ca^{2+}, especially in the mitochondria. This promotes the depletion of ATP with increased Ca^{2+}, leading to cell death. With the return of blood flow, even if it is conducive to the recovery of ATP, a large burst of Ca^{2+} and reactive oxygen species in the mitochondria occurs at the onset of reperfusion, which opens the mitochondrial permeability transition pore and causes further myocardial damage. Thus, reduced ATP and disrupted calcium metabolism eventually lead to myocardial IRI. It has also been identified that Ca^{2+} increase and ATP depletion are involved in the activation of TRPM4, and a link between TRPM4 and myocardial IRI has been reported [36,130–134].

Inhibition of TRPM4 with 9-phenanthrol (9-Phe) has been shown to confer cardioprotective effects against IRI in the rat heart [24]. In the Langendorff-perfused rat heart, the TRPM4 inhibitor 9-Phe produced a dramatic recovery of the damaged left ventricular contractile function caused by experimental IRI. Furthermore, 9-Phe treatment could effectively resist the ventricular fibrillation induced by IRI. This showed that damaged cardiac contractile function caused by IRI could be rescued through the inhibition of TRPM4, which may confer cardioprotection mainly via an anti-arrhythmic effect. After IRI, the infarcted area of myocardium was smaller in the rats treated with 9-Phe, which further elaborated that regulation of TRPM4 is important in reversing the myocardial damage induced by IRI [24].

The relationship between TRPM4 and myocardial IRI has been explored more deeply in vitro as well [23]. In rat ventricular cardiomyocytes H9c2, 9-Phe treatment prevented cellular damage caused by two types of IRI models: one being reactive oxygen species stimulation (ROS) by hydrogen peroxide (H_2O_2) exposure, and the other being hypoxia/reoxygenation (H/R) induction. Moreover, the viability of cardiomyocytes with the TRPM4 knocked down through small interfering RNA (siRNA) transfection was significantly higher than that of the nontransfection group following ROS damage and H/R induction. It can also be suggested that inhibition of TRPM4 protects cardiomyocytes against IRI both in vivo and in vitro, and 9-Phe treatment confers remarkable cardioprotection against oxidative stress injury. Therefore, inhibiting TRPM4 might be promising in treating myocardial IRI for IHD patients [23].

TRPM4 is closely related to intracellular Ca^{2+} dynamic equilibrium, and the mechanism of intracellular Ca^{2+} overload-induced IRI has already been elucidated [8,116,122,135]. Therefore, the role of inhibiting TRPM4 in ameliorating an abrupt increase in intracellular Ca^{2+} during myocardial IRI is being explored.

3.4. TRPM4 and Endothelial Cell Injury and Apoptosis

Endothelial injury is the risk factor and may cause a series of cardiovascular system disorders [136,137]. Due to the research conducted by Gerzanich et al., Becerra et al., and Ding et al., the expression of TRPM4 could be upregulated when the vascular endothelium is damaged under a variety of pathological conditions. For example, TRPM4 expression levels increase by more than 33% in endothelial cells damaged owing to a high-salt diet [138–141]. Moreover, the expression of TRPM4 in both protein and mRNA forms increases in human umbilical vein endothelial cells under hypoxic and ischemic conditions [10,142]. It has also been shown that TRPM4 is involved in lipopolysaccharide-induced vascular endothelial injury [139]. Thus, inhibiting the expression or activity of TRPM4 via 9-Phe and glibenclamide can effectively protect vascular endothelial cells against lipopolysaccharide-induced damage.

In a lipopolysaccharide-treated group, more than 40% of the endothelial cells were apoptotic, whereas the apoptosis in the TRPM4-inhihition group reduced significantly [139]. Lipopolysaccharide induces endothelial cell death because it promotes a rise in intracellular ROS [143]. Furthermore, the expression of TRPM4 is significantly upregulated upon treatment with exogenous ROS (H_2O_2), which results in endothelial cell apoptosis. However, this could be reversed through the inhibition of TRPM4 activity with 9-Phe [138]. Thus, it is implied that the involvement of TRPM4 in endothelial injury is also mediated by ROS [131,133,134,144].

It is clear that under the influence of various vascular injury factors, the upregulation of TRPM4 in vascular endothelial cells produces complete or maximal depolarization, resulting in the continuous influx of sodium ions [137–139]. Soon afterwards, the rise of intracellular Na^+ and Cl^- is able to cause enlargement of osmotic pressure, which drives the influx of H_2O, inducing cell swelling or rupture [140].

4. Conclusions

Overall, TRPM4 is an important nonselective cation channel involved in cellular calcium regulation. a majority of cardiovascular diseases are closely related to calcium homeostasis. As the research on TRPM4 progresses, more functions will be recognized and intrinsic links between TRPM4 and the development of cardiovascular diseases may be discovered.

Author Contributions: Conceptualization: C.W. and K.T.; investigation: C.W. and K.T.; writing—original draft preparation: C.W.; writing—review and editing: K.N. and K.T.; supervision: K.N. and K.T.; project administration: K.T.; funding acquisition: K.T.

Funding: This study was supported by Grant-in-Aid for Scientific Research (C), No. 16K01356.

Acknowledgments: This study was supported by Grant-in-Aid for Scientific Research (C), No. 16K01356.

Conflicts of Interest: The authors declare no conflict of interest.

References

1. Guinamard, R.; Demion, M.; Launay, P. Physiological roles of the trpm4 channel extracted from background currents. *Physiology* **2010**, *25*, 155–164. [CrossRef] [PubMed]
2. Launay, P.; Fleig, A.; Perraud, A.L.; Scharenberg, A.M.; Penner, R.; Kinet, J.P. Trpm4 is a ca2+-activated nonselective cation channel mediating cell membrane depolarization. *Cell* **2002**, *109*, 397–407. [CrossRef]
3. Song, M.Y.; Yuan, J.X. Introduction to trp channels: Structure, function, and regulation. *Adv. Exp. Med. Biol.* **2010**, *661*, 99–108. [PubMed]
4. Fleig, A.; Penner, R. The trpm ion channel subfamily: Molecular, biophysical and functional features. *Trends Pharmacol. Sci.* **2004**, *25*, 633–639. [CrossRef] [PubMed]

5.   Mathar, I.; Jacobs, G.; Kecskes, M.; Menigoz, A.; Philippaert, K.; Vennekens, R. Trpm4. *Handb. Exp. Pharmacol.* **2014**, *222*, 461–487. [PubMed]
6.   Nilius, B.; Mahieu, F.; Prenen, J.; Janssens, A.; Owsianik, G.; Vennekens, R.; Voets, T. The Ca^{2+}-activated cation channel trpm4 is regulated by phosphatidylinositol 4, 5-biphosphate. *EMBO J.* **2006**, *25*, 467–478. [CrossRef] [PubMed]
7.   Zhang, Z.; Okawa, H.; Wang, Y.; Liman, E.R. Phosphatidylinositol 4, 5-bisphosphate rescues trpm4 channels from desensitization. *J. Biol. Chem.* **2005**, *280*, 39185–39192. [CrossRef] [PubMed]
8.   Nilius, B.; Prenen, J.; Tang, J.; Wang, C.; Owsianik, G.; Janssens, A.; Voets, T.; Zhu, M.X. Regulation of the Ca^{2+} sensitivity of the nonselective cation channel trpm4. *J. Biol. Chem.* **2005**, *280*, 6423–6433. [CrossRef] [PubMed]
9.   Nilius, B.; Vennekens, R. From cardiac cation channels to the molecular dissection of the transient receptor potential channel trpm4. *Pflugers Arch.* **2006**, *453*, 313–321. [CrossRef] [PubMed]
10. Vennekens, R.; Nilius, B. Insights into trpm4 function, regulation and physiological role. *Handb. Exp. Pharmacol.* **2007**, *179*, 269–285.
11. Earley, S.; Straub, S.V.; Brayden, J.E. Protein kinase c regulates vascular myogenic tone through activation of trpm4. *Am. J. Physiol. Heart Circ. Physiol.* **2007**, *292*, H2613–H2622. [CrossRef] [PubMed]
12. Watanabe, H.; Murakami, M.; Ohba, T.; Ono, K.; Ito, H. The pathological role of transient receptor potential channels in heart disease. *Circ. J.* **2009**, *73*, 419–427. [CrossRef] [PubMed]
13. Kaneko, Y.; Szallasi, A. Transient receptor potential (trp) channels: a clinical perspective. *Br. J. Pharmacol.* **2014**, *171*, 2474–2507. [CrossRef] [PubMed]
14. Nilius, B. Trp channels in disease. *Biochim. Biophys. Acta* **2007**, *1772*, 805–812. [CrossRef] [PubMed]
15. Cho, C.H.; Lee, Y.S.; Kim, E.; Hwang, E.M.; Park, J.Y. Physiological functions of the trpm4 channels via protein interactions. *BMB Rep.* **2015**, *48*, 1–5. [CrossRef] [PubMed]
16. Voolstra, O.; Huber, A. Post-translational modifications of trp channels. *Cells* **2014**, *3*, 258–287. [CrossRef] [PubMed]
17. Guinamard, R.; Bouvagnet, P.; Hof, T.; Liu, H.; Simard, C.; Salle, L. Trpm4 in cardiac electrical activity. *Cardiovasc. Res.* **2015**, *108*, 21–30. [CrossRef] [PubMed]
18. Liu, H.; El Zein, L.; Kruse, M.; Guinamard, R.; Beckmann, A.; Bozio, A.; Kurtbay, G.; Megarbane, A.; Ohmert, I.; Blaysat, G.; et al. Gain-of-function mutations in trpm4 cause autosomal dominant isolated cardiac conduction disease. *Circ. Cardiovasc. Genet.* **2010**, *3*, 374–385. [CrossRef] [PubMed]
19. Stallmeyer, B.; Zumhagen, S.; Denjoy, I.; Duthoit, G.; Hebert, J.L.; Ferrer, X.; Maugenre, S.; Schmitz, W.; Kirchhefer, U.; Schulze-Bahr, E.; et al. Mutational spectrum in the $Ca^{(2+)}$–Activated cation channel gene trpm4 in patients with cardiac conductance disturbances. *Hum. Mutat.* **2012**, *33*, 109–117. [CrossRef] [PubMed]
20. Liu, H.; Chatel, S.; Simard, C.; Syam, N.; Salle, L.; Probst, V.; Morel, J.; Millat, G.; Lopez, M.; Abriel, H.; et al. Molecular genetics and functional anomalies in a series of 248 brugada cases with 11 mutations in the trpm4 channel. *PLoS ONE* **2013**, *8*. [CrossRef] [PubMed]
21. Duthoit, G.; Fressart, V.; Hidden-Lucet, F.; Simon, F.; Kattygnarath, D.; Charron, P.; Himbert, C.; Aouate, P.; Guicheney, P.; Lecarpentier, Y.; et al. Brugada ecg pattern: a physiopathological prospective study based on clinical, electrophysiological, angiographic, and genetic findings. *Front. Physiol.* **2012**, *3*. [CrossRef] [PubMed]
22. Guinamard, R.; Bois, P. Involvement of transient receptor potential proteins in cardiac hypertrophy. *Biochim. Biophys. Acta* **2007**, *1772*, 885–894. [CrossRef] [PubMed]
23. Piao, H.; Takahashi, K.; Yamaguchi, Y.; Wang, C.; Liu, K.; Naruse, K. Transient receptor potential melastatin-4 is involved in hypoxia-reoxygenation injury in the cardiomyocytes. *PLoS ONE* **2015**, *10*. [CrossRef] [PubMed]
24. Wang, J.; Takahashi, K.; Piao, H.; Qu, P.; Naruse, K. 9-phenanthrol, a trpm4 inhibitor, protects isolated rat hearts from ischemia-reperfusion injury. *PLoS ONE* **2013**, *8*. [CrossRef] [PubMed]
25. Minke, B.; Wu, C.; Pak, W.L. Induction of photoreceptor voltage noise in the dark in drosophila mutant. *Nature* **1975**, *258*, 84–87. [CrossRef] [PubMed]
26. Li, M.; Yu, Y.; Yang, J. Structural biology of trp channels. *Adv. Exp. Med. Biol.* **2011**, *704*, 1–23. [PubMed]
27. Peacock, M. Calcium metabolism in health and disease. *Clin. J. Am. Soc. Nephrol.* **2010**, *5* (Suppl. 1), S23–S30. [CrossRef] [PubMed]

28. Zaichick, S.V.; McGrath, K.M.; Caraveo, G. The role of Ca^{2+} signaling in parkinson's disease. *Dis. Model Mech.* **2017**, *10*, 519–535. [CrossRef] [PubMed]

29. Bronner, F. Extracellular and intracellular regulation of calcium homeostasis. *Sci. World J.* **2001**, *1*, 919–925. [CrossRef] [PubMed]

30. Hennings, H.; Holbrook, K.A. Calcium regulation of cell-cell contact and differentiation of epidermal cells in culture. an ultrastructural study. *Exp. Cell Res.* **1983**, *143*, 127–142. [CrossRef]

31. Kopic, S.; Geibel, J.P. Gastric acid, calcium absorption, and their impact on bone health. *Physiol. Rev.* **2013**, *93*, 189–268. [CrossRef] [PubMed]

32. Campbell, A.K. Calcium as an intracellular regulator. *Proc. Nutr. Soc.* **1990**, *49*, 51–56. [CrossRef] [PubMed]

33. Christakos, S.; Lieben, L.; Masuyama, R.; Carmeliet, G. Vitamin d endocrine system and the intestine. *Bonekey Rep.* **2014**, *3*. [CrossRef] [PubMed]

34. Brown, S.J.; Ruppe, M.D.; Tabatabai, L.S. The parathyroid gland and heart disease. *Methodist. Debakey Cardiovasc. J.* **2017**, *13*, 49–54. [CrossRef] [PubMed]

35. Castaldo, P.; Macri, M.L.; Lariccia, V.; Matteucci, A.; Maiolino, M.; Gratteri, S.; Amoroso, S.; Magi, S. Na$^{(+)}$/Ca^{2+} exchanger 1 inhibition abolishes ischemic tolerance induced by ischemic preconditioning in different cardiac models. *Eur. J. Pharmacol.* **2017**, *794*, 246–256. [CrossRef] [PubMed]

36. Murphy, E.; Steenbergen, C. Mechanisms underlying acute protection from cardiac ischemia-reperfusion injury. *Physiol. Rev.* **2008**, *88*, 581–609. [CrossRef] [PubMed]

37. Potz, B.A.; Sabe, A.A.; Abid, M.R.; Sellke, F.W. Calpains and coronary vascular disease. *Circ. J.* **2016**, *80*, 4–10. [CrossRef] [PubMed]

38. Joseph, L.C.; Subramanyam, P.; Radlicz, C.; Trent, C.M.; Iyer, V.; Colecraft, H.M.; Morrow, J.P. Mitochondrial oxidative stress during cardiac lipid overload causes intracellular calcium leak and arrhythmia. *Heart Rhythm* **2016**, *13*, 1699–1706. [CrossRef] [PubMed]

39. Skioldebrand, E.; Lundqvist, A.; Bjorklund, U.; Sandstedt, M.; Lindahl, A.; Hansson, E.; Hulten, L.M. Inflammatory activation of human cardiac fibroblasts leads to altered calcium signaling, decreased connexin 43 expression and increased glutamate secretion. *Heliyon* **2017**, *3*. [CrossRef] [PubMed]

40. Runte, K.E.; Bell, S.P.; Selby, D.E.; Haussler, T.N.; Ashikaga, T.; LeWinter, M.M.; Palmer, B.M.; Meyer, M. Relaxation and the role of calcium in isolated contracting myocardium from patients with hypertensive heart disease and heart failure with preserved ejection fraction. *Circ. Heart Fail.* **2017**, *10*. [CrossRef] [PubMed]

41. Ramsey, I.S.; Delling, M.; Clapham, D.E. an introduction to trp channels. *Annu. Rev.Physiol.* **2006**, *68*, 619–647. [CrossRef] [PubMed]

42. Prevarskaya, N.; Skryma, R.; Bidaux, G.; Flourakis, M.; Shuba, Y. Ion channels in death and differentiation of prostate cancer cells. *Cell Death Differ.* **2007**, *14*, 1295–1304. [CrossRef] [PubMed]

43. Ciardo, M.G.; Ferrer-Montiel, A. Lipids as central modulators of sensory trp channels. *Biochim. Biophys. Acta* **2017**, *1859*, 1615–1628. [CrossRef] [PubMed]

44. Gees, M.; Colsoul, B.; Nilius, B. The role of transient receptor potential cation channels in Ca^{2+} signaling. *Cold Spring Harb. Perspect. Biol.* **2010**, *2*. [CrossRef] [PubMed]

45. Clapham, D.E.; Runnels, L.W.; Strubing, C. The trp ion channel family. *Nat. Rev. Neurosci.* **2001**, *2*, 387–396. [CrossRef] [PubMed]

46. Nilius, B.; Owsianik, G. The transient receptor potential family of ion channels. *Genome Biol.* **2011**, *12*. [CrossRef] [PubMed]

47. Bouron, A.; Kiselyov, K.; Oberwinkler, J. Permeation, regulation and control of expression of trp channels by trace metal ions. *Pflugers Arch.* **2015**, *467*, 1143–1164. [CrossRef] [PubMed]

48. Gaudet, R. Trp channels entering the structural era. *J. Physiol.* **2008**, *586*, 3565–3575. [CrossRef] [PubMed]

49. Dimke, H.; Hoenderop, J.G.; Bindels, R.J. Molecular basis of epithelial Ca^{2+} and Mg^{2+} transport: Insights from the trp channel family. *J. Physiol.* **2011**, *589*, 1535–1542. [CrossRef] [PubMed]

50. Zheng, J. Molecular mechanism of trp channels. *Compr. Physiol.* **2013**, *3*, 221–242. [PubMed]

51. Nilius, B.; Prenen, J.; Droogmans, G.; Voets, T.; Vennekens, R.; Freichel, M.; Wissenbach, U.; Flockerzi, V. Voltage dependence of the Ca^{2+}-activated cation channel trpm4. *J. Biol. Chem.* **2003**, *278*, 30813–30820. [CrossRef] [PubMed]

52. Nilius, B.; Prenen, J.; Janssens, A.; Owsianik, G.; Wang, C.; Zhu, M.X.; Voets, T. The selectivity filter of the cation channel trpm4. *J. Biol. Chem.* **2005**, *280*, 22899–22906. [CrossRef] [PubMed]

53. Dutta Banik, D.; Martin, L.E.; Freichel, M.; Torregrossa, A.M.; Medler, K.F. Trpm4 and trpm5 are both required for normal signaling in taste receptor cells. *Proc. Natl. Acad. Sci. USA* **2018**, *115*, E772–E781. [CrossRef] [PubMed]

54. Talavera, K.; Yasumatsu, K.; Voets, T.; Droogmans, G.; Shigemura, N.; Ninomiya, Y.; Margolskee, R.F.; Nilius, B. Heat activation of trpm5 underlies thermal sensitivity of sweet taste. *Nature* **2005**, *438*, 1022–1025. [CrossRef] [PubMed]

55. Voets, T.; Droogmans, G.; Wissenbach, U.; Janssens, A.; Flockerzi, V.; Nilius, B. The principle of temperature-dependent gating in cold- and heat-sensitive trp channels. *Nature* **2004**, *430*, 748–754. [CrossRef] [PubMed]

56. Liman, E.R. The Ca$^{(2+)}$-activated trp channels: Trpm4 and trpm5. *Front. Neurosci.* **2007**. [CrossRef]

57. Fonfria, E.; Murdock, P.R.; Cusdin, F.S.; Benham, C.D.; Kelsell, R.E.; McNulty, S. Tissue distribution profiles of the human trpm cation channel family. *J. Recept. Signal Transduct. Res.* **2006**, *26*, 159–178. [CrossRef] [PubMed]

58. Simard, C.; Hof, T.; Keddache, Z.; Launay, P.; Guinamard, R. The trpm4 non-selective cation channel contributes to the mammalian atrial action potential. *J. Mol. Cell. Cardiol.* **2013**, *59*, 11–19. [CrossRef] [PubMed]

59. Demir, T.; Yumrutas, O.; Cengiz, B.; Demiryurek, S.; Unverdi, H.; Kaplan, D.S.; Bayraktar, R.; Ozkul, N.; Bagci, C. Evaluation of trpm (transient receptor potential melastatin) genes expressions in myocardial ischemia and reperfusion. *Mol. Biol. Rep.* **2014**, *41*, 2845–2849. [CrossRef] [PubMed]

60. Guo, J.; She, J.; Zeng, W.; Chen, Q.; Bai, X.C.; Jiang, Y. Structures of the calcium-activated, non-selective cation channel trpm4. *Nature* **2017**, *552*, 205–209. [CrossRef] [PubMed]

61. Winkler, P.A.; Huang, Y.; Sun, W.; Du, J.; Lu, W. Electron cryo-microscopy structure of a human trpm4 channel. *Nature* **2017**, *552*, 200–204. [CrossRef] [PubMed]

62. Autzen, H.E.; Myasnikov, A.G.; Campbell, M.G.; Asarnow, D.; Julius, D.; Cheng, Y. Structure of the human trpm4 ion channel in a lipid nanodisc. *Science* **2018**, *359*, 228–232. [CrossRef] [PubMed]

63. Watschinger, K.; Horak, S.B.; Schulze, K.; Obermair, G.J.; Wild, C.; Koschak, A.; Sinnegger-Brauns, M.J.; Tampe, R.; Striessnig, J. Functional properties and modulation of extracellular epitope-tagged Ca(v)2.1 voltage-gated calcium channels. *Channels* **2008**, *2*, 461–473. [CrossRef] [PubMed]

64. Hammond, G.R.; Dove, S.K.; Nicol, A.; Pinxteren, J.A.; Zicha, D.; Schiavo, G. Elimination of plasma membrane phosphatidylinositol (4,5)-bisphosphate is required for exocytosis from mast cells. *J. Cell Sci.* **2006**, *119*, 2084–2094. [CrossRef] [PubMed]

65. Bulley, S.J.; Clarke, J.H.; Droubi, A.; Giudici, M.L.; Irvine, R.F. Exploring phosphatidylinositol 5-phosphate 4-kinase function. *Adv. Biol. Regul.* **2015**, *57*, 193–202. [CrossRef] [PubMed]

66. Rodriguez-Menchaca, A.A.; Adney, S.K.; Zhou, L.; Logothetis, D.E. Dual regulation of voltage-sensitive ion channels by pip(2). *Front. Pharmacol.* **2012**, *3*. [CrossRef] [PubMed]

67. Macmillan, D.; McCarron, J.G. The phospholipase c inhibitor u-73122 inhibits Ca$^{(2+)}$ release from the intracellular sarcoplasmic reticulum Ca$^{(2+)}$ store by inhibiting Ca$^{(2+)}$ pumps in smooth muscle. *Br. J. Pharmacol.* **2010**, *160*, 1295–1301. [CrossRef] [PubMed]

68. Rohacs, T.; Lopes, C.M.; Michailidis, I.; Logothetis, D.E. Pi(4,5)p2 regulates the activation and desensitization of trpm8 channels through the trp domain. *Nat. Neurosci.* **2005**, *8*, 626–634. [CrossRef] [PubMed]

69. Earley, S. Trpm4 channels in smooth muscle function. *Pflugers Arch.* **2013**, *465*, 1223–1231. [CrossRef] [PubMed]

70. Liu, D.; Liman, E.R. Intracellular Ca^{2+} and the phospholipid pip2 regulate the taste transduction ion channel trpm5. *Proc. Natl. Acad. Sci. USA* **2003**, *100*, 15160–15165. [CrossRef] [PubMed]

71. Bousova, K.; Jirku, M.; Bumba, L.; Bednarova, L.; Sulc, M.; Franek, M.; Vyklicky, L.; Vondrasek, J.; Teisinger, J. Pip2 and pip3 interact with n-terminus region of trpm4 channel. *Biophys. Chem.* **2015**, *205*, 24–32. [CrossRef] [PubMed]

72. Orelle, C.; Dalmas, O.; Gros, P.; Di Pietro, A.; Jault, J.M. The conserved glutamate residue adjacent to the walker-b motif is the catalytic base for atp hydrolysis in the atp-binding cassette transporter bmra. *J. Biol. Chem.* **2003**, *278*, 47002–47008. [CrossRef] [PubMed]

73. Ren, X.Q.; Furukawa, T.; Haraguchi, M.; Sumizawa, T.; Aoki, S.; Kobayashi, M.; Akiyama, S. Function of the abc signature sequences in the human multidrug resistance protein 1. *Mol. Pharmacol.* **2004**, *65*, 1536–1542. [CrossRef] [PubMed]

74. Yao, X.; Kwan, H.Y.; Huang, Y. Regulation of trp channels by phosphorylation. *Neurosignals* **2005**, *14*, 273–280. [CrossRef] [PubMed]

75. Bousova, K.; Herman, P.; Vecer, J.; Bednarova, L.; Monincova, L.; Majer, P.; Vyklicky, L.; Vondrasek, J.; Teisinger, J. Shared cam- and s100a1-binding epitopes in the distal trpm4 n terminus. *FEBS J.* **2018**, *285*, 599–613. [CrossRef] [PubMed]

76. Guinamard, R.; Simard, C.; Del Negro, C. Flufenamic acid as an ion channel modulator. *Pharmacol. Ther.* **2013**, *138*, 272–284. [CrossRef] [PubMed]

77. Demion, M.; Bois, P.; Launay, P.; Guinamard, R. Trpm4, a Ca^{2+}-activated nonselective cation channel in mouse sino-atrial node cells. *Cardiovasc. Res.* **2007**, *73*, 531–538. [CrossRef] [PubMed]

78. Ozhathil, L.C.; Delalande, C.; Bianchi, B.; Nemeth, G.; Kappel, S.; Thomet, U.; Ross-Kaschitza, D.; Simonin, C.; Rubin, M.; Gertsch, J.; et al. Identification of potent and selective small molecule inhibitors of the cation channel trpm4. *Br. J. Pharmacol.* **2018**, *175*, 2504–2519. [CrossRef] [PubMed]

79. Grand, T.; Demion, M.; Norez, C.; Mettey, Y.; Launay, P.; Becq, F.; Bois, P.; Guinamard, R. 9-phenanthrol inhibits human trpm4 but not trpm5 cationic channels. *Br. J. Pharmacol.* **2008**, *153*, 1697–1705. [CrossRef] [PubMed]

80. Burris, S.K.; Wang, Q.; Bulley, S.; Neeb, Z.P.; Jaggar, J.H. 9-phenanthrol inhibits recombinant and arterial myocyte tmem16a channels. *Br. J. Pharmacol.* **2015**, *172*, 2459–2468. [CrossRef] [PubMed]

81. Bethge, K.P. Classification of arrhythmias. *J. Cardiovasc. Pharmacol.* **1991**, *17* (Suppl. 6), S13–S19. [CrossRef] [PubMed]

82. Fu, D.G. Cardiac arrhythmias: Diagnosis, symptoms, and treatments. *Cell Biochem. Biophys.* **2015**, *73*, 291–296. [CrossRef] [PubMed]

83. John, R.M.; Tedrow, U.B.; Koplan, B.A.; Albert, C.M.; Epstein, L.M.; Sweeney, M.O.; Miller, A.L.; Michaud, G.F.; Stevenson, W.G. Ventricular arrhythmias and sudden cardiac death. *Lancet* **2012**, *380*, 1520–1529. [CrossRef]

84. Grace, A.A.; Roden, D.M. Systems biology and cardiac arrhythmias. *Lancet* **2012**, *380*, 1498–1508. [CrossRef]

85. Conway, S.J.; Koushik, S.V. Cardiac sodium-calcium exchanger: a double-edged sword. *Cardiovasc. Res.* **2001**, *51*, 194–197. [CrossRef]

86. Blaustein, M.P.; Lederer, W.J. Sodium/calcium exchange: Its physiological implications. *Physiol. Rev.* **1999**, *79*, 763–854. [CrossRef] [PubMed]

87. Goldhaber, J.I.; Philipson, K.D. Cardiac sodium-calcium exchange and efficient excitation-contraction coupling: Implications for heart disease. *Adv. Exp. Med. Biol.* **2013**, *961*, 355–364. [PubMed]

88. Ottolia, M.; Torres, N.; Bridge, J.H.; Philipson, K.D.; Goldhaber, J.I. Na/ca exchange and contraction of the heart. *J. Mol. Cell. Cardiol.* **2013**, *61*, 28–33. [CrossRef] [PubMed]

89. Giladi, M.; Shor, R.; Lisnyansky, M.; Khananshvili, D. Structure-functional basis of ion transport in sodium-calcium exchanger (ncx) proteins. *Int. J. Mol. Sci.* **2016**, *17*. [CrossRef] [PubMed]

90. Herrmann, S.; Lipp, P.; Wiesen, K.; Stieber, J.; Nguyen, H.; Kaiser, E.; Ludwig, A. The cardiac sodium-calcium exchanger ncx1 is a key player in the initiation and maintenance of a stable heart rhythm. *Cardiovasc. Res.* **2013**, *99*, 780–788. [CrossRef] [PubMed]

91. Voigt, N.; Li, N.; Wang, Q.; Wang, W.; Trafford, A.W.; Abu-Taha, I.; Sun, Q.; Wieland, T.; Ravens, U.; Nattel, S.; et al. Enhanced sarcoplasmic reticulum Ca^{2+} leak and increased Na+- Ca^{2+} exchanger function underlie delayed afterdepolarizations in patients with chronic atrial fibrillation. *Circulation* **2012**, *125*, 2059–2070. [CrossRef] [PubMed]

92. Dobrev, D.; Nattel, S. Calcium handling abnormalities in atrial fibrillation as a target for innovative therapeutics. *J. Cardiovasc. Pharmacol.* **2008**, *52*, 293–299. [CrossRef] [PubMed]

93. Firth, A.L.; Remillard, C.V.; Yuan, J.X. Trp channels in hypertension. *Biochim. Biophys. Acta* **2007**, *1772*, 895–906. [CrossRef] [PubMed]

94. Rosker, C.; Graziani, A.; Lukas, M.; Eder, P.; Zhu, M.X.; Romanin, C.; Groschner, K. Ca^{2+} signaling by trpc3 involves Na^{+} entry and local coupling to the Na^{+}/Ca^{2+} exchanger. *J. Biol. Chem.* **2004**, *279*, 13696–13704. [CrossRef] [PubMed]

95. Doleschal, B.; Primessnig, U.; Wolkart, G.; Wolf, S.; Schernthaner, M.; Lichtenegger, M.; Glasnov, T.N.; Kappe, C.O.; Mayer, B.; Antoons, G.; et al. Trpc3 contributes to regulation of cardiac contractility and arrhythmogenesis by dynamic interaction with ncx1. *Cardiovasc. Res.* **2015**, *106*, 163–173. [CrossRef] [PubMed]

96. Kruse, M.; Schulze-Bahr, E.; Corfield, V.; Beckmann, A.; Stallmeyer, B.; Kurtbay, G.; Ohmert, I.; Brink, P.; Pongs, O. Impaired endocytosis of the ion channel trpm4 is associated with human progressive familial heart block type I. *J. Clin. Investig.* **2009**, *119*, 2737–2744. [CrossRef] [PubMed]

97. Luo, J.; Ashikaga, E.; Rubin, P.P.; Heimann, M.J.; Hildick, K.L.; Bishop, P.; Girach, F.; Josa-Prado, F.; Tang, L.T.; Carmichael, R.E.; et al. Receptor trafficking and the regulation of synaptic plasticity by sumo. *Neuromol. Med.* **2013**, *15*, 692–706. [CrossRef] [PubMed]

98. Irvine, L.A.; Jafri, M.S.; Winslow, R.L. Cardiac sodium channel markov model with temperature dependence and recovery from inactivation. *Biophys. J.* **1999**, *76*, 1868–1885. [CrossRef]

99. Raman, I.M.; Bean, B.P. Inactivation and recovery of sodium currents in cerebellar purkinje neurons: Evidence for two mechanisms. *Biophys. J.* **2001**, *80*, 729–737. [CrossRef]

100. Swynghedauw, B. Molecular mechanisms of myocardial remodeling. *Physiol. Rev.* **1999**, *79*, 215–262. [CrossRef] [PubMed]

101. Wilde, A.A.; Brugada, R. Phenotypical manifestations of mutations in the genes encoding subunits of the cardiac sodium channel. *Circ. Res.* **2011**, *108*, 884–897. [CrossRef] [PubMed]

102. Frey, N.; Katus, H.A.; Olson, E.N.; Hill, J.A. Hypertrophy of the heart: a new therapeutic target? *Circulation* **2004**, *109*, 1580–1589. [CrossRef] [PubMed]

103. McMullen, J.R.; Jennings, G.L. Differences between pathological and physiological cardiac hypertrophy: Novel therapeutic strategies to treat heart failure. *Clin. Exp. Pharmacol. Physiol.* **2007**, *34*, 255–262. [CrossRef] [PubMed]

104. Kecskes, M.; Jacobs, G.; Kerselaers, S.; Syam, N.; Menigoz, A.; Vangheluwe, P.; Freichel, M.; Flockerzi, V.; Voets, T.; Vennekens, R. The Ca^{2+}-activated cation channel trpm4 is a negative regulator of angiotensin ii-induced cardiac hypertrophy. *Basic Res. Cardiol.* **2015**, *110*. [CrossRef] [PubMed]

105. Tham, Y.K.; Bernardo, B.C.; Ooi, J.Y.; Weeks, K.L.; McMullen, J.R. Pathophysiology of cardiac hypertrophy and heart failure: Signaling pathways and novel therapeutic targets. *Arch. Toxicol.* **2015**, *89*, 1401–1438. [CrossRef] [PubMed]

106. Da Rocha, A.L.; Teixeira, G.R.; Pinto, A.P.; de Morais, G.P.; Oliveira, L.D.C.; de Vicente, L.G.; da Silva, L.; Pauli, J.R.; Cintra, D.E.; Ropelle, E.R.; et al. Excessive training induces molecular signs of pathologic cardiac hypertrophy. *J. Cell. Physiol.* **2018**. [CrossRef] [PubMed]

107. Lopez, J.R.; Linares, N.; Brady, P.A.; Terzic, A. Cardiac hypertrophy determines digitalis action on intracellular Ca^{2+} in human myocardium. *Eur. J. Pharmacol.* **1997**, *339*, 161–164. [CrossRef]

108. Vega, R.B.; Bassel-Duby, R.; Olson, E.N. Control of cardiac growth and function by calcineurin signaling. *J. Biol. Chem.* **2003**, *278*, 36981–36984. [CrossRef] [PubMed]

109. Molkentin, J.D.; Lu, J.R.; Antos, C.L.; Markham, B.; Richardson, J.; Robbins, J.; Grant, S.R.; Olson, E.N. a calcineurin-dependent transcriptional pathway for cardiac hypertrophy. *Cell* **1998**, *93*, 215–228. [CrossRef]

110. Nishida, M.; Kurose, H. Roles of trp channels in the development of cardiac hypertrophy. *Naunyn Schmiedebergs Arch. Pharmacol.* **2008**, *378*, 395–406. [CrossRef] [PubMed]

111. Gao, H.; Wang, F.; Wang, W.; Makarewich, C.A.; Zhang, H.; Kubo, H.; Berretta, R.M.; Barr, L.A.; Molkentin, J.D.; Houser, S.R. Ca^{2+} influx through l-type Ca^{2+} channels and transient receptor potential channels activates pathological hypertrophy signaling. *J. Mol. Cell. Cardiol.* **2012**, *53*, 657–667. [CrossRef] [PubMed]

112. Ago, T.; Yang, Y.; Zhai, P.; Sadoshima, J. Nifedipine inhibits cardiac hypertrophy and left ventricular dysfunction in response to pressure overload. *J. Cardiovasc. Transl. Res.* **2010**, *3*, 304–313. [CrossRef] [PubMed]

113. Horiba, M.; Muto, T.; Ueda, N.; Opthof, T.; Miwa, K.; Hojo, M.; Lee, J.K.; Kamiya, K.; Kodama, I.; Yasui, K. T-type Ca^{2+} channel blockers prevent cardiac cell hypertrophy through an inhibition of calcineurin-nfat3 activation as well as l-type Ca^{2+} channel blockers. *Life Sci.* **2008**, *82*, 554–560. [CrossRef] [PubMed]

114. Molkentin, J.D. Calcineurin-nfat signaling regulates the cardiac hypertrophic response in coordination with the mapks. *Cardiovasc. Res.* **2004**, *63*, 467–475. [CrossRef] [PubMed]

115. Takahashi, K.; Kakimoto, Y.; Toda, K.; Naruse, K. Mechanobiology in cardiac physiology and diseases. *J. Cell. Mol. Med.* **2013**, *17*, 225–232. [CrossRef] [PubMed]

116. Minke, B. Trp channels and Ca^{2+} signaling. *Cell Calcium* **2006**, *40*, 261–275. [CrossRef] [PubMed]

117. Wu, X.; Eder, P.; Chang, B.; Molkentin, J.D. Trpc channels are necessary mediators of pathologic cardiac hypertrophy. *Proc. Natl. Acad. Sci. USA* **2010**, *107*, 7000–7005. [CrossRef] [PubMed]

118. Gueffier, M.; Zintz, J.; Lambert, K.; Finan, A.; Aimond, F.; Chakouri, N.; Hedon, C.; Granier, M.; Launay, P.; Thireau, J.; et al. The trpm4 channel is functionally important for the beneficial cardiac remodeling induced by endurance training. *J. Muscle Res. Cell Motil.* **2017**, *38*, 3–16. [CrossRef] [PubMed]

119. Demion, M.; Thireau, J.; Gueffier, M.; Finan, A.; Khoueiry, Z.; Cassan, C.; Serafini, N.; Aimond, F.; Granier, M.; Pasquie, J.L.; et al. Trpm4 gene invalidation leads to cardiac hypertrophy and electrophysiological alterations. *PLoS ONE* **2014**, *9*. [CrossRef] [PubMed]

120. Guinamard, R.; Demion, M.; Magaud, C.; Potreau, D.; Bois, P. Functional expression of the trpm4 cationic current in ventricular cardiomyocytes from spontaneously hypertensive rats. *Hypertension* **2006**, *48*, 587–594. [CrossRef] [PubMed]

121. Collins, H.E.; Zhu-Mauldin, X.; Marchase, R.B.; Chatham, J.C. Stim1/orai1-mediated soce: Current perspectives and potential roles in cardiac function and pathology. *Am. J. Physiol. Heart Circ. Physiol.* **2013**, *305*, H446–H458. [CrossRef] [PubMed]

122. Abriel, H.; Syam, N.; Sottas, V.; Amarouch, M.Y.; Rougier, J.S. Trpm4 channels in the cardiovascular system: Physiology, pathophysiology, and pharmacology. *Biochem. Pharmacol.* **2012**, *84*, 873–881. [CrossRef] [PubMed]

123. Mathar, I.; Vennekens, R.; Meissner, M.; Kees, F.; Van der Mieren, G.; Camacho Londono, J.E.; Uhl, S.; Voets, T.; Hummel, B.; van den Bergh, A.; et al. Increased catecholamine secretion contributes to hypertension in trpm4-deficient mice. *J. Clin. Investig.* **2010**, *120*, 3267–3279. [CrossRef] [PubMed]

124. Mathar, I.; Kecskes, M.; Van der Mieren, G.; Jacobs, G.; Camacho Londono, J.E.; Uhl, S.; Flockerzi, V.; Voets, T.; Freichel, M.; Nilius, B.; et al. Increased beta-adrenergic inotropy in ventricular myocardium from trpm4-/- mice. *Circ. Res.* **2014**, *114*, 283–294. [CrossRef] [PubMed]

125. Bhatnagar, P.; Wickramasinghe, K.; Wilkins, E.; Townsend, N. Trends in the epidemiology of cardiovascular disease in the uk. *Heart* **2016**, *102*, 1945–1952. [CrossRef] [PubMed]

126. Finegold, J.A.; Asaria, P.; Francis, D.P. Mortality from ischaemic heart disease by country, region, and age: Statistics from world health organisation and united nations. *Int. J. Cardiol.* **2013**, *168*, 934–945. [CrossRef] [PubMed]

127. Khera, A.V.; Kathiresan, S. Genetics of coronary artery disease: Discovery, biology and clinical translation. *Nat. Rev. Genet.* **2017**, *18*, 331–344. [CrossRef] [PubMed]

128. Ford, T.J.; Corcoran, D.; Berry, C. Coronary artery disease: Physiology and prognosis. *Eur. Heart J.* **2017**, *38*, 1990–1992. [CrossRef] [PubMed]

129. Cassar, A.; Holmes, D.R., Jr.; Rihal, C.S.; Gersh, B.J. Chronic coronary artery disease: Diagnosis and management. *Mayo Clin. Proc.* **2009**, *84*, 1130–1146. [CrossRef] [PubMed]

130. Carden, D.L.; Granger, D.N. Pathophysiology of ischaemia-reperfusion injury. *J. Pathol.* **2000**, *190*, 255–266. [CrossRef]

131. Cadenas, S. Ros and redox signaling in myocardial ischemia-reperfusion injury and cardioprotection. *Free Radic. Biol. Med.* **2018**, *117*, 76–89. [CrossRef] [PubMed]

132. Frank, A.; Bonney, M.; Bonney, S.; Weitzel, L.; Koeppen, M.; Eckle, T. Myocardial ischemia reperfusion injury: From basic science to clinical bedside. *Semin. Cardiothorac. Vasc. Anesth.* **2012**, *16*, 123–132. [CrossRef] [PubMed]

133. Kalogeris, T.; Baines, C.P.; Krenz, M.; Korthuis, R.J. Cell biology of ischemia/reperfusion injury. *Int. Rev. Cell Mol. Biol.* **2012**, *298*, 229–317. [PubMed]

134. Consolini, A.E.; Ragone, M.I.; Bonazzola, P.; Colareda, G.A. Mitochondrial bioenergetics during ischemia and reperfusion. *Adv. Exp. Med. Biol.* **2017**, *982*, 141–167. [PubMed]

135. Launay, P.; Cheng, H.; Srivatsan, S.; Penner, R.; Fleig, A.; Kinet, J.P. Trpm4 regulates calcium oscillations after t cell activation. *Science* **2004**, *306*, 1374–1377. [CrossRef] [PubMed]

136. Hadi, H.A.; Carr, C.S.; Al Suwaidi, J. Endothelial dysfunction: Cardiovascular risk factors, therapy, and outcome. *Vasc. Health Risk Manag.* **2005**, *1*, 183–198. [PubMed]

137. Widmer, R.J.; Lerman, A. Endothelial dysfunction and cardiovascular disease. *Glob. Cardiol. Sci. Pract.* **2014**, *2014*, 291–308. [CrossRef] [PubMed]

138. Ding, X.Q.; Ban, T.; Liu, Z.Y.; Lou, J.; Tang, L.L.; Wang, J.X.; Chu, W.F.; Zhao, D.; Song, B.L.; Zhang, Z.R. Transient receptor potential melastatin 4 (trpm4) contributes to high salt diet-mediated early-stage endothelial injury. *Cell. Physiol. Biochem.* **2017**, *41*, 835–848. [CrossRef] [PubMed]

139. Becerra, A.; Echeverria, C.; Varela, D.; Sarmiento, D.; Armisen, R.; Nunez-Villena, F.; Montecinos, M.; Simon, F. Transient receptor potential melastatin 4 inhibition prevents lipopolysaccharide-induced endothelial cell death. *Cardiovasc. Res.* **2011**, *91*, 677–684. [CrossRef] [PubMed]

140. Simard, J.M.; Woo, S.K.; Gerzanich, V. Transient receptor potential melastatin 4 and cell death. *Pflugers Arch.* **2012**, *464*, 573–582. [CrossRef] [PubMed]

141. Gerzanich, V.; Woo, S.K.; Vennekens, R.; Tsymbalyuk, O.; Ivanova, S.; Ivanov, A.; Geng, Z.; Chen, Z.; Nilius, B.; Flockerzi, V.; et al. De novo expression of trpm4 initiates secondary hemorrhage in spinal cord injury. *Nat. Med.* **2009**, *15*, 185–191. [CrossRef] [PubMed]

142. Earley, S.; Brayden, J.E. Transient receptor potential channels and vascular function. *Clin. Sci.* **2010**, *119*, 19–36. [CrossRef] [PubMed]

143. Simon, F.; Fernandez, R. Early lipopolysaccharide-induced reactive oxygen species production evokes necrotic cell death in human umbilical vein endothelial cells. *J. Hypertens.* **2009**, *27*, 1202–1216. [CrossRef] [PubMed]

144. Simon, F.; Leiva-Salcedo, E.; Armisen, R.; Riveros, A.; Cerda, O.; Varela, D.; Eguiguren, A.L.; Olivero, P.; Stutzin, A. Hydrogen peroxide removes trpm4 current desensitization conferring increased vulnerability to necrotic cell death. *J. Biol. Chem.* **2010**, *285*, 37150–37158. [CrossRef] [PubMed]

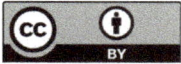

© 2018 by the authors. Licensee MDPI, Basel, Switzerland. This article is an open access article distributed under the terms and conditions of the Creative Commons Attribution (CC BY) license (http://creativecommons.org/licenses/by/4.0/).

Review

The Channel-Kinase TRPM7 as Novel Regulator of Immune System Homeostasis

Wiebke Nadolni and Susanna Zierler *

Walther Straub Institute of Pharmacology and Toxicology, Faculty of Medicine, LMU Munich, Goethestr. 33, 80336 Munich, Germany; wiebke.nadolni@lrz.uni-muenchen.de
* Correspondence: susanna.zierler@lrz.uni-muenchen.de; Tel.: +49-89-2180-75-722

Received: 13 July 2018; Accepted: 13 August 2018; Published: 17 August 2018

Abstract: The enzyme-coupled transient receptor potential channel subfamily M member 7, TRPM7, has been associated with immunity and immune cell signalling. Here, we review the role of this remarkable signalling protein in lymphocyte proliferation, differentiation, activation and survival. We also discuss its role in mast cell, neutrophil and macrophage function and highlight the potential of TRPM7 to regulate immune system homeostasis. Further, we shed light on how the cellular signalling cascades involving TRPM7 channel and/or kinase activity culminate in pathologies as diverse as allergic hypersensitivity, arterial thrombosis and graft versus host disease (G_VHD), stressing the need for TRPM7 specific pharmacological modulators.

Keywords: TRPM7; kinase; inflammation; lymphocytes; calcium signalling; SMAD; TH17; hypersensitivity; regulatory T cells; thrombosis; graft versus host disease

1. Introduction

The melastatin-like TRPM7 channel conducts divalent cations, specifically calcium (Ca^{2+}), magnesium (Mg^{2+}) and zinc (Zn^{2+}) [1–3]. It has been implicated in cellular and systemic Mg^{2+} homeostasis [4–6], Zn^{2+}-mediated toxicity [7,8] and intracellular Ca^{2+} signalling [9–12]. The TRPM7 channel is considered to be constitutively active and its activity to be negatively regulated by intracellular cations (Mg^{2+}, Ba^{2+}, Sr^{2+}, Zn^{2+}, Mn^{2+}), Mg-ATP, polyamines, chloride (Cl^-) and bromide (Br^-) concentrations, low intracellular pH and hydrolysis of the acidic phospholipid phosphatidylinositol 4,5-bisphosphate (PIP_2) [13–16]. Resting free cytosolic Mg^{2+} (0.5–1 mM [Mg^{2+}]$_c$) and Mg-ATP (3–9 mM) concentrations [17] seem to be sufficient to block native TRPM7 channel activity [4,18–20]. TRPM7's unique enzyme encodes a serine-threonine kinase closely related to eukaryotic elongation factor-2 kinase [21], phosphorylating mainly within α-helical loops [22]. A few in vitro TRPM7 kinase substrates have been identified early on, including annexin A1 [23,24], myosin II heavy chain [25] and PLCγ2 [26]. Only recently, with the development of novel mouse models, the first native kinase substrate, SMAD2, was discovered, paving the way for more to follow [11,20,27].

Genetic disruption of TRPM7 in mice ($Trpm7^{-/-}$) is embryonic lethal [4,28]. Deletion of the exons encoding the TRPM7 kinase domain only ($Trpm7^{\Delta k/\Delta k}$) also leads to early embryonic lethality [4]. However, the latter phenotype could be attributed to a reduction in channel activity in this mutant, particularly, as mice bearing a single point mutation at the active site of the kinase (K1646R, $Trpm7^{R/R}$), thus inactivating its catalytic activity, are viable and display no obvious phenotype [29,30]. Heterozygous $Trpm7^{+/\Delta k}$ mice are also viable but develop hypomagnesaemia upon Mg^{2+} restriction [4]. Deletion of the TRPM7 kinase domain at amino acid (aa) 1538 yields in reduced current amplitudes, while caspase-induced deletion at aa 1510 results in enhanced TRPM7 currents [4,31]. Inactivation of kinase activity via the K1646R mutation ($Trpm7^{R/R}$), though, does not affect current development [29,30,32] (Figure 1). However, it was reported to show increased basal current activity right after break-in in macrophages [29]. Recently, it was shown that the Mg^{2+}-sensitivity of the TRPM7 channel is reduced almost two-fold in kinase-deficient *Trpm7*$^{R/R}$ mouse mast cells. The tested Mg^{2+} concentrations, however, suggest that this effect will not influence TRPM7 currents in intact cells with $[Mg^{2+}]_c$ close to 1 mM [20]. Accordingly, how TRPM7 channel and kinase activities affect each other is still incompletely understood. It is thought that they are interdependent in that Mg^{2+} enters through the channel pore and the kinase domain requires Mg^{2+} ions to function [3,22], while the kinase domain rather than the catalytic activity are crucial for channel function [4,29–31].

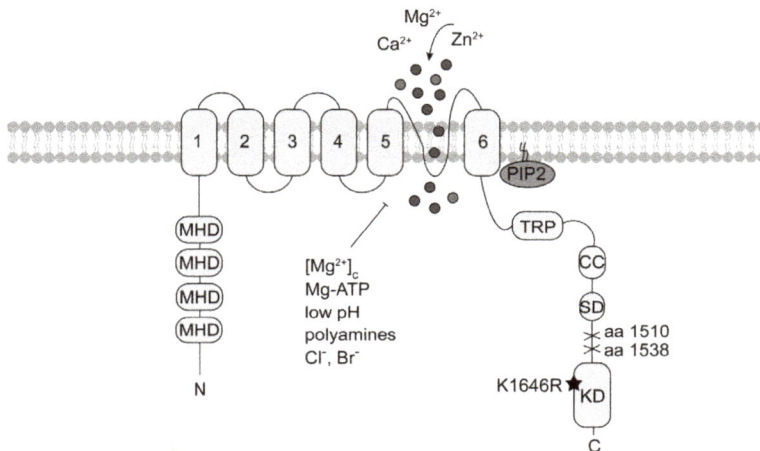

Figure 1. TRPM7 topology. Each TRPM7 protein consists of six transmembrane segments (1 to 6) with the channel pore located between segment 5 and 6. Within the N-terminus are melastatin homology domains (MHD), characteristic for TRPM family members. The cytoplasmic C-terminus contains a transient receptor potential domain (TRP), a coiled-coil domain (CC) and a kinase substrate domain (SD) upstream the atypical α-type serine/threonine protein kinase domain (KD). Mutation at the catalytic side of the kinase (K1646R) abolishes kinase activity without affecting current activity. Deletion of the KD at different amino acids (aa) results in either enhanced or reduced current activity. The black star indicates the location of the point mutation, crosses mark the kinase deletion. TRPM7 is negatively regulated by depletion of phosphatidylinositol 4,5-bisphosphate (PIP$_2$), physiologic free cytosolic magnesium concentrations $[Mg^{2+}]_c$, Mg-ATP, polyamines, low pH and chloride (Cl$^-$) and bromide (Br$^-$) concentrations.

TRPM7 kinase requires Mn^{2+} or Mg^{2+} for its activity and uses mainly Mg-ATP for phosphorylation [22]. Massive auto-phosphorylation of TRPM7 increases kinase activity and substrate recognition [33–36]. Considering the ubiquitous expression of TRPM7, it is not surprising that the protein has a fundamental and non-redundant role in cellular physiology [1,37]. It is involved in processes as diverse as proliferation, growth, migration, apoptosis, differentiation and exocytosis [38]. Tissue-specific deletion of TRPM7 in thymocytes or macrophages, as well as inactivation of the kinase activity (*Trpm7*$^{R/R}$) in mice, highlight the importance of this unique signalling protein for an operating immune system that is still kept in check [20,28,39].

2. The Channel-Kinase TRPM7 in Immune Cell Signalling

2.1. TRPM7 Kinase Regulates Mast Cell Reactivity

Mast cells are associated with the progression of different pathologies such as immediate and delayed hypersensitivity reactions, arthritis, atherosclerosis, heart failure, as well as neuroinflammatory diseases [40–42]. Upon stimulation, mast cells release granules, filled with inflammatory mediators such as histamine, proteases, cytokines and growth factors [43,44]. Mast cells are present in all organs in close proximity to blood vessels, neurons and lymphatic vessels, thus disseminating local inflammatory signals [40]. While classically, mast cells are activated via crosslinking of the IgE receptor ($F_c\varepsilon$RI) upon antigen binding [45], their activation can be triggered by many other stimuli including toll-like receptor (TLR) ligands, complement and neuropeptides. Receptor stimulation in mast cells leads to a network of stimulatory and inhibitory signals [44] encoded via intricate Ca^{2+} signalling events [46,47]. Store operated Ca^{2+} entry is essential for mast cell activation in vitro and in vivo [48,49]. Recently, TRPM7 has been implicated in receptor-induced Ca^{2+} release as well as store-operated Ca^{2+} entry [9,12]. In primary human lung mast cells (HLMCs) and in the human mast cell lines, LAD2 and HMC-1, TRPM7 expression and function was shown to be essential for cell survival. Using adenoviral-mediated knock-down of TRPM7 in HLMC or HMC-1 authors observed enhanced cell death, which was not rescued by extracellular Mg^{2+} supplementation [50]. First indications that TRPM7 is involved in degranulation processes and release of cytokines in rat bone marrow-derived mast cells (BMMCs) were gained in 2014. TRPM7 mRNA expression levels were significantly higher in asthmatic rat BMMCs than in controls. Genetic or pharmacological inhibition of TRPM7 significantly decreased β-hexosaminidase activity and secretion of histamine as well as the release of the pro-inflammatory cytokines IL-6, IL-13 and TNF-α in the asthmatic group compared to the control group. Authors concluded that inhibition of TRPM7 currents reduces mast cell degranulation and cytokine release [51]. However, functional TRPM7 channel or kinase activities were not shown. The pharmacological antagonist used to inhibit TRPM7, 2-Aminoethoxydiphenyl Borate (2-APB), supposedly only blocks channel and not kinase activity but has various off-target effects. Importantly, at the applied concentrations (100–200 μM) 2-APB blocks store operated Ca^{2+} entry (SOCE) via inhibition of Ca^{2+} release activated calcium (CRAC) channels [52]. Thus, it is possible that observed 2-APB effects were in fact not mediated by TRPM7 but SOCE. Authors, however, confirm the reduction in β-hexaminidase activity as well as in histamine and cytokine release, using a lentiviral siRNA-mediated knock-down of TRPM7 in primary BMMCs [51]. Nonetheless, the question remained, whether kinase and/or channel activity were responsible for the observed phenotype. As kinase-deficient *Trpm7*$^{R/R}$ mutant mouse mast cells showed normal current amplitudes but no kinase activity, this model allowed the independent study of TRPM7 channel versus kinase moieties in mast cells [32]. Utilizing the two TRPM7 kinase mutant mouse models (*Trpm7*$^{+/\Delta k}$, *Trpm7*$^{R/R}$), it was shown that the kinase regulated G protein-coupled receptor-activated histamine release, independently of channel activity. TRPM7 kinase activity, moreover, regulated Ca^{2+}-sensitivity of G protein-triggered mast cell degranulation. TRPM7 kinase-deficiency resulted in suppressed IgE-dependent exocytosis and slower cellular degranulation rates. Besides, extracellular Mg^{2+} was necessary to guarantee regulated IgE-induced exocytosis. Authors concluded that the TRPM7 kinase activity controls murine mast cell degranulation and histamine release independently of TRPM7 channel function [32]. Thus, TRPM7 might inflict its immune-modulatory role on mast cells via its kinase domain.

2.2. TRPM7 in Neutrophil Migration

Neutrophils, the most abundant leukocytes in the blood, are one of the key players of the innate immune system, contributing to the clearance of acute inflammation and bacterial infection [53]. During acute inflammation neutrophils are one of the first responding cells. The signalling cascades triggered after neutrophil activation start with migration of neutrophils towards the inflammatory site. The cascade ends with elimination of pathogens via secretion of chemokines, which attract other leukocytes, phagocytosis to maintain tissue homeostasis and degranulation and release of neutrophil extracellular traps (NETs) to prevent the spread of the infection. It is well established that Ca^{2+} signalling is pivotal for the recruitment cascade and activation of neutrophils, highlighting the importance of ion channels for neutrophil function [54,55]. TRPM7 channel activity has been implicated as a regulator of cell migration by facilitating Ca^{2+} oscillations [56–58]. Using a human neutrophil cell line, it was shown that TRPM7 is recruited into lipid rafts in a CD147-dependent manner. Knock-down of CD147, a glycoprotein required for neutrophil recruitment and chemotaxis, caused significant decrease in lipid raft localization of TRPM7. Thus, TRPM7 was suggested to be involved in the CD147-triggered Ca^{2+}-induced chemotaxis, adhesion and invasiveness of human neutrophils [59]. However, Wang and colleagues did not show functional TRPM7 ion channel activity and one needs to keep in mind that neutrophil-like cell lines are controversially discussed regarding their comparability to primary neutrophils [53]. During acute lung injury (ALI), the permeability of the alveolar-capillary membrane is increased, which in turn can lead to migration of neutrophils [60]. A septic rat model treated with salvianolic B showed that sepsis-induced ALI was reduced due to decreased levels of TRMP6 and TRPM7 mRNA in lung tissue, potentially linking TRPM7 to neutrophil migration and infiltration [61]. As patients with inherited neutrophil deficiencies suffer from severe infections that are often fatal, underscoring the importance of this cell type in immune defence, it is critical to gain a better understanding of the role of TRPM7 channel and kinase activities in the signalling cascades triggering neutrophil migration [53].

2.3. TRPM7 Guides Macrophage Activation and Polarization

Blood monocytes and tissue macrophages are major components of innate immunity, strategically positioned throughout the body tissues to orchestrate inflammatory processes. Similar to neutrophils, they maintain tissue homeostasis via phagocytosis of dead cells, debris or potentially harmful pathogens. As antigen presenting cells they are able to activate and coordinate the adaptive immune system [62,63]. Various TRP proteins have been associated with macrophage-mediated inflammatory responses [64]. TRPM7 has also been linked to the activation and proliferation of monocytes and macrophages [29,65–68]. However, controversies on the role of TRPM7 for macrophage activation in response to LPS remain [39,68]. On the one hand, TRPM7 channel activity was suggested to be essential for macrophage proliferation and polarization into the alternate or anti-inflammatory M2-subtype [68]. LPS and co-stimulatory cytokines IFN-γ (pro-inflammatory M1-type) or IL-4 and IL-13 (anti-inflammatory M2-type) trigger the polarization of macrophages [69,70]. Interestingly, the activity of TRPM7 increased significantly in response to stimulation with IL-4. The TRPM7 inhibitor NS8593 [71] blocked IL-4 and M-CSF induced proliferation and reduced the inhibitory effect of IL-4 or M-CSF on the LPS-induced expression of the pro-inflammatory cytokine TNF-α, thus, counteracting the differentiation into the M2 subtype [68]. On the other hand, more recently, TRPM7 channel activity has been implicated in macrophage activation in response to LPS and LPS-induced peritonitis [39]. In TRPM7-deficient macrophages (*Trpm7$^{fl/fl}$*(LysM Cre)) IL-1β secretion was significantly reduced and also the gene expression upon LPS stimulation was altered, indicating a key function of TRPM7 in the activation process of macrophages. In addition, it was found that TRPM7 is pivotal for the endocytosis of LPS-TLR4-CD14 signalling complexes with TRPM7-deficient macrophages showing significantly reduced internalization of TLR4 and CD14. Schappe et al. demonstrated that these defects upon LPS stimulation were due to diminished TRPM7-mediated Ca^{2+} influx. They speculate that TRPM7 not only controls TLR4 internalization but also regulates downstream IRF3 and NFκB signalling by mediating cytosolic Ca^{2+} elevations. Moreover, in a LPS-dependent model of peritonitis, *Trpm7$^{fl/fl}$* (LysM Cre) mice had decreased serum cytokine levels after LPS treatment, preventing pathological inflammation. Specifically, the expression levels of *Tnfa* and *Il1b* were significantly reduced, resulting in a diminished recruitment of immune cells into the peritoneum. Thus, *Trpm7$^{fl/fl}$* (LysM Cre) mice were protected from the development of LPS-induced peritonitis. Consequently, it was suggested that TRPM7 channel blockade could be beneficial for the treatment of chronic infections or septic shock [39]. The difference in the macrophage response to LPS might depend on different protocols used. However, to date there is no consensus, whether LPS induces Ca^{2+} elevations resulting in macrophage activation. Several studies have found no changes in cytosolic Ca^{2+} concentrations in response to LPS treatment in macrophages [72,73].

The role of TRPM7 kinase activity in macrophage or dendritic cell function is far less understood. TRPM7 kinase-deficient mice (*Trpm7$^{R/R}$*) show no defects in percentages of macrophages [29]. Also,

Trpm7$^{R/R}$ CD11c$^+$ dendritic cells develop normally and display regular major histocompatibility complex II (MHCII) and integrin expression [20].

2.4. TRPM7 Affects Lymphocyte Functions

Lymphocytes forming the adaptive or acquired immune response are activated and regulated by cells of the innate immune system, that is, macrophages and provide immunologic memory [74]. Antigen specific lymphocytes respond to pathogens with activation induced proliferation and clonal expansion. This temporal proliferative burst is terminated with a return to cell quiescence and eventual cell death. The autonomous timing of proliferation ensures an appropriate response magnitude whilst preventing uncontrolled expansion. Thus, a detailed understanding of the regulatory principles governing lymphocyte activation, proliferation, differentiation and survival is essential to a cohesive picture of the immune system homeostasis [75].

2.4.1. TRPM7 Kinase Regulates Intracellular Calcium Signals and Proliferation in Lymphocytes

Upon T cell receptor (TCR) or B cell receptor (BCR) stimulation, phospholipase C (PLC) is activated, catalysing the hydrolysis of PIP$_2$ into diacylglycerol (DAG) and inositol (1,4,5) triphosphate (IP$_3$). Subsequently, IP$_3$ triggers Ca^{2+}-release from the endoplasmatic reticulum (ER) Ca^{2+}-store via the IP$_3$-receptor (IP$_3$R). Upon depletion of Ca^{2+} from the ER lumen, the stromal interaction molecule (STIM) translocates to the plasma membrane and triggers SOCE via CRAC channels. This prolonged increase in intracellular Ca^{2+} concentrations is essential for the nuclear factor of activated T cells (NFAT) to translocate into the nucleus and induce transcription of genes essential for cell proliferation and clonal expansion (Figure 2) [38].

Recently, Romagnani et al. revealed that TRPM7 kinase-dead (*Trpm7$^{R/R}$*) CD4$^+$ T cells show slightly but significantly decreased Ca^{2+} signals upon stimulation with plate-bound anti-CD3/CD28 antibodies, whereas basal cytosolic Ca^{2+} concentrations ([Ca^{2+}]$_c$) were unaltered [20]. These experiments were performed using extracellular 2 mM Ca^{2+} concentrations. Similarly, Beesetty et al. showed that receptor-mediated Ca^{2+} signalling was significantly diminished in *Trpm7$^{R/R}$* T cells using anti-CD3 crosslinking in 0.4 mM extracellular Ca^{2+} levels, and differences in 2 mM Ca^{2+} concentrations were even more pronounced. Nevertheless, basal [Ca^{2+}]$_c$ was also unchanged. In addition, SOCE was decreased in *Trpm7$^{R/R}$* splenocytes upon pre-treatment with phorbol 12-myristate 13-acetate (PMA) and ionomycin, while there was no difference in ER-store Ca^{2+} content. Basal [Ca^{2+}]$_c$, however, were lower in PMA and ionomycin pre-activated *Trpm7$^{R/R}$* T cells compared to wild-type (WT) [10]. These results are in line with recent studies, suggesting that TRPM7 regulates store-operated Ca^{2+} entry. Faouzi et al. linked TRPM7 channel and kinase moieties to direct involvement in SOCE. *Trpm7*-deficient chicken B lymphocytes exhibited down-regulation of SOCE, which was mainly attributed to missing kinase activity [12]. Moreover, it was shown that TRPM7 channels seem to be essential to sustain the Ca^{2+} content of intracellular stores in resting cells. Authors speculate that TRPM7 kinase may directly phosphorylate STIM2, thereby influencing Ca^{2+} entry via SOCE, yet found no effect on phosphorylation of STIM1 or STIM2 [12]. The first indication that TRPM7 activity is involved in SOCE was found in 2005. Matsushita and colleagues reported that SOCE, in response to thapsigargin-induced store depletion, was increased in HEK293 cells transfected with WT TRPM7 but did not change in cells transfected with a kinase domain-deleted *TRPM7$^{\Delta KD}$* (aa 1-1599) mutant construct, compared to mock transfected controls. However, the described *TRPM7$^{\Delta KD}$* mutant displayed almost no current activity, leaving the question of the role of TRPM7 channel versus kinase moieties unanswered [76]. Also, the impact of TRPM7 kinase activity on T cell proliferation efficiency, following Ca^{2+} signalling events, remains controversial. While Romagnani et al. discovered that *Trpm7$^{R/R}$* T cells proliferate independently of their kinase activity in response to TCR stimulation (plate-bound anti-CD3/CD28) [20], Beesetty et al. showed a reduced T cell proliferation, in response to PMA and ionomycin treatment during the first 24 hours, which was compensated for after 48 and 72 hours [10]. As the reported reduction in Ca^{2+} signalling was very small, using plate-bound anti-CD3/CD28 antibodies, it is not surprising that *Trpm7R/R* T cell proliferation was not altered [20]. The decrease in SOCE upon pre-treatment with PMA ionomycin in *Trpm7R/R* splenocytes however, was much more pronounced, resulting in reduced proliferation [10]. The combination of PMA—directly activating protein kinase C—with the calcium ionophore ionomycin, which increases $[Ca^{2+}]_c$, is a fast and powerful stimulus, circumventing classical receptor activation. Thus the observed alterations in proliferation depend on the experimental conditions used, suggesting that TRPM7 kinase might influence proliferation depending on the stimuli and that receptor-operated mechanisms might be compensating [10,20]. Summarizing, these studies highlight a potential role of TRPM7 kinase activity in regulating Ca^{2+} signalling and subsequent activation processes in T cells and suggest TRPM as key regulator of the temporal proliferative burst. However, how exactly TRPM7 channel and kinase activities interplay to regulate Ca^{2+} signalling and subsequent proliferation in T lymphocytes still needs further investigation.

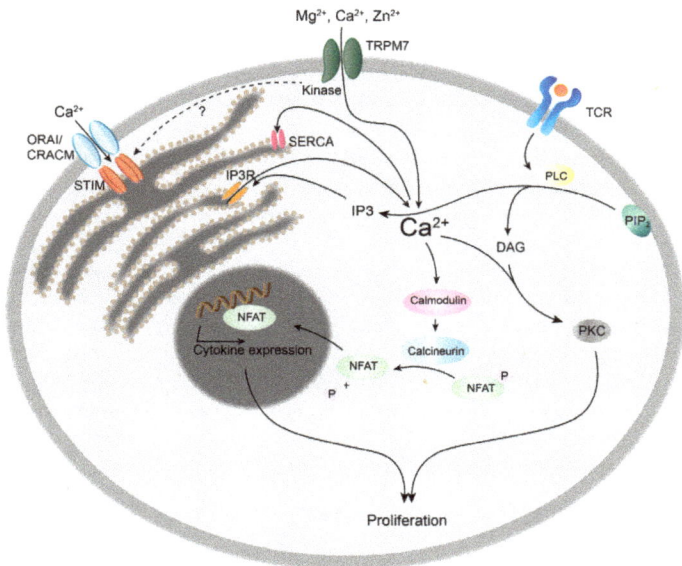

Figure 2. Role of TRPM7 kinase in calcium signalling and proliferation of T cells. Upon T cell receptor (TCR) binding, phospholipase C (PLC) is activated and hydrolyses phosphatidylinositol 4,5-biphosphate (PIP$_2$) to inositol 1,4,5-triphosphate (IP$_3$) and diacylglycerol (DAG). DAG in conjunction with Ca^{2+} activates protein kinase C (PKC), thus inducing cell proliferation. IP$_3$ induces Ca^{2+} release from the endoplasmic reticulum (ER) via IP$_3$ receptor (IP$_3$R), followed by the translocation of the stromal interaction molecule (STIM) to the plasma membrane. STIM triggers Ca^{2+} influx from the extracellular space via ORAI/CRACM channels. Ca^{2+} is rapidly removed from the cytosol by the sarco/endoplasmic reticulum Ca^{2+}-ATPase (SERCA), refilling the ER Ca^{2+} stores. The prolonged increase in cytosolic Ca^{2+} concentrations leads to the activation of calcineurin, resulting in the dephosphorylation and nuclear translocation of nuclear factor of activated T cells (NFAT) and subsequent cytokine expression, e.g., interleukin 2 (IL-2), triggering clonal expansion of T cells.

2.4.2. TRPM7 in Cell Growth, Activation and Development of B Cells

A *Trpm7*-deficient B-lymphocyte cell line (chicken DT40 cells) exhibits a selective defect to proliferate in regular media but can do so in media supplemented with 10 mM Mg^{2+}. After 24 h in regular media, TRPM7-deficient B cells accumulated in the G0/G1 phase of the cell cycle and were reduced in average cell size. Authors conclude that TRPM7-deficient cells display a defect in growth, failing to increase in size and mass. This defect was attributed to the lack of signalling downstream of phosphoinositide 3-kinase (PI3-K) with impaired mammalian target of rapamycin complex 1 (mTORC1) signalling, ribosomal S6 kinase (S6K) and Akt activation, whereas ERK phosphorylation was unaltered. Interestingly, overexpression of constitutively active AKT was not sufficient to overcome this growth defect. However, provision of a heterologous sustained PI3K signal, utilizing a constitutively active form of the catalytic subunit of PI3K, p110α, counteracted the failure of TRPM7-deficient cells to grow and proliferate in regular media. Thus TRPM7 was positioned alongside PI3K signalling as a central regulator of lymphocyte growth [77]. Moreover, TRPM7 was shown to be essential for cell-cycle progression, as *Trpm7*-deficient DT40 B cells showed an up-regulation of $p27^{kip}$, a key cell cycle regulator which blocks the transition from G_0 to S phase. The quiescence was reversible and rescued by Mg^{2+} supplementation or TRPM7 overexpression [78]. Utilizing the same *Trpm7*-deficient DT40 B cell line and a DT40 cell line expressing the kinase-dead mutant (K1648R), it was recently shown that TRPM7 is essential for early events of B cell activation through both kinase and channel activities. TRPM7 channel activity controlled antigen uptake and presentation to T cells [27]. Previously, TRPM7 kinase has been suggested to regulate non-muscle myosin IIA filament stability as well as actomyosin contractility by phosphorylating myosin IIA heavy chain [25], while the Mg^{2+} influx through the channel was also correlated with maintenance of myosin II-dependent cytoskeletal organization [79]. TIRF microscopy revealed that expression of TRPM7 in B cells controlled actin dynamics and slowed antigen internalization, resulting in prolonged B cell signalling. Authors conclude that TRPM7 signalling is essential for B cell affinity maturation and antibody production [27]. Moreover, recent findings indicate that TRPM7 expression is required for murine B cell development. Mice with tissue specific deletion of TRPM7 in B cells failed to generate peripheral B cells due to a developmental defect at the pro-B cell stage and increased apoptosis of B cell precursors in the bone marrow. In vitro the development of *Trpm7*-deficient B cells could be rescued via Mg^{2+}-supplementation. Whereas, TRPM7 kinase-deficiency did not affect the development of B cells in the bone marrow or the percentage of peripheral B cells. Interestingly, the deletion of the entire TRPM7 protein in B cells lead to increased percentages of neutrophils, eosinophils and monocytes in the spleen of mutant mice, compared to WT which could be attributed to the primary lack of B cells [80]. Thus, TRPM7 channel and kinase activities seem unique and non-redundant for proper B cell function.

2.4.3. TRPM7 in Murine T Cell Development, Differentiation and Transcriptional Regulation

In murine T lymphocytes TRPM7 is required for thymic development and thymopoiesis. Conditional knock-out of *Trpm7* in the T cell lineage was shown to disrupt thymopoiesis, with thymocytes remaining in the double negative ($CD4^-CD8^-$) state and resulted in altered chemokine and cytokine expression profiles [28], indicating that TRPM7 channel and/or kinase are important for T cell function. Using the homozygous kinase-dead *Trpm7*$^{R/R}$ mouse model, recently it was shown that TRPM7 kinase activity is not essential for thymopoiesis [10,20]. However, the enzymatic activity of TRPM7 is required for intra-epithelial T cell homeostasis. *Trpm7*$^{R/R}$ mice almost completely lack gut intraepithelial T lymphocytes (IELs) [20]. Intestinal IELs represent a first line of defence within the largest immune organ of our body [81]. Numerous effector T lymphocytes differentiate in the intestine, from where they migrate into the periphery [82,83]. Thus, understanding the gut immune system, harbouring ~70% of the total lymphocytes in the human body, is of utmost importance [81,84] for regulating of immune homeostasis. Analysis of the percentage of remaining *TRPM7*$^{R/R}$ IELs revealed a significant reduction in pro-inflammatory T_H17 cell subsets, while the percentage of anti-inflammatory T_{reg} cells was unaffected compared to WT. Consistently, the in vitro differentiation of naïve *Trpm7*$^{R/R}$ T cells into T_H17 cells was also compromised, while the T_{reg} cell differentiation proceeded unperturbed. These findings were coherent with the robust reduction of IL-17 concentration in serum from *Trpm7*$^{R/R}$ mice [20]. As TGF-β/SMAD pathways are crucial for the polarization of $CD4^+$ T cells into T_H17 cells [85], it is likely that the TGF-β/SMAD signalling pathway is affected by TRPM7 kinase activity (Figure 3). Notably, Western Blot analysis of *Trpm7*$^{R/R}$ naïve $CD4^+$

T cells treated with TGF-β1 revealed a significant reduction in SMAD2 phosphorylation, while SMAD3 phosphorylation was unaltered. Analysis of the TGF-β1-induced SMAD2 translocation was also significantly reduced in *Trpm7$^{R/R}$* naïve CD4$^+$ T cells. Thus, authors conclude that the TRPM7 kinase regulates T$_H$17 cell differentiation via TGF-β/SMAD2 dependent pathways. An in vitro kinase assay using highly purified recombinant TRPM7 kinase, SMAD2, as well as C-terminally truncated SMAD2 revealed that TRPM7 phosphorylates SMAD2 in a dose dependent manner but fails to phosphorylate the truncated SMAD2. Thus, the C-terminal Ser465/467-motif of SMAD2 was identified as a novel substrate for the TRPM7 kinase [20]. The upregulation of the integrin αE, also known as CD103, enables T cells to migrate into the gut epithelium [86,87] and is dependent on SMAD2 TGF-β/SMAD2 signalling cascades [88], which was significantly impaired in TGF-β-treated *Trpm7$^{R/R}$* T cells. Using a chromatin immunoprecipitation (ChIP) assay, the authors demonstrated a defective binding of SMAD2 to the *Itgae* (CD103) promoter in *Trpm7$^{R/R}$* T cells in response to TGF-β. Consequently, the expression of the gene encoding for CD103, *Itgae*, was also significantly reduced in primary *Trpm7$^{R/R}$* IELs as well as in response to TGF-β and T cell receptor co-stimulation in naïve *Trpm7$^{R/R}$* T cells. Consistently, the expression of the signature transcription factor for T$_H$17 cells, *Rorc*, as well as the cytokine IL-17, which both depend on SMAD2 phosphorylation and translocation into the nucleus, were also impaired in *Trpm7$^{R/R}$* T cells (Figure 3). Interestingly, the CD103 expression in *Trpm7$^{R/R}$* CD11c$^+$ dendritic cells was normal, compared to WT [20]. If or how TRPM7 kinase is triggered via TGF-β stimulation in T cells is still under investigation. One emerging concept, however, could involve a constitutively active TRPM7 kinase that phosphorylates SMAD2 once it is anchored to the plasma membrane following TGF-β receptor activation (Figure 3). Importantly, this selective defect of SMAD2 signalling in T cells culminating in reduced pro-inflammatory T$_H$17 cell differentiation, while leaving anti-inflammatory T$_{reg}$ cell differentiation unaffected (Figure 4A,B), highlights the essential function of TRPM7 kinase in immune homeostasis [20]. These results suggest that TRPM7 kinase might serve as molecular switch from pro-inflammatory to anti-inflammatory milieu and highlights the potential of TRPM7 kinase inhibition for the treatment of pro-inflammatory diseases.

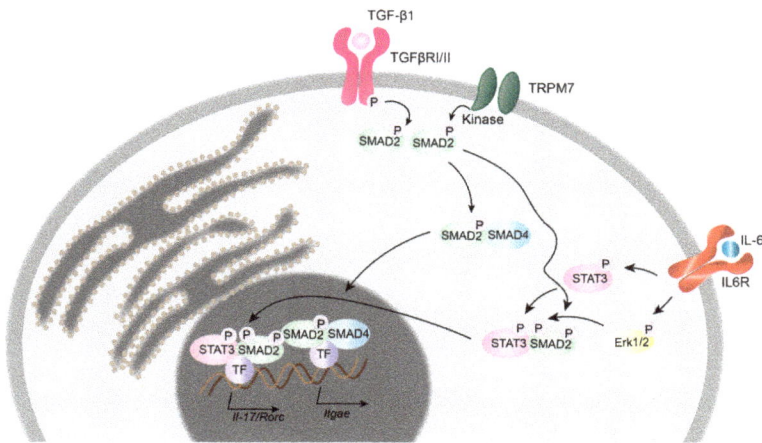

Figure 3. TRPM7 kinase in T cell signalling and transcriptional regulation. Upon binding of tumour growth factor β1 (TGF-β1), the TGF-β receptor complex (TGFβRI/II) initiates the phosphorylation of the c-terminal SXS-motif of SMAD2. Results gained from TRPM7 kinase deficient murine T cells suggest an additional mechanism by which the TRPM7 kinase phosphorylates SMAD2 directly, once it is anchored to the plasma membrane. Phosphorylated SMAD2 interacts with SMAD4 and promotes the transcription of *Itgae*, *Il-17* and *Rorc* genes. The interleukin 6 (IL-6) dependent STAT3 as well as Erk1/2 phosphorylation pathway is unaltered in TRPM7 kinase deficient murine T cells.

To date, very little is known regarding the role of TRPM7 in human lymphocytes. Pharmacological inhibition of TRPM7 in a human T cell line results in growth arrest and reduced proliferation [89]. TRPM7 was suggested to be involved in the migration of activated human T cells, where it is located in the uropod, in conjunction with the calcium-activated potassium channel, $K_{Ca}3.1$, facilitating T cell migration. Knock-down via siRNA resulted in a significant reduction in number and velocity of migrating cells [90]. Moreover, TRPM7 was associated with TNF-α-induced necroptosis in T cells. Knock-down of TRPM7 in a T cell line protected it from necroptosis [91]. Nonetheless, it will be necessary to determine if the observed crucial functions of TRPM7 kinase and channel moieties in murine lymphocytes also applies to human counterparts.

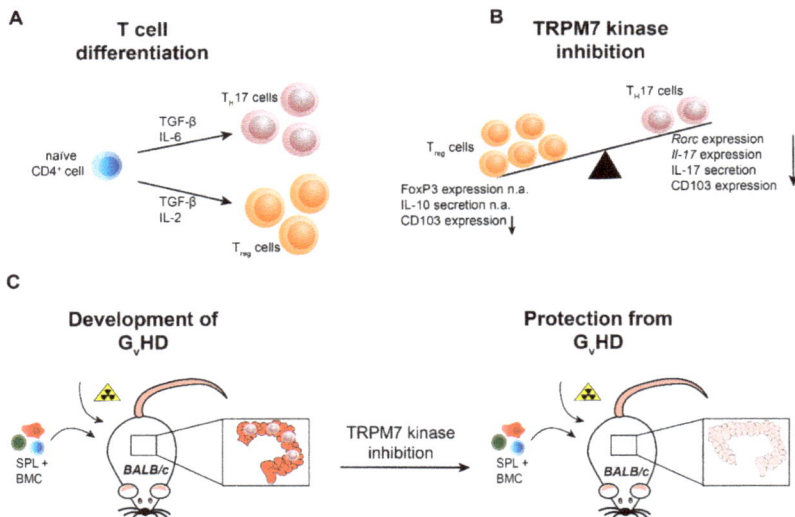

Figure 4. TRPM7 kinase is essential for T cell differentiation into the pro-inflammatory T_H17 cell type and the development of graft versus host disease. (**A**) Naïve CD4$^+$ T cells differentiate into pro-inflammatory T_H17 cells in the presence of TGF-β and IL-6. For the differentiation into anti-inflammatory regulatory T cells (T_{regs}), the cytokines TGF-β and IL-2 are required. (**B**) Genetic inactivation of TRPM7 kinase activity (*Trpm7$^{R/R}$*) results in reduced T_H17 cell differentiation, indicated via diminished *Rorc* and *Il-17* mRNA expression as well as IL-17 serum levels, while T_{reg} cell differentiation, evident via FoxP3 expression and IL-10 serum levels, is unaltered. In addition, integrin αE (CD103) expression is reduced in TRPM7 kinase deficient T cells. (**C**) Transplantation of bone marrow cells (BMC, C57BL/6) in conjunction with splenocytes (SPL, C57BL/6) triggers the development of graft versus host disease (G_VHD) in lethally irradiated mice with different genetic background (BALB/c), manifesting in massive tissue destruction of the intestine but also lung and skin tissues. TRPM7 kinase deficient BMC and SPL transplantation does not induce inflammation in the intestine and ameliorates or even prevents disease progression, suggesting TRPM7 kinase inhibition as valid tool for the treatment of G_VHD. n.a. (not altered).

3. TRPM7-Mediated Hematologic and Inflammatory Diseases

3.1. Hypomagnesaemia and TRPM7 Kinase in Delayed-Type Hypersensitivity Reactions

Mg^{2+} is a vital mineral macronutrient. Considering that low serum Mg^{2+} levels have also been linked to memory decline, neurodegenerative diseases, decrease in muscle performance, heart failure, certain cancers, autoimmune diseases and allergic reactions, it is of critical importance to further identify the mechanisms regulating the availability of this macronutrient [92,93]. Recently, it was shown that TRPM7, in conjunction with its sister channel TRPM6, regulates systemic Mg^{2+} homeostasis via absorption of Mg^{2+} in the intestine [94]. The interconnection between nutrient metabolism and the immune system occurs at many levels, ranging from endocrine signalling to direct sensing of nutrients by immune cells [95]. Interestingly, adult *Trpm6*-deficient mice suffered from hypomagnesaemia and displayed a degeneration of many lymphoid organs. The thymus of mutant mice was only rudimentary present with an essentially undistinguishable cortex region. Also, the red pulp of the spleens of *Trpm6*-deficient mice was substantially reduced. Dietary Mg^{2+} supplementation rescued these phenotypes, indicating that indeed hypomagnesaemia was responsible for the observed deficits [94].

While homozygous genetic deletion of the ubiquitously expressed TRPM7 kinase domain in mice leads to early embryonic lethality, heterozygous *Trpm7+/Δk* mice are viable and develop a severe hypomagnesaemia upon Mg^{2+} restriction, leading to increased mortality, susceptibility to seizures as well as prevalence for allergic hypersensitivity [4]. It is known that low, systemic Mg^{2+} levels correlate with cell-extrinsic enhancement of systemic inflammatory and allergic responses [96]. To evaluate the level of delayed-type hypersensitivity responses in *Trpm7+/Δk* mice, oxazolone sensitization experiments were performed. *Trpm7+/Δk* mice displayed an elevated oxazolone-induced contact hypersensitivity, compared to WT [4]. Interestingly, homozygous mice with genetic inactivation of TRPM7 kinase activity, via a point mutation within the active site of the kinase, *Trpm7R/R*, were viable and did not develop hypomagnesaemia or hypersensitivity responses. In fact, they even displayed reduced oxazolone-induced delayed type hypersensitivity responses [30]. Their systemic Mg^{2+} and Ca^{2+} levels were similar to WT, as the channel function was not affected by the point mutation [29,30,32]. Since allergic reactions are triggered by mast cell-mediated histamine release, the role of TRPM7 in mast cell degranulation and histamine release was studied using *Trpm7+/+*, *Trpm7+/Δk* and *Trpm7R/R* mice. As reported, degranulation and histamine release proceeded independently of TRPM7 channel function. However, as extracellular Mg^{2+} was essential to control unperturbed IgE-DNP-dependent exocytosis and removal of Mg^{2+} exaggerated histamine release, the observed differences in hypersensitivity responses could be attributed to the different systemic Mg^{2+} levels in *Trpm7+/Δk* versus *Trpm7R/R* mice. G-protein-coupled receptor stimulation revealed strong suppression of histamine release in both kinase-deficient mast cells (*Trpm7+/Δk* and *Trpm7R/R*), whereas removal of extracellular Mg^{2+} caused the phenotype to revert, suggesting that the TRPM7 kinase activity regulates murine mast cell degranulation by changing its sensitivity to intracellular Ca^{2+} and extracellular Mg^{2+} concentrations [32]. Thus, TRPM7 might inflict its immune-modulatory role by sensing cations via its kinase domain. To date, little is known about activation mechanisms or physiologic substrates of TRPM7 kinase.

3.2. The TRPM7 Channel-Kinase in Arterial Thrombosis and Stroke

TRPM7 kinase has been suggested to regulate myosin IIB filament stability as well as actomyosin contractility by phosphorylating myosin IIA [25]. Recently, it was shown that TRPM7 channel activity also affects myosin IIA activity independently of kinase function. In conditional *Trpm7*-deficient mice (*Trpm7fl/fl-Pf4Cre*), TRPM7 modulates platelet function via regulation of cellular Mg^{2+} homeostasis and cytoskeletal myosin IIA activity. Members of a human pedigree with mutations in *TRPM7* (p.C721G), causing disrupted channel activity, suffer from macrothrombocytopenia and arterial fibrosis. The defect in platelet biogenesis is mainly caused by cytoskeletal alterations resulting in impaired pro-platelet formation by *TRPM7*-deficient megakaryocytes, which is rescued by Mg^{2+} supplementation [79]. In contrast, homozygous kinase-dead *TRPM7R/R* mice show normal platelet counts, size and morphology, thus suggesting that the lack of TRPM7 channel rather than its kinase activity accounts for the macrothrombocytopenia in *Trpm7fl/fl-Pf4Cre* mice [79]. However, the kinase controls platelet function in arterial thrombosis via regulation of Ca^{2+} responses, Syk and PLCγ2 activity. Bone marrow (BM) chimeras revealed that the kinase is not only relevant for platelet function, as both, recipients of WT BM as well as WT recipient of *Trpm7R/R* BM, developed reduction in infarct size and improvement of neurological and motoric functions in an in vivo transient middle cerebral artery occlusion (tMCAO) model. Thus, TRPM7 kinase activity in neurons and glial cells may also be critical for the progression of ischemic brain infarction [11]. These findings highlight TRPM7 kinase as a potential target for the treatment of thrombosis thus protecting from stroke or myocardial infarction.

3.3. TRPM7 Kinase Signalling Supports Graft versus Host Reactions

Graft versus host disease (G$_V$HD) is the most common side effect of an allogeneic hematopoietic stem cell transplantation (HCST). In this immune reaction the donor T cells recognize the patients human leukocyte antigen (HLA) as foreign, causing an inflammatory cascade [97]. G$_V$HD can be divided into acute and chronic, depending on the time of diagnosis [98]. In acute G$_V$HD the pre-transplant radiation may cause tissue damage in the host, leading to the activation of antigen presenting cells followed by activation of the donor T cells. This can lead to severe damage of liver, skin, mucosa and the gastrointestinal tract [99]. All in all, G$_V$HD causes 15–30% of death after HCST, highlighting the importance of enhancing the understanding of this disease and finding improved treatments. Recently, it was shown that TRPM7 kinase activity promotes gut colonization by T cells in acute G$_V$HD. During this process, naïve donor CD4$^+$ T cells recognize alloantigens on antigen presenting cells in target organs, including the intestine (Figure 4C).

The role of different T$_H$ subsets and signalling pathways in the pathogenesis of G$_V$HD is incompletely understood. To address whether defective intestinal colonization by CD4$^+$ T cells lacking TRPM7 kinase activity could affect acute G$_V$HD, the bone marrow (BM) of BALB/c WT mice was lethally irradiated and replaced by bone marrow (BM) cells from WT C57BL/6 mice together with WT or *TRPM7$^{R/R}$* splenocytes. As expected, injection of WT splenocytes resulted in massive intestinal damage and most mice died within 35 days after transplantation. In contrast, injection of *TRPM7$^{R/R}$* splenocytes did not cause intestinal damage and resulted in a dramatically increased survival of these mice within the first 60 days after transplantation [20]. These results unravel a fundamental role of TRPM7 kinase in T cell function and suggest a therapeutic potential of kinase inhibitors in averting acute G$_V$HD.

4. Conclusions

The involvement of TRPM7 in the pathogenesis of deregulated immune responses highlights the necessity for novel pharmacological tools. TRPM7 represents a new promising drug target for the treatment of pro-inflammatory diseases and hypersensitivity. It is tempting to speculate that pharmacological modulation of TRPM7 may reinstate immune system homeostasis. Particularly appealing is the fact that TRPM7 kinase-deficiency in mice does not result in an obvious phenotype and only moderately affects haemostasis. Thus, TRPM7 kinase inhibition should not cause major side effects. Therefore, new TRPM7 kinase inhibitors and novel kinase substrates have to be identified.

Author Contributions: W.N. performed literature search, wrote sections of the original draft, prepared the figures and edited the manuscript. S.Z. wrote the original draft, designed the figures and edited the manuscript.

Funding: S.Z. was supported by the Deutsche Forschungsgemeinschaft (TRR 152) and a Marie-Curie Fellowship (REA) FP7-PEOPLE-2012-CIG.

Acknowledgments: We thank Lynda Addington for critical reading of the manuscript. Images were designed using Adobe Illustrator CC.

Conflicts of Interest: The authors declare no conflict of interest.

References

1. Nadler, M.J.; Hermosura, M.C.; Inabe, K.; Perraud, A.L.; Zhu, Q.; Stokes, A.J.; Kurosaki, T.; Kinet, J.P.; Penner, R.; Scharenberg, A.M.; et al. LTRPC7 is a Mg.ATP-regulated divalent cation channel required for cell viability. *Nature* **2001**, *411*, 590–595. [CrossRef] [PubMed]
2. Monteilh-Zoller, M.K.; Hermosura, M.C.; Nadler, M.J.; Scharenberg, A.M.; Penner, R.; Fleig, A. TRPM7 provides an ion channel mechanism for cellular entry of trace metal ions. *J. Gen. Physiol.* **2003**, *121*, 49–60. [CrossRef] [PubMed]

3. Runnels, L.W.; Yue, L.; Clapham, D.E. TRP-PLIK, a bifunctional protein with kinase and ion channel activities. *Science* **2001**, *291*, 1043–1047. [CrossRef] [PubMed]

4. Ryazanova, L.V.; Rondon, L.J.; Zierler, S.; Hu, Z.; Galli, J.; Yamaguchi, T.P.; Mazur, A.; Fleig, A.; Ryazanov, A.G. TRPM7 is essential for Mg^{2+} homeostasis in mammals. *Nat. Commun.* **2010**, *1*, 109. [CrossRef] [PubMed]

5. Schmitz, C.; Perraud, A.L.; Johnson, C.O.; Inabe, K.; Smith, M.K.; Penner, R.; Kurosaki, T.; Fleig, A.; Scharenberg, A.M. Regulation of vertebrate cellular Mg^{2+} homeostasis by TRPM7. *Cell* **2003**, *114*, 191–200. [CrossRef]

6. He, Y.; Yao, G.; Savoia, C.; Touyz, R.M. Transient receptor potential melastatin 7 ion channels regulate magnesium homeostasis in vascular smooth muscle cells: Role of angiotensin II. *Circ. Res.* **2005**, *96*, 207–215. [CrossRef] [PubMed]

7. Abiria, S.A.; Krapivinsky, G.; Sah, R.; Santa-Cruz, A.G.; Chaudhuri, D.; Zhang, J.; Adstamongkonkul, P.; DeCaen, P.G.; Clapham, D.E. TRPM7 senses oxidative stress to release Zn^{2+} from unique intracellular vesicles. *Proc. Natl. Acad. Sci. USA* **2017**, *114*, E6079–E6088. [CrossRef] [PubMed]

8. Inoue, K.; Branigan, D.; Xiong, Z.G. Zinc-induced neurotoxicity mediated by transient receptor potential melastatin 7 channels. *J. Biol. Chem.* **2010**, *285*, 7430–7439. [CrossRef] [PubMed]

9. Suzuki, S.; Lis, A.; Schmitz, C.; Penner, R.; Fleig, A. The TRPM7 kinase limits receptor-induced calcium release by regulating heterotrimeric G-proteins. *Cell. Mol. Life Sci.* **2018**, *75*, 3069–3078. [CrossRef] [PubMed]

10. Beesetty, P.; Wieczerzak, K.B.; Gibson, J.N.; Kaitsuka, T.; Luu, C.T.; Matsushita, M.; Kozak, J.A. Inactivation of TRPM7 kinase in mice results in enlarged spleens, reduced T-cell proliferation and diminished store-operated calcium entry. *Sci. Rep.* **2018**, *8*, 3023. [CrossRef] [PubMed]

11. Gotru, S.K.; Chen, W.; Kraft, P.; Becker, I.C.; Wolf, K.; Stritt, S.; Zierler, S.; Hermanns, H.M.; Rao, D.; Perraud, A.L.; et al. TRPM7 Kinase Controls Calcium Responses in Arterial Thrombosis and Stroke in Mice. *Arterioscler. Thromb. Vasc. Biol.* **2018**, *38*, 344–352. [CrossRef] [PubMed]

12. Faouzi, M.; Kilch, T.; Horgen, F.D.; Fleig, A.; Penner, R. The TRPM7 channel kinase regulates store-operated calcium entry. *J. Physiol.* **2017**, *595*, 3165–3180. [CrossRef] [PubMed]

13. Demeuse, P.; Penner, R.; Fleig, A. TRPM7 channel is regulated by magnesium nucleotides via its kinase domain. *J. Gen. Physiol.* **2006**, *127*, 421–434. [CrossRef] [PubMed]

14. Kozak, J.A.; Matsushita, M.; Nairn, A.C.; Cahalan, M.D. Charge screening by internal pH and polyvalent cations as a mechanism for activation, inhibition, and rundown of TRPM7/MIC channels. *J. Gen. Physiol.* **2005**, *126*, 499–514. [CrossRef] [PubMed]

15. Runnels, L.W.; Yue, L.; Clapham, D.E. The TRPM7 channel is inactivated by PIP_2 hydrolysis. *Nat. Cell Biol.* **2002**, *4*, 329–336. [CrossRef] [PubMed]

16. Yu, H.; Zhang, Z.; Lis, A.; Penner, R.; Fleig, A. TRPM7 is regulated by halides through its kinase domain. *Cell. Mol. Life Sci.* **2013**, *70*, 2757–2771. [CrossRef] [PubMed]

17. Romani, A.M. Cellular magnesium homeostasis. *Arch. Biochem. Biophys.* **2011**, *512*, 1–23. [CrossRef] [PubMed]

18. Chubanov, V.; Ferioli, S.; Gudermann, T. Assessment of TRPM7 functions by drug-like small molecules. *Cell Calcium* **2017**, *67*, 166–173. [CrossRef] [PubMed]

19. Ferioli, S.; Zierler, S.; Zaisserer, J.; Schredelseker, J.; Gudermann, T.; Chubanov, V. TRPM6 and TRPM7 differentially contribute to the relief of heteromeric TRPM6/7 channels from inhibition by cytosolic Mg^{2+} and Mg.ATP. *Sci. Rep.* **2017**, *7*, 8806. [CrossRef] [PubMed]

20. Romagnani, A.; Vettore, V.; Rezzonico-Jost, T.; Hampe, S.; Rottoli, E.; Nadolni, W.; Perotti, M.; Meier, M.A.; Hermanns, C.; Geiger, S.; et al. TRPM7 kinase activity is essential for T cell colonization and alloreactivity in the gut. *Nat. Commun.* **2017**, *8*, 1917. [CrossRef] [PubMed]

21. Yamaguchi, H.; Matsushita, M.; Nairn, A.C.; Kuriyan, J. Crystal structure of the atypical protein kinase domain of a TRP channel with phosphotransferase activity. *Mol. Cell* **2001**, *7*, 1047–1057. [CrossRef]

22. Ryazanova, L.V.; Dorovkov, M.V.; Ansari, A.; Ryazanov, A.G. Characterization of the protein kinase activity of TRPM7/ChaK1, a protein kinase fused to the transient receptor potential ion channel. *J. Biol. Chem.* **2004**, *279*, 3708–3716. [CrossRef] [PubMed]

23. Dorovkov, M.V.; Ryazanov, A.G. Phosphorylation of annexin I by TRPM7 channel-kinase. *J. Biol. Chem.* **2004**, *279*, 50643–50646. [CrossRef] [PubMed]

24. Dorovkov, M.V.; Kostyukova, A.S.; Ryazanov, A.G. Phosphorylation of annexin A1 by TRPM7 kinase: A switch regulating the induction of an alpha-helix. *Biochemistry* **2011**, *50*, 2187–2193. [CrossRef] [PubMed]

25. Clark, K.; Middelbeek, J.; Dorovkov, M.V.; Figdor, C.G.; Ryazanov, A.G.; Lasonder, E.; van Leeuwen, F.N. The alpha-kinases TRPM6 and TRPM7, but not eEF-2 kinase, phosphorylate the assembly domain of myosin IIA, IIB and IIC. *FEBS Lett.* **2008**, *582*, 2993–2997. [CrossRef] [PubMed]

26. Deason-Towne, F.; Perraud, A.L.; Schmitz, C. Identification of Ser/Thr phosphorylation sites in the C2-domain of phospholipase C γ2 (PLCγ2) using TRPM7-kinase. *Cell Signal.* **2012**, *24*, 2070–2075. [CrossRef] [PubMed]

27. Krishnamoorthy, M.; Wasim, L.; Buhari, F.H.M.; Zhao, T.; Mahtani, T.; Ho, J.; Kang, S.; Deason-Towne, F.; Perraud, A.L.; Schmitz, C.; et al. The channel-kinase TRPM7 regulates antigen gathering and internalization in B cells. *Sci. Signal.* **2018**, *11*, eaah6692. [CrossRef] [PubMed]

28. Jin, J.; Desai, B.N.; Navarro, B.; Donovan, A.; Andrews, N.C.; Clapham, D.E. Deletion of Trpm7 disrupts embryonic development and thymopoiesis without altering Mg^{2+} homeostasis. *Science* **2008**, *322*, 756–760. [CrossRef] [PubMed]

29. Kaitsuka, T.; Katagiri, C.; Beesetty, P.; Nakamura, K.; Hourani, S.; Tomizawa, K.; Kozak, J.A.; Matsushita, M. Inactivation of TRPM7 kinase activity does not impair its channel function in mice. *Sci. Rep.* **2014**, *4*, 5718. [CrossRef] [PubMed]

30. Ryazanova, L.V.; Hu, Z.; Suzuki, S.; Chubanov, V.; Fleig, A.; Ryazanov, A.G. Elucidating the role of the TRPM7 alpha-kinase: TRPM7 kinase inactivation leads to magnesium deprivation resistance phenotype in mice. *Sci. Rep.* **2014**, *4*, 7599. [CrossRef] [PubMed]

31. Desai, B.N.; Krapivinsky, G.; Navarro, B.; Krapivinsky, L.; Carter, B.C.; Febvay, S.; Delling, M.; Penumaka, A.; Ramsey, I.S.; Manasian, Y.; et al. Cleavage of TRPM7 releases the kinase domain from the ion channel and regulates its participation in Fas-induced apoptosis. *Dev. Cell* **2012**, *22*, 1149–1162. [CrossRef] [PubMed]

32. Zierler, S.; Sumoza-Toledo, A.; Suzuki, S.; Duill, F.O.; Ryazanova, L.V.; Penner, R.; Ryazanov, A.G.; Fleig, A. TRPM7 kinase activity regulates murine mast cell degranulation. *J. Physiol.* **2016**, *594*, 2957–2970. [CrossRef] [PubMed]

33. Kim, T.Y.; Shin, S.K.; Song, M.Y.; Lee, J.E.; Park, K.S. Identification of the phosphorylation sites on intact TRPM7 channels from mammalian cells. *Biochem. Biophys. Res. Commun.* **2012**, *417*, 1030–1034. [CrossRef] [PubMed]

34. Clark, K.; Middelbeek, J.; Morrice, N.A.; Figdor, C.G.; Lasonder, E.; van Leeuwen, F.N. Massive autophosphorylation of the Ser/Thr-rich domain controls protein kinase activity of TRPM6 and TRPM7. *PLoS ONE* **2008**, *3*, e1876. [CrossRef] [PubMed]

35. Brandao, K.; Deason-Towne, F.; Zhao, X.; Perraud, A.L.; Schmitz, C. TRPM6 kinase activity regulates TRPM7 trafficking and inhibits cellular growth under hypomagnesic conditions. *Cell. Mol. Life Sci.* **2014**, *71*, 4853–4867. [CrossRef] [PubMed]

36. Cai, N.; Bai, Z.; Nanda, V.; Runnels, L.W. Mass Spectrometric Analysis of TRPM6 and TRPM7 Phosphorylation Reveals Regulatory Mechanisms of the Channel-Kinases. *Sci. Rep.* **2017**, *7*, 42739. [CrossRef] [PubMed]

37. Fonfria, E.; Murdock, P.R.; Cusdin, F.S.; Benham, C.D.; Kelsell, R.E.; McNulty, S. Tissue distribution profiles of the human TRPM cation channel family. *J. Recept. Signal Transduct.* **2006**, *26*, 159–178. [CrossRef] [PubMed]

38. Zierler, S.; Hampe, S.; Nadolni, W. TRPM channels as potential therapeutic targets against pro-inflammatory diseases. *Cell Calcium* **2017**, *67*, 105–115. [CrossRef] [PubMed]

39. Schappe, M.S.; Szteyn, K.; Stremska, M.E.; Mendu, S.K.; Downs, T.K.; Seegren, P.V.; Mahoney, M.A.; Dixit, S.; Krupa, J.K.; Stipes, E.J.; et al. Chanzyme TRPM7 Mediates the Ca^{2+} Influx Essential for Lipopolysaccharide-Induced Toll-Like Receptor 4 Endocytosis and Macrophage Activation. *Immunity* **2018**, *48*, 59–74. [CrossRef] [PubMed]

40. Siebenhaar, F.; Redegeld, F.A.; Bischoff, S.C.; Gibbs, B.F.; Maurer, M. Mast Cells as Drivers of Disease and Therapeutic Targets. *Trends Immunol.* **2017**, *39*, 151–162. [CrossRef] [PubMed]

41. Kempuraj, D.; Selvakumar, G.P.; Thangavel, R.; Ahmed, M.E.; Zaheer, S.; Raikwar, S.P.; Iyer, S.S.; Bhagavan, S.M.; Beladakere-Ramaswamy, S.; Zaheer, A. Mast Cell Activation in Brain Injury, Stress, and Post-traumatic Stress Disorder and Alzheimer's Disease Pathogenesis. *Front. Neurosci.* **2017**, *11*, 703. [CrossRef] [PubMed]

42. Skaper, S.D.; Facci, L.; Zusso, M.; Giusti, P. Neuroinflammation, Mast Cells, and Glia: Dangerous Liaisons. *Neuroscientist* **2017**, *23*, 478–498. [CrossRef] [PubMed]

43. Lindstedt, K.A.; Kovanen, P.T. Isolation of mast cell granules. *Curr. Protoc. Cell Biol.* **2006**, *29*, 3–16. [CrossRef] [PubMed]

44. Bulfone-Paus, S.; Nilsson, G.; Draber, P.; Blank, U.; Levi-Schaffer, F. Positive and Negative Signals in Mast Cell Activation. *Trends Immunol.* **2017**, *38*, 657–667. [CrossRef] [PubMed]

45. Evans, D.P.; Thomson, D.S. Histamine release from rat mast cells passively sensitised with homocytotropic (IgE) antibody. *Int. Arch. Allergy Appl. Immunol.* **1972**, *43*, 217–231. [CrossRef] [PubMed]

46. Chen, Y.C.; Chang, Y.C.; Chang, H.A.; Lin, Y.S.; Tsao, C.W.; Shen, M.R.; Chiu, W.T. Differential Ca^{2+} mobilization and mast cell degranulation by FcepsilonRI- and GPCR-mediated signaling. *Cell Calcium* **2017**, *67*, 31–39. [CrossRef] [PubMed]

47. Gaudenzio, N.; Sibilano, R.; Marichal, T.; Starkl, P.; Reber, L.L.; Cenac, N.; McNeil, B.D.; Dong, X.; Hernandez, J.D.; Sagi-Eisenberg, R.; et al. Different activation signals induce distinct mast cell degranulation strategies. *J. Clin. Investig.* **2016**, *126*, 3981–3998. [CrossRef] [PubMed]

48. Baba, Y.; Nishida, K.; Fujii, Y.; Hirano, T.; Hikida, M.; Kurosaki, T. Essential function for the calcium sensor STIM1 in mast cell activation and anaphylactic responses. *Nat. Immunol.* **2008**, *9*, 81–88. [CrossRef] [PubMed]

49. Vig, M.; DeHaven, W.I.; Bird, G.S.; Billingsley, J.M.; Wang, H.; Rao, P.E.; Hutchings, A.B.; Jouvin, M.H.; Putney, J.W.; Kinet, J.P. Defective mast cell effector functions in mice lacking the CRACM1 pore subunit of store-operated calcium release-activated calcium channels. *Nat. Immunol.* **2008**, *9*, 89–96. [CrossRef] [PubMed]

50. Wykes, R.C.; Lee, M.; Duffy, S.M.; Yang, W.; Seward, E.P.; Bradding, P. Functional transient receptor potential melastatin 7 channels are critical for human mast cell survival. *J. Immunol.* **2007**, *179*, 4045–4052. [CrossRef] [PubMed]

51. Huang, L.; Ng, N.M.; Chen, M.; Lin, X.; Tang, T.; Cheng, H.; Yang, C.; Jiang, S. Inhibition of TRPM7 channels reduces degranulation and release of cytokines in rat bone marrow-derived mast cells. *Int. J. Mol. Sci.* **2014**, *15*, 11817–11831. [CrossRef] [PubMed]

52. DeHaven, W.I.; Smyth, J.T.; Boyles, R.R.; Bird, G.S.; Putney, J.W., Jr. Complex actions of 2-aminoethyldiphenyl borate on store-operated calcium entry. *J. Biol. Chem.* **2008**, *283*, 19265–19273. [CrossRef] [PubMed]

53. Amulic, B.; Cazalet, C.; Hayes, G.L.; Metzler, K.D.; Zychlinsky, A. Neutrophil function: From mechanisms to disease. *Annu. Rev. Immunol.* **2012**, *30*, 459–489. [CrossRef] [PubMed]

54. Dixit, N.; Simon, S.I. Chemokines, selectins and intracellular calcium flux: Temporal and spatial cues for leukocyte arrest. *Front. Immunol.* **2012**, *3*, 188. [CrossRef] [PubMed]

55. Immler, R.; Simon, S.I.; Sperandio, M. Calcium signalling and related ion channels in neutrophil recruitment and function. *Eur. J. Clin. Investig.* **2018**, e12964. [CrossRef] [PubMed]

56. Abed, E.; Moreau, R. Importance of melastatin-like transient receptor potential 7 and magnesium in the stimulation of osteoblast proliferation and migration by PDGF. *Am. J. Physiol. Cell Physiol.* **2009**, *297*, C360–C368. [CrossRef] [PubMed]

57. Chen, J.P.; Luan, Y.; You, C.X.; Chen, X.H.; Luo, R.C.; Li, R. TRPM7 regulates the migration of human nasopharyngeal carcinoma cell by mediating Ca^{2+} influx. *Cell Calcium* **2010**, *47*, 425–432. [CrossRef] [PubMed]

58. Wei, C.; Wang, X.; Chen, M.; Ouyang, K.; Song, L.S.; Cheng, H. Calcium flickers steer cell migration. *Nature* **2009**, *457*, 901–905. [CrossRef] [PubMed]

59. Wang, C.H.; Rong, M.Y.; Wang, L.; Ren, Z.; Chen, L.N.; Jia, J.F.; Li, X.Y.; Wu, Z.B.; Chen, Z.N.; Zhu, P. CD147 up-regulates calcium-induced chemotaxis, adhesion ability and invasiveness of human neutrophils via a TRPM-7-mediated mechanism. *Rheumatology* **2014**, *53*, 2288–2296. [CrossRef] [PubMed]

60. Johnson, E.R.; Matthay, M.A. Acute lung injury: Epidemiology, pathogenesis, and treatment. *J. Aerosol Med. Pulm. Drug Deliv.* **2010**, *23*, 243–252. [CrossRef] [PubMed]

61. Yang, C.W.; Liu, H.; Li, X.D.; Sui, S.G.; Liu, Y.F. Salvianolic acid B protects against acute lung injury by decreasing TRPM6 and TRPM7 expressions in a rat model of sepsis. *J. Cell. Biochem.* **2018**, *119*, 701–711. [CrossRef] [PubMed]

62. Iwasaki, A.; Medzhitov, R. Control of adaptive immunity by the innate immune system. *Nat. Immunol.* **2015**, *16*, 343–353. [CrossRef] [PubMed]

63. Varol, C.; Mildner, A.; Jung, S. Macrophages: Development and tissue specialization. *Annu. Rev. Immunol.* **2015**, *33*, 643–675. [CrossRef] [PubMed]

64. Santoni, G.; Morelli, M.B.; Amantini, C.; Santoni, M.; Nabissi, M.; Marinelli, O.; Santoni, A. "Immuno-Transient Receptor Potential Ion Channels": The Role in Monocyte- and Macrophage-Mediated Inflammatory Responses. *Front. Immunol.* **2018**, *9*, 1273. [CrossRef] [PubMed]

65. Lee, Y.K.; Im, Y.J.; Kim, Y.L.; Im, D.S. Characterization of Ca^{2+} influx induced by dimethylphytosphingosine and lysophosphatidylcholine in U937 monocytes. *Biochem. Biophys. Res. Commun.* **2006**, *348*, 1116–1122. [CrossRef] [PubMed]

66. Wuensch, T.; Thilo, F.; Krueger, K.; Scholze, A.; Ristow, M.; Tepel, M. High glucose-induced oxidative stress increases transient receptor potential channel expression in human monocytes. *Diabetes* **2010**, *59*, 844–849. [CrossRef] [PubMed]

67. Li, Y.; Jiang, H.; Ruan, C.; Zhong, J.; Gao, P.; Zhu, D.; Niu, W.; Guo, S. The interaction of transient receptor potential melastatin 7 with macrophages promotes vascular adventitial remodeling in transverse aortic constriction rats. *Hypertens. Res.* **2014**, *37*, 35–42. [CrossRef] [PubMed]

68. Schilling, T.; Miralles, F.; Eder, C. TRPM7 regulates proliferation and polarisation of macrophages. *J. Cell Sci.* **2014**, *127*, 4561–4566. [CrossRef] [PubMed]

69. Murray, P.J.; Wynn, T.A. Protective and pathogenic functions of macrophage subsets. *Nat. Rev. Immunol.* **2011**, *11*, 723–737. [CrossRef] [PubMed]

70. Martinez, F.O.; Helming, L.; Gordon, S. Alternative activation of macrophages: An immunologic functional perspective. *Annu. Rev. Immunol.* **2009**, *27*, 451–483. [CrossRef] [PubMed]

71. Chubanov, V.; Mederos y Schnitzler, M.; Meissner, M.; Schafer, S.; Abstiens, K.; Hofmann, T.; Gudermann, T. Natural and synthetic modulators of SK (Kca2) potassium channels inhibit magnesium-dependent activity of the kinase-coupled cation channel TRPM7. *Br. J. Pharmacol.* **2012**, *166*, 1357–1376. [CrossRef] [PubMed]

72. Vaeth, M.; Zee, I.; Concepcion, A.R.; Maus, M.; Shaw, P.; Portal-Celhay, C.; Zahra, A.; Kozhaya, L.; Weidinger, C.; Philips, J.; et al. Ca^{2+} Signaling but Not Store-Operated Ca^{2+} Entry Is Required for the Function of Macrophages and Dendritic Cells. *J. Immunol.* **2015**, *195*, 1202–1217. [CrossRef] [PubMed]

73. Haslberger, A.; Romanin, C.; Koerber, R. Membrane potential modulates release of tumor necrosis factor in lipopolysaccharide-stimulated mouse macrophages. *Mol. Biol. Cell* **1992**, *3*, 451–460. [CrossRef] [PubMed]

74. Yatim, K.M.; Lakkis, F.G. A brief journey through the immune system. *Clin. J. Am. Soc. Nephrol.* **2015**, *10*, 1274–1281. [CrossRef] [PubMed]

75. Heinzel, S.; Marchingo, J.M.; Horton, M.B.; Hodgkin, P.D. The regulation of lymphocyte activation and proliferation. *Curr. Opin. Immunol.* **2018**, *51*, 32–38. [CrossRef] [PubMed]

76. Matsushita, M.; Kozak, J.A.; Shimizu, Y.; McLachlin, D.T.; Yamaguchi, H.; Wei, F.Y.; Tomizawa, K.; Matsui, H.; Chait, B.T.; Cahalan, M.D.; et al. Channel function is dissociated from the intrinsic kinase activity and autophosphorylation of TRPM7/ChaK1. *J. Biol. Chem.* **2005**, *280*, 20793–20803. [CrossRef] [PubMed]

77. Sahni, J.; Scharenberg, A.M. TRPM7 ion channels are required for sustained phosphoinositide 3-kinase signaling in lymphocytes. *Cell Metab.* **2008**, *8*, 84–93. [CrossRef] [PubMed]

78. Sahni, J.; Tamura, R.; Sweet, I.R.; Scharenberg, A.M. TRPM7 regulates quiescent/proliferative metabolic transitions in lymphocytes. *Cell Cycle* **2010**, *9*, 3565–3574. [CrossRef] [PubMed]

79. Stritt, S.; Nurden, P.; Favier, R.; Favier, M.; Ferioli, S.; Gotru, S.K.; van Eeuwijk, J.M.; Schulze, H.; Nurden, A.T.; Lambert, M.P.; et al. Defects in TRPM7 channel function deregulate thrombopoiesis through altered cellular Mg^{2+} homeostasis and cytoskeletal architecture. *Nat. Commun.* **2016**, *7*, 11097. [CrossRef] [PubMed]

80. Krishnamoorthy, M.; Buhari, F.H.M.; Zhao, T.; Brauer, P.M.; Burrows, K.; Cao, E.Y.; Moxley-Paquette, V.; Mortha, A.; Zuniga-Pflucker, J.C.; Treanor, B. The ion channel TRPM7 is required for B cell lymphopoiesis. *Sci. Signal.* **2018**, *11*, eaan2693. [CrossRef] [PubMed]

81. Van Wijk, F.; Cheroutre, H. Mucosal T cells in gut homeostasis and inflammation. *Expert Rev. Clin. Immunol.* **2010**, *6*, 559–566. [CrossRef] [PubMed]

82. Kamada, N.; Nunez, G. Role of the gut microbiota in the development and function of lymphoid cells. *J. Immunol.* **2013**, *190*, 1389–1395. [CrossRef] [PubMed]

83. Campbell, D.J.; Butcher, E.C. Rapid acquisition of tissue-specific homing phenotypes by $CD4^+$ T cells activated in cutaneous or mucosal lymphoid tissues. *J. Exp. Med.* **2002**, *195*, 135–141. [CrossRef] [PubMed]

84. Qiu, Y.; Wang, W.; Xiao, W.; Yang, H. Role of the intestinal cytokine microenvironment in shaping the intraepithelial lymphocyte repertoire. *J. Leukoc. Biol.* **2015**, *97*, 849–857. [CrossRef] [PubMed]

85. Veldhoen, M.; Hocking, R.J.; Atkins, C.J.; Locksley, R.M.; Stockinger, B. TGFbeta in the context of an inflammatory cytokine milieu supports de novo differentiation of IL-17-producing T cells. *Immunity* **2006**, *24*, 179–189. [CrossRef] [PubMed]

86. Habtezion, A.; Nguyen, L.P.; Hadeiba, H.; Butcher, E.C. Leukocyte Trafficking to the Small Intestine and Colon. *Gastroenterology* **2016**, *150*, 340–354. [CrossRef] [PubMed]

87. Schon, M.P.; Arya, A.; Murphy, E.A.; Adams, C.M.; Strauch, U.G.; Agace, W.W.; Marsal, J.; Donohue, J.P.; Her, H.; Beier, D.R.; et al. Mucosal T lymphocyte numbers are selectively reduced in integrin alpha E (CD103)-deficient mice. *J. Immunol.* **1999**, *162*, 6641–6649. [PubMed]

88. Mokrani, M.; Klibi, J.; Bluteau, D.; Bismuth, G.; Mami-Chouaib, F. Smad and NFAT pathways cooperate to induce CD103 expression in human CD8 T lymphocytes. *J. Immunol.* **2014**, *192*, 2471–2479. [CrossRef] [PubMed]

89. Zierler, S.; Yao, G.; Zhang, Z.; Kuo, W.C.; Porzgen, P.; Penner, R.; Horgen, F.D.; Fleig, A. Waixenicin A inhibits cell proliferation through magnesium-dependent block of transient receptor potential melastatin 7 (TRPM7) channels. *J. Biol. Chem.* **2011**, *286*, 39328–39335. [CrossRef] [PubMed]

90. Kuras, Z.; Yun, Y.H.; Chimote, A.A.; Neumeier, L.; Conforti, L. KCa3.1 and TRPM7 channels at the uropod regulate migration of activated human T cells. *PLoS ONE* **2012**, *7*, e43859. [CrossRef] [PubMed]

91. Cai, Z.; Jitkaew, S.; Zhao, J.; Chiang, H.C.; Choksi, S.; Liu, J.; Ward, Y.; Wu, L.G.; Liu, Z.G. Plasma membrane translocation of trimerized MLKL protein is required for TNF-induced necroptosis. *Nat. Cell Biol.* **2014**, *16*, 55–65. [CrossRef] [PubMed]

92. Wolf, F.; Hilewitz, A. Hypomagnesaemia in patients hospitalised in internal medicine is associated with increased mortality. *Int. J. Clin. Pract.* **2014**, *68*, 111–116. [CrossRef] [PubMed]

93. Trapani, V.; Wolf, F.I.; Scaldaferri, F. Dietary magnesium: The magic mineral that protects from colon cancer? *Magnes. Res.* **2015**, *28*, 108–111. [CrossRef] [PubMed]

94. Chubanov, V.; Ferioli, S.; Wisnowsky, A.; Simmons, D.G.; Leitzinger, C.; Einer, C.; Jonas, W.; Shymkiv, Y.; Bartsch, H.; Braun, A.; et al. Epithelial magnesium transport by TRPM6 is essential for prenatal development and adult survival. *eLife* **2016**, *5*, e20914. [CrossRef] [PubMed]

95. Kau, A.L.; Ahern, P.P.; Griffin, N.W.; Goodman, A.L.; Gordon, J.I. Human nutrition, the gut microbiome and the immune system. *Nature* **2011**, *474*, 327–336. [CrossRef] [PubMed]

96. Malpuech-Brugere, C.; Nowacki, W.; Daveau, M.; Gueux, E.; Linard, C.; Rock, E.; Lebreton, J.; Mazur, A.; Rayssiguier, Y. Inflammatory response following acute magnesium deficiency in the rat. *Biochim. Biophys. Acta* **2000**, *1501*, 91–98. [CrossRef]

97. Ferrara, J.L.; Reddy, P. Pathophysiology of graft-versus-host disease. *Semin. Hematol.* **2006**, *43*, 3–10. [CrossRef] [PubMed]

98. Filipovich, A.H.; Weisdorf, D.; Pavletic, S.; Socie, G.; Wingard, J.R.; Lee, S.J.; Martin, P.; Chien, J.; Przepiorka, D.; Couriel, D.; et al. National Institutes of Health consensus development project on criteria for clinical trials in chronic graft-versus-host disease: I. Diagnosis and staging working group report. *Biol. Blood Marrow Transplant.* **2005**, *11*, 945–956. [CrossRef] [PubMed]

99. Ferrara, J.L.; Levine, J.E.; Reddy, P.; Holler, E. Graft-versus-host disease. *Lancet* **2009**, *373*, 1550–1561. [CrossRef]

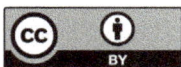

© 2018 by the authors. Licensee MDPI, Basel, Switzerland. This article is an open access article distributed under the terms and conditions of the Creative Commons Attribution (CC BY) license (http://creativecommons.org/licenses/by/4.0/).

Article

Bioavailable Menthol (Transient Receptor Potential Melastatin-8 Agonist) Induces Energy Expending Phenotype in Differentiating Adipocytes

Pragyanshu Khare [1,2,3,†], Aakriti Chauhan [1,†], Vibhu Kumar [1], Jasleen Kaur [1], Neha Mahajan [1,4], Vijay Kumar [1,5], Adam Gesing [6], Kanwaljit Chopra [2], Kanthi Kiran Kondepudi [1] and Mahendra Bishnoi [1,*]

[1] National Agri-Food Biotechnology Institute (NABI), Knowledge City-Sector 81, SAS Nagar, Punjab 140603, India; khare.pragyanshu@gmail.com (P.K.); chauhanaakriti11@gmail.com (A.C.); vibhu.kumar99@gmail.com (V.K.); jasleen.820@gmail.com (J.K.); mahajan23neha@gmail.com (N.M.); 2210.vijay@gmail.com (V.K.); kiran@nabi.res.in (K.K.K.)
[2] Pharmacology Division, University Institute of Pharmaceutical Sciences (UIPS), Panjab University, Chandigarh 160014, India; dr_chopra_k@yahoo.com
[3] Department of Pharmacology & Toxicology, National Institute of Pharmaceutical Education and Research (NIPER)-Raebareli, Transit campus Lucknow, Uttar Pradesh 226301, India
[4] Regional Centre for Biotechnology, Faridabad-Gurgaon expressway, Faridabad, Haryana 121001, India
[5] Department of Biotechnology, Panjab University, Sector-25, Chandigarh 160014, India
[6] Department of Endocrinology of Ageing, Medical University of Lodz, Zeligowski St, No 7/9, 90-752 Lodz, Poland; adges7@yahoo.com
* Correspondence: mbishnoi@nabi.res.in; Tel.: +91(172)5221261
† These authors contributed equally to this work.

Received: 31 December 2018; Accepted: 19 March 2019; Published: 26 April 2019

Abstract: Recent evidence supports the role of menthol, a TRPM8 agonist, in enhanced energy expenditure, thermogenesis and BAT-like activity in classical WAT depots in a TRPM8 dependent and independent manner. The present study was designed to analyse whether oral and topical administration of menthol is bioavailable at subcutaneous adipose tissue and is sufficient to directlyinduce desired energy expenditure effects. GC-FID was performed to study menthol bioavailability in serum and subcutaneous white adipose tissue following oral and topical administration. Further, 3T3L1 adipocytes were treated with bioavailable menthol doses and different parameters (lipid accumulation, "*browning/brite*" and energy expenditure gene expression, metal analysis, mitochondrial complex's gene expression) were studied. No difference was observed in serum levels but significant difference was seen in the menthol concentration on subcutaneous adipose tissues after oral and topical application. Menthol administration at bioavailable doses significantly increased "*browning/brite*" and energy expenditure phenotype, enhanced mitochondrial activity related gene expression, increased metal concentration during adipogenesis but did not alter the lipid accumulation as well as acute experiments were performed with lower dose of menthol on mature adipocytes In conclusion, the present study provides evidence that bioavailable menthol after single oral and topical administration is sufficient to induce "*brite*" phenotype in subcutaneous adipose tissue However, critical dose characterization for its clinical utility is required.

Keywords: adipose tissue; bioavailable; menthol; topical; TRPM8

---

1. Introduction

The imbalance between energy intake and energy expenditure is a well-known aspect of the escalating prevalence of obesity throughout the world as a major nutritional challenge [1,2]. Multiple factors like physical activity, dietary energy intake, basal metabolic rate, variation in environmental and body temperature are reported to influence energy expenditure [3,4]. Enhancement of energy expenditure is one of the cardinal approach toward prevention of body weight gain and obesity [5]. Numerous studies have reported the direct relation of cold exposure with non-shivering thermogenesis, followed by reduction in body fat [6–8]. Interestingly, clinical studies have also reported a vital link between cold-exposure and elevated energy expenditure through adaptive thermogenesis [9]. Studies on adipocytes have also reported a relationship between cold receptor, TRPM8 and energy expenditure showing upregulated expression of UCP-1 and PGC-1α owing to TRPM8 activation [10].

Complex physiology of the body makes it difficult to understand the exact mechanisms involved in energy expenditure. Transient receptor potential cation channel subfamily Melastatin member 8 (TRPM8) is a thermoreceptor present on the sensory nerve endings innervating the gut and skin [11–13] that senses non-noxious cold stimuli ranging from 18–25 °C, hence making it attractive target for cold mimicking. Involvement of TRPM8 dependent and independent pathways in mediating cold-induced energy expenditure is well reported. Recently we have published that anti-obesity effect of menthol, a TRPM8 agonist is mediated through glucagon dependent mechanisms particularly in adipose tissues [14]. Activation of TRPM8 receptors in the gut and skin by oral and topical administration of menthol leads to increase in serum glucagon levels, thus activating several downstream catabolic processes like glycogenolysis, gluconeogenesis, *browning* of white adipose tissue (WAT) and activation of energy expenditure markers in WAT and brown adipose tissue (BAT) [14]. This is supposedly an indirect action of menthol on adipose tissue wherein presence of TRPM8 is not essential. On the other hand, studies from our laboratory provide a strong evidence of significant expression of TRPM8 in undifferentiated (pre-adipocytes) and differentiated (adipocytes) 3T3-L1 cells suggesting its significance in adipogenesis [15]. Also, TRPM8 is functionally expressed in rodent WAT [16] and BAT [17] as well as human WAT [18]. Alternatively, Ma et al. showed that the mouse BAT expresses TRPM8 receptor which upon activation by menthol, significantly increased the levels of p-PKA that further phosphorylates the transcription factor cyclic AMP-responsive element-binding protein (CREB), ultimately leading to enhanced UCP1 expression [17,19]. Thus, chronic dietary menthol increased thermogenesis, core body temperature, prevented diet-induced obesity and the abnormal glucose homeostasis in wild-type mice but not in UCP1$^{(-/-)}$ and TRPM8$^{(-/-)}$ mice [17], suggesting TRPM8 receptor presence on adipose tissue is essential. Other studies also demonstrated the induction of white-to-brown-like phenotype through TRPM8 activation on human WAT [18,20], summarizing the importance of the presence of TRPM8 on adipose tissue.

We hypothesize that different TRPM8 dependent and independent actions are contributing to the anti-obesity effect of menthol. The present study is an attempt to reveal whether topical (10% *w/v*) or oral (200 mg/kg, p.o.) administration of menthol used during acute studies in our previous work is bioavailable at subcutaneous adipose tissue (direct or through serum). Further, using in-vitro 3T3L1 cell line model, we attempted to study that whether bioavailable menthol at subcutaneous adipose tissue is sufficient to induce direct effect on "*browning*" and mitochondrial energy metabolism followed by enhanced energy expenditure effects. Furthermore, this manuscript endeavours to elucidate the presence of metal ions and their role in mitochondrial electron transport chain for significant elevation in energy expenditure owing to the menthol treatment.

2. Materials and Methods

2.1. Chemicals

Mouse 3T3-L1 preadipocytes were obtained from National Centre for Cell Science (NCCS, Pune, India). Dulbecco's Modified Eagle Medium (DMEM), Foetal Bovine Serum (FBS), Penicillin-Streptomycin and Phosphate-Buffered Saline (PBS) was procured from Lonza Inc. (Walkersville, MD, USA). Menthol, AMTB hydrate, Isopropyl alcohol (IPA), 3-isobutyl-1-methylxanthine (IBMX), Dexamethasone (DMS), Insulin, Oil-Red-O (ORO) powder, 3-(4,5-dimethylthiazol-2-yl)-2,5-diphenyl-2*H*-tetrazolium bromide

(MTT)and Dimethyl Sulfoxide (DMSO) were obtained from Sigma Aldrich Co. (St. Louis, MO, USA). GeneZol RNA Extraction Reagent was obtained from Genetix Biotech Asia Pvt. Ltd. (New Delhi, India). Absolute Ethanol (Biotechnology grade) was procured from Amresco Inc. (Cochran Road, Solon, OH, USA). Nitric acid (Trace Metal Grade) was obtained from Fisher Scientific UK Limited (Bishop Meadow Road, Loughborough, Leicestershire, UK) and Dichloromethane (DCM) was procured from Central Drug House (New Delhi, India). All other reagents used were of analytical grade and were procured from local supplier.

2.2. Animal Treatment

21 Swiss Male Albino mice (25–30 g) bred in Central Animal Facility of National Institute of Pharmaceutical Education and Research (NIPER), Mohali, Punjab, India were used for the experiment. 3 mice per cage were housed on a 12 h light/dark cycle with ad libitum food and water supply. The experiment was approved by the Institutional Animal Ethical Committee, NIPER, Mohali, Punjab, India. All the experiments were conducted in accordance with the Committee for the Purpose of Control and Supervision in Experiments on Animals (CPCSEA) guidelines on the use and care of experimental animals. Mice were randomly divided into 3 different groups consisting 3 animals for control group, 9 animals for oral administration of menthol and 9 animals for topical administration of menthol. Oral administration of menthol was given at the dose of 200 mg/Kg in 0.1% tween-80, while topical administration of menthol was given on abdominal area by 1 mL topical application of 10% menthol in 0.1% tween 80. Animals were euthanized after 30, 60 and 120 min of menthol administration by cervical dislocation, blood was collected by cardiac puncture for serum isolation and subcutaneous white adipose tissues were collected for pharmacokinetic profiling of menthol [14].

2.3. Gas Chromatography-Flame Ionization Detector (GC-FID) for Menthol Bioavailability in Serum and Subcutaneous WAT

2.3.1. Extraction Procedure

Both serum and adipose tissue samples were extracted fromDCM containing 200 ng/mL of thymol as internal standard. The samples were continuously vortexed for 3 min and centrifuged at 6000 rpm for next 3 min. After centrifugation, the supernatant was isolated and again extracted in DCM as discussed above. The supernatant finally obtained was used for the pharmacokinetic evaluation of menthol both in serum and adipose tissue.

2.3.2. GC-FID Protocol

Separation and detection was done by injecting 1 μL of target analyte in gas chromatograph (Agilent 7890B) equipped with split less injector system and flame ionization detector. Ultra-pure nitrogen gas was passed through a molecular sieve and oxygen trap and was used as carrier gas with flow rate of 1 mL/min. The injection port was held at 240 °C operated at split less mode. Separation was done using DB5 capillary column (Agilent Technologies) with dimension 30 m × 320 μm × 1 μm with oven temperature kept at 40 °C and then increased to 250 °C at the rate of 10 °C/min, hold time for 2 min. and sample run time for 23 min. the FID temperature was maintained at 280 °C for detection. Flow of hydrogen gas used for FID was at the rate of 30 mL/min. The flow of air for FID was 300 mL/min along with makeup flow at the rate of 25 mL/min. Calculations were done using EZ Chrome Software (Menlo Park, CA, USA).

2.4. 3T3-L1 Cell Culture

Mouse 3T3-L1 pre-adipocytes were allowed to culture in basal medium comprising DMEM supplemented with 10% *v/v* FBS and 1% penicillin-streptomycin. Whole cell culture was maintained at 37 °C in a humidified incubator along with continuous supply of 95% O_2 and 5% CO_2. At 60% confluency, cellular differentiation from 3T3-L1 pre-adipocytes to adipocytes was induced using differentiation medium containing basal medium supplemented with 0.1 mM IBMX, 0.1 µM DMS and 1 µg/mL insulin for 48 h. Stock solutions of 0.1 µM DMS and 0.1 mM IBMX were prepared in absolute ethanol and DMSO respectively and were directly supplemented to DMEM culture medium. Further, the cells were shifted to maintenance medium (basal medium with 1 µg/mL insulin) for 10 days with medium replacement on every alternate day. Working solutions of 1, 50, 100, 200 and 300 µM menthol for the treatment were also prepared in absolute ethanol and directly supplemented to culture (differentiation/maintenance) medium during adipogenesis. Dose selection of menthol for in-vitro study was done on the basis of in-vivo pharmacokinetic profile of menthol in serum and adipose tissues. Two different sets of experiments were performed, (A) Effect of menthol administration at different doses (1, 10, 30 and 50 µM during adipogenesis. (B) Effect of menthol administration (1 µM) on matured adipocytes after 1 h of treatment. The entire cell culturing experiments were carried out as per American Type Culture Collection (ATCC) guidelines.

2.5. Cell Viability Assay

Cell cytotoxicity was assessed using MTT assay. Undifferentiated 3T3-L1 preadipocyte cells were seeded in a 96 well plate at density of 1×10^4 cells/well and incubated with varying concentrations (50, 100 and 300 µM) of menthol dissolved in <0.001% ethanol at 37 °C for 24 h. For control, undifferentiated pre-adipocytes treated with ethanol (<0.001%) were taken. After 24 h, media was replaced with MTT as per the instructions by manufacturer (Sigma Aldrich Co., St. Louis, MO, USA). Formazan crystals formed by live cells are solubilized in isopropanol and absorbance was measured at 570 nm using microplate reader (Spectra max M5e, Molecular Devices LLC, San Jose, CA, USA) [21].

2.6. Oil-Red-O Staining

A stock solution of 0.5% *w/v* of ORO was prepared IPA and was stored at room temperature. A working solution of ORO stain was prepared by diluting the stock solution with distilled water in the ratio 3:2. For staining, the supernatant in the culture plates after treatment with varying concentrations of menthol (1, 50 and 200 µM) was removed and cells were washed using PBS. After washing, mature adipocytes were fixed with 10% *v/v* formaldehyde in PBS and kept for 30 min at room temperature followed by three subsequent washing with PBS. Then, the PBS was aspirated and 60% of IPA was added followed by incubation for 5 min. Further, the cells were stained in ORO working solution filled in culture plates to completely cover the plate bottom (1.25 mL per well for 6-well culture plate) and kept for incubation for 10 min. The cells were then washed with 60% IPA to rinse away excess ORO dye followed by final elution of dye in 100% IPA (2.5 mL per well for 6-well culture plate). The plates were again kept for incubation at room temperature for 10 min. Now, 200 µL of each eluate was added to a 96 well microtiter plate. Also, 200 µL of 100 % IPA was filled on the same microtiter plate as blank. Finally, intracellular lipid content was quantified after extracting ORO bound cells with 100% IPA and absorbance was taken at 570nm using Nano Quant–Infinite M200 Pro (Tecan, Switzerland) [22,23].

2.7. ICP-MS for Metal Analysis

Cells from control and test samples (1, 50 and 200 µM administration of menthol during differentiation) were pellet down and digested with nitric acid using Microwave Reaction System (Mars 6, CEM Corporation, Matthews, NC, USA). The concentration of different elements was estimated in the digested samples using standard protocol for inductively coupled plasma mass spectrometry (ICP-MS:77006, Agilent Technologies, Santa Clara, CA, USA) [14].

2.8. qRT-PCR for Browning/Energy Expenditure Genes

Total RNA from both control and treated adipocytes was extracted after 10 days of treatment using Acid guanidinium thiocyanate-phenol-chloroform extraction method with GeneZol RNA Extraction Reagent, IPA, Chloroform and was reversely transcribed to cDNA from 1 µg of RNA using iScript cDNA Synthesis Kit (Bio-Rad Laboratories Inc., Hercules, CA, USA). Quantitative real time-polymerase chain reaction (qRT-PCR) was performed with the cDNA as templates in 40 cycles using Custom RT^2 PCR Array Kit (CLAM 30615C, Qiagen Lifesciences, Waltham, MA, USA) and RT^2 SYBR Green ROX qPCR Mastermix (Qiagen Lifesciences) keeping GAPDH as internal control and 7 gene specific primers for adipogenesis including *TNFRSF9, PPARGC1A, PRDM16, CIDEA, TLE3, HOXC10* and *NRIP1*. The qRT-PCR process was performed by programming thermocycler (CFX96 Touch Real-Time PCR Detection System (Bio-Rad Laboratories Inc., Hercules, CA, USA)) to apply initial cycle for denaturation at 95 °C for 2 min, followed by 40 cycles of annealing and elongation at 60 °C for 30 s and denaturation at 95 °C for 5 s. The complete experiment was performed using three biological replicates [14]. Analysis of relative gene expression was done using $2^{-\Delta\Delta ct}$ method [24] and values were expressed in the terms of fold change with reference to control [14].

2.9. Gene Expression Analysis of Mitochondrial Energy Metabolism

Total RNA from both control and treated adipocytes was extracted after 10 days of treatment using Acid guanidinium thiocyanate-phenol-chloroform extraction method with GeneZol RNA Extraction Reagent, IPA, Chloroform and was reversely transcribed to cDNA from 5 µg of RNA using RT^2 first strand kit (Qiagen Lifesciences). qRT-PCR was performed using RT^2 Profiler PCR Array Kit for Mouse Mitochondrial Energy Metabolism (PAMM 008ZC-12, Qiagen Lifesciences, Waltham, MA, USA) and RT^2 SYBR Green ROX qPCR Mastermix (Qiagen Lifesciences). The thermocycler (Applied Biosystem 7500F Real Time PCR System (Applied Biosystems, Fosters City, CA, USA)) was programmed to apply initial cycle for denaturation at 95 °C for 10 min, followed by 40 cycles of annealing and elongation at 60 °C for 1 min and denaturation at 95 °C for 15 s. Three biological replicates were used for this experiment [14]. Analysis of relative gene expression was done using $2^{-\Delta\Delta ct}$ method [24] and values were expressed in the terms of fold change with reference to control [14].

2.10. Statistical Analysis

All the values are expressed as mean ± SEM. A group comparison in in-vivo study was carried out using unpaired student t-test and two-way ANOVA followed by Tukey's post-hoc test. Group comparison in-vitro study was done using unpaired student t-test and one-way ANOVA followed by Tukey's post-hoc test. Pearson correlation was performed and representative matrix was made using Gitools 2.3.1. (San Fernando Rd, Burbank, CA, USA). $p \leq 0.05$ was considered statistically significant. Correlation matrix and clustering was done by k-means ++ Manhattan distance clusters 6.

3. Results

3.1. Pharmacokinetic Profile of Acute Oral Administration and Topical Application of TRPM8 Agonist (Menthol) in Mice

Serum menthol concentration after oral (200 mg/kg) and topical administration (10% *w/v*) was determined at different time intervals of 0, 30, 60 and 120 min. The peak plasma concentration after oral and topical administration was attained at 30 and 60 min respectively. Bioavailable concentration of menthol in serum after oral administration at 30, 60 and 120 min was found to be 3.28 µg/mL (20.4 µM), 1.51 µg/mL (9.66 µM) and 0.76 µg/mL (4.86 µM) respectively. Serum concentration after topical administration at 30, 60 and 120 min was found to be 1.60 µg/mL (10.23 µM), 2.71 µg/mL (17.28 µM) and 0.82 µg/mL (5.2 µM) respectively (Figure 1A). Area under the curve of concentration and time graph was also determined and no significant difference was observed in serum metal concentration between oral and topical administration (Figure 1B).

Similarly, menthol concentration in the adipose tissue was also determined at the same time intervals. The peak concentration after oral and topical administration was attained at 30 min. Concentration of menthol after oral administration at 30, 60 and 120 min was found to be 28.33 µg/mL (181.09 µM), 17.38 µg/mL (111.2 µM) and 12.51 µg/mL (79.98 µM) respectively. Menthol concentration in the adipose tissue after topical administration at 30, 60 and 120 min was found to be 53.09 µg/mL

(339.74 µM), 28.94 µg/mL (185.19 µM) and 20.11 µg/mL (128.69 µM) respectively (Figure 1C). Area under the curve of concentration and time graph for topical administration was significantly higher than the oral administration which signifies that higher amount of menthol was available in the adipose tissue after topical administration (Figure 1D).

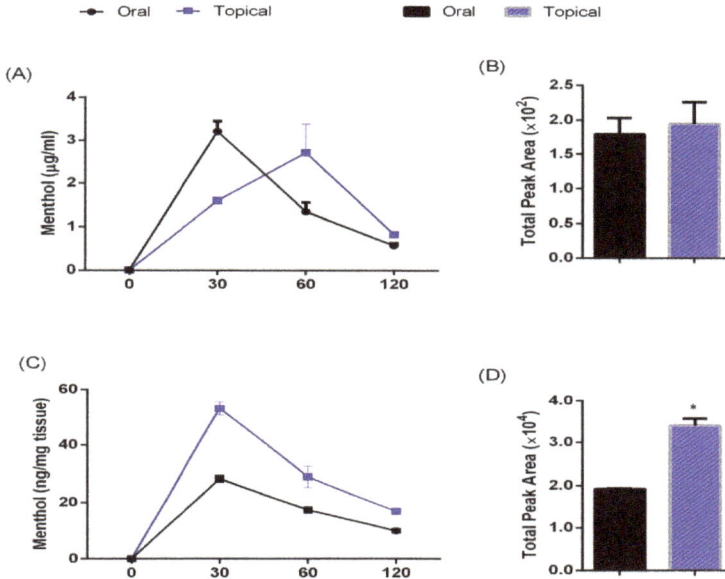

Figure 1. Pharmacokinetic of menthol administration upon oral and topical administration(**A**) Time dependent changes in serum concentration of menthol; (**B**) Area under the time-concentration curve in serum of menthol treated mouse; (**C**) Time dependent changes in concentration of menthol in subcutaneous adipose tissue; (**D**) Area under the time-concentration curve in subcutaneous adipose tissue of menthol treated mice. Oral- Single dose of oral menthol administration at 200 mg/kg. Topical-Single dose of topical menthol application at 10% concentration (300 µL/animal). $n = 3$. All the values are expressed as mean ± S.E.M; * $p < 0.05$.

3.2. Menthol Treatment Did Not Affect Cellular Differentiation, Lipid Accumulation and Cell Viability in 3T3-L1 Cells In-Vitro

No change in cell viability was observed with menthol treatment in comparison to the vehicle treated group up to 300 µM dose (Figure 2A). Oil red O staining is used as a quantitative method to analyse the difference in the degree of differentiation and lipid accumulation in adipocytes in cell culture. The effect of varying concentrations of menthol (1 µM, 50 µM, 100 µM and 200 µM) was evaluated during adipogenesis. Slight decrease in lipid accumulation was observed with menthol 1 µM dose as compared to vehicle treated group and no change was observed with 50 and 200 µM doses (Figure 2B). No significant difference in cellular differentiation of 3T3-L1 cells was observed between the vehicle and menthol treated cells (Figure 2C).

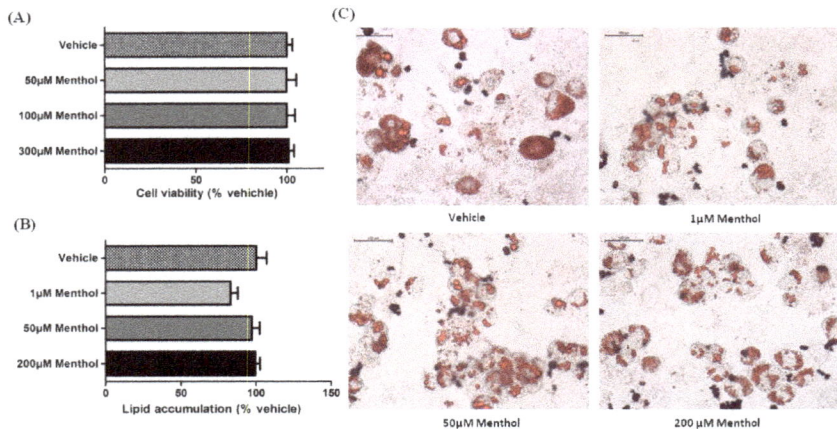

Figure 2. Effect of menthol on adipogenesis in 3T3-L1 cells. (**A**) Cell viability in pre-adipocytes treated with menthol for 24 h. (**B**) Effect of menthol on lipid accumulation in 3T3-L1 cells. (**C**) Effect of various concentration of menthol on differentiation of 3T3-L1 cells. Red spots in images represents area stained by Oil Red O dye. All values are expressed as mean ± S.E.M. (*n* = 3). One-way ANOVA followed by Tukey's multiple comparison post hoc test was applied. * each vs. vehicle.

3.3. Menthol Treatment Altered Metal Concentration and Browning Gene Markers in 3T3-L1 Pre-Adipocytes In-Vitro

The effect of 1, 50 and 200 (data not shown) μM concentrations of menthol treatment during the adipogenesis process on different concentrations of metals in matured adipocytes was evaluated by ICP-MS. Significant increase in the concentrations of iron and copper was observed after 1 μM menthol treatment as compared to their respective controls. Similar pattern was also observed with 50 μM menthol treatment, showing marked elevation in levels of iron, copper and zinc as compared to their corresponding controls. However, significant reduction in cobalt metal levels was observed with both doses of menthol (1 and 50 μM) as compared to vehicle treated group. No significant change in the level of metals like calcium and magnesium was observed with both doses of menthol (Figure 3A,B). There was no significant difference in metal concentrations at 50 μM and 200 μM doses of menthol, hence we used 1 and 50 μM for further studies.

Treatment with 1, 10, 30 and 50 μM concentrations of menthol was given during the process of adipogenesis to check the mRNA expression of *browning* markers. At 1 μM menthol increase in the mRNA expression of *browning* markers that is, Peroxisome proliferator-activated receptor gamma (*PPARCG1A*), Homeobox C10 (*HOXC10*), Tumour necrosis factor receptor superfamily member 9 (*TNFRSF9*) and Uncoupling protein (*UCP1*) was observedas compared to vehicle treated group. A marked reduction in the mRNA expression of Transducin like enhancer of split 3 (*TLE3*) and no change was observed in PR domain containing16 (*PRDM16*), Cell Death inducing DFFA like effector A (*CIDEA*) and Nuclear receptor-interacting protein 1 (*NRIP1*) at 1 μM menthol treatment. At 10 μM, there was a significant reduction in gene expression of *CIDEA*, *NRIP1*, *TLE3* and *TNFRSF9*. No significant change in levels of *PRDM16*, *HOXC10*, *UCP1* and *PPARGC1A*, similar pattern of change in levels of gene expression was observed at 30 μM. Although at 50 μM menthol treatment significantly reduced the mRNA expression of *CIDEA* only. There was no significant difference observed in expression of *HOXC10*, *PRDM16*, *UCP1*, *NRIP1* and *PPARGC1A* as compared to control (Figure 4A). Acute experiment was performed at 1 μM concentration of menthol for 1 h on mature adipocytes. Significant increase in the gene expression of *browning* markers that is, *PRDM16*, *PPARGC1A*, *TNFRSF9*, *TMEM26* and *UCP1* was observed (Figure 4B).

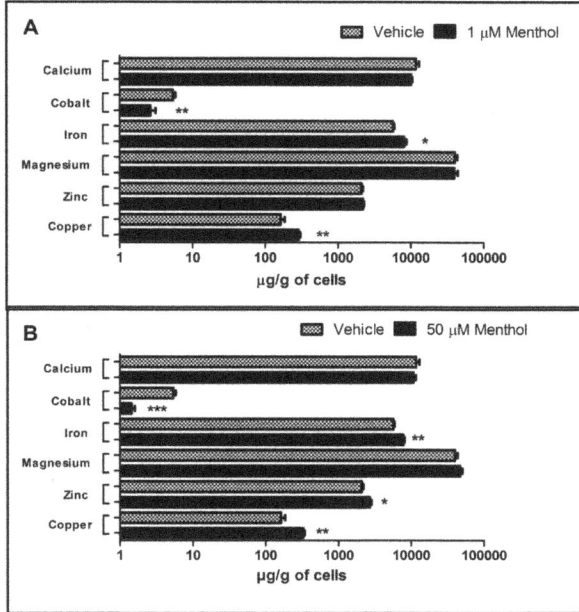

Figure 3. Effect of menthol treatment on. (**A**) Metal concentration (Ca, Co, Fe, Mg, Zn, Cu) in 3T3-L1 cells at 1 µM dose; (**B**) Metal concentration (Ca, Co, Fe, Mg, Zn, Cu) in 3T3-L1 cells at 50 µM dose; n = 3–5; All the values are expressed as mean ± S.E.M; Analysis was carried out by student unpaired t-test; * $p < 0.05$, ** $p < 0.01$, *** $p < 0.001$.

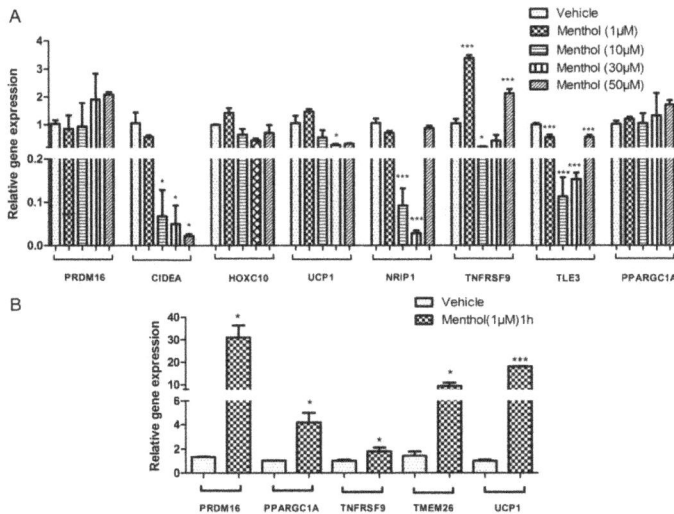

Figure 4. Effect of menthol treatment on: (**A**) Relative expression of energy expenditure genes in 3T3-L1 cells at 1 µM, 10 µM, 30 µM and 50 µM menthol treatment; (**B**)Relative expression of energy expenditure genes in 3T3-L1 cells at 1 µM menthol treatment for 1 h. n = 3–5; All the values are expressed as mean ± S.E.M; Analysis was carried out by student paired t-test and one-way ANOVA followed by Tukey's multiple comparison; * $p < 0.05$, ** $p < 0.01$, *** $p < 0.001$.

3.4. Menthol Treatment Modulated Mitochondrial Activity Gene Markers for Energy Metabolism in 3T3-L1 Pre-Adipocytes In-Vitro

The effect of 1 μM and 50 μM of menthol treatment on different mitochondrial genes was studied. In the NADH dehydrogenase (Complex I), significant increase in the gene expression of *Ndufa1*, *Ndufb2*, *Ndufc1*, *Ndufc2*, *Ndufa6*, *Ndufb3*, *Ndufb5*, *Ndufs6* was observed as compared to vehicle treated group. Significant increase in expression of *Uqcrq* gene in cytochrome c reductase (complex III) was observed as compared to vehicle treated group. In the cytochrome c oxidase (complex IV) significant increase in expression of *Cox6a1*, *Cox6c* genes were also observed. In the F-Type ATP synthase (complex V) significant elevation in the *Atp5j* gene expression was also observed as compared to vehicle treated group (Figure 5A,B). Although, 50 μM menthol supplementation also displayed a modulatory effect over gene expressions for mitochondrial energy metabolism, however, the change observed was insignificant in comparison to vehicle treated group (Figure 5A).

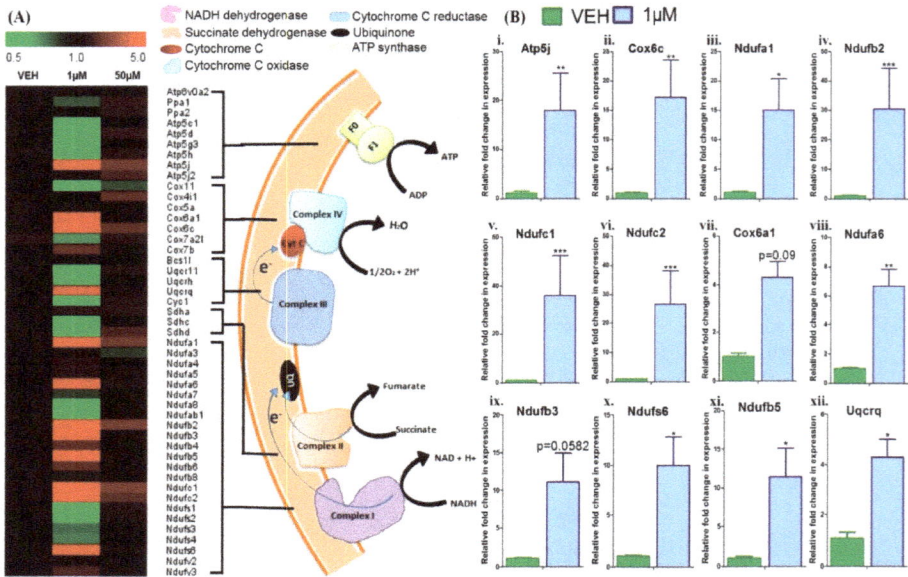

Figure 5. Heat map analysis of gene expression; and genes with statistically significant differential expression in 1 μM menthol treated group. (**A**) Heat map shows gene expression in vehicle, 1 μM and 50 μM menthol treated 3T3-L1 cells (*n* = 3 each). Colour from red to green indicates high to low expression. (**B**) Comparative analysis of selected genes in 1 μM menthol treated group. Normalization was done with reference gene B2M (β-2-microglobulin). The relative fold change in gene expression for mitochondrial biogenesis genes was compared in the three groups. Statistical analysis was done for genes i-vi using two-way ANOVA and for genes vii-xii using two-tailed unpaired t-test. * *p* <0.05, ** *p* <0.01, *** *p* <0.001, each vs vehicle treated group.

4. Discussion

In our recently published manuscript, we have shown that the oral and topical administration of menthol, a TRPM8 agonist, has anti-obesity potential through a TRPM8 mediated glucagon dependent mechanism [14]. We provided evidence that TRPM8 mediated increase in serum glucagon and resultant increase in "glucagon machinery" in liver and adipose tissue is the signature of global shift from "fat storing state" to "fat burning state" in response to menthol administration [14]. During this work, we could suggest that the presence of TRPM8 receptor on adipose tissue is not required and the effect is selective to the glucagon receptor present on adipose tissue, hence we may say that it is an indirect action of menthol on adipose tissue. Also, recent paper by Clemmemsen and colleagues suggested that icilin, a TRPM8 agonist, effect on BAT energy expenditure cannot be explained by direct effects of icilin on adipocytes suggesting indirect actions to increase thermogenesis, likely through induction of sympathetic tone [25]. However, the literature provide evidence for the presence of functional TRPM8 receptors on mouse and human adipose tissue, both white and brown [16–18,26] and adipocyte cell lines [15]. These studies have mentioned that menthol induced increase in calcium influx in adipose tissue, mitochondrial activation and enhanced gene expression is mediated by TRPM8 receptors present on adipose tissue. The doses used in these studies are not based on the bioavailability profile of menthol, hence to establish a link between bioavailable doses of menthol and its functional effects on adipocytes is warranted. In this work, we tend to answer the question that at the acute doses showing anti-obesity effect [14], how much of menthol was bioavailable in serum and subcutaneous WAT. Also, whether this bioavailable menthol has any direct action on adipose tissue mediated through TRPM8 or others to induce energy expenditure.

Menthol was bioavailable to adipose tissues via both routes, oral and topical, through serum and direct absorption, respectively. Serum concentration of menthol reached a maximum at 30 min and 60 min respectively in the case of oral and topical administration; however, the total area reached under the curve/peak concentration was similar over a period of 2 h. The concentration of menthol in subcutaneous WAT reached a maximum at 30 min in the case of both oral and topical administration, with a maximum peak concentration significantly higher in the case of topical administration. We can easily argue that due to proximity of subcutaneous WAT to the site of application (topical), we see a significantly higher concentration. Menthol is lipophilic in nature and its partitioning in adipose tissue through topical application is significantly higher as compared to oral administration. We understand that partitioning in rodent adipose tissue is positively predictive of partitioning in human adipose tissue [27], hence we suggest that this data has clinical utility through the direct effect of menthol on adipose tissue [14]. Previous literature also supports that L-menthol administration increases metabolic rate and thermogenesis in humans [27]. In the same study, authors have concluded that these effects are minor in oral administration as compared to topical administration due to faster metabolism of menthol (glucoronidation) and higher values of menthol glucuronides levels in blood [27]. Summarizing, route of administration is important for the action of menthol on subcutaneous adipose tissue whereas in serum both oral and topical are similarly bioavailable.

Now, the question is whether bioavailable menthol after topical administration is enough to show the desired effects in adipose tissue, may be directly. We used pharmacokinetic based mathematical calculations to convert the bioavailable concentration of menthol in µM concentrations. We calculated that there is a range of concentration that is, 1 µM to 200 µM which will sufficiently cover the bioavailable amount of menthol on adipose tissues after topical administration. At these concentrations of menthol, 3T3L1 cells were viable as assessed by MTT assay. Also, at these doses there was no significant change in the accumulation of fat in differentiating adipose cells as shown by ORO staining. There was minor observation that some of cells were of smaller sizes.

There is lot of recent literature linking adipose tissue metal concentration with adipose tissue health, differentiation and *"browning"* of white adipose tissue. Specifically, in this regard, iron and copper has major significance [28,29]. Iron and copper are essential components of the mitochondrial inner membrane complexes constituting the electron transport chain, therefore, the involvement of copper and iron in energy metabolism via their involvement in mitochondrial function (brown adipose tissue activation) is not surprising [29]. We performed metal analysis in differentiated adipocytes after treating cells with 1, 50 and 200 µM of menthol during differentiation. We selected few important one based on their importance to adipose tissue health (calcium and cobalt), adipose tissue inflammation (zinc, calcium and iron), mitochondrial activation (iron and copper), cell toxicity (cobalt), glucose utilization and transport (zinc and magnesium), initiation of *"brite"* phenotype in white adipose tissue (iron and copper) for analysis [28,30–35]. Menthol administration during differentiation significantly increased the levels of iron and copper at 1 μM whereas there was no significant change in the levels of magnesium, calcium and zinc. Cobalt concentration was significantly decreased in menthol treated differentiated adipocytes. However, at higher doses, 50 and 200 μM (data not shown) there was significant increase in the levels of iron, copper, zinc and magnesium whereas significant decrease in cobalt concentration with no change in calcium concentration. Looking into the metal concentration profile after menthol administration during differentiation of pre-adipocyte to adipocytes, we could suggest that menthol caused mitochondrial activation and increase in *"brite"* phenotype. This data further supports our previous finding where we linked HFD, metal concentration in adipose tissue and menthol administration in an in-vivo model of obesity [14].

Based on metal concentration changes, we selected 1 and 50 μM (both 50 and 200 μM had similar metal concentration profile) for further gene expression studies. We studied the change in expression of energy expenditure and *"browning"* related genes in differentiating adipose tissue. By critically looking into the gene expression data we could understand that (a) at 1 μM, menthol administration significantly modulated these genes which is very well corroborated with the existing literature [16], (b) these changes are not dose dependent, as at higher doses 10, 30 and 50 μM of the effect was reversed, although not dose dependently in some of the genes. Although we have not done these experiments but we may speculate that it may be due to desensitization of TRPM8 at this dose due to chronic presence of menthol during the process of adipogenesis. Further, we suggest that menthol at higher concentration might be acting through either TRPM8 dependent or independent mechanisms. There are numerous other actions of menthol which has link with energy expenditure phenomenon like its action of other excitatory or inhibitory channels, its role in TRPM8 independent increase in intracellular calcium, its role in oxidative effects [36]. Importantly at higher doses menthol acts on TRPV3 [37] and TRPA1 channels [38] which are closely related to adipogenesis, glucose utilization, hormone release and *"browning."* This should be further explored to understand numerous actions of menthol. Based on these effects, we studied the effect of menthol on the mitochondrial activity complexes genes using PCR arrays (84 gene array). The effect on mitochondrial activation genes (approx. 40/84 genes) was positively correlated with energy expenditure genes, significantly higher at 1 μM and at 50 μM, it was decreased, which can be attributed to possible desensitization. In our previous study with TRPV1 agonist, capsaicin, we did see the same phenomenon increase in *"browning"* at 1 μM and decrease at 50 μM, which was correlated to the combination of desensitization and increase in the levels of PPAR-γ at higher doses [23]. We cannot rule out this kind of mechanism with menthol given that both these channels are calcium permeable and in homogenous matrix their agonists can show similar effects. At 1 μM, the changes in metal concentration, especially iron and copper, energy expenditure genes and mitochondrial complex genes are positively correlated (Figure 6). We may say that at 1 μM menthol induces energy expenditure and mitochondrial activation, hence *"brite"* phenotype in differentiating adipocytes. Linking our bioavailable menthol with *"brite"* phenotype induction in differentiating adipocytes, we can suggest that even the topical dose less than 10%, may be 2% or 5% will be sufficient to induce this effect.

There are some limitations of this study. We could have included further experiments to have a clear picture of desensitization or any other mechanisms responsible for the decrease in effect at 50 μM. We are planning extensive studies along these lines to establish the role of TRPM8 (using pharmacological antagonism), other TRP channels (TRPV3 or TRPA1) or non-TRP channels (calcium channels, GABA/glycine receptors) in menthol's action. Further about the toxicity of menthol, there are number of human studies both as oral administration as well as topical application (patch) [39–41]. Orally LD50 of menthol for rodents was observed approx. 3000 mg/kg of body weight and in canine it is approx. 1 g/kg in cats. The dose which we have used is quite less as compared to these [42]. However, further characterization will enable us to finalize the dose both topically and orally. Also, topical administration at multiple doses should be done to clearly establish cause and effect relationship. These studies will help us to develop topical menthol application as a therapeutic/preventive strategy against obesity and related co-morbidities.

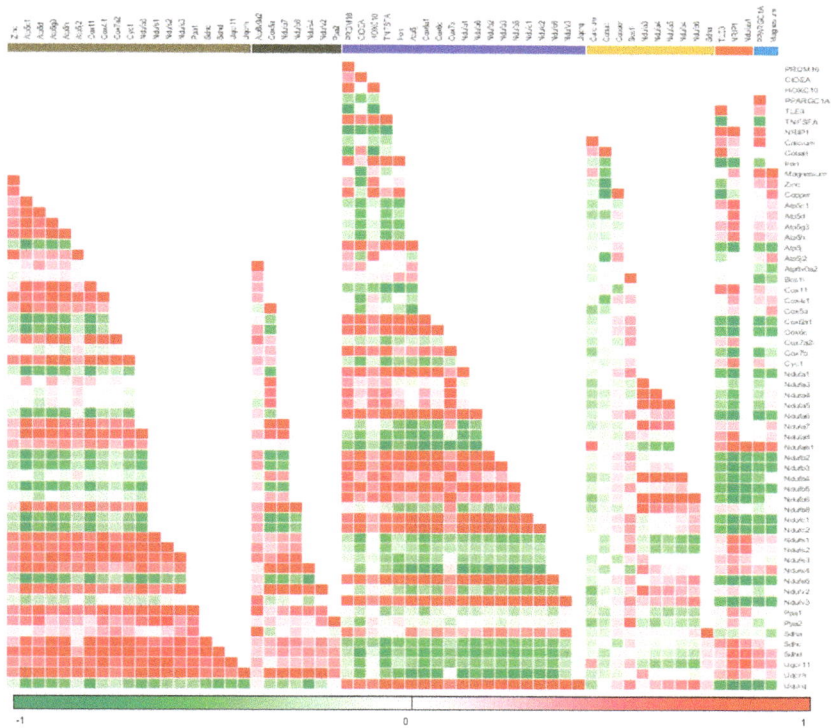

Figure 6. Correlation matrix and clustering of all the data generated through the experiments. The correlation matrix using K-means and Manhattan distance algorithms was drawn, which showed the clustered genes/parameters with respect to each other. Intensity of colours green and red indicate the negative or positive correlation respectively. Genes/parameters along X-axis are clustered using Manhattan distance plot, colour bars showing nearest related groups of genes/parameters.

5. Conclusions

Over all, summarizing this study, we have provided evidence that a single dose of menthol is sufficiently bioavailable to induce energy expanding *"brite"* phenotype in differentiating adipocytes which is dependent on TRPM8 at a lower concentration (Figure 7). These findings can be further exploited to devise dietary (mint based nutraceuticals) or non-dietary (cold mimicking) approaches to combat obesity and type-2 diabetes.

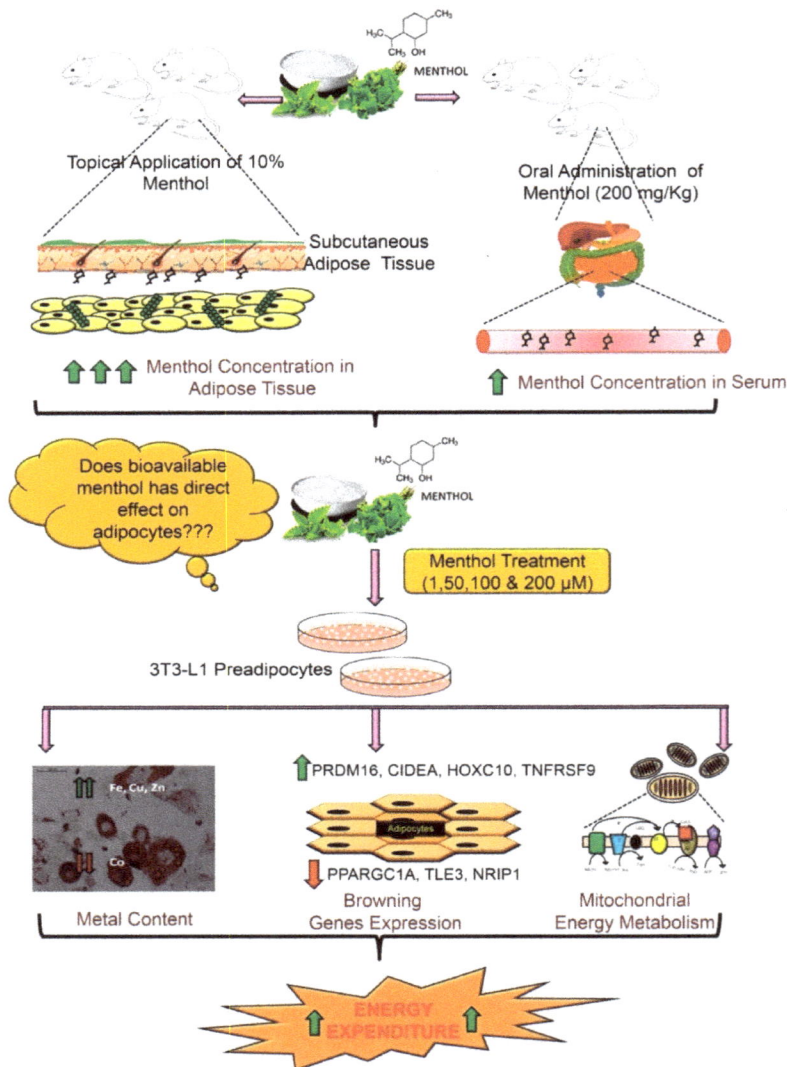

Figure 7. Summary of effect of bioavailable menthol on adipose tissue using in-vitro model. Using the bioavailable concentrations of menthol in adipose tissue and serum upon oral/topical administration, the dosage were decided for in-vitro menthol treatment and effect was checked on expression of genes involved in adipogenesis, *browning*, mitochondrial biogenesis and energy expenditure. The results showed enhanced energy expenditure markers, which indicates improved negative energy balance leading to reduction in obese phenotype.

Author Contributions: M.B., A.G. and P.K. generated the hypothesis. M.B., K.C., P.K., K.K.K. designed the experiments and wrote the manuscript. P.K., A.C., V.K. (Vijay Kumar), N.M., V.K. (Vibhu Kumar) performed the experiments and data calculation. J.K., V.K. (Vijay Kumar) and V.K. (Vibhu Kumar) helped in data presentation and correlation analysis.

Funding: Department of Science and Technology (DST/INT/PLO/P-22/2016/G), Government of India under Indo-Polish Bilateral program.

Acknowledgments: Authors would like to thank Department of Science and Technology (DST/INT/PLO/P-22/2016/G), Government of India for research grant given to National Agri-Food Biotechnology Institute (NABI) and Mahendra Bishnoi under Indo-Polish Bilateral program.

Conflicts of Interest: The authors declare no conflict of interest.

References

1. WHO. Obesity: Preventing and Managing the Global Epidemic. Available online: https://www.who.int/nutrition/publications/obesity/WHO_TRS_894/en/ (accessed on 16 December 2018).
2. Mitchell, N.S.; Catenacci, V.A.; Wyatt, H.R.; Hill, J.O. Obesity: Overview of an epidemic. *Psychiatr. Clin.* **2011**, *34*, 717–732. [CrossRef] [PubMed]
3. Christiansen, E.; Garby, L. Prediction of body weight changes caused by changes in energy balance. *Eur. J. Clin. Investig.* **2002**, *32*, 826–830. [CrossRef]
4. Donahoo, W.T.; Levine, J.A.; Melanson, E.L. Variability in energy expenditure and its components. *Curr. Opin. Clin. Nutr. Metab. Care* **2004**, *7*, 599–605. [CrossRef] [PubMed]
5. Michlig, S.; Merlini, J.M.; Beaumont, M.; Ledda, M.; Tavenard, A.; Mukherjee, R.; Camacho, S.; Le Coutre, J. Effects of TRP channel agonist ingestion on metabolism and autonomic nervous system in a randomized clinical trial of healthy subjects. *Sci. Rep.* **2016**, *6*, 20795. [CrossRef] [PubMed]
6. Saito, M.; Okamatsu-Ogura, Y.; Matsushita, M.; Watanabe, K.; Yoneshiro, T.; Nio-Kobayashi, J.; Iwanaga, T.; Miyagawa, M.; Kameya, T.; Nakada, K. High incidence of metabolically active brown adipose tissue in healthy adult humans: Effects of cold exposure and adiposity. *Diabetes* **2009**, *58*, 1526–1531. [CrossRef]
7. van der Lans, A.A.; Hoeks, J.; Brans, B.; Vijgen, G.H.; Visser, M.G.; Vosselman, M.J.; Hansen, J.; Jörgensen, J.A.; Wu, J.; Mottaghy, F.M. Cold acclimation recruits human brown fat and increases nonshivering thermogenesis. *J. Clin. Investig.* **2013**, *123*, 3395–3403. [CrossRef]
8. van Marken Lichtenbelt, W.; Kingma, B.; Van Der Lans, A.; Schellen, L. Cold exposure–an approach to increasing energy expenditure in humans. *Trends Endocrinol. Metab.* **2014**, *25*, 165–167. [CrossRef]
9. Romu, T.; Vavruch, C.; Dahlqvist-Leinhard, O.; Tallberg, J.; Dahlström, N.; Persson, A.; Heglind, M.; Lidell, M.E.; Enerbäck, S.; Borga, M. A randomized trial of cold-exposure on energy expenditure and supraclavicular brown adipose tissue volume in humans. *Metabolism* **2016**, *65*, 926–934. [CrossRef]
10. Li, C.; Li, J.; Xiong, X.; Liu, Y.; Lv, Y.; Qin, S.; Liu, D.; Wei, R.; Ruan, X.; Zhang, J. TRPM8 activation improves energy expenditure in skeletal muscle and exercise endurance in mice. *Gene* **2018**, *641*, 111–116. [CrossRef]
11. McKemy, D.D.; Neuhausser, W.M.; Julius, D. Identification of a cold receptor reveals a general role for TRP channels in thermosensation. *Nature* **2002**, *416*, 52–58. [CrossRef]
12. Peier, A.M.; Moqrich, A.; Hergarden, A.C.; Reeve, A.J.; Andersson, D.A.; Story, G.M.; Earley, T.J.; Dragoni, I.; McIntyre, P.; Bevan, S. A TRP channel that senses cold stimuli and menthol. *Cell* **2002**, *108*, 705–715. [CrossRef]
13. Bautista, D.M.; Siemens, J.; Glazer, J.M.; Tsuruda, P.R.; Basbaum, A.I.; Stucky, C.L.; Jordt, S.-E.; Julius, D. The menthol receptor TRPM8 is the principal detector of environmental cold. *Nature* **2007**, *448*, 204–208. [CrossRef]
14. Khare, P.; Mangal, P.; Baboota, R.K.; Jagtap, S.; Kumar, V.; Singh, D.P.; Boparai, R.K.; Sharma, S.S.; Khardori, R.; Bhadada, S.K. Involvement of glucagon in preventive effect of menthol against high fat diet induced obesity in mice. *Front. Pharmacol.* **2018**, *9*. [CrossRef]
15. Bishnoi, M.; Kondepudi, K.K.; Gupta, A.; Karmase, A.; Boparai, R.K. Expression of multiple Transient Receptor Potential channel genes in murine 3T3-L1 cell lines and adipose tissue. *Pharmacol. Rep.* **2013**, *65*, 751–755. [CrossRef]
16. Jiang, C.; Zhai, M.; Yan, D.; Li, D.; Li, C.; Zhang, Y.; Xiao, L.; Xiong, D.; Deng, Q.; Sun, W. Dietary menthol-induced TRPM8 activation enhances WAT "browning" and ameliorates diet-induced obesity. *Oncotarget* **2017**, *8*, 75114. [CrossRef]
17. Ma, S.; Yu, H.; Zhao, Z.; Luo, Z.; Chen, J.; Ni, Y.; Jin, R.; Ma, L.; Wang, P.; Zhu, Z. Activation of the cold-sensing TRPM8 channel triggers UCP1-dependent thermogenesis and prevents obesity. *J. Mol. Cell Biol.* **2012**, *4*, 88–96. [CrossRef]
18. Rossato, M.; Granzotto, M.; Macchi, V.; Porzionato, A.; Petrelli, L.; Calcagno, A.; Vencato, J.; De Stefani, D.; Silvestrin, V.; Rizzuto, R. Human white adipocytes express the cold receptor TRPM8 which activation induces UCP1 expression, mitochondrial activation and heat production. *Mol. Cell. Endocrinol.* **2014**, *383*, 137–146. [CrossRef]

19. Vögler, O.; Lopez-Bellan, A.; Alemany, R.; Tofé, S.; González, M.; Quevedo, J.; Pereg, V.; Barcelo, F.; Escriba, P. Structure–effect relation of C18 long-chain fatty acids in the reduction of body weight in rats. *Int. J. Obes.* **2008**, *32*, 464–473. [CrossRef]

20. Goralczyk, A.; van Vijven, M.; Koch, M.; Badowski, C.; Yassin, M.S.; Toh, S.-A.; Shabbir, A.; Franco-Obregón, A.; Raghunath, M. TRP channels in brown and white adipogenesis from human progenitors: New therapeutic targets and the caveats associated with the common antibiotic, streptomycin. *FASEB J.* **2017**, *31*, 3251–3266. [CrossRef]

21. Khare, P.; Jagtap, S.; Jain, Y.; Baboota, R.K.; Mangal, P.; Boparai, R.K.; Bhutani, K.K.; Sharma, S.S.; Premkumar, L.S.; Kondepudi, K.K. Cinnamaldehyde supplementation prevents fasting-induced hyperphagia, lipid accumulation, and inflammation in high-fat diet-fed mice. *Biofactors* **2016**, *42*, 201–211.

22. Yang, M.T.; Fu, J.; Wang, Y.-K.; Desai, R.A.; Chen, C.S. Assaying stem cell mechanobiology on microfabricated elastomeric substrates with geometrically modulated rigidity. *Nat. Protoc.* **2011**, *6*, 187–213. [CrossRef] [PubMed]

23. Baboota, R.K.; Singh, D.P.; Sarma, S.M.; Kaur, J.; Sandhir, R.; Boparai, R.K.; Kondepudi, K.K.; Bishnoi, M. Capsaicin induces "brite" phenotype in differentiating 3T3-L1 preadipocytes. *PLoS ONE* **2014**, *9*, e103093. [CrossRef]

24. Livak, K.J.; Schmittgen, T.D. Analysis of relative gene expression data using real-time quantitative PCR and the $2^{-\Delta\Delta CT}$ method. *Methods* **2001**, *25*, 402–408. [CrossRef] [PubMed]

25. Clemmensen, C.; Jall, S.; Kleinert, M.; Quarta, C.; Gruber, T.; Reber, J.; Sachs, S.; Fischer, K.; Feuchtinger, A.; Karlas, A. Coordinated targeting of cold and nicotinic receptors synergistically improves obesity and type 2 diabetes. *Nat. Commun.* **2018**, *9*, 4304. [CrossRef]

26. Moraes, M.N.; de Assis, L.V.M.; dos Santos Henriques, F.; Batista, M.L., Jr.; Güler, A.D.; de Lauro Castrucci, A.M. Cold-sensing TRPM8 channel participates in circadian control of the brown adipose tissue. *Biochim. Biophys. Acta (BBA) Mol. Cell Res.* **2017**, *1864*, 2415–2427. [CrossRef] [PubMed]

27. Valente, A.; Carrillo, A.E.; Tzatzarakis, M.N.; Vakonaki, E.; Tsatsakis, A.M.; Kenny, G.P.; Koutedakis, Y.; Jamurtas, A.Z.; Flouris, A.D. The absorption and metabolism of a single L-menthol oral versus skin administration: Effects on thermogenesis and metabolic rate. *Food Chem. Toxicol.* **2015**, *86*, 262–273. [CrossRef]

28. Zhao, L.; Zhang, X.; Shen, Y.; Fang, X.; Wang, Y.; Wang, F. Obesity and iron deficiency: A quantitative meta-analysis. *Obes. Rev.* **2015**, *16*, 1081–1093. [CrossRef] [PubMed]

29. Wang, C.; Liang, X.; Tao, C.; Yao, X.; Wang, Y.; Wang, Y.; Li, K. Induction of copper and iron in acute cold-stimulated brown adipose tissues. *Biochem. Biophys. Res. Commun.* **2017**, *488*, 496–500. [CrossRef]

30. Severson, D.L.; Denton, R.M.; Pask, H.T.; Randle, P.J. Calcium and magnesium ions as effectors of adipose-tissue pyruvate dehydrogenase phosphate phosphatase. *Biochem. J.* **1974**, *140*, 225–237. [CrossRef]

31. Zemel, M.B.; Shi, H.; Greer, B.; Dirienzo, D.; Zemel, P.C. Regulation of adiposity by dietary calcium. *FASEB J.* **2000**, *14*, 1132–1138. [CrossRef]

32. Yanoff, L.; Menzie, C.; Denkinger, B.; Sebring, N.; McHugh, T.; Remaley, A.; Yanovski, J. Inflammation and iron deficiency in the hypoferremia of obesity. *Int. J. Obes.* **2007**, *31*, 1412. [CrossRef]

33. Prasad, A.S.; Beck, F.W.; Bao, B.; Fitzgerald, J.T.; Snell, D.C.; Steinberg, J.D.; Cardozo, L.J. Zinc supplementation decreases incidence of infections in the elderly: Effect of zinc on generation of cytokines and oxidative stress. *Am. J. Clin. Nutr.* **2007**, *85*, 837–844. [CrossRef]

34. Kazi, T.G.; Afridi, H.I.; Kazi, N.; Jamali, M.K.; Arain, M.B.; Jalbani, N.; Kandhro, G.A. Copper, chromium, manganese, iron, nickel, and zinc levels in biological samples of diabetes mellitus patients. *Biol. Trace Elem. Res.* **2008**, *122*, 1–18. [CrossRef] [PubMed]

35. Kawakami, T.; Hanao, N.; Nishiyama, K.; Kadota, Y.; Inoue, M.; Sato, M.; Suzuki, S. Differential effects of cobalt and mercury on lipid metabolism in the white adipose tissue of high-fat diet-induced obesity mice. *Toxicol. Appl. Pharmacol.* **2012**, *258*, 32–42. [CrossRef]

36. Oz, M.; El Nebrisi, E.G.; Yang, K.-H.S.; Howarth, F.C.; Al Kury, L.T. Cellular and Molecular Targets of Menthol Actions. *Front. Pharmacol.* **2017**, *8*, 472. [CrossRef]

37. Macpherson, L.J.; Hwang, S.W.; Miyamoto, T.; Dubin, A.E.; Patapoutian, A.; Story, G.M. More than cool: Promiscuous relationships of menthol and other sensory compounds. *Mol. Cell. Neurosci.* **2006**, *32*, 335–343. [CrossRef]

38. Karashima, Y.; Damann, N.; Prenen, J.; Talavera, K.; Segal, A.; Voets, T.; Nilius, B. Bimodal action of menthol on the transient receptor potential channel TRPA1. *J. Neurosci.* **2007**, *27*, 9874–9884. [CrossRef] [PubMed]

39. Gelal, A.; Jacob, P.; Yu, L.; Benowitz, N.L. Disposition Kinetics and Effects of Menthol*. *Clin. Pharmacol. Ther.* **1999**, *66*, 128–135. [CrossRef] [PubMed]

40. Kaffenberger, R.M.; Doyle, M.J. Determination of Menthol and Menthol Glucuronide in Human Urine by Gas Chromatography Using an Enzyme-Sensitive Internal Standard and Flame Ionization Detection. *J. Chromatogr. B. Biomed. Sci. App.* **1990**, *527*, 59–66. [CrossRef]

41. Martin, D.; Valdez, J.; Boren, J.; Mayersohn, M. Dermal Absorption of Camphor, Menthol, and Methyl Salicylate in Humans. *J. Clin. Pharmacol.* **2004**, *44*, 1151–1157. [CrossRef] [PubMed]

42. JECFA. Menthol. In *Evaluation of certain food additives and contaminants: forty-second report of the Joint FAO/WHO Expert Committee on Food Additives*; World Health Organizaton: Geneva, Switzerland, 1999; pp. 57–76.

© 2019 by the authors. Licensee MDPI, Basel, Switzerland. This article is an open access article distributed under the terms and conditions of the Creative Commons Attribution (CC BY) license (http://creativecommons.org/licenses/by/4.0/).

cells

Article

TRPV1-Like Immunoreactivity in the Human Locus K, a Distinct Subregion of the Cuneate Nucleus

Marina Del Fiacco [1], Maria Pina Serra [1], Marianna Boi [1], Laura Poddighe [1], Roberto Demontis [2], Antonio Carai [2] and Marina Quartu [1,*]

[1] Department of Biomedical Sciences, University of Cagliari, Cittadella Universitaria di Monserrato, 09042 Monserrato (CA), Italy; marina.delfiacco@gmail.com (M.D.F.); mpserra@unica.it (M.P.S.); marianna.boi@unica.it (M.B.); laura.poddighe@gmail.com (L.P.)

[2] Department of Medical Sciences and Public Health, University of Cagliari, Cittadella Universitaria di Monserrato, 09042 Monserrato (CA), Italy; demrob@unica.it (R.D.); acarai@medicina.unica.it (A.C.)

* Correspondence: quartu@unica.it; Tel.: +39-070-675-4084

Received: 29 April 2018; Accepted: 5 July 2018; Published: 8 July 2018

Abstract: The presence of transient receptor potential vanilloid type-1 receptor (TRPV1)-like immunoreactivity (LI), in the form of nerve fibres and terminals, is shown in a set of discrete gray matter subregions placed in the territory of the human cuneate nucleus. We showed previously that those subregions share neurochemical and structural features with the protopathic nuclei and, after the ancient name of our town, collectively call them Locus Karalis, and briefly Locus K. TRPV1-LI in the Locus K is codistributed, though not perfectly overlapped, with that of the neuropeptides calcitonin gene-related peptide and substance P, the topography of the elements immunoreactive to the three markers, in relation to each other, reflecting that previously described in the caudal spinal trigeminal nucleus. Myelin stainings show that myelinated fibres, abundant in the cuneate, gracile and trigeminal magnocellular nuclei, are scarce in the Locus K as in the trigeminal substantia gelatinosa. Morphometric analysis shows that cell size and density of Locus K neurons are consistent with those of the trigeminal substantia gelatinosa and significantly different from those of the magnocellular trigeminal, solitary and dorsal column nuclei. We propose that Locus K is a special component of the human dorsal column nuclei. Its functional role remains to be determined, but TRPV1 appears to play a part in it.

Keywords: human medulla oblongata; cuneate nucleus; dorsal column nuclei; TRPV1; calcitonin gene-related peptide; substance P

1. Introduction

The transient receptor potential vanilloid type-1 receptor (TRPV1) is a polymodal ion channel expressed in primary sensory neurons, critically involved in the perception of mechanical and thermal stimuli as well as in pain modulation, and in allodynia and hyperalgesia in neuropathic pain [1–7]. Temperature (over 42 °C), low extracellular pH and capsaicin represent TRPV1 activators often used in experimental studies. To date, TRPV1 is viewed as a molecular integrator of different stimuli in the peripheral polymodal nociceptors; thus, it is activated by noxious heat, acidic and basic pH, voltage, endogenous lipid-derived compounds, and a variety of substances, among which the agonist resiniferatoxin is the best known [1,2,4,8–11]. In rodents, TRPV1 is expressed by a subset of peripheral sensory neurons involved in pain sensation [12–22]. Available studies on human tissue show the occurrence of TRPV1 in neurons of dorsal root ganglia (DRG) [15,23–28] and trigeminal ganglion (TG) [29,30], and their central and peripheral endings [25,31–33]. TRPV1, in addition to Calcitonin Gene-Related Peptide (CGRP) and Substance P (SP), is localized in primary sensory neurons and, in particular, in those of small and medium size, with poorly myelinated or unmyelinated small calibre fibres, responsible for the reception of nociceptive protopathic stimuli. It has been shown that, in primary sensory neurons, TRPV1 activation triggers the release of CGRP and SP [11,33–37], typical markers of the capsaicin-sensitive sensory neurons [8]. The neuropeptides in turn activate their effector cell receptors, leading to neurogenic inflammation and sensitization of nociceptors [8,11]. The aberrant activation of TRPV1 has been implicated in different neuropathological conditions including inflammation [38–43], neuropathic pain [26,27,31,43], visceral pain [40,41,43–45], nerve injury [43,46,47] and migraine [33]. In humans, the local injection of capsaicin has been shown to cause sensitization of the cutaneous afferents [48–50], release of CGRP from peripheral nerve endings [11,51,52] and pain in the deep somatic tissues [53–56].

Classically, the dorsal column nuclear complex consists of the larger cuneate, gracile and external cuneate nuclei, and of the smaller medial and lateral pericuneate nuclei, nucleus Z and nucleus X of Pompeiano and Brodal [57]. For the most part, they receive large myelinated primary afferent fibres conveying somatic epicritic, kinesthetic and proprioceptive sensation from the trunk and limbs, and relay to the thalamus and cerebellum. Several substances have been identified as synaptic neurotransmitters in the dorsal column nuclei. Thus, glutamate and glycine and gamma-aminobutyric acid act as excitatory and inhibitory neurotransmitters [58–66], and other molecules, such as adenosine triphosphate, acetylcholine, and monoamines, may also function as transmitters and/or modulators [58,67–69]. As a general rule, neuropeptide immunoreactive elements are less abundant in dorsal column nuclei than in regions that relay protopathic and nociceptive stimuli, namely the spinal dorsal horn and the spinal trigeminal and solitary nuclei, both in humans [70–75] and in laboratory animals [76–91]. Recently, we have formally defined additional distinctive subdivisions of the human dorsal column nuclei, evident from prenatal to old life [92]. Extending early observations on the presence of gray matter areas that are strongly immunoreactive to SP in the territory of the human cuneate nucleus and adjacent fascicle [70,71], we have shown that the cuneate nucleus fields rich in SP also host neural structures immunoreactive to the neuropeptides CGRP, methionine- and leucine-enkephalin, peptide histidine-isoleucine, somatostatin and galanin, the trophin glial cell line-derived neurotrophic factor, and the neuroplasticity proteins polysialylated neural cell adhesion molecule and growth-associated protein-43 [92] and references therein. Moreover, the topographical distribution of the structures immunoreactive to all those markers in relation to each other clearly showed that the neurochemistry of those cuneate nucleus gray matter fields, at variance with the remaining nuclear territory, was strikingly similar to that of the spinal cord dorsal horn and the spinal nucleus of the trigeminal nerve [70,71,92–97]. As a tribute to the place where M.D.F. first observed and described those discrete cuneate nucleus subregions, after the ancient name of our town, Cagliari, we collectively call them Locus Karalis and briefly Locus K [98,99].

With the aim of further describing the capsaicin-sensitive component of the human nervous system, here we show that the Locus K, identified by its immunoreactivity to SP and CGRP, also contains TRPV1-like immunoreactivity (LI) in specimens from prenatal and neonatal life to adult age. Furthermore, we show that the cyto- and myeloarchitecture of the Locus K also harmonize with those of the protopathic and nociceptive sensory nuclei.

2. Materials and Methods

2.1. Tissue Sampling

Specimens of medulla oblongata were obtained at autopsy from subjects with no signs of neuropathology, at age ranging 21 gestation weeks to 88 years (Table 1). The sampling and handling of human specimens conformed to the guidelines of the local Ethics Committee of the National Health System and complied with the principles enunciated in the Declaration of Helsinki. R.D. and A.C. collected the human tissues and R.D. was the only one to have access to identifying information about the autopsied subjects. The used specimens had been stored as part of the standardized procedure for autopsy samples at the section of Forensic Medicine of the Department of Public Health, Clinical and Molecular Medicine. The Ethics Committee formally stated that the present study complied with the ethical principles and does not need approval because all the used specimens were processed anonymously (Report No. 9, 15/07/2015). Fixation in 4%, freshly prepared phosphate-buffered formaldehyde, pH 7.3, for 4–6 h at 4 °C, was followed by overnight rinsing in 0.1 M phosphate buffer (PB), pH 7.3, containing 5–20% sucrose.

Table 1. List of specimens.

Case	Age	Sex	Primary Cause of Death	Post-Mortem Hours
1	Fetus 21 w.g.	F	Cardiorespiratory failure	29
2	Pre-term newborn 6 d (25 w.g.)	F	Pneumonitis	25
3	Pre-term newborn 1 d (34 w.g.)	M	Cardiorespiratory failure	29
4	Pre-term newborn (38 w.g.)	M	Cardiorespiratory failure	38
5	Full-term newborn (40 w.g.)	M	Cardiorespiratory failure	28
6	Full-term newborn 1 d	M	Cardiorespiratory failure	24
7	Full-term newborn 2 d	F	Persistence of fetal circulation	38
8	Full-term newborn 7 d	F	Cardiorespiratory failure	27
9	Adult 44 y	M	Stabbing	40
10	Adult 53 y	F	Cardiorespiratory failure	31
11	Adult 56 y	F	Cardiomyopathy	34
12	Adult 71 y	M	Renal failure	25

F, female; d, days; h, hours; M, male; y, years; w.g., weeks of gestation (calculated from the 1st day of the latest menstrual cycle).

2.2. Immunohistochemistry and Histology

Adjacent transverse slices of the medulla oblongata were cut with a cryostat at 10–14 or 30 µm and collected in series on chrome alum-gelatin coated slides. The avidin–biotin-peroxidase complex (ABC) immunostaining technique was used. Slides were treated with 0.1% phenylhydrazine (Sigma Aldrich, St Louis, MO, USA) in phosphate buffered saline (PBS) containing 0.2% Triton X-100 (PBS/T) to block the endogenous peroxidase activity, and successively with 20% of normal goat serum (Vector Labs Inc., Burlingame, CA, USA) to minimize non-specific staining. Rabbit polyclonal antibodies against TRPV1 (Thermo Scientific, Waltham, MA, USA), diluted 1:500, and against CGRP (Chemicon, Temecula, CA, USA), diluted 1:1000, and a guinea-pig polyclonal antibody against SP (AbCam, Cambridge, UK), diluted 1:1200, were used as primary antibody. Biotin-conjugated goat anti-rabbit and anti-guinea-pig sera (Vector), both diluted 1:400, were used as secondary antiserum. The immunoreaction was revealed with 30 min of incubation with the ABC (BioSpa Div. Milan, Italy), diluted 1:250, and followed by incubation with a solution of 0.1 M phosphate buffer (PB), pH 7.3, containing 0.05% 3, 3'-diaminobenzidine (Sigma Aldrich, St Louis, MO, USA), 0.04% nickel ammonium sulfate and 0.01% hydrogen peroxide. All antisera and ABC were diluted in PBS/T. The specificity of the TRPV1 antibody has been validated by Western blot analysis on protein samples of human pre-term and adult TG and caudal medulla oblongata, and reported in a previous work [30]. Negative control preparations were obtained either by incubating tissue sections with the diluted primary antibody preabsorbed with 10 mM of the respective peptide for 24 h at 4 °C or by omitting the primary antibody. Cresyl violet, Black-Gold II staining kit (Biosensis, Thebarton, Australia) and/or Klüver–Barrera techniques were used as Nissl and myelin stainings. Observations and photographs were made with a photomicroscope Olympus BX61 (Hamburg, Germany), and with a slide scanner Nanozoomer 2.0-RS (Hamamatsu).

2.3. Morphometric Analysis

Morphometric analysis was performed on cuneate nucleus, gracile nucleus, external cuneate nucleus, Locus K, caudal spinal trigeminal nucleus substantia gelatinosa and magnocellular part, and solitary nucleus. Cell size analysis was performed on digital images captured with a 20× objective magnification. Cell mean diameters were automatically measured by Leica Application

Suite Advanced Fluorescence (LAS AF) Software; statistical parameters (mean, minimum, maximum, S.D.) and histograms of the cell sizes were obtained by the Statistica 7 software (Version 7.0.61.0; StatSoft Inc., Palo Alto, CA, USA). Cell density (number of cells/mm^2) was measured on digital images captured with a 10× objective magnification; statistical analysis was performed with One-way analysis of variance (ANOVA) and the Tukey's *post-hoc* test by means of the software GraphPad Prism 6 for Windows (GraphPad Software, La Jolla, San Diego, CA, USA)

3. Results

In the human caudal medulla oblongata of all examined specimens, from fetal and neonatal age (Figure 1a,b and Figure 2a) to adult life (Figure 3a,b), at levels between the pyramidal decussation and the obex, the territory of the cuneate nucleus contains distinct areas of gray matter that include TRPV1 strongly positive networks of varicose filaments and dot-like structures, interpreted as nerve fibres and terminals. By contrast, the remaining territory of the cuneate nucleus hosts scarce immunoreactivity. No evidence of immunoreactive cell bodies was found. Compared to the outcome in newborn tissue, the density of TRPV1-like immunoreactive structures appears reduced in adult specimens. No gender differences were observed. Immunostaining for CGRP and SP in adjacent sections allows for ascertaining that the TRPV1-LI is localized to the Locus K (Figures 1a–d and 2a,b). However, though codistributed, the immunoreactivity for the receptor and the neuropeptides do not strictly overlap. In fact, though present in the superficial dorsal edge of the gray area, the bulk of TRPV1-LI, compared with the CGRP- and SP-LI, occupies a deeper zone of the Locus K (Figures 1a–d and 2a,b). This is congruent with the previously described localization of the three markers in the substantia gelatinosa of the caudal spinal trigeminal nucleus [27]. As described for the neuropeptides [67,68,89], TRPV1-like immunoreactive fibres, either isolated or in thin bundles, are detectable within the cuneate fascicle (Figure 3c). No positive labelling is detectable at levels rostral to the obex. Alternate sections immunolabelled for TRPV1 and the neuropeptides, and histochemically stained for myelin (Figures 1 and 2) effectively contribute to demonstrate the topographical localization of the TRPV1-LI of the Locus K and show its myeloarchitectural organization. In particular, analysis of myelin stained sections shows that the cuneate nucleus subregions with strong immunoreactivity to TRPV1 and the two neuropeptides contain rare myelinated fibres, whereas numerous stained fibres can be seen running across the territory of the main cuneate nucleus (Figures 1–3). As previously described for the other markers, at certain levels, two distinct components of the Locus K, both containing TRPV1-LI, are detectable in the horizontal plane (Figure 2). The two regions are both located along the dorsal boundary of the cuneate nucleus, one in a dorsal and/or medial position, and the other one lateral to the cuneate nucleus and medial to the dorsomedial end of the caudal spinal trigeminal nucleus substantia gelatinosa (Figure 2). The medially located region may show a triangular, oval or arched profile, whereas the lateral one is round-shaped and the immunoreactivity is mostly confined to its crescent-shaped dorsal border (Figure 2). The histochemical stainings show that myelinated fibres, abundant in the cuneate nucleus, gracile nucleus, and caudal spinal trigeminal nucleus magnocellular part, conversely are scarce in both the Locus K and caudal spinal trigeminal nucleus substantia gelatinosa (Figure 1c,d, Figures 2c and 3a,b).

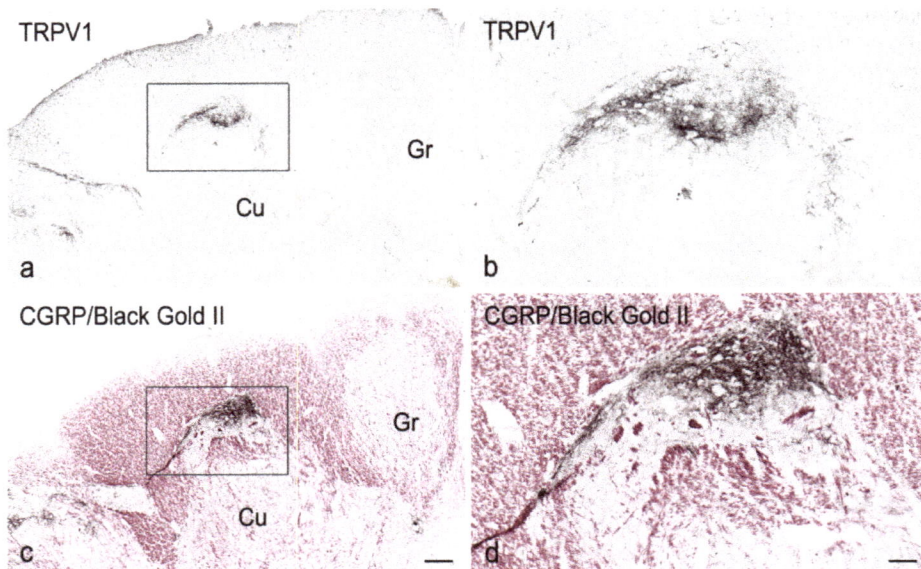

Figure 1. Full-term newborn, case 6. Left side dorsal quadrant in two consecutive sections of the caudal medulla oblongata immunostained for TRPV1 (**a,b**) and for CGRP followed by myelin Black Gold II counterstaining (**c,d**). Strongly TRPV1- and CGRP-like immunoreactive areas, along the dorsal border of the cuneate nucleus (Cu), are located in the Locus K (box in (**a,c**)) and are shown at higher magnification in (**b,d**), respectively. Gr, gracile nucleus. Scale bar: (**a**) = (**c**): 250 µm; (**b**) = (**d**): 50 µm.

Nissl staining performed on adult tissue sections (Figure 4) indicates that, in the LK, the cells are smaller and more closely packed (Figure 4g,h and Figure 5) than in the cuneate nucleus (Figure 4e,f and Figure 5), the histological aspect of the Locus K appearing rather similar to that of the caudal spinal trigeminal nucleus substantia gelatinosa (Figure 4i,j and Figure 5). The obvious tissue structure differences are proved by the analysis of cell size (histograms in Figure 4) and density (Figure 5). In the Locus K, as in the trigeminal substantia gelatinosa, the measured neurons show mean cell diameters between 5 and 18 µm (mean 8.55 and 8.68 µm, respectively), whereas, in the magnocellular part of the caudal spinal trigeminal nucleus, the mean diameters range 5 to 35 µm (mean 11.7 µm) and in the solitary nucleus 5 to 26 µm (mean 11.4 µm). In dorsal column nuclei, namely cuneate, external cuneate and gracile nuclei, the cell size is definitely larger, the mean cell diameter ranging 5 to 32 µm (mean 15 µm) in the cuneate and gracile nuclei, and 13 to 38 µm (mean 22 µm) in the external cuneate nucleus. As for the cell density (Figure 5), the mean value is $872.37/mm^2$ in Locus K, $579.63/mm^2$ in the substantia gelatinosa of caudal spinal trigeminal nucleus, $257.7/mm^2$ in the magnocellular part of caudal spinal trigeminal nucleus, $323.09/mm^2$ in the solitary nucleus, and between 125 and $159/mm^2$ in the dorsal column nuclei (cuneate, external cuneate and gracile nuclei). One-way ANOVA showed that scored differences in density are statistically significant ($p < 0.0001$); single p-values adjusted for multiple comparisons among the seven examined nuclear regions are reported in Table 2.

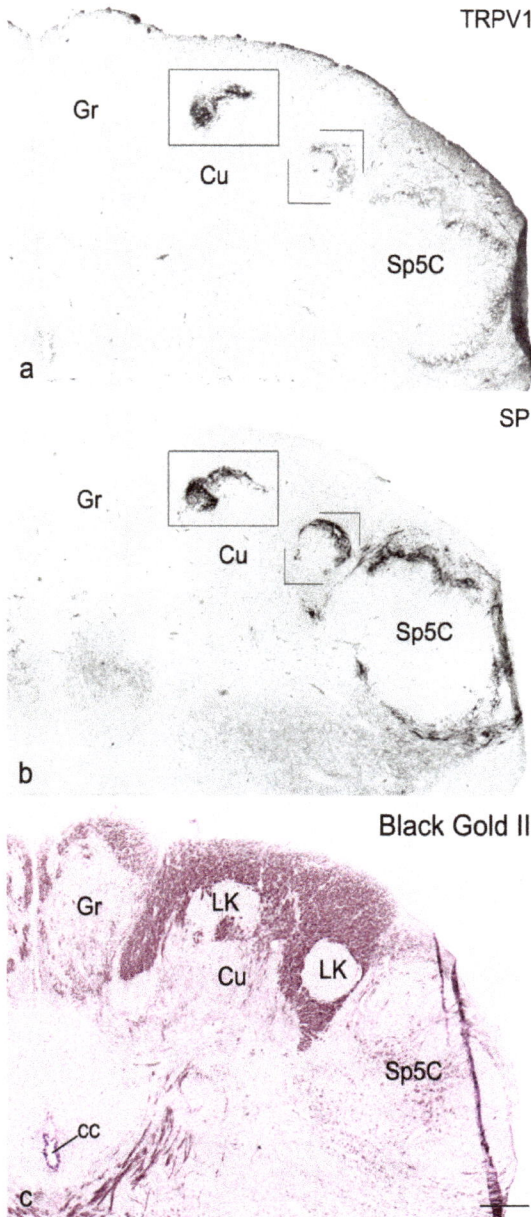

Figure 2. Full-term newborn, case 6. (**a–c**): right dorsal quadrant of three consecutive sections of the caudal medulla oblongata immunostained for TRPV1 (**a**) and SP (**b**), and stained for myelin with Black Gold II (**c**). TRPV1-LI (boxes in (**a**)) and SP-LI (boxes in (**b**)) are codistributed in a parallel way in the Locus K (LK) and in the spinal trigeminal nucleus (Sp5C) substantia gelatinosa. cc, central canal; Cu, cuneate nucleus; Gr, gracile nucleus. Scale bar: (**a**,**b**) = (**c**) 250 µm.

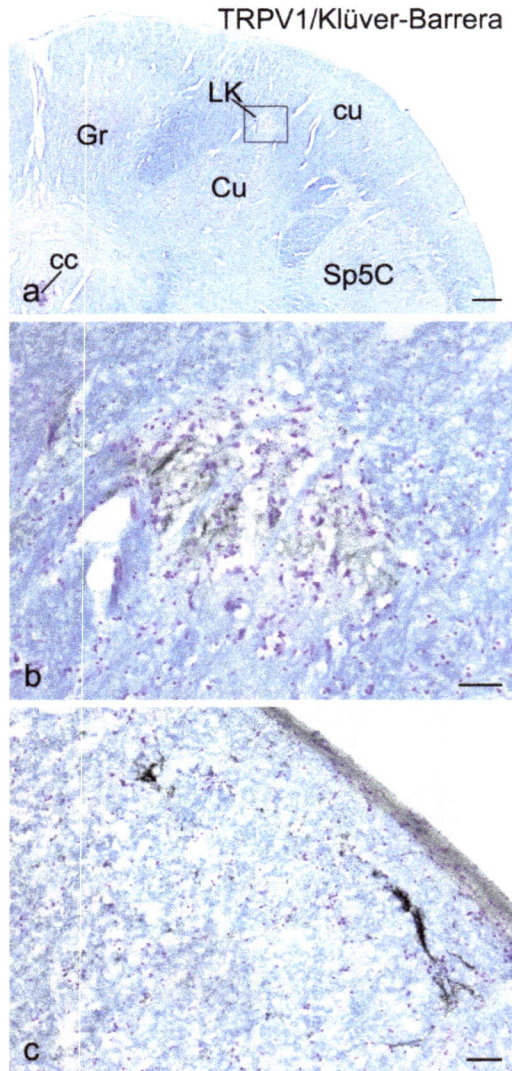

Figure 3. Adult, case 9. Right dorsal quadrant of caudal medulla oblongata immunostained for TRPV1 and counterstained with Klüver–Barrera (**a**). Locus K (LK) containing TRPV1-LI (box in (**a**)) is shown in (**b**) at higher magnification. **c**: thin fibre bundles in the dorsolateral fasciculus cuneatus (cu). cc, central canal; Cu, cuneate nucleus; Gr, gracile nucleus; Sp5C, caudal spinal trigeminal nucleus. Scale bar: (**a**) 250 μm; (**b**,**c**) 20 μm.

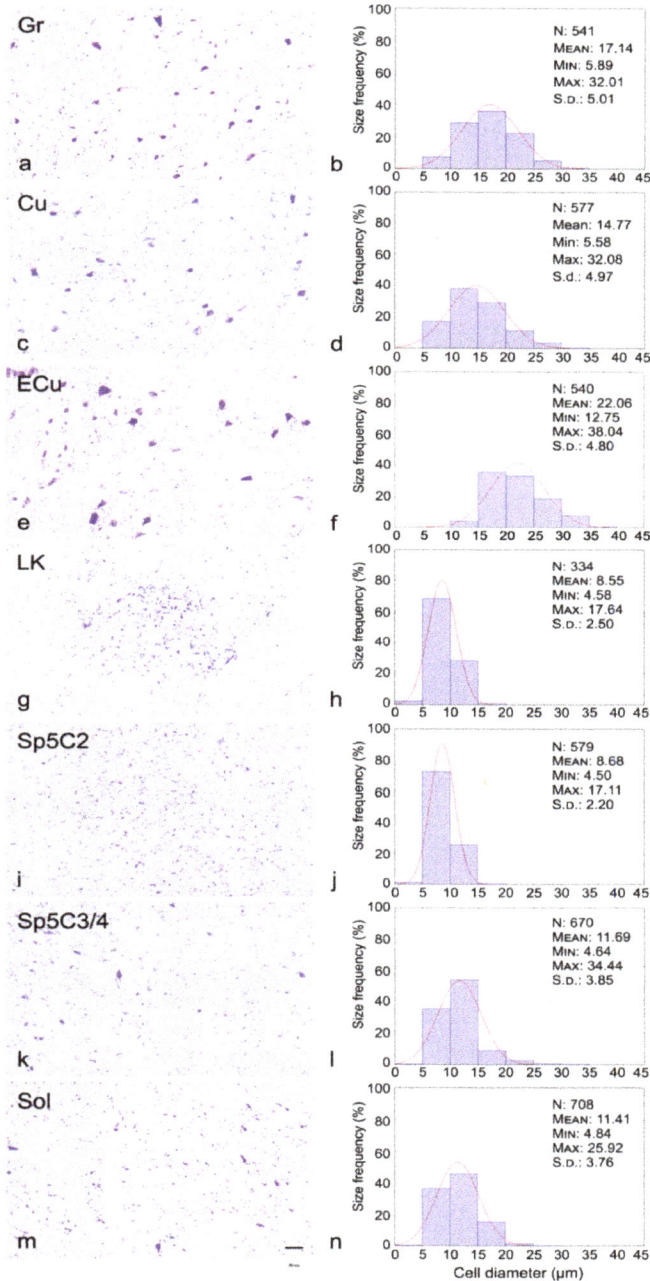

Figure 4. Adult, case 9. Nissl stained gracile nucleus (Gr), cuneate nucleus (Cu), external cuneate nucleus (ECu), Locus K (LK), caudal spinal trigeminal nucleus substantia gelatinosa (Sp5C2) and magnocellular region (Sp5C3/4), solitary nucleus (Sol) and relative size frequency histograms. In histograms, x-axis values represent the mean cell diameters expressed in µm, y-axis values report the relative percent frequency. Curves superimposed on the histograms represent the theoretical normal distribution. Scale bar: (**a, c, e, g, i, k**) = (**m**) 50 µm.

Cell density

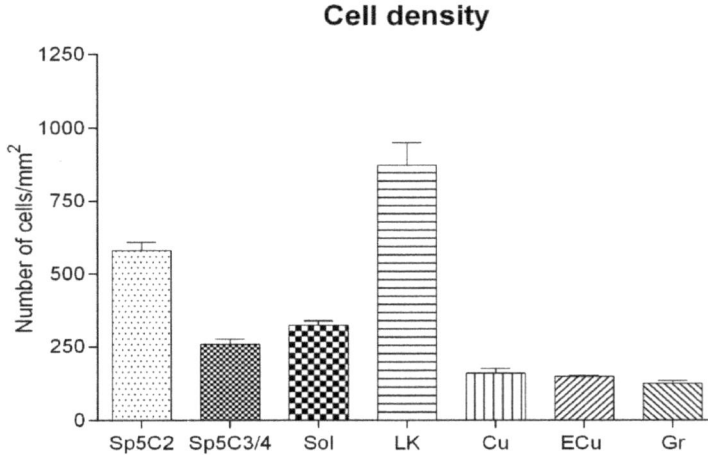

Figure 5. Adult, case 9. Histogram of mean cell density in the Locus K (LK) as compared to protopathic sensory nuclei and dorsal column nuclei of the human medulla oblongata. Differences in density among the seven regions are statistically significant (see Table 2). Caudal spinal trigeminal nucleus substantia gelatinosa (Sp5C2) and magnocellular region (Sp5C3/4), solitary nucleus (Sol), cuneate nucleus (Cu), external cuneate nucleus (ECu) and gracile nucleus (Gr).

Table 2. *P*-values, calculated by means of one way ANOVA followed by Tukey's *post-hoc* test, relevant to pair-wise contrasts between mean cell densities of Locus K (LK) and those of protopathic sensory and dorsal column nuclei in the human medulla oblongata (see histogram in Figure 5). Each *p*-value is adjusted to account for multiple comparison (significance level: 0.05; confidence level: 95%). Caudal spinal trigeminal nucleus substantia gelatinosa (Sp5C2) and magnocellular region (Sp5C3/4), solitary nucleus (Sol), cuneate nucleus (Cu), external cuneate nucleus (ECu) and gracile nucleus (Gr).

Nuclei	Summary	Adjusted *p*-Value
Sp5C3/4 vs. Sol	*	0.0267
Sp5C3/4 vs. LK	**	0.0033
Sp5C2 vs. LK	****	<0.0001
Sp5C2 vs. Cu	ns	0.5456
Sp5C2 vs. ECu	****	<0.0001
Sp5C2 vs. Gr	ns	0.1186
Sp5C3/4 vs. Cu	****	<0.0001
Sp5C3/4 vs. ECu	****	<0.0001
Sp5C3/4 vs. Gr	****	<0.0001
Sol vs. LK	****	<0.0001
Sol vs. Cu	****	<0.0001
Sol vs. ECu	****	<0.0001
Sol vs. Gr	****	<0.0001
LK vs. Cu	****	<0.0001
LK vs. ECu	****	<0.0001
LK vs. Gr	****	<0.0001
Cu vs. ECu	ns	0.9998
Cu vs. Gr	ns	0.9203
ECu vs. Gr	ns	0.9771

*, $p < 0.05$; **, $p < 0.005$, ****, $p < 0.0001$; ns, not significant.

4. Discussion

The results obtained provide evidence for the presence of TRPV1-LI, in the form of a network of nerve fibres and terminals, within a set of distinct subnuclear areas located in the territory of the human cuneate nucleus, which we designate as Locus Kalaris or, briefly, Locus K. In a previous study, we provided a three-dimensional reconstruction of those areas [92], showing that the Locus K spans longitudinally from the pyramidal decussation to the obex level, first appearing caudally at the level of the cuneate nucleus caudal pole, and being located along the dorsal border of the cuneate nucleus. Similarly to several other markers, such as neuropeptides and molecules indicative of trophism and neuroplasticity [70,71,92–97], TRPV1-LI is detectable in the Locus K throughout life, from fetal to adult age. The present study also provides the first description of the morphometric features of the Locus K and a comparative analysis between Locus K and a number of the human medulla oblongata sensory nuclei. Among them, the mean cell size shows the lowest values in the Locus K and in the spinal trigeminal nucleus substantia gelatinosa, is somewhat higher in the spinal trigeminal nucleus magnocellular part and solitary nucleus, and is by far larger in the cuneate, gracile and external cuneate nuclei. A similar, though reversed, trend among the same nuclei is maintained with regard to the mean cell density, which shows the highest value in the Locus K followed by the spinal trigeminal nucleus substantia gelatinosa, whereas it lessens in the spinal trigeminal nucleus magnocellular part and solitary nucleus, and is greatly reduced in the cuneate, external cuneate and gracile nuclei. Thus, the concurrent immunohistochemical labelling for TRPV1 and the neuropeptides CGRP and SP (this study), which in turn are codistributed with several other markers [92], and the outcome of the cyto- and myeloarchitectural analysis, display the remarkable similarity in the neurochemical and structural arrangement between the Locus K and the protopathic sensory nuclei of the human medulla oblongata. Moreover, the pattern of immunolabeling and relative distribution of TRPV1-, CGRP- and SP-LI uphold the possibility that the Locus K is structurally organized in a laminar pattern, likewise the spinal trigeminal nucleus substantia gelatinosa. All of these observations induce consideration of a role in protopathic sensory neurotransmission for the Locus K and a functional involvement of TRPV1 in it, similar to that proposed in the spinal dorsal horn and, more generally, in the protopathic sensory nuclei. Ample evidence on the neurochemical anatomy of the somatosensory system in different animal species, including man, shows that immunoreactivity to several neuropeptides is concentrated in the superficial laminae of the spinal dorsal horn, in the caudal spinal trigeminal nucleus substantia gelatinosa, and in the solitary nucleus, being generally scarce to absent in the dorsal column nuclei [92] (and references therein), [100,101]. In a similar way, at a central level, the majority of TRPV1-containing structures occur in the superficial laminae of the rat spinal cord dorsal horn [22,102–105], in the rat [106] and human trigeminal substantia gelatinosa [27], and have a recognized role in transduction and transmission of noxious stimuli. In these territories, TRPV1 has been localized to unmyelinated (C) or thinly myelinated (Adelta) primary sensory afferents [1,11,14,102,106] that terminate mostly in lamina I and the inner part of lamina II of the rat spinal cord dorsal horn [102,103]. We showed a similar distribution in the human spinal trigeminal nucleus substantia gelatinosa [30]. However, postsynaptic TRPV1 has also been reported in the rodent superficial dorsal horn [103,107–109]. Moreover, together with that in somatic pain perception, TRPV1 appears to play an important role in visceral pain. In fact, at L4-S1 levels of the spinal cord dorsal horn [104,110] and sacral dorsal commissural nucleus [111], TRPV1 expression has been associated with visceral afferents innervating the urinary bladder and other pelvic organs, and TRPV1-bearing terminals have been shown in the solitary nucleus [112,113].

The existence of a region with the neurochemical and structural characteristics as the Locus K in the territory of the dorsal column nuclei, as well as the occurrence of TRPV1-LI in it, may sound in marked contrast with the classical functional role of those nuclei, which is epicritic sensibility. However, in keeping with a role in pain and protopathic perception, the dorsal columns, largely composed of thick myelinated fibres involved in the transmission of fine touch, vibratory sense and proprioception, also include a large proportion of thin and unmyelinated fibres [114–116], which may reach up to 25% in the human sacral spinal cord [117]. In the rat, these fibres have been identified as primary afferents and many of them are immunoreactive to CGRP and SP [117–121]. Additionally, nociceptive second order sensory fibres run in the dorsal column, composing the post-synaptic dorsal column (PSDC) pathway. The latter originates from neurons located in the central area of the spinal cord [122–124] and includes neuropeptidergic fibres [125]. The PSDC pathway carries visceral nociceptive information and clinical reports show that its surgical interruption effectively relieves intractable visceral pain in cancer patients [124,126,127]. Thus, on the one hand, the main involvement in sensory neurotransmission for TRPV1 and several neuropeptides, namely CGRP and SP, remains related to the protopathic sensory perception. On the other hand, the possibility that these molecules play a role in the epicritic sensibility classically attributed to the dorsal column nuclei may also be taken into account. In fact, at both peripheral and central level, TRPV1 may also contribute to mechanotransmission, especially after injury [108,128–131], and TRPV1-immunostaining has been detected in laminae III-V of the spinal cord dorsal horn, receiving, among others, primary afferents involved in proprioception [104]. Moreover, TRPV1- [132] and CGRP-positive fibres [128] have been shown to innervate light touch mechanoreceptor Meissner's corpuscles in monkey and rat, respectively, and SP-positive fibres also occur in human and rat Meissner's corpuscles and other mechanoreceptors [133–135]. We did not detect TRPV1-positive cell bodies in the LK. However, besides the likely prospect that the TRPV1-like immunoreactive fibres of the LK belong to neurons composing a sensory pathway, the possibility that, at least in part, they represent processes of local neurons or glial cells can not be ruled out, as shown in the rat spinal cord, with a role for the receptor in the control of pain transmission and onset of neuropathic pain disfunctions, such as hyperalgesia and allodynia [22,107,109]. Finally, the possibility should also be considered that the TRPV1-like immunoreactive fibres in the LK belong, at least in part, to descending projections. In fact, experimental evidence underlines the role of supraspinal TRPV1 in pain modulation, the rostral-ventrolateral medulla (RVM), periaqueductal grey (PAG), amygdala, solitary tract nucleus, locus coeruleus, somatosensory and anterior cingulated cortex, and insula being the territories most involved in this functional meaning [15,136–142]. Although the knowledge of the TRPV1 role in most of these systems is still incomplete, the TRPV1-mediated activation of the PAG-RVM antinociceptive pain pathway has drawn attention as a possible pharmacological target for some types of intractable pain [142].

At the present time, the possible functional involvement of the Locus K remains a matter of speculation. The localization pattern of TRPV1-, CGRP- and SP-LI in it shows that the elements containing the three markers do not overlap perfectly. This agrees with our findings on the substantia gelatinosa of the spinal trigeminal nucleus [30] and suggests that, especially in the deep part of the Locus K, the TRPV1-LI may reside in non peptidergic [13,14] and perhaps in non presynaptic [102,143] elements.

In conclusion, the Locus K is still a "Nucleus in Search of a Function". However, on a positive note, TRPV1 must be considered one of the Characters playing in it.

Author Contributions: Conceptualization, M.D.F. and M.Q.; Formal analysis, M.P.S.; Funding acquisition, M.D.F., M.P.S. and M.Q.; Investigation, M.D.F., M.P.S., M.B., L.P. and M.Q.; Project administration, M.D.F. and M.Q.; Resources, R.D. and A.C.; Validation, M.D.F., M.P.S., M.B. and M.Q.; Visualization, M.D.F., M.P.S., M.B. and M.Q.; Writing—Original draft, M.D.F. and M.Q.; Writing—Review and editing, M.D.F. and M.Q.

Funding: The study was supported by grants from the Regione Autonoma della Sardegna (P.O.R. F.S.E. 2007–2013) and the University of Cagliari (Progetti di Ricerca di Interesse Dipartimentale, PRID 2015; Fondo Integrativo per la Ricerca, FIR 2016, 2017).

Conflicts of Interest: The authors declare no conflict of interest. The founding sponsors had no role in the design of the study; in the collection, analyses, or interpretation of data; in the writing of the manuscript, and in the decision to publish the results.

References

1. Caterina, M.J.; Schumacher, M.A.; Tominaga, M.; Rosen, T.A.; Levine, J.D.; Julius, D. The capsaicin receptor: A heat-activated ION channel in the pain pathway. *Nature* **1997**, *389*, 816–824. [CrossRef] [PubMed]
2. Szallasi, A.; Cortright, D.N.; Blum, C.A.; Eid, S.R. The vanilloid receptor TRPV1: 10 years from channel cloning to antagonist proof-of-concept. *Nat. Rev. Drug Discov.* **2007**, *6*, 357–372. [CrossRef] [PubMed]

3. Gao, Y.; Cao, E.; Julius, D.; Cheng, Y. TRPV1 structures in nanodiscs reveal mechanisms of ligand and lipid action. *Nature* **2016**, *534*, 347–351. [CrossRef] [PubMed]

4. Carnevale, V.; Rohacs, T. TRPV1: A Target for Rational Drug Design. *Pharmaceuticals* **2016**, *9*, 52. [CrossRef] [PubMed]

5. Kanai, Y.; Nakazato, E.; Fujiuchi, A.; Hara, T.; Imai, A. Involvement of an increased spinal TRPV1 sensitization through its up-regulation in mechanical allodynia of CCI rats. *Neuropharmacology* **2005**, *49*, 977–984. [CrossRef] [PubMed]

6. Basso, L.; Altier, C. Transient Receptor Potential Channels in neuropathic pain. *Curr. Opin. Pharmacol.* **2017**, *32*, 9–15. [CrossRef] [PubMed]

7. Wang, C.; Gu, L.; Ruan, Y.; Gegen, T.; Yu, L.; Zhu, C.; Yang, Y.; Zhou, Y.; Yu, G.; Tang, Z. Pirt together with TRPV1 is involved in the regulation of neuropathic pain. *Neural Plast.* **2018**, *2018*, 4861491. [CrossRef] [PubMed]

8. Szallasi, A.; Blumberg, P.M. Vanilloid (capsaicin) receptors and mechanisms. *Pharmacol. Rev.* **1999**, *51*, 159–212. [PubMed]

9. Hwang, S.W.; Cho, H.; Kwak, J.; Lee, S.Y.; Kang, C.J.; Kang, C.J.; Jung, J.; Cho, S.; Min, K.H.; Suh, Y.G.; et al. Direct activation of capsaicin receptors by products of lipoxygenases: Endogenous capsaicin-like substances. *Proc. Natl. Acad. Sci. USA* **2000**, *97*, 6155–6160. [CrossRef] [PubMed]

10. Bölcskei, K.; Helyes, Z.; Szabó, A.; Sándor, K.; Elekes, K.; Németh, J. Investigation of the role of TRPV1 receptors in acute and chronic nociceptive processes using gene-deficient mice. *Pain* **2005**, *117*, 368–376. [CrossRef] [PubMed]

11. Holzer, P. The pharmacological challenge to tame the transient receptor potential vanilloid-1 (TRPV1) nocisensor. *Br. J. Pharmacol.* **2008**, *155*, 1145–1162. [CrossRef] [PubMed]

12. Helliwell, R.J.; McLatchie, L.M.; Clarke, M.; Winter, J.; Bevan, S.; McIntyre, P. Capsaicin sensitivity is associated with the expression of the vanilloid (capsaicin) receptor (VR1) mRNA in adult rat sensory ganglia. *Neurosci. Lett.* **1998**, *250*, 177–180. [CrossRef]

13. Tominaga, M.; Caterina, M.J.; Malmberg, A.B.; Rosen, T.A.; Gilbert, H.; Skinner, K.; Raumann, B.E.; Basbaum, A.I.; Julius, D. The cloned capsaicin receptor integrates multiple pain-producing stimuli. *Neuron* **1998**, *21*, 531–543. [CrossRef]

14. Michael, G.J.; Priestley, J.V. Differential expression of the mRNA for the vanilloid receptor subtype 1 in cells of the adult rat dorsal root and nodose ganglia and its downregulation by axotomy. *J. Neurosci.* **1999**, *19*, 1844–1854. [CrossRef] [PubMed]

15. Mezey, E.; Tóth, Z.E.; Cortright, D.N.; Arzubi, M.K.; Krause, J.E.; Elde, R.; Guo, A.; Blumberg, P.M.; Szallasi, A. Distribution of mRNA for vanilloid receptor subtype 1 (VR1), and VR1-like immunoreactivity, in the central nervous system of the rat and human. *Proc. Natl. Acad. Sci. USA* **2000**, *97*, 3655–3660. [CrossRef] [PubMed]

16. Matsumoto, I.; Emori, Y.; Ninomiya, Y.; Abe, K. A comparative study of three cranial sensory ganglia projecting into the oral cavity: In situ hybridization analyses of neurotrophin receptors and thermosensitive cation channels. *Mol. Brain Res.* **2001**, *93*, 105–112. [CrossRef]

17. Ichikawa, H.; Fukunaga, T.; Jin, H.W.; Fujita, M.; Takano-Yamamoto, T.; Sugimoto, T. VR1-, VRL-1- and P2X3 receptor-immunoreactive innervation of the rat temporomandibular joint. *Brain Res.* **2004**, *1008*, 131–136. [CrossRef] [PubMed]

18. Ichikawa, H.; Sugimoto, T. The co-expression of VR1 and VRL-1 in the rat vagal sensory ganglia. *Brain Res.* **2003**, *980*, 293–296. [CrossRef]

19. Dinh, Q.T.; Groneberg, D.A.; Peiser, C.; Springer, J.; Joachim, R.A.; Arck, P.C.; Klapp, B.F.; Fischer, A. Nerve growth factor-induced substance P in capsaicin-insensitive vagal neurons innervating the lower mouse airway. *Clin. Exp. Allergy* **2004**, *34*, 1474–1479. [CrossRef] [PubMed]

20. Damann, N.; Rothermel, M.; Klupp, B.G.; Mettenleiter, T.C.; Hatt, H.; Wetzel, C.H. Chemosensory properties of murine nasal and cutaneous trigeminal neurons identified by viral tracing. *BMC Neurosci.* **2006**, *7*, 46. [CrossRef] [PubMed]

21. Bevan, S.; Quallo, T.; Andersson, D.A. TRPV1. In *Handbook of Experimental Pharmacology*; Springer: Berlin/Heidelberg, Germany, 2014; Volume 222, pp. 207–245.

22. Quartu, M.; Carozzi, V.A.; Dorsey, S.G.; Serra, M.P.; Poddighe, L.; Picci, C.R.; Boi, M.A.; Melis, T.I.; Del Fiacco, M.; Meregalli, C.R.; et al. Bortezomib treatment produces nocifensive behavior and changes in the expression of TRPV1, CGRP, and substance P in the rat DRG, spinal cord, and sciatic nerve. *BioMed Res. Int.* **2014**, 180428. [CrossRef] [PubMed]

23. Cortright, D.N.; Crandall, M.; Sanchez, J.F.; Zou, T.; Krause, J.E.; White, G. The tissue distribution and functional characterization of human VR1. *Biochem. Biophys. Res. Commun.* **2001**, *281*, 1183–1189. [CrossRef] [PubMed]

24. Holzer, P. TRPV1 and the gut: From a tasty receptor for a painful vanilloid to a key player in hyperalgesia. *Eur. J. Pharmacol.* **2004**, *500*, 231–241. [CrossRef] [PubMed]

25. Morgan, C.R.; Rodd, H.D.; Clayton, N.; Davis, J.B.; Boissonade, F.M. Vanilloid receptor 1 expression in human tooth pulp in relation to caries and pain. *J. Orofac. Pain* **2005**, *19*, 248–260. [PubMed]

26. Lauria, G.; Morbin, M.; Lombardi, R.; Capobianco, R.; Camozzi, F.; Pareyson, D.; Manconi, M.; Geppetti, P. Expression of capsaicin receptor immunoreactivity in human peripheral nervous system and in painful neuropathies. *J. Peripher. Nerv. Syst.* **2006**, *11*, 262–271. [CrossRef] [PubMed]

27. Facer, P.; Smith, G.D.; Benham, C.D.; Chessell, I.P.; Bountra, C.; Sinisi, M.; Birch, R.; Anand, P. Differential expression of the capsaicin receptor TRPV1 and related novel receptors TRPV3, TRPV4 and TRPM8 in normal human tissues and changes in traumatic and diabetic neuropathy. *BMC Neurol.* **2007**, *7*, 11. [CrossRef] [PubMed]

28. Anand, U.; Otto, W.R.; Bountra, C.; Chessell, I.; Sinisi, M.; Birch, R.; Anand, P. Cytosine arabinoside affects the heat and capsaicin receptor TRPV1 localisation and sensitivity in human sensory neurons. *J. Neurooncol.* **2008**, *89*, 1–7. [CrossRef] [PubMed]

29. Hou, M.; Uddman, R.; Tajti, J.; Kanje, M.; Edvinsson, L. Capsaicin receptor immunoreactivity in the human trigeminal ganglion. *Neurosci. Lett.* **2002**, *330*, 223–226. [CrossRef]

30. Quartu, M.; Serra, M.P.; Boi, M.; Poddighe, L.; Picci, C.; Demontis, R.; Del Fiacco, M. TRPV1 receptor in the human trigeminal ganglion and spinal nucleus: Immunohistochemical localization and comparison with the neuropeptides CGRP and SP. *J. Anat.* **2016**, *229*, 755–767. [CrossRef] [PubMed]

31. Yilmaz, Z.; Renton, T.; Yiangou, Y.; Zakrzewska, J.; Chessell, I.P.; Bountra, C.; Anand, P. Burning mouth syndrome as a trigeminal small fibre neuropathy: Increased heat and capsaicin receptor TRPV1 in nerve fibres correlates with pain score. *J. Clin. Neurosci.* **2007**, *14*, 864–871. [CrossRef] [PubMed]

32. Shinoda, M.; Takeda, M.; Honda, K.; Maruno, M.; Katagiri, A.; Satoh-Kuriwada, S.; Shoji, N.; Tsuchiya, M.; Iwata, K. Involvement of peripheral artemin signaling in tongue pain: Possible mechanism in burning mouth syndrome. *Pain* **2015**, *156*, 2528–2537. [CrossRef] [PubMed]

33. Del Fiacco, M.; Quartu, M.; Boi, M.; Serra, M.P.; Melis, T.; Boccaletti, R.; Shevel, E.; Cianchetti, C. TRPV1, CGRP and SP in scalp arteries of patients suffering from chronic migraine. *J. Neurol. Neurosurg. Psychiatry* **2015**, *86*, 393–397. [CrossRef] [PubMed]

34. Trevisani, M.; Smart, D.; Gunthorpe, M.J.; Tognetto, M.; Barbieri, M.; Campi, B.; Amadesi, S.; Gray, J.; Jerman, J.C.; Brough, S.J.; et al. Ethanol elicits and potentiates nociceptor responses via the vanilloid receptor-1. *Nat. Neurosci.* **2002**, *5*, 546–551. [CrossRef] [PubMed]

35. Grant, A.D.; Gerard, N.P.; Brain, S.D. Evidence of a role for NK1 and CGRP receptors in mediating neurogenic vasodilatation in the mouse ear. *Br. J. Pharmacol.* **2002**, *135*, 356–362. [CrossRef] [PubMed]

36. Chizh, B.A.; O'Donnell, M.B.; Napolitano, A.; Wang, J.; Brooke, A.C.; Aylott, M.C.; Bullman, J.N.; Gray, E.J.; Lai, R.Y.; Williams, P.M.; et al. The effects of the TRPV1 antagonist SB-705498 on TRPV1 receptor-mediated activity and inflammatory hyperalgesia in humans. *Pain* **2007**, *132*, 132–141. [CrossRef] [PubMed]

37. Starr, A.; Graepel, R.; Keeble, J.; Schmidhuber, S.; Clark, N.; Grant, A.; Shah, A.M.; Brain, S.D. A reactive oxygen species-mediated component in neurogenic vasodilatation. *Cardiovasc. Res.* **2008**, *78*, 139–147. [CrossRef] [PubMed]

38. Park, C.K.; Kim, M.S.; Fang, Z.; Li, H.Y.; Jung, S.J.; Choi, S.Y.; Lee, S.J.; Park, K.; Kim, J.S.; Oh, S.B. Functional expression of thermo-transient receptor potential channels in dental primary afferent neurons: Implication for tooth pain. *J. Biol. Chem.* **2006**, *281*, 17304–17311. [CrossRef] [PubMed]

39. Akbar, A.; Yiangou, Y.; Facer, P.; Walters, J.R.; Anand, P.; Ghosh, S. Increased capsaicin receptor TRPV1-expressing sensory fibres in irritable bowel syndrome and their correlation with abdominal pain. *Gut* **2008**, *57*, 923–929. [CrossRef] [PubMed]

40. Holzer, P. Transient receptor potential (TRP) channels as drug targets for diseases of the digestive system. *Pharmacol. Ther.* **2011**, *131*, 142–170. [CrossRef] [PubMed]
41. Holzer, P.; Izzo, A.A. The pharmacology of TRP channels. *Br. J. Pharmacol.* **2014**, *171*, 2469–2473. [CrossRef] [PubMed]
42. Chung, M.-K.; Lee, J.; Duraes, G.; Ro, J.Y. Lipopolysaccharide-induced pulpitis up-regulates TRPV1 in trigeminal ganglia. *J. Dent. Res.* **2011**, *90*, 1103–1107. [CrossRef] [PubMed]
43. Brandt, M.R.; Beyer, C.E.; Stahl, S.M. TRPV1 Antagonists and Chronic Pain: Beyond Thermal Perception. *Pharmaceuticals* **2012**, *5*, 114–132. [CrossRef] [PubMed]
44. Sikandar, S.; Dickenson, A.H. Visceral pain: The ins and outs, the ups and downs. *Curr. Opin. Support. Palliat. Care* **2012**, *6*, 17–26. [CrossRef] [PubMed]
45. Kondo, E.; Jinnouchi, O.; Nakano, S.; Ohnishi, H.; Kawata, I.; Okamoto, H.; Takeda, N. Aural stimulation with capsaicin ointment improved swallowing function in elderly patients with dysphagia: A randomized, placebo-controlled, double-blind, comparative study. *Clin. Interv. Aging* **2017**, *12*, 1921–1928. [CrossRef] [PubMed]
46. Urano, H.; Ara, T.; Fujinami, Y.; Hiraoka, B.Y. Aberrant TRPV1 expression in heat hyperalgesia associated with trigeminal neuropathic pain. *Int. J. Med. Sci.* **2012**, *9*, 690–697. [CrossRef] [PubMed]
47. Zakir, H.M.; Mostafeezur, R.M.; Suzuki, A.; Hitomi, S.; Suzuki, I.; Maeda, T.; Seo, K.; Yamada, Y.; Yamamura, K.; Lev, S.; et al. Expression of TRPV1 channels after nerve injury provides an essential delivery tool for neuropathic pain attenuation. *PLoS ONE* **2012**, *7*, e44023. [CrossRef] [PubMed]
48. Gazerani, P.; Pedersen, N.S.; Staahl, C.; Drewes, A.M.; Arendt-Nielsen, L. Subcutaneous Botulinum toxin type A reduces capsaicin-induced trigeminal pain and vasomotor reactions in human skin. *Pain* **2009**, *141*, 60–69. [CrossRef] [PubMed]
49. Aykanat, V.; Gentgall, M.; Briggs, N.; Williams, D.; Yap, S.; Rolan, P. Intradermal capsaicin as a neuropathic pain model in patients with unilateral sciatica. *Br. J. Clin. Pharmacol.* **2012**, *73*, 37–45. [CrossRef] [PubMed]
50. Silberberg, A.; Moeller-Bertram, T.; Wallace, M.S. A randomized, double-blind, crossover study to evaluate the depth response relationship of intradermal capsaicin-induced pain and hyperalgesia in healthy adult volunteers. *Pain Med.* **2015**, *16*, 745–752. [CrossRef] [PubMed]
51. Fehrenbacher, J.C.; Sun, X.X.; Locke, E.E.; Henry, M.A.; Hargreaves, K.M. Capsaicin-evoked CGRP release from human dental pulp: A model system for the study of peripheral neuropeptide secretion in normal healthy tissue. *Pain* **2009**, *144*, 253–261. [CrossRef] [PubMed]
52. Burns, L.E.; Ramsey, A.A.; Emrick, J.J.; Janal, M.N.; Gibbs, J.L. Variability in Capsaicin-stimulated Calcitonin Gene-related Peptide Release from Human Dental Pulp. *J. Endod.* **2016**, *42*, 542–546. [CrossRef] [PubMed]
53. Witting, N.; Svensson, P.; Gottrup, H.; Arendt-Nielsen, L.; Jensen, T.S. Intramuscular and intradermal injection of capsaicin: A comparison of local and referred pain. *Pain* **2000**, *84*, 407–412. [CrossRef]
54. Arendt-Nielsen, L.; Yarnitsky, D. Experimental and clinical applications of quantitative sensory tsting applied to skin, muscles and viscera. *J. Pain* **2009**, *10*, 556–572. [CrossRef] [PubMed]
55. Sohn, M.K.; Graven-Nielsen, T.; Arendt-Nielsen, L.; Svensson, P. Inhibition of motor unit firing during experimental muscle pain in humans. *Muscle Nerv.* **2000**, *23*, 1219–1226. [CrossRef]
56. O'Neill, J.; Brock, C.; Olesen, A.E.; Andresen, T.; Nilsson, M.; Dickenson, A.H. Unravelling the mystery of capsaicin: A tool to understand and treat pain. *Pharmacol. Rev.* **2012**, *64*, 939–971. [CrossRef] [PubMed]
57. Pompeiano, O.; Brodal, A. Spinovestibular fibers in the cat; an experimental study. *J. Comp. Neurol.* **1957**, *108*, 353–381. [CrossRef] [PubMed]
58. Galindo, A.; Krnjević, K.; Schwartz, S. Micro-iontophoretic studies on neurones in the cuneate nucleus. *J. Physiol.* **1967**, *192*, 359–377. [CrossRef] [PubMed]
59. Roberts, P.J. The release of amino acids with proposed neurotransmitter function from the cuneate and gracile nuclei of the rat in vivo. *Brain Res.* **1974**, *67*, 419–428. [CrossRef]
60. Rustioni, A.; Schmechel, D.E.; Cheema, S.; Fitzpatrick, D. Glutamic acid decarboxylase-containing neurons in the dorsal column nuclei of the cat. *Somatosens. Res.* **1984**, *1*, 329–357. [CrossRef] [PubMed]
61. Westman, J. Light and electron microscopical studies of the GABA innervation of the dorsal column nuclei and the lateral cervical nucleus in the primate species *Macaca fascicularis* and *Papio anubis*. *Upsala J. Med. Sci.* **1989**, *94*, 255–270. [CrossRef] [PubMed]
62. De Biasi, S.; Rustioni, A. Ultrastructural immunocytochemical localization of excitatory amino acids in the somatosensory system. *J. Histochem. Cytochem.* **1990**, *38*, 1745–1754. [CrossRef] [PubMed]

63. Heino, R.; Westman, J. Quantitative analysis of the feline dorsal column nuclei and their GABAergic and non-GABAergic neurons. *Anat. Embryol.* **1991**, *184*, 181–193. [CrossRef] [PubMed]

64. De Biasi, S.; Vitellaro-Zuccarello, L.; Bernardi, P.; Valtschanoff, J.G.; Weinberg, R.J. Ultrastructural and immunocytochemical characterization of primary afferent terminals in the rat cuneate nucleus. *J. Comp. Neurol.* **1994**, *347*, 275–287. [CrossRef] [PubMed]

65. Popratiloff, A.; Valtschanoff, J.G.; Rustioni, A.; Weinberg, R.J. Colocalization of GABA and glycine in the rat dorsal column nuclei. *Brain Res.* **1996**, *706*, 308–312. [CrossRef]

66. Lue, J.H.; Chen, S.H.; Shieh, J.Y.; Wen, C.Y. Afferent synaptic contacts on glycine-immunoreactive neurons in the rat cuneate nucleus. *Synapse* **2001**, *41*, 139–149. [CrossRef] [PubMed]

67. Henderson, Z.; Sherriff, F.E. Distribution of choline acetyltransferase immunoreactive axons and terminals in the rat and ferret brainstem. *J. Comp. Neurol.* **1991**, *314*, 147–163. [CrossRef] [PubMed]

68. Blomqvist, A.; Broman, J. Serotoninergic innervation of the dorsal column nuclei and its relation to cytoarchitectonic subdivisions: An immunohistochemical study in cats and monkeys (*Aotus trivirgatus*). *J. Comp. Neurol.* **1993**, *327*, 584–596. [CrossRef] [PubMed]

69. Maqbool, A.; Batten, T.F.; Berry, P.A.; McWilliam, P.N. Distribution of dopamine-containing neurons and fibres in the feline medulla oblongata: A comparative study using catecholamine-synthesizing enzyme and dopamine immunohistochemistry. *Neuroscience* **1993**, *53*, 717–733. [CrossRef]

70. Del Fiacco, M.; Dessi, M.L.; Atzori, M.G.; Levanti, M.C. Substance P in the human brainstem. Preliminary results of its immunohistochemical localization. *Brain Res.* **1983**, *264*, 142–147. [CrossRef]

71. Del Fiacco, M.; Dessì, M.L.; Levanti, M.C. Topographical localization of substance P in the human post-mortem brainstem. An immunohistochemical study in the newborn and adult tissue. *Neuroscience* **1984**, *12*, 591–611. [CrossRef]

72. Chigr, F.; Najimi, M.; Leduque, P.; Charnay, Y.; Jordan, D.; Chayvialle, J.A.; Tohyama, M.; Kopp, N. Anatomical distribution of somatostatin immunoreactivity in the infant brainstem. *Neuroscience* **1989**, *29*, 615–628. [CrossRef]

73. Unger, J.W.; Lange, W. Immunohistochemical mapping of neurophysins and calcitonin gene-related peptide in the human brainstem and cervical spinal cord. *J. Chem. Neuroanat.* **1991**, *4*, 299–309. [CrossRef]

74. Coveñas, R.; Martin, F.; Belda, M.; Smith, V.; Salinas, P.; Rivada, E.; Gonzalez-Baron, S. Mapping of neurokinin-like immunoreactivity in the human brainstem. *BMC Neurosci.* **2003**, *4*, 3. [CrossRef]

75. Coveñas, R.; Martín, F.; Salinas, P.; Rivada, E.; Smith, V.; Aguilar, L.A.; Díaz-Cabiale, Z.; Narváez, J.A.; Tramu, G. An immunocytochemical mapping of methionine-enkephalin-Arg(6)-Gly(7)-Leu(8) in the human brainstem. *Neuroscience* **2004**, *128*, 843–859. [CrossRef] [PubMed]

76. Simantov, R.; Kuhar, M.J.; Uhl, G.R.; Snyder, S.H. Opioid peptide enkephalin: Immunohistochemical mapping in rat central nervous system. *Proc. Natl. Acad. Sci. USA* **1977**, *74*, 2167–2171. [CrossRef] [PubMed]

77. Cuello, A.C.; Kanazawa, I. The distribution of substance P immunoreactive fibers in the rat central nervous system. *J. Comp. Neurol.* **1978**, *178*, 129–156. [CrossRef] [PubMed]

78. Ljungdahl, A.; Hökfelt, T.; Nilsson, G. Distribution of substance P-like immunoreactivity in the central nervous system of the rat—I. Cell bodies and nerve terminals. *Neuroscience* **1978**, *3*, 861–943. [CrossRef]

79. Haber, S.; Elde, R. The distribution of enkephalin immunoreactive fibers and terminals in the monkey central nervous system: An immunohistochemical study. *Neuroscience* **1982**, *7*, 1049–1095. [CrossRef]

80. Conrath-Verrier, M.; Dietl, M.; Arluison, M.; Cesselin, F.; Bourgoin, S.; Hamon, M. Localization of Met-enkephalin-like immunoreactivity within pain-related nuclei of cervical spinal cord, brainstem and midbrain in the cat. *Brain Res. Bull.* **1983**, *11*, 587–604. [CrossRef]

81. Johansson, O.; Hökfelt, T.; Elde, R.P. Immunohistochemical distribution of somatostatin-like immunoreactivity in the central nervous system of the adult rat. *Neuroscience* **1984**, *13*, 265–339. [CrossRef]

82. Kawai, Y.; Takami, K.; Shiosaka, S.; Emson, P.C.; Hillyard, C.J.; Girgis, S.; MacIntyre, I.; Tohyama, M. Topographic localization of calcitonin gene-related peptide in the rat brain: An immunohistochemical analysis. *Neuroscience* **1985**, *15*, 747–763. [CrossRef]

83. Vincent, S.R.; McIntosh, C.H.; Buchan, A.M.; Brown, J.C. Central somatostatin systems revealed with monoclonal antibodies. *J. Comp. Neurol.* **1985**, *238*, 169–186. [CrossRef] [PubMed]

84. Skofitsch, G.; Jacobowitz, D.M. Immunohistochemical mapping of galanin-like neurons in the rat central nervous system. *Peptides* **1985**, *6*, 509–546. [CrossRef]

85. Skofitsch, G.; Jacobowitz, D.M. Calcitonin gene-related peptide: Detailed immunohistochemical distribution in the central nervous system. *Peptides* **1985**, *6*, 721–745. [CrossRef]

86. Taber-Pierce, E.; Lichtenstein, E.; Feldman, S.C. The somatostatin systems of the guinea-pig brainstem. *Neuroscience* **1985**, *15*, 215–235. [CrossRef]

87. Melander, T.; Hökfelt, T.; Rökaeus, A. Distribution of galanin-like immunoreactivity in the rat central nervous system. *J. Comp. Neurol.* **1986**, *248*, 475–517. [CrossRef] [PubMed]

88. Kruger, L.; Sternini, C.; Brecha, N.C.; Mantyh, P.W. Distribution of calcitonin gene-related peptide immunoreactivity in relation to the rat central somatosensory projection. *J. Comp. Neurol.* **1988**, *273*, 149–162. [CrossRef] [PubMed]

89. Kordower, J.H.; Le, H.K.; Mufson, E.J. Galanin immunoreactivity in the primate central nervous system. *J. Comp. Neurol.* **1992**, *319*, 479–500. [CrossRef] [PubMed]

90. Zhang, X.; Meister, B.; Elde, R.; Verge, V.M.; Hökfelt, T. Large calibre primary afferent neurons projecting to the gracile nucleus express neuropeptide Y after sciatic nerve lesions: An immunohistochemical and in situ hybridization study in rats. *Eur. J. Neurosci.* **1993**, *5*, 1510–1519. [CrossRef] [PubMed]

91. Van Rossum, D.; Hanisch, U.K.; Quirion, R. Neuroanatomical localization, pharmacological characterization and functions of CGRP, related peptides and their receptors. *Neurosci. Biobehav. Rev.* **1997**, *21*, 649–678. [CrossRef]

92. Del Fiacco, M.; Quartu, M.; Serra, M.P.; Boi, M.; Demontis, R.; Poddighe, L.; Picci, C.; Melis, T. The human cuneate nucleus contains discrete subregions whose neurochemical features match those of the relay nuclei for nociceptive information. *Brain Struct. Funct.* **2014**, *219*, 2083–2101. [CrossRef] [PubMed]

93. Del Fiacco, M.; Quartu, M.; Serra, M.P.; Follesa, P.; Lai, M.L.; Bachis, A. Topographical localization of glial cell line-derived neurotrophic factor in the human brain stem: An immunohistochemical study of prenatal, neonatal and adult brains. *J. Chem. Neuroanat.* **2002**, *23*, 29–48. [CrossRef]

94. Quartu, M.; Lai, M.L.; Del Fiacco, M. GAP-43 in the spinal trigeminal and dorsal column nuclei of the newborn and adult man: Immunohistochemical distribution and comparison with that of the neuropeptides SP and CGRP. *Ital. J. Anat. Embryol.* **1995**, *100*, 205–211. [PubMed]

95. Quartu, M.; Serra, M.P.; Boi, M.; Ferretti, M.T.; Lai, M.L.; Del Fiacco, M. Tissue distribution of Ret, GFRalpha-1, GFRalpha-2 and GFRalpha-3 receptors in the human brainstem at fetal, neonatal and adult age. *Brain Res.* **2007**, *1173*, 36–52. [CrossRef] [PubMed]

96. Quartu, M.; Serra, M.P.; Boi, M.; Sestu, N.; Lai, M.L.; Del Fiacco, M. Tissue distribution of neurturin, persephin and artemin in the human brainstem at fetal, neonatal and adult age. *Brain Res.* **2007**, *1143*, 102–115. [CrossRef] [PubMed]

97. Quartu, M.; Serra, M.P.; Boi, M.; Ibba, V.; Melis, T.; Del Fiacco, M. Polysialylated-neural cell adhesion molecule (PSA-NCAM) in the human trigeminal ganglion and brainstem at prenatal and adult ages. *BMC Neurosci.* **2008**, *9*, 108. [CrossRef] [PubMed]

98. Serra, M.P.; Quartu, M.; Poddighe, L.; Picci, C.; Melis, T.; Del Fiacco, M. Locus K: A novel territory of the human dorsal column nuclei. In Proceedings of the 23th National Congress of Gruppo Italiano per lo S tudio della Neuromorfologia, Cagliari, Italy, 22–23 November 2013; PAGE Press: Pavia, Italy, 2013; p. 13.

99. Serra, M.P.; Quartu, M.; Boi, M.; Poddighe, L.; Melis, T.; Picci, C.; Del Fiacco, M. Locus K: Cuneate subnuclear regions in human dorsal column nuclei with neurochemical, cyto- and myeloarchitectural features of protopathic sensory nuclei. In Proceedings of the 9th FENS Forum of Neuroscience, Milan, Italy, 5–9 July 2014; Volume 7, p. 2773.

100. Rustioni, A.; Weinberg, R.J. The somatosensory system. In *Handbook of Chemical Neuroanatomy, Integrated Systems of the CNS, Part II*; Björklund, A., Hökfelt, T., Swanson, L.W., Eds.; Elsevier Science Publishers B.V. (Biomedical Division): Amsterdam, Holland, 1989; Volume 7, pp. 219–321. ISBN 0444812326, 9780444812322.

101. Broman, J. Neurotransmitters in subcortical somatosensory pathways. *Anat. Embryol.* **1994**, *189*, 181–214. [CrossRef] [PubMed]

102. Guo, A.; Vulchanova, L.; Wang, J.; Li, X.; Elde, R. Immunocytochemical localization of the vanilloid receptor 1 (VR1): Relationship to neuropeptides, the P2X3 purinoceptor and IB4 binding sites. *Eur. J. Neurosci.* **1999**, *11*, 946–958. [CrossRef] [PubMed]

103. Valtschanoff, J.G.; Rustioni, A.; Guo, A.; Hwang, S.J. Vanilloid receptor VR1 is both presynaptic and postsynaptic in the superficial laminae of the rat dorsal horn. *J. Comp. Neurol.* **2001**, *436*, 225–235. [CrossRef] [PubMed]

104. Hwang, S.J.; Oh, J.M.; Valtschanoff, J.G. Expression of the vanilloid receptor TRPV1 in rat dorsal root ganglion neurons supports different roles of the receptor in visceral and cutaneous afferents. *Brain Res.* **2005**, *1047*, 261–266. [CrossRef] [PubMed]

105. Špicarová, D.; Paleček, J. The role of spinal cord vanilloid (TRPV1) receptors in pain modulation. *Physiol. Res.* **2008**, *57* (Suppl. 3), S69–S77. [PubMed]

106. Bae, Y.C.; Oh, J.M.; Hwang, S.J.; Shigenaga, Y.; Valtschanoff, J.G. Expression of vanilloid receptor TRPV1 in the rat trigeminal sensory nuclei. *J. Comp. Neurol.* **2004**, *478*, 62–71. [CrossRef] [PubMed]

107. Doly, S.; Fischer, J.; Salio, C.; Conrath, M. The vanilloid receptor-1 is expressed in rat spinal dorsal horn astrocytes. *Neurosci. Lett.* **2004**, *357*, 123–126. [CrossRef] [PubMed]

108. Chen, Y.; Willcockson, H.H.; Valtschanoff, J.G. Influence of the vanilloid receptor TRPV1 on the activation of spinal cord glia in mouse models of pain. *Exp. Neurol.* **2009**, *220*, 383–390. [CrossRef] [PubMed]

109. Kim, Y.H.; Back, S.K.; Davies, A.J.; Jeong, H.; Jo, H.J.; Chung, G.; Na, H.S.; Bae, Y.C.; Kim, S.J.; Kim, J.S.; et al. TRPV1 in GABAergic interneurons mediates neuropathic mechanical allodynia and disinhibition of the nociceptive circuitry in the spinal cord. *Neuron* **2012**, *74*, 640–647. [CrossRef] [PubMed]

110. Hwang, S.J.; Valtschanoff, J.G. Vanilloid receptor VR1-positive afferents are distributed differently at different levels of the rat lumbar spinal cord. *Neurosci. Lett.* **2003**, *349*, 41–44. [CrossRef]

111. Yang, K. Postnatal excitability development and innervation by functional transient receptor potential vanilloid 1 (TRPV1) terminals in neurons of the rat spinal sacral dorsal commissural nucleus: An electrophysiological study. *Mol. Neurobiol.* **2016**, *53*, 6033–6042. [CrossRef] [PubMed]

112. Mandadi, S.; Roufogalis, B.D. ThermoTRP channels in nociceptors: Taking a lead from capsaicin receptor TRPV1. *Curr. Neuropharmacol.* **2008**, *6*, 21–38. [CrossRef] [PubMed]

113. Peters, J.H.; McDougall, S.J.; Fawley, J.A.; Andresen, M.C. TRPV1 marks synaptic segregation of multiple convergent afferents at the rat medial solitary tract nucleus. *PLoS ONE* **2011**, *6*, e25015. [CrossRef] [PubMed]

114. Langford, L.A.; Coggeshall, R.E. Unmyelinated axons in the *Posterior funiculi*. *Science* **1981**, *211*, 176–177. [CrossRef] [PubMed]

115. Chung, K.S.; Coggeshall, R.E. Unmyelinated primary afferent fibers in dorsal funiculi of cat sacral spinal cord. *J. Comp. Neurol.* **1985**, *238*, 365–369. [CrossRef] [PubMed]

116. Chung, K.; Langford, L.A.; Coggeshall, R.E. Primary afferent and propriospinal fibers in the rat dorsal and dorsolateral funiculi. *J. Comp. Neurol.* **1987**, *263*, 68–75. [CrossRef] [PubMed]

117. McNeill, D.L.; Chung, K.; Carlton, S.M.; Coggeshall, R.E. Calcitonin gene-related peptide immunostained axons provide evidence for fine primary afferent fibers in the dorsal and dorsolateral funiculi of the rat spinal cord. *J. Comp. Neurol.* **1988**, *272*, 303–308. [CrossRef] [PubMed]

118. Tamatani, M.; Senba, E.; Tohyama, M. Calcitonin gene-related peptide- and substance P-containing primary afferent fibers in the dorsal column of the rat. *Brain Res.* **1989**, *495*, 122–130. [CrossRef]

119. Patterson, J.T.; Coggeshall, R.E.; Lee, W.T.; Chung, K. Long ascending unmyelinated primary afferent axons in the rat dorsal column: Immunohistochemical localizations. *Neurosci. Lett.* **1990**, *108*, 6–10. [CrossRef]

120. Noguchi, K.; Kawai, Y.; Fukuoka, T.; Senba, E.; Miki, K. Substance P induced by peripheral nerve injury in primary afferent sensory neurons and its effect on dorsal column nucleus neurons. *J. Neurosci.* **1995**, *15*, 7633–7643. [CrossRef] [PubMed]

121. Miki, K.; Fukuoka, T.; Tokunaga, A.; Noguchi, K. Calcitonin gene-related peptide increase in the rat spinal dorsal horn and dorsal column nucleus following peripheral nerve injury: Up-regulation in a subpopulation of primary afferent sensory neurons. *Neuroscience* **1998**, *82*, 1243–1252. [CrossRef]

122. Rustioni, A. Spinal neurons project to the dorsal column nuclei of rhesus monkeys. *Science* **1976**, *196*, 656–658. [CrossRef]

123. Willis, W.D.; Coggeshall, R.E. *Sensory Mechanisms of the Spinal Cord*; Kluwer Academic/Plenum Publishers: New York, NY, USA, 2004.

124. Wang, Y.; Mu, X.; Liu, Y.; Zhang, X.; Wu, A.; Yue, Y. NK-1-receptor-mediated lesion of spinal post-synaptic dorsal column neurons might improve intractable visceral pain of cancer origin. *Med. Hypotheses* **2011**, *76*, 102–104. [CrossRef] [PubMed]

125. Conti, F.; De Biasi, S.; Giuffrida, R.; Rustioni, A. Substance P containing projections in the dorsal columns of rats and cats. *Neuroscience* **1990**, *34*, 607–621. [CrossRef]

126. Becker, R.; Gatscher, S.; Sure, U.; Bertalanffy, H. The punctate midline myelotomy concept for visceral cancer pain control–case report and review of the literature. *Acta Neurochir. Suppl.* **2002**, *79*, 77–78. [CrossRef] [PubMed]

127. Paleček, J. The Role of Dorsal Columns Pathway in Visceral Pain. *Physiol. Res.* **2004**, *53* (Suppl. 1), S125–S130. [PubMed]

128. Pomonis, J.D.; Harrison, J.E.; Mark, L.; Bristol, D.R.; Valenzano, K.J.; Walker, K. N-(4-Tertiarybutylphenyl)-4-(3-cholorphyridin-2-yl)tetrahydropyrazine-1 (2H)-carbox-amide (BCTC), a novel, orally effective vanilloid receptor 1 antagonist with analgesic properties: II. In vivo characterization in rat models of inflammatory and neuropathic pain. *J. Pharmacol. Exp. Ther.* **2003**, *306*, 387–393. [CrossRef] [PubMed]

129. Cui, M.; Honore, P.; Zhong, C.; Gauvin, D.; Mikusa, J.; Hernandez, G.; Chandran, P.; Gomtsyan, A.; Brown, B.; Bayburt, E.K.; et al. TRPV1 receptors in the CNS play a key role in broad-spectrum analgesia of TRPV1 antagonists. *J. Neurosci.* **2006**, *26*, 9385–9393. [CrossRef] [PubMed]

130. Culshaw, A.J.; Bevan, S.; Christiansen, M.; Copp, P.; Davis, A.; Davis, C.; Dyson, A.; Dziadulewicz, E.K.; Edwards, L.; Eggelte, H.; et al. Identification and biological characterization of 6-aryl-7-isopropylquinazolinones as novel TRPV1 antagonists that are effective in models of chronic pain. *J. Med. Chem.* **2006**, *49*, 471–474. [CrossRef] [PubMed]

131. McGaraughty, S.; Chu, K.L.; Brown, B.S.; Zhu, C.Z.; Zhong, C.; Joshi, S.K.; Honore, P.; Faltynek, C.R.; Jarvis, M.F. Contributions of central and peripheral TRPV1 receptors to mechanically evoked and spontaneous firing of spinal neurons in inflamed rats. *J. Neurophysiol.* **2008**, *100*, 3158–3166. [CrossRef] [PubMed]

132. Paré, M.; Elde, R.; Mazurkiewicz, J.E.; Smith, A.M.; Rice, F.L. The Meissner corpuscle revised: A multiafferented mechanoreceptor with nociceptor immunochemical properties. *J. Neurosci.* **2001**, *21*, 7236–7246. [CrossRef] [PubMed]

133. Ishida-Yamamoto, A.; Senba, E.; Tohyama, M. Calcitonin gene-related peptide- and substance P-immunoreactive nerve fibers in Meissner's corpuscles of rats: An immunohistochemical analysis. *Brain Res.* **1988**, *453*, 362–366. [CrossRef]

134. Dalsgaard, C.J.; Jonsson, C.E.; Hökfelt, T.; Cuello, A.C. Localization of substance P-immunoreactive nerve fibers in the human digital skin. *Experientia* **1983**, *39*, 1018–1020. [CrossRef] [PubMed]

135. Ide, K.; Yasumasa, S.; Hiromoto, I.; Hironubu, I. Sensory nerve supply in the human subacromial bursa. *J. Shoulder Elb. Surg.* **1996**, *5*, 371–382. [CrossRef]

136. Cristino, L.; de Petrocellis, L.; Pryce, G.; Baker, D.; Guglielmotti, V.; Di Marzo, V. Immunohistochemical localization of cannabinoid type 1 and vanilloid transient receptor potential vanilloid type 1 receptors in the mouse brain. *Neuroscience* **2006**, *139*, 1405–1415. [CrossRef] [PubMed]

137. Liapi, A.; Wood, J.N. Extensive co-localization and heteromultimer formation of the vanilloid receptor-like protein TRPV2 and the capsaicin receptor TRPV1 in the adult rat cerebral cortex. *Eur. J. Neurosci.* **2005**, *22*, 825–834. [CrossRef] [PubMed]

138. Maione, S.; Bisogno, T.; de Novellis, V.; Palazzo, E.; Cristino, L.; Valenti, M.; Petrosino, S.; Guglielmotti, V.; Rossi, F.; Di Marzo, V. Elevation of endocannabinoid levels in the ventrolateral periaqueductal grey through inhibition of fatty acid amide hydrolase affects descending nociceptive pathways via both cannabinoid receptor type 1 and transient receptor potential vanilloid type-1 receptors. *J. Pharmacol. Exp. Ther.* **2006**, *316*, 969–982. [CrossRef] [PubMed]

139. Roberts, J.C.; Davis, J.B.; Benham, C.D. [^{3}H]Resiniferatoxin autoradiography in the CNS of wild-type and TRPV1 null mice defines TRPV1 (VR-1) protein distribution. *Brain Res.* **2004**, *995*, 176–183. [CrossRef] [PubMed]

140. Nagy, I.; Sántha, P.; Jancsó, G.; Urbán, L. The role of the vanilloid (capsaicin) receptor (TRPV1) in physiology and pathology. *Eur. J. Pharmacol.* **2004**, *500*, 351–369. [CrossRef] [PubMed]

141. Palazzo, E.; Rossi, F.; Maione, S. Role of TRPV1 receptors in descending modulation of pain. *Mol. Cell. Endocrinol.* **2008**, *286* (Suppl. 1), S79–S83. [CrossRef] [PubMed]

142. Tóth, A.; Boczán, J.; Kedei, N.; Lizanecz, E.; Bagi, Z.; Papp, Z.; Édes, I.; Csiba, L.; Blumberg, P.M. Expression and distribution of vanilloid receptor 1 (TRPV1) in the adult rat brain. *Mol. Brain Res.* **2005**, *135*, 162–168. [CrossRef] [PubMed]

143. Aoki, Y.; Ohtori, S.; Takahashi, K.; Ino, H.; Douya, H.; Ozawa, T.; Saito, T.; Moriya, H. Expression and co-expression of VR1, CGRP, and IB4-binding glycoprotein in dorsal root ganglion neurons in rats: Differences between the disc afferents and the cutaneous afferents. *Spine* **2005**, *30*, 1496–1500. [CrossRef] [PubMed]

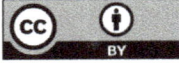

© 2018 by the authors. Licensee MDPI, Basel, Switzerland. This article is an open access article distributed under the terms and conditions of the Creative Commons Attribution (CC BY) license (http://creativecommons.org/licenses/by/4.0/).

cells

MDPI

Article

Expression Profiling of the Transient Receptor Potential Vanilloid (TRPV) Channels 1, 2, 3 and 4 in Mucosal Epithelium of Human Ulcerative Colitis

Theodoros Rizopoulos, Helen Papadaki-Petrou and Martha Assimakopoulou *

Department of Anatomy, Histology and Embryology, School of Medicine, University of Patras, Rion 26504, Greece; thodrizop@gmail.com (T.R.); elenipetroo2000@yahoo.gr (H.P.-P.)
* Correspondence: massim@upatras.gr; Tel.: +30-261-096-9186 or +30-261-096-9195

Received: 30 April 2018; Accepted: 14 June 2018; Published: 15 June 2018

Abstract: The Transient Receptor Potential (TRP) family of selective and non-selective ion channels is well represented throughout the mammalian gastrointestinal track. Several members of the Transient Receptor Potential Vanilloid (TRPV) subfamily have been identified in contributing to modulation of mobility, secretion and sensitivity of the human intestine. Previous studies have focused on the detection of TRPV mRNA levels in colon tissue of patients with inflammatory bowel disease (IBD) whereas little information exists regarding TRPV channel expression in the colonic epithelium. The aim of this study was to evaluate the expression levels of TRPV1, TRPV2, TRPV3 and TRPV4 in mucosa epithelial cells of colonic biopsies from patients with ulcerative colitis (UC) in comparison to colonic resections from non-IBD patients (control group). Immunohistochemistry, using specific antibodies and quantitative analyses of TRPV-immunostained epithelial cells, was performed in semi-serial sections of the samples. TRPV1 expression was significantly decreased whereas TRPV4 expression was significantly increased in the colonic epithelium of UC patients compared to patients in the control group ($p < 0.05$). No significant difference for TRPV2 and TRPV3 expression levels between UC and control specimens was detected ($p > 0.05$). There was no correlation between TRPV channel expression and the clinical features of the disease ($p > 0.05$). Further investigation is needed to clarify the role of TRPV channels in human bowel inflammatory response.

Keywords: TRPV1; TRPV2; TRPV3; TRPV4; mucosal epithelium; ulcerative colitis; inflammatory bowel disease

---

1. Introduction

The importance of the Transient Receptor Potential family (TRP) of selective and non-selective cation channels in cellular homeostasis via regulation of calcium and magnesium ions levels has been well documented [1]. TRPC (Canonical), TRPV (Vanilloid), TRPM (Melastatin), TRPA (Ankyrin), TRPN (no mechanoreceptor potential C-NOMPC), TRPP (Polycystin) and TRPML (Mucolipin) are TRP subfamilies [2]. Certain TRP channels serve as "cellular sensors" for a wide range of extracellular stimuli such as changes in temperature, osmotic pressure and pH [3]. Additionally, members of the TRP family appear to be important for the temperature-dependent formation of normal epithelial tight junctions and thus, in the control of cell proliferation and growth. Besides their well-documented role in the cell surface, TRP channels are reported to be present in intracellular membranes and are implicated in the trafficking of interactive proteins [3]. TRP activation in nerve cells enhances cell excitability leading to increased release of neurotransmitters whereas in peripheral cells (e.g., epithelial cells, immune cells), it results in increased expression of inflammatory mediators [1–3].

TRPV1, TRPV2, TRPV3, and TRPV4 along with TRPM8 and TRPA1 constitute the thermo-TRPion channels [4]. In particular, the highest levels of ion permeability of TRPV1 channels are achieved when they are exposed to temperatures higher than 42 °C. TRPV1 can also be activated by physical stimuli including acidic pH, mechanic distention and high membrane electric potential. Exogenous substances (e.g., capsaicin) as well as endogenous derivates like endocannabinoids (e.g., anandamide) and palmitoylethanolamide augment TRPV1 channel activity. TRPV1 expression has been found in many parts of the nervous system where it plays a crucial role in clinical conditions such as migraines, schizophrenia, myasthenia gravis, Alzheimer disease and depression [1–6]. Furthermore, TRPV1 is implicated in neurogenic inflammation, a process which involves perception of pain and both vasodilation and plasma extravasation aroused from the release of two vasoactive neuropeptides, calcitonin gene-related polypeptide (CGRP) and substance P (SP), from a subpopulation of peptidergic neurons which highly express TRPV1 [5]. TRPV2 channels share 50% domain similarity to TRPV1. They respond to noxious heat with an activation threshold of >52 °C, to changes in osmolarity and to membrane stretch. Accumulating data provide evidence that TRPV2 might participate in neurogenic inflammation [7]. TRPV3 protein produced by the translation of the same with TRPV1 gene, reaches the highest levels of its permeability when exposed to temperatures of 33–39 °C and chemical stimuli like menthol, carvacol, camphor, and eugenol. Activation of TRPV3 has been associated with cellular release of IL-1, a pro-inflammatory cytokine [8]. Temperatures of 27–34 °C, low osmolarity, acidic pH, and mechanical stress are some of the physical stimuli that increase the TRPV4 channel permeability. Certain epoxyeichosatetraenoic acid derivatives are endogenous TRPV4 agonists and phytochemical bisandrographolide A, the phorbol ester 4α-phorbol 12,13-didecanoate (4α-PDD), cannabidivarin and tetrahydrocannabivarin are exogenous TRPV4 agonists [9]. Inflammatory mediators are known to augment TRPV1 and TRPV4 activity by sensitization. Experimental data implicate TRPV1 and TRPV4 channel contribution in allodynia, thermal hyperalgesia and visceral hypersensitivity [10–13].

Ulcerative colitis (UC), Crohn's disease (CD) and indeterminate colitis are the constituents of the inflammatory bowel disease (IBD). UC mainly affects the mucosa of the colon and rectum and is characterized by usually long-term remissions between flares and mild to severe exacerbations of abdominal pain and bloody diarrhea to weight loss, fever and anemia. During a colonoscopy, small ulcers on the colon's lining and pseudopolyps may be revealed but the microscopic evaluation of tissue biopsies is crucial for a definite diagnosis. Increased inflammatory cells in the lamina propria, alteration of crypt architecture or even crypt abscesses and ulcers are some of the typical histopathological features of UC tissue specimens [14,15]. Despite the slightly elevated risk of colorectal cancer and the life-threatening complications of severe exacerbations, no difference in mortality rates between patients with UC and the background population has been revealed [16,17].

The impact on the quality of patients' life with IBD on the health care system and society is of great importance and this partly explains the growing interest in involving new molecules for the treatment of the disease [18]. To that point is the investigation of TRPV1–4 channel expression in IBD patients. Previous studies have detected increased TRPV1 [19–27] and TRPV4 [28–31] expression in sensory fibers which was correlated with visceral hypersensitivity and hyperalgesia in inflamed human and mouse bowel. Quantitation of mRNA levels for TRPV1 [24,26,27] and TRPV4 channels [29,30] has been also assessed in colon biopsies from IBD patients and healthy controls. Recent data in experimental animals implicate TRPV2 in the development of colitis [32] whereas contribution of TRPV4 to intestinal inflammation via chemokine release has been reported [29]. The expression of TRPV1 and TRPV4 in epithelial cells of the human colon [26,29], and TRPV3 presence in distal mouse colon epithelium has been documented [33]. These findings contribute to current knowledge of nociceptive signals generated in the intestine by exciting sensitized nociceptors as a result of mechanical stimulation or distension implying that targeting TRPV channels could be a new therapeutic opportunity for treating patients with IBD [34–37].

Given the histological changes in the mucosa of patients with IBD and the involvement of TRPV channels in intestinal inflammation, we aimed to assess the immunohistochemical quantification of TRPV1, TRPV2, TRPV3, and TRPV4 channel expression in the mucosal epithelium of colonic biopsies from patients with UC compared with colonic resections from non-IBD patients (control group).

The relationship between channel expression and patients' clinical manifestations of the disease was also investigated.

2. Materials and Methods

2.1. Patients

A total of 52 Greek patients of mean age about 49.17 ($\pm$17.96) years old either treated for an exacerbation of UC or proto-diagnosed with this type of IBD (26 active, 24 quiescent and 2 with dysplasia) in the Department of Internal Medicine of "Agios Andreas" Hospital, Patras, Greece, from 1996 to 2014, were included in this study. The corresponding tissue blocks were retrieved from archival files of the Department of Pathology of "Agios Andreas" Hospital, Patras. The control group comprised of gut tissue samples from non-IBD patients ($n = 12$; mean age, 75.25 years, range, 68–83 years) excluded due to colon cancer (retrieved up to 5 cm away from the tumor's edge), postoperative ileus, and lipomatosis of the ileocecal valve. The control tissue samples were collected from the same department, during the same period. The use of the human specimens was in accordance with the University of Patras Ethics Commission. All research protocols were conducted, and patients were treated in accordance with the tenets of the Declaration of Helsinki.

2.2. Immunohistochemistry

All tissues were prepared in formalin and embedded in liquid paraffin. Semi-serial sections of 4 μm collected on poly-L-lysine slides, deparaffinized in xylene and dehydrated using graded alcohol diluents up to water were used for antigen retrieval which was performed by microwaving the slides in 0.01 M citrate buffer (pH 6). Endogenous peroxidase activity was quenched by treatment with 1% hydrogen peroxide solution for 20 min. Incubation at room temperature with 1% bovine serum albumin (SERVA, Heidelberg, Germany) in Tris-HCL-buffered saline was performed for 10 min. Tissue sections were subsequently incubated with primary antibodies overnight at 4 °C for TRPV1, TRPV2, TRPV3 and 2 h RT for TRPV4. Detection of the TRPV1, TRPV2, TRPV3 and TRPV4 channels was performed using the polyclonal rabbit anti-TRPV1 antibody (cat. no. NBP1-71774; dilution 1:200; Novus Biologicals, Ltd., Cambridge, UK), polyclonal rabbit anti-TRPV2 (cat. no. TA317464; dilution 1:200, Acris Antibodies GmbH, Herford, Germany), monoclonal mouse anti-TRPV3 antibody (cat. no. AM20072PU-N; dilution 1:300, Acris Antibodies GmbH, Herford, Germany), and the rabbit polyclonal to TRPV4 (cat. no. ab39260; dilution 1:200) (Abcam, Cambridge, UK). These antibodies have been used to detect human TRPV channels in previous studies [38–41]. After three rinses in buffer, the slides were incubated with the un-avidin-biotin complex technique named Envision (Dako Cytomation; Agilent Technologies, Inc., Santa Clara, CA, USA). Tissue staining was visualized with 3,3'-diaminobenzidine (DAB) as a chromogen (which yielded brown reaction products). Slides were counterstained with Mayer's hematoxylin solution, dehydrated and mounted. To ensure antibody specificity, negative controls included the omission of primary antibody and substitution with non-immune serum. Control slides were invariably negative for immunostaining. Renal tissue was used as positive control for TRPV1, TRPV3, and TRPV4 antibodies and ophthalmic pterygium for TRPV2 antibody [42,43].

2.3. Scoring

All immunohistochemical sections were assessed blindly and independently by two observers (TR and MA), followed by a joint review for resolution of any differences. The expression of proteins was determined as the mean percentage of positive mucosa epithelial cells, manually counted, with the aid of an ocular grid, in ten non-overlapping, random fields (total magnification, $\times$400) for each case (labeling index, LI; % labeled cells). Immunopositively stained endothelial and lamina propria cells were excluded from the cell counts. Expression of proteins included in this study was examined in adjacent (semi-serial) sections of each sample. Microphotographs were obtained using a Nikon

DXM 1200C digital camera mounted on a Nikon Eclipse 80i microscope and ACT-1C software (Nikon Instruments Inc., Melville, NY, USA).

2.4. Statistical Analysis

Non-parametric methods were used for the statistical analysis of the results. Median comparisons were performed with Wilcoxon's Rank-Sum test (equivalent to the Mann–Whitney U test) and the Kruskal–Wallis test. Correlation analysis was performed by utilizing Kendall's τ (or Spearman's ρ) rank correlation to assess the significance of associations between LIs. *p* values of <0.05 were considered to indicate a statistically significant difference. Statistical analyses were carried out using the SPSS package (version 23.0; SPSS, Inc., Chicago, IL, USA).

3. Results

3.1. Immunolocalization of Transient Receptor Potential Vanilloid Channels in Ulcerative Colitis and Control Non-IBD Samples

Cytoplasmic TRPV1 immunostaining was detected predominantly in the upper layer of the epithelium in 98% of UC specimens. All epithelial layers in UC cases demonstrated TRPV2, TRPV3, and TRPV4 cytoplasmic immunoreactivity, 71%, 89%, and 94% respectively. Strong cytoplasmic immunoreactivities for TRPV1, weak for TRPV2, moderate for TRPV3, and weak to moderate for TRPV4 channels were observed in epithelium of all (100%) control tissues. TRPV4 nuclear immunostaining was also noticed in certain epithelial cells. Scattered cells in the lamina propria, vascular endothelium, muscularis mucosa, and enteric nervous system displayed immunopositivity for all TRPV channels (Figures 1–3).

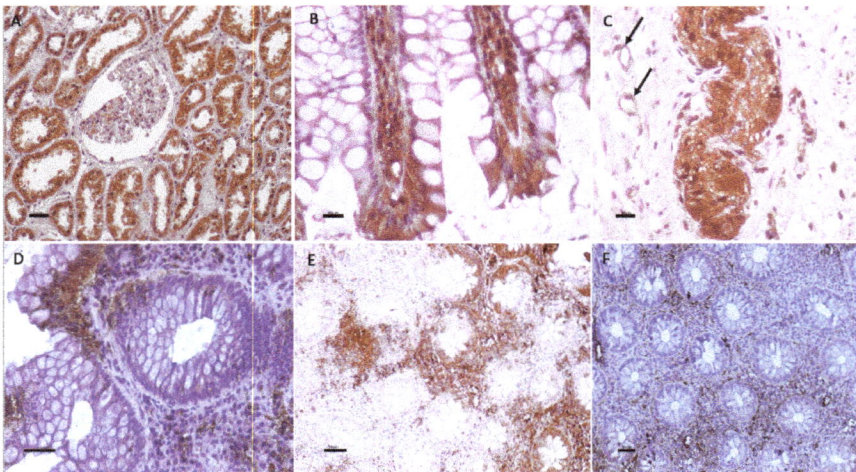

Figure 1. TRPV1 immunolocalization in UC and control non-IBD samples (**A–E**) and TRPV3 nerve fiber immunolabeling in UC (**F**). (**A**) Renal tissue sections were used as positive control for TRPV1-immunostaining; (**B**) Strong cytoplasmic TRPV1 immunoreactivity in mucosal epithelium of control group. Note TRPV1-immunostained cells in lamina propria; (**C**) Cells in enteric nervous system display strong TRPV1 immunopositivity. Furthermore, endothelial cells are TRPV1-immunoreactive (arrows); (**D**) Strong cytoplasmic TRPV1 immunostaining in a few superficial mucosa cells of this UC specimen; (**E**) Heterogeneity in TRPV1 in epithelium of UC sample. Note TRPV1-immunonegative mucosa cells nearby to TRPV1-immunopositive mucosa cells (LI = 50). (**F**) TRPV3 immunoreactivity in nerve fibers in UC. Counterstain, hematoxylin; original magnification, ×400 (**A–D,F**), ×200 (**E**); scale bar, 50 μm.

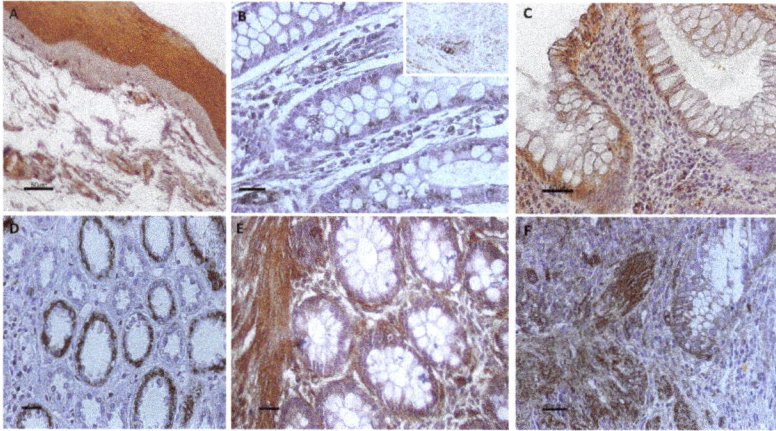

Figure 2. Panel presenting expression patterns of TRPV2 (**B**,**C**) and TRPV3 (**D**,**F**) in UC and control samples; (**A**) Ophthalmic pterygium tissue samples were used as positive controls for TRPV2 immunoreactivity; (**B**) TRPV2-immunostaining in intestinal epithelial cells of control colon. ((**B**), insert) Cells in enteric nervous system display strong TRPV2-immunopositivity; (**C**) Moderate cytoplasmic TRPV2 staining in numerous mucosa cells in UC specimen. Several TRPV2-immunopositive cells are observed in lamina propria cells; (**D**) Renal tissue sections were used as positive control for TRPV3-immunostaining; (**E**) Aberrant cytoplasmic TRPV3-immunostaining in epithelial cells of control sample. Note the strong-immunostained smooth muscle cells in muscularis mucosa; (**F**) Cytoplasmic expression of TRPV3 in epithelium and muscularis mucosa of UC sample. Counterstain, hematoxylin; original magnification, ×400; scale bar, 50 μm.

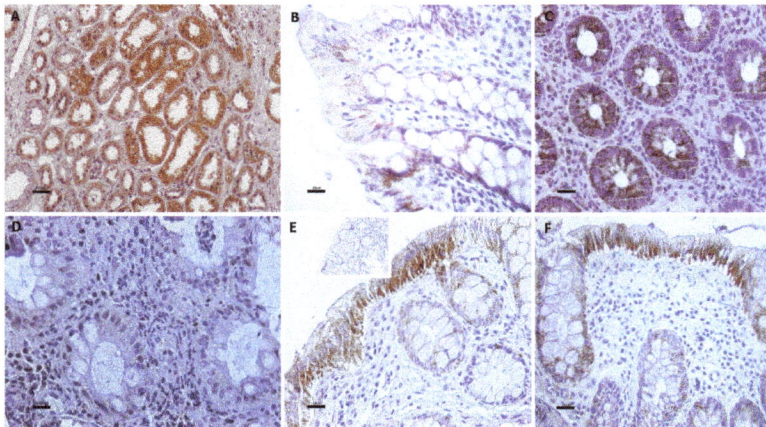

Figure 3. Panel depicting the cellular distribution of TRPV4 in UC and control intestine specimens. (**A**) Renal tissue sections were used as positive control for TRPV4-immunostaining. (**B**) Weak TRPV4-immunostaining in intestinal epithelial cells of control colon. (**C**) Granular cytoplasmic TRPV4-immunoexpression is identified in the cytoplasm of numerous mucosa cells in UC. (**D**) Nuclei of mucosa cells display TRPV4 immunostaining in this UC sample. (**E**,**F**) Strong granular cytoplasmic TRPV4 immunolocalization in superficial mucosa cells and goblet cells whereas there are mucosa cells with weak immunostaining of UC samples. ((**E**), insert) Immunostaining is absent in negative control sections. Counterstain, hematoxylin; original magnification, ×400; scale bar, 50 μm.

3.2. Quantitative Analyses of the Immunohistochemical Findings

Immunohistochemical findings are illustrated in Table 1. TRPV1 expression levels were significantly decreased whereas TRPV4 expression levels were significantly increased in UC specimens compared with control non-IBD samples. In contrast, no significant difference was identified for TRPV2 and TRPV3 LIs between UC and control group (Figure 4). A significant correlation was found between TRPV1 and TRPV3 expression levels (Spearman's rho = 0.462; p = 0.002) and between TRPV3 and TRPV4 expression levels (Spearman's rho = 0.357; p = 0.01) in UC. Finally, TRPV1–4 channel expression was independent of the extent of colon inflammation, the clinical features and the symptoms of the disease as well as patients' age and gender ($p \geq 0.05$.)

Table 1. Immunohistochemical expression of TRPV1, TRPV2, TRPV3, and TRPV4 channels in colonic epithelium of human UC and non-IBD control samples. The (non-parametric) Wilcoxon's Rank-Sum test was performed and the level of significant was defined as $p < 0.05$.

TRPV LIs	Ulcerative Colitis (n = 52)	Control Group (n = 12)
TRPV1 LIs Mean ± SD, % (range)	68.333 ± 28.28 [a,b,c] (0–100)	88.33 ± 16.07 [f,g,h] (70–100)
TRPV2 LIs Mean ± SD, % (range)	18.52 ± 23.77 [d,e] (0–80)	15.00 ± 13.22 [i] (0–25)
TRPV3 LIs Mean ± SD, % (range)	51.00 ± 36.19 (0–100)	60.66 ± 51.78 [k] (2–100)
TRPV4 LIs Mean ± SD, % (range)	47.80 ± 33.09 (0–100)	22.50 ± 15.00 (10–40)

LI, the percentage of positive-labeled cells from the total number of epithelial cells counted; Mean, mean labeling index; SD, standard deviation; [a] $p < 0.001$ vs. TRPV2 expression in UC; [b] $p = 0.01$ vs. TRPV3 expression in UC; [c] $p = 0.002$ vs. TRPV4 expression in UC; [d] $p < 0.001$ vs. TRPV3 expression in UC; [e] $p < 0.001$ vs. TRPV4 expression in UC; [f] $p < 0.001$ vs. TRPV2 expression in control group; [g] $p < 0.02$ vs. TRPV3 expression in control group; [h] $p < 0.001$ vs. TRPV4 expression in control group; [i] $p < 0.001$ vs. TRPV3 expression in control group; [k] $p = 0.01$ vs. TRPV4 expression in control group.

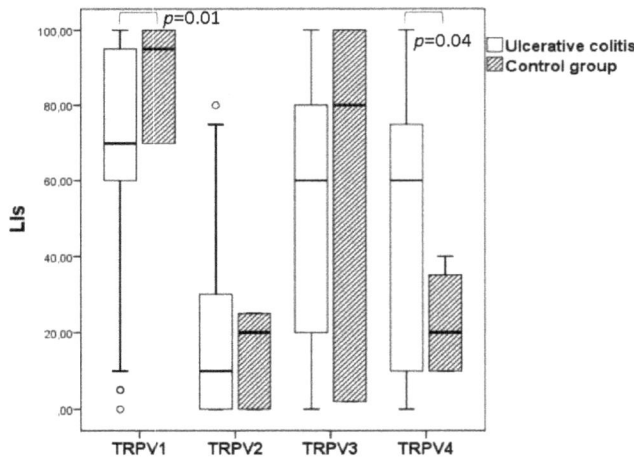

Figure 4. Comparison of TRPV channel expression in mucosa epithelial cells of UC and non-IBD control samples. Significant differences between UC and non-IBD group for TRPV1 and TRPV4 expression was detected ($p < 0.05$). No significant difference was observed regarding TRPV2 and TRPV3 expression ($p > 0.05$).

4. Discussion

Previous studies have focused on quantitation of mRNA levels for TRPV channels in IBD. Thus, Kun et al. [26] demonstrated a decreased TRPV1 gene expression in UC patients and downregulation of TRPV1 transcripts in Trpa1 KO animals parallel to the enhanced inflammation upon DSS treatment. In contrast, Keszthelyi et al. [24] found no changes in mRNA levels of TRPV1 in UC patients in remission. Additionally, Fichna et al. [30] showed that TRPV4 mRNA expression was significantly elevated in patients with UC compared with healthy subjects whereas D'Aldebert et al. [29] reported no significant difference for TRPV4 mRNA quantitative expression in UC. Considering that colonic nerve fibers in IBD patients highly express TRPV1 and TRPV4 channels [19,22,28], it is obvious that these neurons largely contribute to the TRPV mRNA levels detected in colonic samples.

In the present study, TRPV channel immune-expression was quantitated in mucosal epithelium of UC and non-inflamed intestine samples (control group). The percentage of positively (labeled) cells out of the total number of epithelial cells was counted and the data was statistically analyzed. UC patients showed statistically decreased TRPV1 expression and statistically increased TRPV4 expression compared with the control group. Vinuesa et al. [44] have shown increased carcinogenesis in mice genetically deficient in TRPV1 which was strongly related to inflammation. Therefore, TRPV1 decreased expression in epithelium of UC samples may be associated with the exacerbated colon inflammation and consequently with the loss of the protective role of TRPV1 against colon cancer. However, in a similar study of Luo et al. [45] a significant upregulation of TRPV1 in colonic epithelium was observed in active IBD patients. Future investigations would clarify the involvement of epithelial TRPV1 channels in pathogenesis of IBD.

Activation of TRPV4 channels in mouse intestinal epithelial cells has been implicated in paracellular epithelial cell permeability, increased intracellular calcium concentrations and maintenance of chronic inflammation via chemokine release and recruitment of monocytes, macrophages, neutrophils and Th1 cells [29]. The increased TRPV4 expression in human mucosa epithelial cells of patients with UC may indicate a possible role of this channel in the inflammation process and provides TRPV4 as an attractive therapeutic target for human IBD. It is worthy to note that TRPV4 staining was mainly localized in the cytoplasm but there were cases in which TRPV4 immunostaining was present in the nucleus of epithelial cells. The feature of TRPV4 localization only in the nucleus has been also shown in myocardium of neonatal mice [46]. Although TRPV1 and TRPV4 were differentially expressed in inflamed bowel tissues, there was no significant correlation with clinical features of the patients and disease severity. Furthermore, the apparent difference in mean age between control and diseased groups did not influenced the data.

Low expression levels of TRPV2 were identified in both UC and normal intestine tissue and there are no published data referring to the contribution of TRPV2 in human ulcerative colitis. However, previous knowledge indicates the possible involvement of TRPV2 in experimental colitis [32]. Additionally, the role of TRPV3 in the human alimentary canal has not been well investigated. TRPV3 levels were slightly decreased in patients with ulcerative colitis in this study. It has been reported that, TRPV3 channels are important for the integrity of the epidermal barrier [8]. It would be interesting to define the contribution of TRPV3 channels in gastrointestinal inflammation and maintenance of the mucus integrity. Statistical analyses revealed the existence of positive correlation between TRPV1 and TRPV3 expression levels and between TRPV3 and TRPV4 expression levels in UC samples. Since, the heterotetramerization of TRPV1 and TRPV3 has already been documented [5], the effects of co-expression of TRPV3 and TRPV4 should be studied.

It is important to note that a variety of cells in the lamina propria exhibited TRPV immunoreactivity. Accumulating data show the presence of TRPV1 and TRPV4 in inflammatory cells including macrophages, leukocytes [26,30]. Furthermore, blood vessels demonstrated strong immunopositivity for all TRP channels. It is known that in endothelial cells, TRPV1 is activated by endocannabinoids, TRPV3 by dietary agonists, and TRPV4 by shear stress, epoxyeicosatrienoic acids and downstream of Gq-coupled receptor activation. Ca^{2+} entry through endothelial TRPV channels triggers NO$^-$ and EDHF-dependent vasodilation [47,48]. Specifically, TRPV4 activation and Ca^{2+} entry may occur by mechanical stimulation of the endothelium by increased fluid viscosity and thus shear stress [49]. It would be interesting to define the role of endothelial TRPV channels in angiogenesis and carcinogenesis as recent published data implies that TRPV3, TRPV4, TRPV5, TRPM4 and TRPC6 may be thought of as potential genes contributing to colorectal cancer tumorigenesis [50]. Further investigation is needed for the TRPV channels' involvement in IBD and any possible correlation between the expression levels of these channels and the presence of dysplasia as well as the patients' complications and treatment, in large-scale studies.

Author Contributions: T.R. carried out the immunostaining, T.R. and M.A. conceived and designed the experiments, performed the analyses of immunohistochemical findings and statistical analyses, and wrote the manuscript, H.P.-P. carried out the pathological evaluation of the specimens and reviewed the manuscript.

Acknowledgments: The authors would like to thank the Department of Pathology of "Agios Andreas" Hospital, Patras for providing gut tissue samples.

Conflicts of Interest: The authors declare that they have no conflict of interest.

References

1. Venkatachalam, K.; Montell, C. TRP Channels. *Annu. Rev. Biochem.* **2007**, *76*, 387–417. [CrossRef] [PubMed]
2. Pedersen, S.F.; Owsianik, G.; Nilius, B. TRP channels: An overview. *Cell Calcium* **2005**, *38*, 233–252. [CrossRef] [PubMed]
3. Nilius, B. TRP channels in disease. *Biochim. Biophys. Acta* **2007**, *1772*, 805–812. [CrossRef] [PubMed]
4. Vay, L.; Gu, C.H.; McNaughton, P.A. The thermo-TRP ion channel family: Properties and therapeutic implications. *Br. J. Pharmacol.* **2012**, *165*, 787–801. [CrossRef] [PubMed]
5. Kaneko, Y.; Szallasi, A. Transient receptor potential (TRP) channels: A clinical perspective. *Br. J. Pharmacol.* **2014**, *171*, 2474–2507. [CrossRef] [PubMed]
6. Nilius, B.; Szallasi, A. Transient receptor potential channels as drug targets: From the science of basic research to the art of medicine. *Pharmacol. Rev.* **2014**, *66*, 676–814. [CrossRef] [PubMed]
7. Perálvarez-Marín, A.; Doñate-Macian, P.; Gaudet, R. What do we know about the transient receptor potential vanilloid 2 (TRPV2) ion channel? *FEBS J.* **2013**, *280*, 5471–5487. [CrossRef] [PubMed]
8. Nilius, B.; Biró, T.; Owsianik, G. TRPV3: Time to decipher a poorly understood family member! *J. Physiol.* **2014**, *592*, 295–304. [CrossRef] [PubMed]
9. Everaerts, W.; Nilius, B.; Owsianik, G. The vanilloid transient receptor potential channel TRPV4: From structure to disease. *Prog. Biophys. Mol. Biol.* **2010**, *103*, 2–17. [CrossRef] [PubMed]
10. Chatter, R.; Cenac, N.; Roussis, V.; Kharrat, R.; Vergnolle, N. Inhibition of sensory afferents activation and visceral pain by a brominated algal diterpene. *Neurogastroenterol. Motil.* **2012**, *24*, e336–e343. [CrossRef] [PubMed]
11. Grant, A.D.; Cottrell, G.S.; Amadesi, S.; Trevisani, M.; Nicoletti, P.; Materazzi, S.; Altier, C.; Cenac, N.; Zamponi, G.W.; Bautista-Cruz, F.; et al. Protease-activated receptor 2 sensitizes the transient receptor potential vanilloid 4 ion channel to cause mechanical hyperalgesia in mice. *J. Physiol.* **2007**, *578 Pt 3*, 715–733. [CrossRef] [PubMed]
12. Cenac, N.; Altier, C.; Chapman, K.; Liedtke, W.; Zamponi, G.; Vergnolle, N. Transient receptor potential vanilloid-4 has a major role in visceral hypersensitivity symptoms. *Gastroenterology* **2008**, *135*, 937–946. [CrossRef] [PubMed]
13. Vermeulen, W.; De Man, J.G.; Pelckmans, P.A.; De Winter, B.Y. Neuroanatomy of lower gastrointestinal pain disorders. *World J. Gastroenterol.* **2014**, *20*, 1005–1020. [CrossRef] [PubMed]
14. Feakins, R.M. Inflammatory bowel disease biopsies: Updated British Society of Gastroenterology reporting guidelines. *J. Clin. Pathol.* **2013**, *66*, 1005–1026. [CrossRef] [PubMed]
15. Sobczak, M.; Fabisiak, A.; Murawska, N.; Wesołowska, E.; Wierzbicka, P.; Wlazłowski, M.; Wójcikowska, M.; Zatorski, H.; Zwolińska, M.; Fichna, J. Current overview of extrinsic and intrinsic factors in etiology and progression of inflammatory bowel diseases. *Pharmacol. Rep.* **2014**, *66*, 766–775. [CrossRef] [PubMed]

16. Barral, M.; Dohan, A.; Allez, M.; Boudiaf, M.; Camus, M.; Laurent, V.; Hoeffel, C.; Soyer, P. Gastrointestinal cancers in inflammatory bowel disease: An update with emphasis on imaging findings. *Crit. Rev. Oncol. Hematol.* **2016**, *97*, 30–46. [CrossRef] [PubMed]

17. Triantafillidis, J.K.; Nasioulas, G.; Kosmidis, P.A. Colorectal cancer and inflammatory bowel disease: Epidemiology, risk factors, mechanisms of carcinogenesis and prevention strategies. *Anticancer Res.* **2009**, *29*, 2727–2737. [PubMed]

18. D'Haens, G.R.; Panaccione, R.; Higgins, P.D.; Vermeire, S.; Gassull, M.; Chowers, Y.; Hanauer, S.B.; Herfarth, H.; Hommes, D.W.; Kamm, M.; et al. The London Position Statement of the World Congress of Gastroenterology on Biological Therapy for IBD with the European Crohn's and Colitis Organization: When to start, when to stop, which drug to choose, and how to predict response? *Am. J. Gastroenterol.* **2011**, *106*, 199–212. [CrossRef] [PubMed]

19. Yiangou, Y.; Facer, P.; Dyer, N.H.; Chan, C.L.; Knowles, C.; Williams, N.S.; Anand, P. Vanilloid receptor 1 immunoreactivity in inflamed human bowel. *Lancet* **2001**, *357*, 1338–1339. [CrossRef]

20. Akbar, A.; Yiangou, Y.; Facer, P.; Walters, J.R.; Anand, P.; Ghosh, S. Increased capsaicin receptor TRPV1-expressing sensory fibres in irritable bowel syndrome and their correlation with abdominal pain. *Gut* **2008**, *57*, 923–929. [CrossRef] [PubMed]

21. Ravnefjord, A.; Brusberg, M.; Kang, D.; Bauer, U.; Larsson, H.; Lindström, E.; Martinez, V. Involvement of the transient receptor potential vanilloid 1 (TRPV1) in the development of acute visceral hyperalgesia during colorectal distension in rats. *Eur. J. Pharmacol.* **2009**, *611*, 85–91. [CrossRef] [PubMed]

22. Akbar, A.; Yiangou, Y.; Facer, P.; Brydon, W.G.; Walters, J.R.; Anand, P.; Ghosh, S. Expression of the TRPV1 receptor differs in quiescent inflammatory bowel disease with or without abdominal pain. *Gut* **2010**, *59*, 767–774. [CrossRef] [PubMed]

23. Engel, M.A.; Khalil, M.; Mueller-Tribbensee, S.M.; Becker, C.; Neuhuber, W.L.; Neurath, M.F.; Reeh, P.W. The proximodistal aggravation of colitis depends on substance P released from TRPV1-expressing sensory neurons. *J. Gastroenterol.* **2012**, *47*, 256–265. [CrossRef] [PubMed]

24. Keszthelyi, D.; Troost, F.J.; Jonkers, D.M.; Helyes, Z.; Hamer, H.M.; Ludidi, S.; Vanhoutvin, S.; Venema, K.; Dekker, J.; Szolcsányi, J.; et al. Alterations in mucosal neuropeptides in patients with irritable bowel syndrome and ulcerative colitis in remission: A role in pain symptom generation? *Eur. J. Pain.* **2013**, *17*, 1299–1306. [CrossRef] [PubMed]

25. De Fontgalland, D.; Brookes, S.J.; Gibbins, I.; Sia, T.C.; Wattchow, D.A. The neurochemical changes in the innervation of human colonic mesenteric and submucosal blood vessels in ulcerative colitis and Crohn's disease. *Neurogastroenterol. Motil.* **2014**, *26*, 731–744. [CrossRef] [PubMed]

26. Kun, J.; Szitter, I.; Kemény, A.; Perkecz, A.; Kereskai, L.; Pohóczky, K.; Vincze, A.; Gódi, S.; Szabó, I.; Szolcsányi, J.; et al. Upregulation of the transient receptor potential ankyrin 1 ion channel in the inflamed human and mouse colon and its protective roles. *PLoS ONE* **2014**, *9*, e108164. [CrossRef] [PubMed]

27. Van Wanrooij, S.J.; Wouters, M.M.; Van Oudenhove, L.; Vanbrabant, W.; Mondelaers, S.; Kollmann, P.; Kreutz, F.; Schemann, M.; Boeckxstaens, G.E. Sensitivity testing in irritable bowel syndrome with rectal capsaicin stimulations: Role of TRPV1 upregulation and sensitization in visceral hypersensitivity? *Am. J. Gastroenterol.* **2014**, *109*, 99–109. [CrossRef] [PubMed]

28. Brierley, S.M.; Page, A.J.; Hughes, P.A.; Adam, B.; Liebregts, T.; Cooper, N.J.; Holtmann, G.; Liedtke, W.; Blackshaw, L.A. Selective role for TRPV4 ion channels in visceral sensory pathways. *Gastroenterology* **2008**, *134*, 2059–2069. [CrossRef] [PubMed]

29. D'Aldebert, E.; Cenac, N.; Rousset, P.; Martin, L.; Rolland, C.; Chapman, K.; Selves, J.; Alric, L.; Vinel, J.P.; Vergnolle, N. Transient receptor potential vanilloid 4 activated inflammatory signals by intestinal epithelial cells and colitis in mice. *Gastroenterology* **2011**, *140*, 275–285. [CrossRef] [PubMed]

30. Fichna, J.; Mokrowiecka, A.; Cygankiewicz, A.I.; Zakrzewski, P.K.; Małecka-Panas, E.; Janecka, A.; Krajewska, W.M.; Storr, M.A. Transient receptor potential vanilloid 4 blockade protects against experimental colitis in mice: A new strategy for inflammatory bowel diseases treatment? *Neurogastroenterol. Motil.* **2012**, *24*, e557–e560. [CrossRef] [PubMed]

31. McGuire, C.; Boundouki, G.; Hockley, J.R.F.; Reed, D.; Cibert-Goton, V.; Peiris, M.; Kung, V.; Broad, J.; Aziz, Q.; Chan, C.; et al. Ex vivo study of human visceral nociceptors. *Gut* **2018**, *67*, 86–96. [CrossRef] [PubMed]

32. Issa, C.M.; Hambly, B.D.; Wang, Y.; Maleki, S.; Wang, W.; Fei, J.; Bao, S. TRPV2 in the development of experimental colitis. *Scand. J. Immunol.* **2014**, *80*, 307–312. [CrossRef] [PubMed]

33. Ueda, T.; Yamada, T.; Ugawa, S.; Ishida, Y.; Shimada, S. TRPV3, a thermosensitive channel is expressed in mouse distal colon epithelium. *Biochem. Biophys. Res. Commun.* **2009**, *383*, 130–134. [CrossRef] [PubMed]

34. Boesmans, W.; Owsianik, G.; Tack, J.; Voets, T.; Vanden Berghe, P. TRP channels in neurogastroenterology: Opportunities for therapeutic intervention. *Br. J. Pharmacol.* **2011**, *162*, 18–37. [CrossRef] [PubMed]

35. Vergnolle, N. TRPV4: New therapeutic target for inflammatory bowel diseases. *Biochem. Pharmacol.* **2014**, *89*, 157–161. [CrossRef] [PubMed]

36. Parenti, A.; De Logu, F.; Geppetti, P.; Benemei, S. What is the evidence for the role of TRP channels in inflammatory and immune cells? *Br. J. Pharmacol.* **2016**, *173*, 953–969. [CrossRef] [PubMed]

37. Beckers, A.B.; Weerts, Z.Z.R.M.; Helyes, Z.; Masclee, A.A.M.; Keszthelyi, D. Review article: Transient receptor potential channels as possible therapeutic targets in irritable bowel syndrome. *Aliment. Pharmacol. Ther.* **2017**, *46*, 938–952. [CrossRef] [PubMed]

38. Samivel, R.; Kim, D.W.; Son, H.R.; Rhee, Y.H.; Kim, E.H.; Kim, J.H.; Bae, J.S.; Chung, Y.J.; Chung, P.S.; Raz, E.; et al. The role of TRPV1 in the CD4$^+$ T cell-mediated inflammatory response of allergic rhinitis. *Oncotarget* **2016**, *7*, 148–160. [CrossRef] [PubMed]

39. Fusi, C.; Materazzi, S.; Minocci, D.; Maio, V.; Oranges, T.; Massi, D.; Nassini, R. Transient receptor potential vanilloid 4 (TRPV4) is downregulated in keratinocytes in human non-melanoma skin cancer. *J. Invest. Dermatol.* **2014**, *134*, 2408–2417. [CrossRef] [PubMed]

40. Yang, Y.S.; Cho, S.I.; Choi, M.G.; Choi, Y.H.; Kwak, I.S.; Park, C.W.; Kim, H.O. Increased expression of three types of transient receptor channels (TRPA1, TRPV4 and TRPV3) in burn scars with post-burn pruritus. *Acta Derm. Venereol.* **2015**, *95*, 20–24. [CrossRef] [PubMed]

41. Sterle, I.; Zupančič, D.; Romih, R. Correlation between urothelial differentiation and sensory proteins P2X3, P2X5, TRPV1, and TRPV4 in normal urothelium and papillary carcinoma of human bladder. *Biomed. Res. Int.* **2014**, *2014*, 1–9. [CrossRef] [PubMed]

42. Kassmann, M.; Harteneck, C.; Zhu, Z.; Nürnberg, B.; Tepel, M.; Gollasch, M. Transient receptor potential vanilloid 1 (TRPV1), TRPV4, and the kidney. *Acta Physiol.* **2013**, *207*, 546–564. [CrossRef] [PubMed]

43. Assimakopoulou, M.; Pagoulatos, D.; Nterma, P.; Pharmakakis, N. Immunolocalization of cannabinoid receptor type 1 and CB2 cannabinoid receptors, and transient receptor potential vanilloid channels in pterygium. *Mol. Med. Rep.* **2017**, *16*, 5285–5293. [CrossRef] [PubMed]

44. Vinuesa, A.G.; Sancho, R.; García-Limones, C.; Behrens, A.; Ten Dijke, P.; Calzado, M.A.; Muñoz, E. Vanilloid receptor-1 regulates neurogenic inflammation in colon and protects mice from colon cancer. *Cancer Res.* **2012**, *72*, 1705–1716. [CrossRef] [PubMed]

45. Luo, C.; Wang, Z.; Mu, J.; Zhu, M.; Zhen, Y.; Zhang, H. Upregulation of the transient receptor potential vanilloid 1 in colonic epithelium of patients with active inflammatory bowel disease. *Int. J. Clin. Exp. Pathol.* **2017**, *10*, 11335–11344.

46. Zhao, Y.; Huang, H.; Jiang, Y.; Wei, H.; Liu, P.; Wang, W.; Niu, W. Unusual localization and translocation of TRPV4 protein in cultured ventricular myocytes of the neonatal rat. *Eur. J. Histochem.* **2012**, *56*, e32. [CrossRef] [PubMed]

47. Baylie, R.L.; Brayden, J.E. TRPV channels and vascular function. *Acta Physiol.* **2011**, *203*, 99–116. [CrossRef] [PubMed]

48. Köhler, R.; Heyken, W.T.; Heinau, P.; Schubert, R.; Si, H.; Kacik, M.; Busch, C.; Grgic, I.; Maier, T.; Hoyer, J. Evidence for a functional role of endothelial transient receptor potential V4 in shear stress-induced vasodilatation. *Arterioscler. Thromb. Vasc. Biol.* **2006**, *26*, 1495–1502. [CrossRef] [PubMed]

49. Hoyer, J.; Köhler, R.; Distler, A. Mechanosensitive Ca^{2+} oscillations and STOC activation in endothelial cells. *FASEB J.* **1998**, *12*, 359–366. [CrossRef] [PubMed]

50. Sozucan, Y.; Kalender, M.E.; Sari, I.; Suner, A.; Oztuzcu, S.; Arman, K.; Yumrutas, O.; Bozgeyik, I.; Cengiz, B.; Igci, Y.Z.; et al. TRP genes family expression in colorectal cancer. *Exp. Oncol.* **2015**, *37*, 208–212. [PubMed]

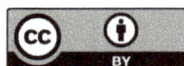

© 2018 by the authors. Licensee MDPI, Basel, Switzerland. This article is an open access article distributed under the terms and conditions of the Creative Commons Attribution (CC BY) license (http://creativecommons.org/licenses/by/4.0/).

![cells logo] *cells*

MDPI

Article

Purification of Functional Human TRP Channels Recombinantly Produced in Yeast

Liying Zhang [1], Kaituo Wang [1], Dan Arne Klaerke [2], Kirstine Calloe [2], Lillian Lowrey [2], Per Amstrup Pedersen [3], Pontus Gourdon [1,*] and Kamil Gotfryd [1,*]

[1] Department of Biomedical Sciences, University of Copenhagen, Nørre Allé 14, DK-2200 Copenhagen N, Denmark; liying.zhang@sund.ku.dk (L.Z.); kaituo@sund.ku.dk (K.W.)
[2] Department of Veterinary and Animal Sciences, University of Copenhagen, Dyrlægevej 100, DK-1870 Frederiksberg C, Denmark; dak@sund.ku.dk (D.A.K.); kirstinec@sund.ku.dk (K.C.); lillianclowrey@gmail.com (L.L.)
[3] Department of Biology, University of Copenhagen, Universitetsparken 13, DK-2100 Copenhagen OE, Denmark; papedersen@bio.ku.dk
* Correspondence: pontus@sund.ku.dk (P.G.); kamil@sund.ku.dk (K.G.); Tel.: +45-50-33-99-90 (P.G.); +45-41-40-28-69 (K.G.)

Received: 3 January 2019; Accepted: 3 February 2019; Published: 11 February 2019

Abstract: (1) Background: Human transient receptor potential (TRP) channels constitute a large family of ion-conducting membrane proteins that allow the sensation of environmental cues. As the dysfunction of TRP channels contributes to the pathogenesis of many widespread diseases, including cardiac disorders, these proteins also represent important pharmacological targets. TRP channels are typically produced using expensive and laborious mammalian or insect cell-based systems. (2) Methods: We demonstrate an alternative platform exploiting the yeast *Saccharomyces cerevisiae* capable of delivering high yields of functional human TRP channels. We produce 11 full-length human TRP members originating from four different subfamilies, purify a selected subset of these to a high homogeneity and confirm retained functionality using TRPM8 as a model target. (3) Results: Our findings demonstrate the potential of the described production system for future functional, structural and pharmacological studies of human TRP channels.

Keywords: ion channels; overproduction; production platform; protein purification; *Saccharomyces cerevisiae*; sensors; transient receptor potential (TRP) channels; yeast

1. Introduction

Transient receptor potential (TRP) channels constitute one of the largest families of ion channels and serve as cellular sensors that permeate cations, such as calcium, magnesium and sodium, in response to physical or chemical stimuli. Human TRP channels are widely expressed throughout the body, including brain, heart, liver, lung, small and large intestine, skeletal muscle, skin, pancreas, as well as in inflammatory and immune cells [1,2]. Changes of temperature, pH, the concentration of chemicals or membrane potential modulate TRP channel activity, highlighting their essential physiological roles in the sensation of thermal shifts [3], pain [4], taste [5] and pressure [6]. Malfunction of TRP channels significantly contributes to the development of many pathological conditions, including bipolar disorder, diabetes mellitus, various types of cancer, coronary heart disease and muscular dystrophia [7]. Consequently, TRP channels represent attractive pharmacological targets and indeed several TRP-modulating compounds currently undergoing clinical trials [8].

Based on sequence homology, topology and function, human TRP channels are divided into six subfamilies (Figure 1A): TRPC (canonical), TRPV (vanilloid), TRPM (melastatin), TRPA (ankyrin), TRPP (polycystin) and TRPML (mucolipin). Moreover, two additional subfamilies, i.e., TRPN and

TRPY have been identified in *Drosophila melanogaster* and yeast, respectively. Structurally, TRP channels assemble as homo- or hetero-tetramers with a single pore formed in the center. Each subunit consists of intracellular N- and C-termini, six transmembrane helices (TM1-TM6) interconnected by relatively short loops, with a pore forming loop (P) inserted between the TM5 and TM6 (Figure 1B,C) [9,10]. Currently, several structures are available for the TRP family (Table 1), including TRPA [11], TRPPP2-3 [12,13], TRPV1-6 [14–19], TRPC3-6 [20–24], TRPML1 and 3 [25,26], as well as TRPM2, 4 [27,28] and 7-8 [29,30] from different species. In addition to revealing the overall architectures, the gathered structural information provided mechanistic insights explaining fundamental regulatory and functional mechanisms [9,31], as well as facilitated drug development, with, e.g., TRPV1 being a highly medically relevant target [32].

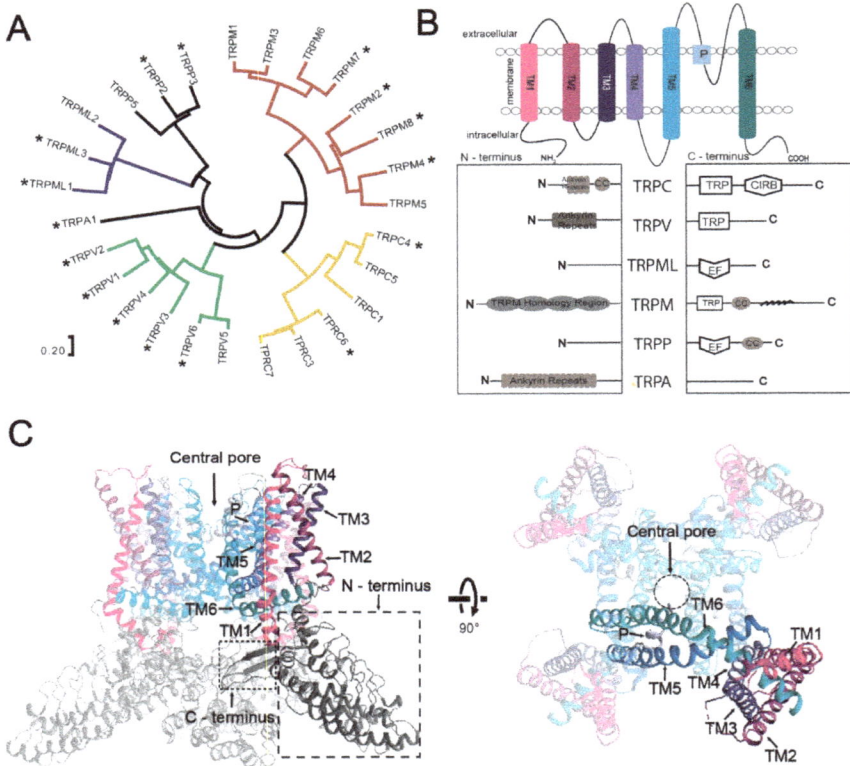

Figure 1. Human transient receptor potential (TRP) channels. (**A**) Phylogenetic distribution of the human TRP channel family including six subfamilies comprising proteins with distinct channel properties. Protein sequences were aligned using MEGA7 (https://www.megasoftware.net/). Structurally determined channels are highlighted with stars (not all structures were of protein with human origin, see also Table 1). (**B**) Topology of TRP channels showing in detail distinct architecture of the intracellular N- and C-termini across TRP channel subfamilies. (**C**) Overall structure of TRP channels with three out of the four monomers shown in pale colors (the structure of TRPV1, PDB-ID: 3J5P [14], was used as a model). TRP channel monomers consist of six transmembrane helices (TM1 to TM6) that assemble as tetramers with a single ion conducting central pore in the center formed by TM5, TM6 and the interconnecting pore-loop (P).

Being membrane proteins, many types of studies of TRP channels are nevertheless hindered by the difficulty of producing protein samples of sufficient quantity and quality in an economically sustainable manner. Systematic analysis of heterologous expression systems utilized for production of TRP channels for structural studies reveals that mammalian and insect cell-based platforms are the most commonly used (Table 1). TRPV1 [14], TRPM2 [27] and TRPV3 [16] channels were isolated from modified human HEK cells, whereas TRPML3 was overproduced using an insect (*Sf9*) cell-based platform [26]. To our knowledge, yeast, i.e., *Saccharomyces cerevisiae*, has been exploited to deliver the structures of two TRP channels only, namely TRPV2 from *Rattus norvegicus* [15] and TRPV5 from *Oryctolagus cuniculus* [18], whereas no structure is available originating from a bacterial host, despite attempts [33].

For many researchers, the primary expression system, also for the production of integral membrane proteins, has traditionally been *Escherichia coli*, due to the ease of genetic manipulation, availability of optimized expression plasmids, high-speed of growth and low cost [34,35]. However, generation of many proteins from higher sources frequently requires a eukaryotic expression system, such as insect, mammalian or yeast as hosts [36]. Compared to *E. coli*, the establishment of insect or mammalian cell-derived expression is nevertheless cost- and time-consuming. In this context, *S. cerevisiae* has advantages as it offers a cheap and robust large-scale production of properly-folded proteins with post-translational modifications combined with user-friendly genetic manipulations and simple culture conditions [36–38]. Hence, yeast represents an attractive complement for synthesis of high-quality protein, which has potential to permit in-depth biophysical and biochemical characterization, as well as drug discovery of many important targets, including TRP channels, for basic and applied sciences.

Here, we describe the development of an economic and effective method to isolate purified, functional human TRP channels applying a previously described robust *S. cerevisiae* membrane protein production platform [34,36,37]. Briefly, we approached 11 selected human TRP members belonging to 4 different subfamilies and produced these as full-length channels C-terminally fused to green fluorescent protein (GFP). We proceeded further with one member from each subfamily, i.e., TRPC4, TRPV3, TRPML2 and TRPM8, screened for suitable detergents for membrane extraction and assessed the quality of the solubilized samples by florescence-detection size-exclusion chromatography (F-SEC). Subsequently, we performed large-scale purification using affinity chromatography and investigated homogeneity of the samples employing SEC. Finally, for TRPM8, a medically significant target for the development of drugs to treat cold-associated respiratory disorders [39] and prostate cancer, respectively [40], we confirmed retained channel function following reconstitution into artificial lipid bilayers. Overall, our results suggest that *S. cerevisiae* is suitable for obtaining large-scales of active human TRP channels for numerous down-stream applications.

Table 1. Structurally determined TRP channels. TRP channels produced in *Saccharomyces cerevisiae* are framed. Targets included in this study are indicated in colors (yellow, green, blue and red represent TRPC, TRPV, TRPML and TRPM subfamilies, respectively). Boxes indicate the recombinant proteins produced in yeast, targets purified in this study are shown in bold. Additional information about constructs, structure determination method and obtained resolution are also shown.

Target	Organism	Expression System	Full Length	Truncation	Structure Determination Method	Resolution Å
TRPC3	Homo sapiens	Homo sapiens (AD-HEK293)	x		cryo-EM	4.4
TRPC4	Mus musculus	Spodoptera frugiperda		x	cryo-EM	3.3
TRPC5	Mus musculus	Homo sapiens (HEK293S)		x	cryo-EM	2.9
TRPC6	Mus musculus	Spodoptera frugiperda		x	cryo-EM	3.8
TRPC6	Homo sapiens	Homo sapiens (AD-HEK293)	x		cryo-EM	3.8
TRPV1	Rattus norvegicus	Homo sapiens (HEK293S)		minimal function	cryo-EM	4.2
TRPV2	Rattus norvegicus	Saccharomyces cerevisiae	x		cryo-EM	4.4
TRPV2	Oryctolagus cuniculus	Spodoptera frugiperda	x		cryo-EM	3.8
TRPV2	Oryctolagus cuniculus	Spodoptera frugiperda		minimal function	X-ray	3.9
TRPV3	Mus musculus	Homo sapiens (HEK293S)	x		cryo-EM	4.3
TRPV4	Xenopus tropicalis	Pichia pastoris		x	cryo-EM	3.8
TRPV5	Oryctolagus cuniculus	Saccharomyces cerevisiae	x		cryo-EM	3.9
TRPV6	Rattus norvegicus	Homo sapiens (HEK293S)		x	X-ray	3.2
TRPV6	Homo sapiens	Homo sapiens (HEK293S)	x		cryo-EM	3.6
TRPML1	Homo sapiens	Homo sapiens (HEK293S)	x		cryo-EM	3.7
TRPML3	Callithrix jacchus	Spodoptera frugiperda	x		cryo-EM	2.9
TRPM2	Danio rerio	Homo sapiens (HEK293S)	x		cryo-EM	3.3
TRPM4	Homo sapiens	Homo sapiens (HEK293F)	x		cryo-EM	3.2
TRPM7	Mus musculus	Homo sapiens (HEK293S)		x	cryo-EM	3.3
TRPM8	Ficedula albicollis	Homo sapiens (HEK293S)	x		cryo-EM	4.1
TRPA1	Homo sapiens	Homo sapiens (HEK293)	x		cryo-EM	4.2
TRPP2	Homo sapiens	Homo sapiens (HEK293S)		x	cryo-EM	4.2
TRPP3	Homo sapiens	Homo sapiens (HEK293S)	x		cryo-EM	3.1

2. Materials and Methods

2.1. Cloning and Construction of Plasmids

All cDNAs encoding full-length human TRP channels were codon-optimized for *S. cerevisiae* and purchased from GenScript (New Jersey, NJ, USA). Codon-optimization algorithm involves adjustment of a variety of parameters, including codon adaptability, mRNA structure, and various cis-elements critical in transcription and translation. TRP channel cDNAs and GFP were PCR amplified with AccuPol DNA polymerase (Amplicon, Odense, Denmark) and the primers listed in Supplementary Table S1. Each TRP channel-GFP-His8 fusion was generated by homologous recombination by co-transforming the *S. cerevisiae* PAP1500 strain [41] with a TRP PCR fragment, a GFP PCR fragment, as well as BamHI, HindIII and SalI digested pEMBLyex4 vector [42]. The PCR primers were designed to encode a Tobacco Etch Virus (TEV) protease cleavage site (GENLYFQ↓SQF) between the TRP channel and the GFP-octa-histidine (His8)-tag. Transformants were selected on agar plates containing synthetic defined (SD) medium with leucine (60 mg L^{-1}) and lysine (30 mg L^{-1}). The accuracy of all constructs was confirmed by DNA sequencing.

2.2. Small-Scale Expression of TRP Channels and Live Cell Bioimaging

All TEV-GFP-His8-fusions were expressed in the *S. cerevisiae* strain PAP1500 essentially as previously described [43]. Briefly, transformants were inoculated in 5 mL of SD media [44] containing glucose (20 g L^{-1}), leucine (60 mg L^{-1}) and lysine (30 mg L^{-1}), and grown overnight at 30 °C. The following day, 200 μL of the culture was transferred to 5 mL of the same media lacking leucine and grown for 24 h at 30 °C to increase plasmid copy number upon leucine deprivation. Subsequently, 5 mL of the culture was scaled up to 50 mL in the same medium for another 24 h and used to inoculate 2 L of media supplemented with amino acid (alanine (20 mg L^{-1}), arginine (20 mg L^{-1}), aspartic acid (100 mg L^{-1}), cysteine (20 mg L^{-1}), glutamic acid (100 mg L^{-1}), histidine (20 mg L^{-1}), lysine (30 mg L^{-1}), methionine (20 mg L^{-1}), phenylalanine 50 mg L^{-1}), proline (20 mg L^{-1}), serine (375 mg L^{-1}), threonine (200 mg L^{-1}), tryptophan (20 mg L^{-1}), tyrosine (30 mg L^{-1}) and valine (150 mg L^{-1})), glucose (10 g L^{-1}) and glycerol (3% *v/v*). Following glucose consumption, protein expression was induced by adding galactose to a final concentration of 2% and allowed for 48 h at 15 °C until the cells were harvested. Obtained material typically yielded in ~10 g of wet cell pellet.

Localization of expressed TEV-GFP-His8-fused TRP channels was performed by bioimaging of GFP fluorescence in vivo using the Nikon Eclipse E600 microscope (Nikon, Japan) equipped with a Optronics MagnaFire camera (Optronics, Muskogee, OK, USA).

2.3. Membrane Preparation, Detergent Screens and F-SEC

S. cerevisiae cells were homogenized mechanically (BioSpec, Bartlesville, OK, USA) using glass beads and crude membranes were prepared as previously described [45]. Briefly, following ultracentrifugation (205,000× *g*, 3 h, 4 °C), membranes were resuspended in ice-cold solubilization buffer (SB; 20 mM Tris-NaOH pH 7.5, 500 M NaCl, 10% glycerol, 1 mM EDTA, 1 mM EGTA) supplemented with SIGMAFAST protease inhibitor cocktail (Sigma, St. Louis Missouri, MO, USA), 1 mM PMSF (Sigma) and 2 mM 2-mercaptoethanol (Sigma), and stored at −80 °C until further use. Isolated membranes from yeast overexpressing the respective TRP channel were subjected to detergent screening to test solubilization efficacy. Briefly, solubilization was performed at vigorous rotation (2 h, 4 °C) in SB in the presence of n-dodecyl-D-maltoside (DDM; Anatrace, Maumee, OH, USA), n-decyl-D-maltoside (DM; Anatrace) or 2,2-didecylpropane-1,3-bis-β-D-maltopyranoside (LMNG; Anatrace) in a final concentration of 2% (1:1 detergent-to-membrane mass ratio) or n-dodecylphosphocholine (FC-12; Anatrace) or n-heksadecylphosphocholine (FC-16; Anatrace) in a final concentration of 1% (1:2 detergent-to-membrane mass ratio). Insoluble material was removed by ultracentrifugation (50,000× *g*, 20 min, 4 °C) and 20 μL of the supernatant was used to measure GFP fluorescence (excitation 485 nm, emission 520 nm) to estimate detergent extraction efficacy.

The remaining material was loaded on Superose 6 HR 10/30 column (GE Healthcare, Copenhagen, Denmark) equilibrated with buffer composed of 20 mM Tris-NaOH pH 7.5, 150 mM NaCl and 0.03% DDM, and subjected to F-SEC performed on ÄKTA Pure system (GE Healthcare) equipped with a Prominence RF-20A fluorescence detector (Shimadzu, Kyoto, Japan).

2.4. Large-Scale Protein Production, TEV Protease Cleavage and SEC

Large-scale expression of selected TRP channels was performed in 15-L bioreactors essentially as previously reported [42]. Briefly, 50 mL of the yeast culture described above was scaled up to 1 L in the same medium and grown overnight at 30 °C. The following day, the culture was used to inoculate 10 L of identical medium supplemented with 3% glucose, 3% glycerol, amino acids (excluding leucine), inorganic salts and vitamins, and the growth was performed in Applikon fermenters connected to an ADI 1030 Bio Controller (Applikon Biotechnology, Delft, Netherlands) with the automated maintenance of culture pH at 6.0. Approximately 18 h after inoculation, 1 L of 20% glucose was added to further increase the growth of cells. Following glucose consumption, protein expression was induced by adding galactose to a final concentration of 2% and allowed for 96 h at 15 °C until the cells were harvested. Obtained material typically yielded in ~150–200 g of wet cell pellet.

Large-scale protein purification was performed using immobilized metal ion affinity chromatography (IMAC) with crude membranes isolated from 40 g of fermenter-grown yeast cells (obtained from ~3 L of cell culture). Membranes were solubilized by vigorous rotation (3 h, 4 °C) in SB containing the detergent of interest in a final concentration of 2% (DDM or DM) or 1% (FC-16). Insoluble material was removed by centrifugation (35,000× g, 1 h, 4 °C) and the supernatant was loaded onto a HisTrap HP column (GE Healthcare), washed with 50 mL of IMAC buffer (20 mM Tris-NaOH pH 7.5, 500 mM NaCl, 10% glycerol and 3 × CMC of the respective detergent). Subsequently, bound protein was eluted in IMAC buffer supplemented with step-wise (60, 250 and 500 mM) imidazole gradient. Top IMAC fractions were pooled, concentrated on Vivaspin concentrators (MWCO 100 kDa; Sartorius, Göttingen, Germany) and the GFP-His8-tag was cleaved with TEV-His10-tagged protease (home source; 16 h, 4 °C) mixed with the protein sample in a ratio of 1:10 (*w/w*). Treatment with TEV protease was performed with concomitant dialysis against IMAC buffer supplemented with 20 mM imidazole performed in MWCO 10 kDa dialysis bags (ThermoScientific, Waltham, MA, USA). Following cleavage with TEV protease, reverse IMAC (RIMAC) was performed to rebind un-cleaved TEV-GFP-His8-fusions, free GFP-His8-tag and TEV-His10-tagged protease. Briefly, samples were loaded onto a HisTrap HP column (GE Healthcare) equilibrated with 15 mL of IMAC buffer containing 20 mM imidazole, and the flow through was collected and concentrated to ~5 mg mL^{-1} as already described. Subsequently, RIMAC- or IMAC-pure samples were loaded onto a Superose 6 HR 10/30 column (GE Healthcare) equilibrated with SEC buffer (20 mM Tris-NaOH pH 7.5, 150 mM NaCl, 10% glycerol and 3 × CMC of the respective detergent). Following each SEC run, fractions corresponding to the main elution peak were pooled and concentrated to ~1 mg mL^{-1} as already described.

2.5. Measurements of Single Channel Ion Conductance

Single channel ion conductance was measured in lipid bilayers using an Orbit Mini workstation (Nanion Technologies, München, Germany) with 50 μm MECA4 recording chips with 4 microelectrode cavities (Ionera Technologies, Freiburg, Germany) as previously described [46]. Voltage was controlled by the EDR 3 software (Elements, Cesena, Italy). 150 μL of the recording solution (10 mM HEPES pH 7.2, 200 mM KCl, 100 mM NaCl and 0.2 mM CaCl$_2$) was added to the cavity of the chip and electrical contact was established between the electrodes. Lipid planar membranes were formed over the electrode using 10 mM of 1,2-diphytanoyl-sn-glycero-3-phosphocholine (DPhPc; Avanti Polar Lipids, Alabaster, AL, USA) and 1 mM cholesterol in n-nonane (Avanti Polar Lipids). DDM-solubilized SEC-purified TRPM8 sample (0.2 μL of 6.34 μg μL^{-1}) was added to recording solution close to the bilayers on the cis-side of the chip. Voltage was switched between positive and negative values, increasing by 20-mV intervals to stimulate protein insertion into the membrane. To activate TRPM8, 1.0 μL of icilin (Sigma) was added to a final concentration of 0.2 μM. Once channel activity was detected, voltage steps to −20, −40, −80, −100, 20, 40, 60, 80 and 100 mV were applied. If no activity was observed after more than 2.5 min, the solution was gently mixed, and if still no activity, an additional 0.2 μL of protein sample was added. All recordings were obtained at room temperature (20–22 °C).

Recordings were low-pass filtered at 0.5 kHz and analyzed using Clampfit 10.7 software (Molecular Devices, San Jose, CA, USA). For single channel events current amplitude was determined. Single channel current was plotted as a function of voltage (I/V curve) using Prism 7 software (GraphPad, San Diego, CA, USA) and slope conductance was determined by linear regression.

3. Results

3.1. Selected TRP-Channel Targets and The Expression System

To investigate the capacity of *S. cerevisiae* to serve as a host for production of human TRP channels, we selected 11 human members belonging to 4 of the main subfamilies, hence, representing targets with a variety of distinct structural (e.g., N- and C-termini) and functional features. Specifically, the portfolio included the following members: TRPC3, TRPC4, TRPC5, TRPV1, TRPV3, TRPV4, TRPML1, TRPML2, TRPML3, TRPM1 and TRPM8. Each expression plasmid encompassed full-length sequences codon-optimized for *S. cerevisiae* with C-terminal TEV-GFP-His8-tag fusions (Figure 2A) to enable visualization, affinity purification and quality control of generated targets. Constructs were designed to employ the hybrid promoter (CG-P) of the pEMBLyex4 vector, enhanced by the PAP1500 yeast production strain overexpressing the GAL4p transcriptional activator (Figure 2B) [42]. The potency of the system is further increased through selection for leucine autotrophy that significantly increases the plasmid copy number prior to induction of the protein of interest [47].

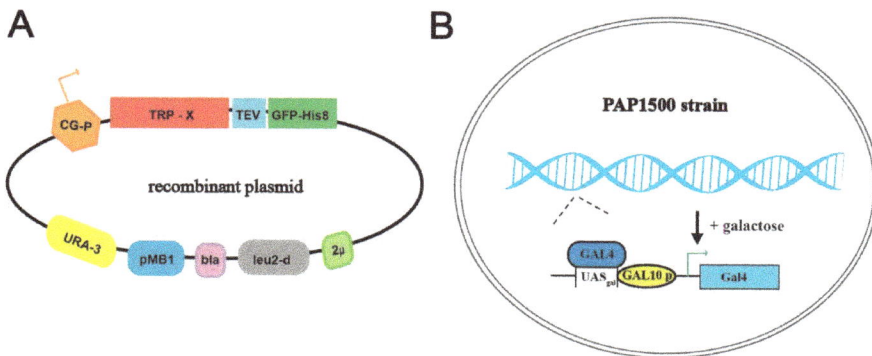

Figure 2. Schematic overview of the yeast production system. (**A**) Map of the employed plasmid encoding the respective TRP channels fused C-terminally with a Tobacco Etch Virus, TEV, protease cleavage site followed by green fluorescent protein sequence, GFP, attached to an octa-histidine stretch, His8-tag (TEV-GFP-His8-tag). Other critical elements of the plasmid include 2μ (yeast 2 micron origin of replication), leu2-d (poorly expressed allele of the β-iso-propyl-malate dehydrogenase gene), bla (β-lactamase gene), pMB1 (pMB1 origin of replication), URA3 (yeast orotidine-5′-phosphate decarboxylase gene) and CG-P (hybrid promoter of GAL10 upstream activating sequence and 5′ non-translated leader of cytochrome-1 gene). (**B**) The *Saccharomyces cerevisiae* protein production strain PAP1500 overexpresses the Gal4 transcriptional activator in the presence of galactose. Gal4 is the limiting factor for expression from galactose regulated promoter. GAL10 p, UASgal, a specific DNA binding site for GAL4 activator.

3.2. Small-Scale Production and Localization in S. cerevisiae

As low protein yields obstruct most types of downstream studies, the obtained quantity of the targets is critical to evaluate. Taking advantage of GFP detection of target accumulation permitted by the fusion tag, we determined the produced levels of the 11 human TRP channels following 2-day induction in 2-L cultures. By measuring whole-cell GFP fluorescence [48] and a GFP standard [49], we estimated the target levels to range from 2.4 to 5.2 mg of protein per liter cell culture (Figure 3A), representing rather promising yields for further optimization to produce samples for biophysical, structural and drug discovery efforts. The highest protein levels were achieved for TRPC4, whereas TRPML1 expressed the lowest, but still with encouraging yields.

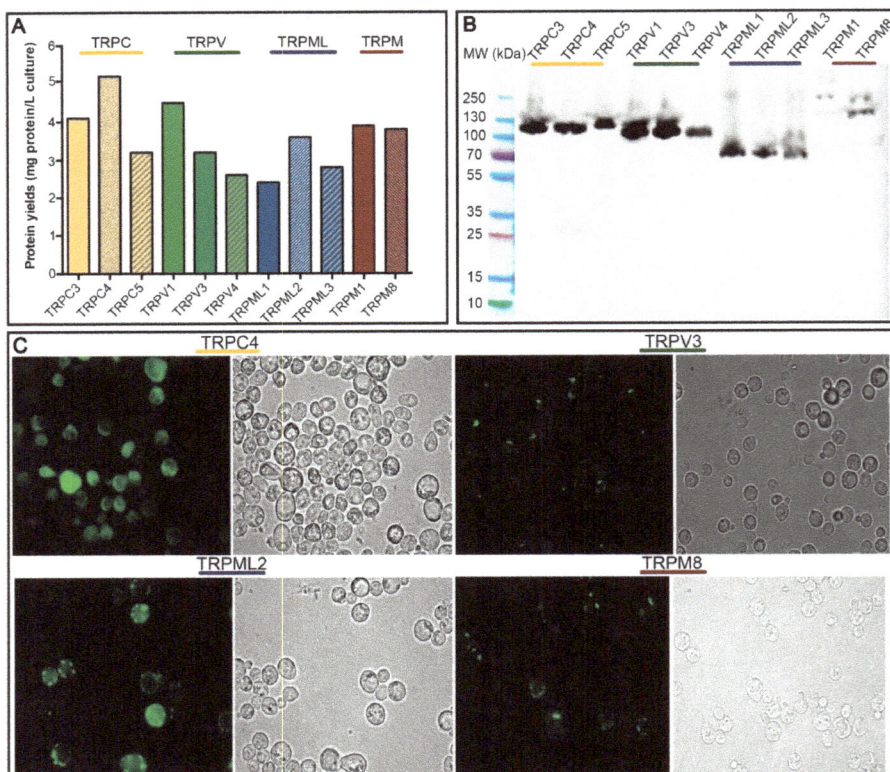

Figure 3. Expression and localization of human TRP channels. Data are shown for *S. cerevisiae* cell cultures grown in 2-L scale for 48 h at 15 °C. (**A**) Estimates of protein production levels of 11 human TRP-channels. Measured whole-cell GFP fluorescence was converted to the protein amount and the predicted yield is shown as mg per liter cell of culture. (**B**) In-gel GFP fluorescence of SDS-PAGE-separated crude membranes containing the different TRP channel targets. The image includes all samples separated on the same gel. (**C**) Live cell bioimaging of yeast cells expressing selected TRP channels. For each target GFP fluorescence and differential interference contrast micrographs are shown. Magnification: 1000×.

Subsequently, we took advantage of yet another useful feature of correctly-folded GFP, i.e., its SDS-resistance, and employed in-gel GFP fluorescence (visible following SDS-PAGE), to visualize the targets in crude membrane preparations (Figure 3B). Encouragingly, all the assessed 11 human TRP channels accumulated in the membranes in the full-length form. The electrophoretic mobility correlated well with the predicted molecular weight, with TRPM1 representing the heaviest target (wild-type MW of 198.7 kDa) and TRPML3 the lightest (wild-type MW of 57.7 kDa), respectively. For TRPC4 and TRPM1, an additional weak fluorescent band of lower molecular mass was observed, indicating marginal protein degradation. TRPM8 migrated as two fluorescent bands, reflecting monomeric and higher oligomeric (here dimeric) forms. In addition, the appearance of an additional blurred and smeary band for TRPM8 may indicate posttranslational glycosylation as previously reported for this protein [50]. However, as we achieved acceptable expression levels for this target, we did not attempt further optimization by removing glycosylation sites that were previously reported to enhance protein secretion [51].

Based on these highly promising production levels and indicative sample quality, as well as the fact that *S. cerevisiae*-based heterologous expression of well-behaving TRPV1 channel has been reported [52], we decided to narrow our target portfolio to characterize further one selected member from each subfamily, i.e., TRPC4, TRPV3, TRPML2 and TRPM8.

We then evaluated the localization of the produced human TRP channels in *S. cerevisiae* (Figure 3C). As seen from live cell bioimaging fluorescent micrographs, TRPC4 and TRPML2 accumulate mainly in the plasma membrane, whereas TRPV3 and TRPM8 reside in intra-cellular compartments. Such target-specific compartmental differences in the protein accumulation are frequently observed and do not affect the final quality of the produced samples [53].

3.3. Solubilization Screen and F-SEC

Successful chromatography purification of membrane proteins necessitates detergent(s) to enable membrane extraction and stabilization in solution [54]. To identify the most suitable detergents for solubilization of TRPC4, TRPV3, TRPML2 and TRPM8, we assessed several non-ionic (typically milder) and zwitterionic (harsher) surfactants, but the majority displayed only partial extraction of the targets (Supplementary Table S2). Overall, non-ionic DDM and DM (tested at a concentration of 2% w/w), and zwitterionic FC-12 and FC-16 (1%) were the most efficient (Figure 4A), with the latter being able to extract 4 TRP targets with at least 44% efficacy as observed for TRPML2. Interestingly, although used at higher concentration, milder non-ionic DDM and DM were less effective, but still provided fair solubilization, with only TRPM8 channel being extracted at lower, i.e., 20% efficacy, whereas the yield for both TRPC4 and TRPV3 exceeded 40%. However, TRPML2 resisted solubilization with non-ionic detergents and was only extracted with FC-12 and FC-16.

As already mentioned, an ideal extraction detergent should also maintain protein stability, an essential factor for obtaining high-quality samples for most biochemical, biophysical and biomedical applications. To evaluate protein behavior following exposure to detergent, we again took advantage of the TEV-GFP-His8-tag and conducted F-SEC (Figure 4B–E) in presence of 0.03% DDM to minimize aggregation of tested samples, where the SEC profile of the resulting solubilized fusion protein was monitored by the fluorescence spectroscopy [55]. For each target two F-SEC runs were performed to compare the profiles after solubilization with different detergents. In case of FC-16 all obtained F-SEC profiles were sharp and symmetrical, suggesting that the TRP channels were monodispersed in this detergent. Only for TRPC4 (Figure 4B) a small fraction of the protein eluted in the void volume of the column, indicating partial aggregation. TRPC4 exhibited almost identical behavior in DDM (Figure 4B), whereas the F-SEC profile for DDM-solubilized TRPM8 was broader, but devoid of aggregation (Figure 4E). DM solubilization of TRPV3 revealed marginal aggregation and a main peak elution across a relatively large volume span, suggesting partial disruption of the tetramer (Figure 4C). The F-SEC profile of FC-12-solubilized TRPML2 demonstrated two major fluorescence peaks, indicating dissociation of the oligomeric state towards a lower oligomeric (or monomeric) state (Figure 4D).

Considering the findings from the solubilization screen and F-SEC analysis, as well as previous reports demonstrating that fos-cholines can be detrimental to membrane proteins [55,56], and the fact that both DDM and DM are popular detergents for structural and functional studies (also of TRP channels) [9,57], we decided to use primarily these milder surfactants for the subsequent large-scale purifications.

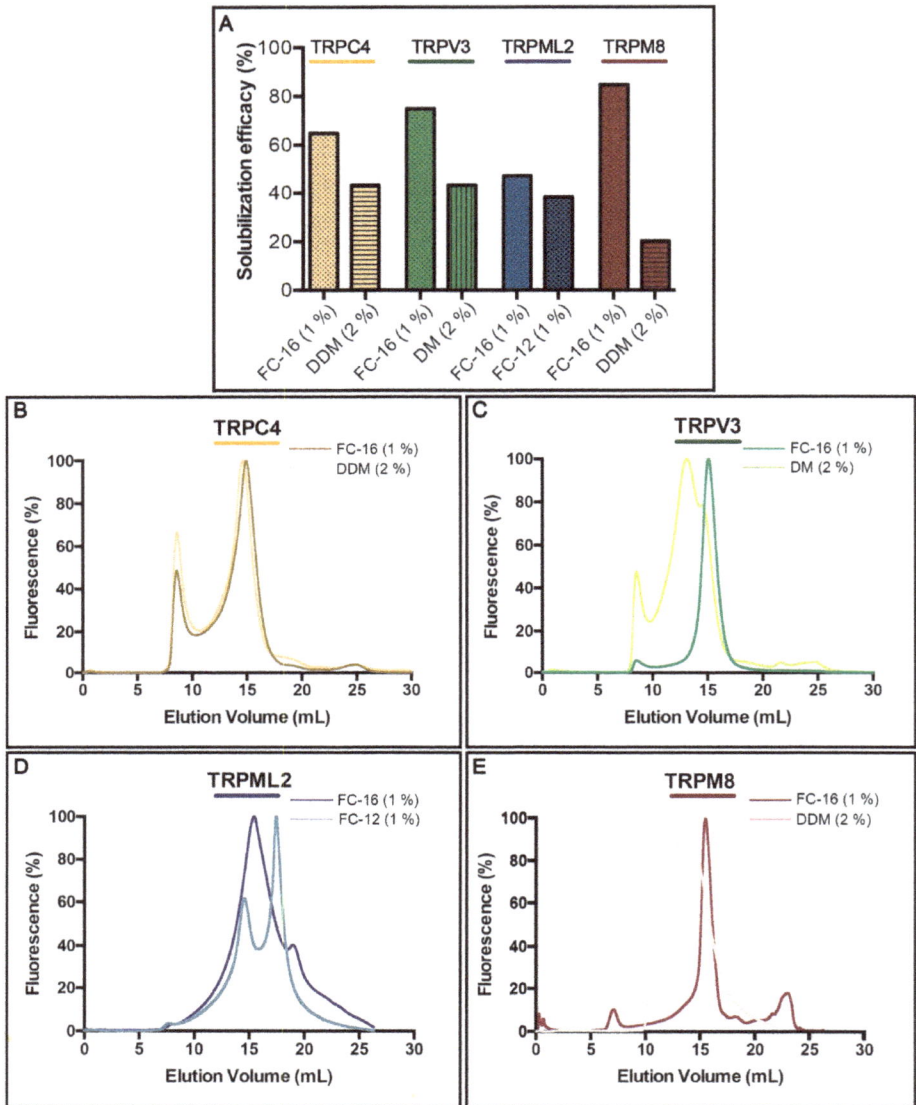

Figure 4. Solubilization and fluorescence-detection size-exclusion chromatography (F-SEC) of selected human TRP channels. (**A**) Solubilization efficacy in FC-12 (at a concentration of 1%), FC-16 (1%), DDM (2%) and DM (2%) of crude *S. cerevisiae* membranes for selected TRP channels. Solubilization was performed for 2 h at 4 °C and GFP fluorescence of the solubilized material (supernatant following ultracentrifugation) was used to calculate the percentage of extraction. (**B–E**) F-SEC analysis of the detergent-solubilized samples. Concentrations of the corresponding detergents used during solubilization are indicated. Normalized F-SEC profiles were obtained for solubilized material separated on Superose 6 HR 10/30 column where GFP fluorescence was monitored. The void volume of the column (Superose 6 HR 10/30) is ~8 mL.

3.4. Purification

Affinity purification of the selected 4 targets was performed based on crude membranes isolated from 40 g fermenter-grown *S. cerevisiae* cells (obtained from ~3 L of cell culture) induced for 96 h at 15 °C (Figure 5A–D). Membranes were solubilized for 3 h at 4 °C with the detergents indicated in the respective panels of Figure 4, based on the prior F-SEC analysis. As observed from the respective chromatograms, all TRP channels eluted at imidazole concentrations of ~250 mM. The total yield of the purified protein ranged from 0.5 to 1.5 mg per liter cell culture (for TRPM8 and TRPV3, respectively) and the overall purity already following the initial purification step was fair (see insets with Coomassie-stained SDS-PAGE gels). We subsequently concentrated the top fractions and attempted TEV protease facilitated removal of the GFP-His8-tag. However, only the TRPC4- and TRPV3-fusions were successfully cleaved, whereas TRPML2 and TRPM8 remained refractory to the TEV treatment (data not shown). This likely reflects poor accessibility of the C-termini in the two latter constructs, preventing proteolytic activity. For TRPC4 and TRPV3, we performed reverse affinity purification (R-IMAC), and obtained samples of higher purity as contaminants rebound to the resin (data not shown).

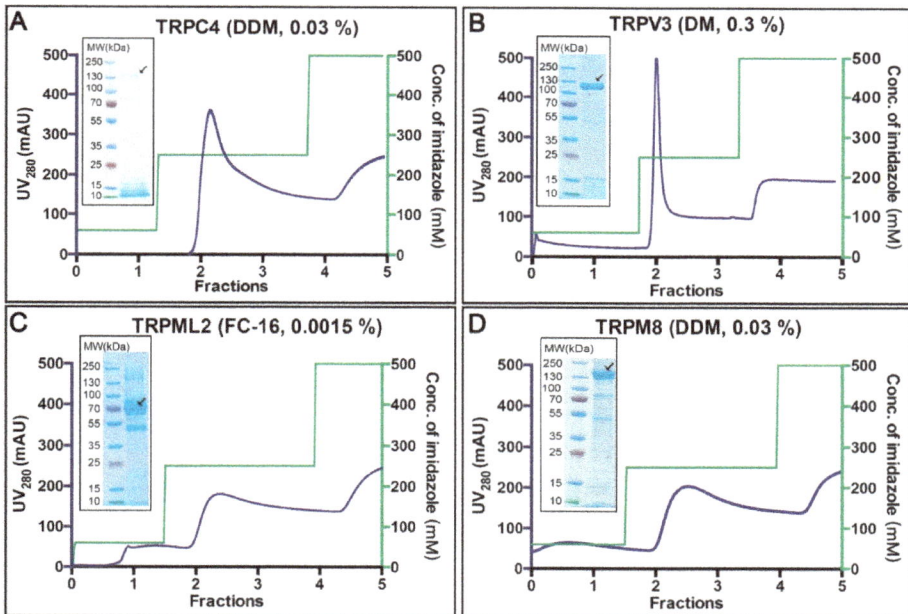

Figure 5. Purification of selected human TRP channels. (**A–D**) Selected targets were purified from crude *S. cerevisiae* membranes isolated from 40 g of fermenter-grown cells (obtained from ~3 L of cell culture) induced for 96 h at 15 °C. Membranes were solubilized with the indicated detergents for 3 h at 4 °C. Affinity protein purification was performed using immobilized metal ion affinity chromatography (IMAC). Concentrations of the corresponding detergents used for protein elution are indicated. IMAC profiles display UV$_{280}$ signal for eluted protein (blue) and the corresponding imidazole gradients used for elution (green). Insets: Coomassie-stained SDS-PAGE gels with concentrated affinity-purified samples. Black arrows indicate the MW for the corresponding fusion protein.

The (reverse) affinity-purified TRP channels were subjected to SEC run with 3 × CMC of the corresponding detergents used for solubilization, to further verify the sample quality (Figure 6A–D). Tag-free TRPC4 eluted as a symmetric peak, indicating a high degree of homogeneity (Figure 6A).

Similarly, although the SEC analysis of TRPV3 displayed some signs of aggregation, the overall shape and proportion suggested mono-dispersity of the sample (Figure 6B). We also obtained an acceptable SEC profile for TRPML2, however, the main peak was preceded by a significant shoulder, indicating the presence of higher oligomers (or even aggregation) in the sample (Figure 6C). The generated SEC profile for TRPM8 was symmetric overall, hinting again at a high homogeneity of the purified protein (Figure 6D).

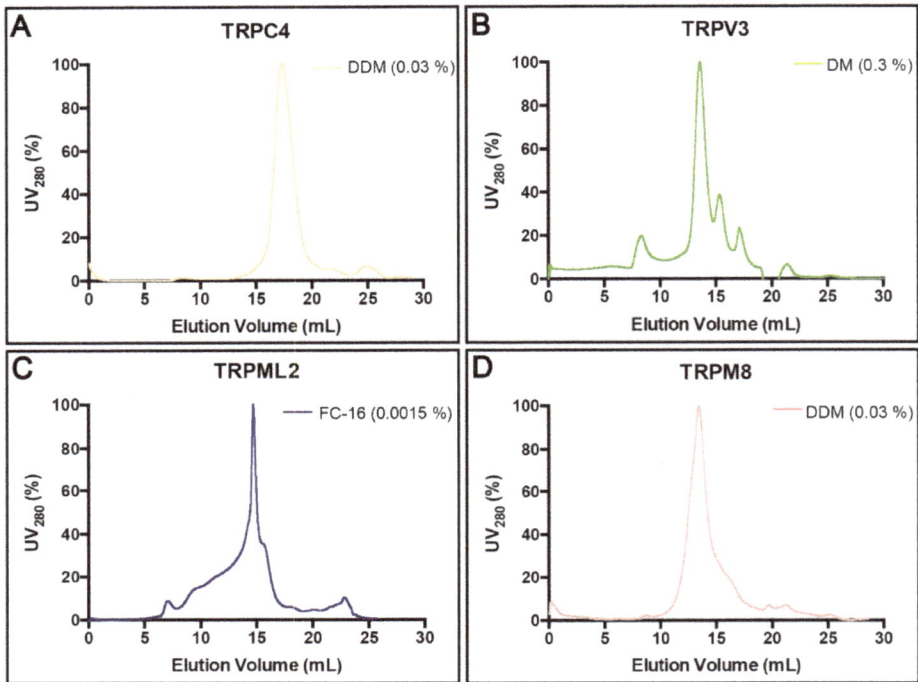

Figure 6. Size-exclusion chromatography (SEC) of selected human TRP channels. (**A–D**) Normalized SEC profiles for protein samples previously purified using reverse (TRPC4, A and TRPV3, B) or direct (TRPML2, C and TRPM8, D) affinity chromatography (immobilized metal ion affinity chromatography, IMAC). Concentrations of the corresponding detergents used during SEC are indicated. The void volume of the column (Superose 6 HR 10/30) is ~8 mL.

3.5. Single Channel Current Recordings of DDM-Solubilized TRPM8

Considering the relatively high predicted molecular weight, possible glycosylation, the lowest extraction efficacy in milder detergents, hence the obtained protein yield, as well as its high medical relevance, we nominated TRPM8 channel for functional characterization efforts. Current amplitude was determined (Figure 7A,B) and plotted as a function of voltage (Vm) and a linear regression was made to determine slope conductance, as shown in Figure 7C. The single channel conductance of purified TRPM8 channels was determined to 56.9 ± 3.2 pS.

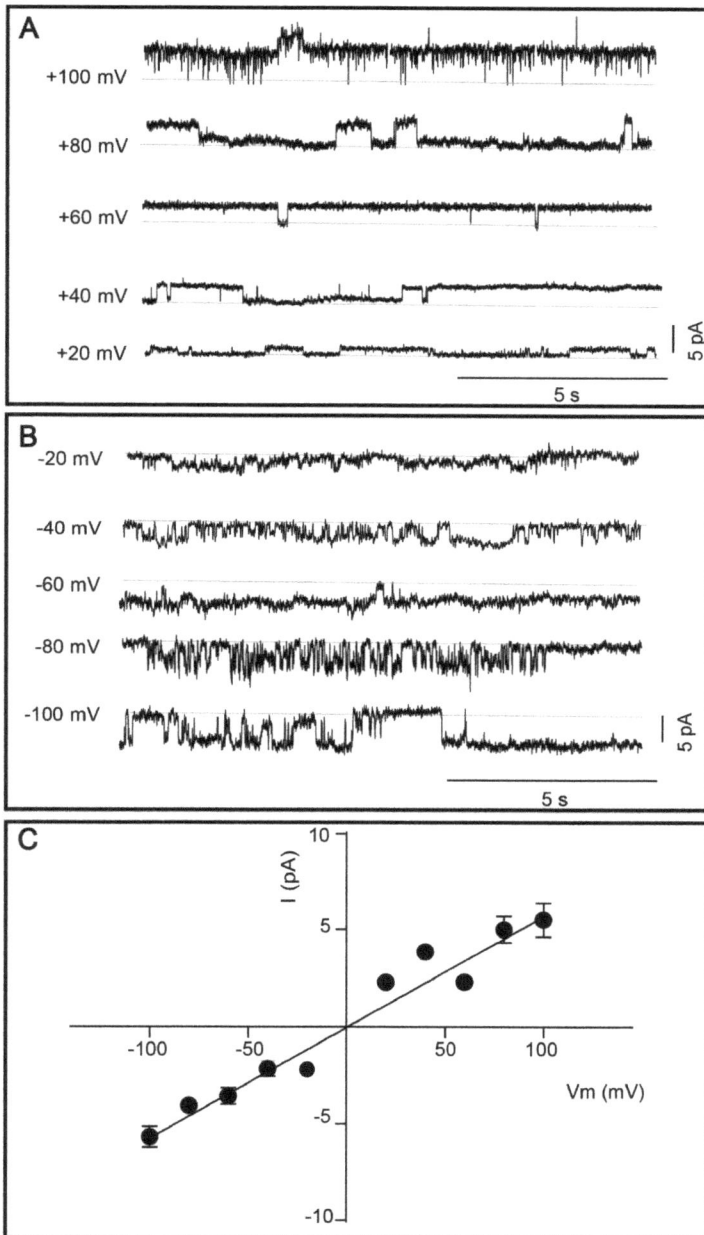

Figure 7. Single channel activity of affinity and size-exclusion chromatography purified TRPM8. (**A–B**) Representative single channel currents of TRPM8 reconstituted in the planar lipid bilayer membranes. Currents were elicited by positive (**A**) and negative (**B**) voltage steps. Channel activity is observed at all applied voltages. Zero current is indicated by the blue lines. (**C**) Current (I) was plotted as a function of voltage (V) and a linear regression was fitted to the data to determine the slope conductance (56.9 ± 3.2 pS). Results are shown as mean ± SEM, each data point was based on 2–52 single channel events.

4. Discussion

Membrane proteins, especially those of human origin, remain poorly understood relative to their soluble counterparts and are underrepresented in protein structure databases, largely due to difficulties in generation of prime-quality samples required for downstream efforts [58]. Furthermore, membrane proteins represent very attractive drug targets, and thus, cheap, high-efficiency, easy-to-handle and reproducible heterologous expression platforms capable of delivering large yields of recombinant human membrane proteins are still highly demanded.

The most widely exploited system for production of TRP channels from higher organisms is undoubtedly mammalian cell-based platforms that have provided several targets, including TRPV1 [14], TRPV6 [19], TRPC3 [20], TRPC4 [22], TRPM2 [27], TRPM4 [28], TRPM8 [30], TRPML1 [25], TRPA [11] and TRPPP2 [12]. However, complex growth requirements, high costs and modest yields leave room for alternative approaches [35]. Nevertheless, hitherto only two of the available structures of mammalian TRP channels, but none of human origin, originate from the protein produced in *S. cerevisiae* [15,18]. Compared to the mammalian expression systems, *S. cerevisiae* offers higher proteins yields, simpler culture conditions and significantly lower costs [59]. Importantly, as yeast can commonly contaminate mammalian cell cultures, implementation of careful aseptic routines is, however, necessary in laboratories culturing concomitantly these two types of cells [60].

In this study, we present a novel approach towards overproduction of human TRP channels employing an *S. cerevisiae*-based heterologous expression system. This platform was already successfully used for generation of several classes of membrane proteins, including the human ether-à-go-go-related (ERG) channel [49] and aquaporins [61], and even sample that yielded the first crystal structure of a human aquaglyceroporin [62]. Here, we approached the production of the challenging human TRP channels in a systematic way, starting from design of suitable plasmids, yield assessments, localization tests and solubilization screens, to affinity-based purification, SEC-based analysis and functional characterization of one selected target.

The first critical step in the optimization of recombinant protein overproduction is to assemble suitable expression plasmids [63]. Here, our strategy was based on the employment of full-length human TRP channel sequences that were codon-optimized for *S. cerevisiae*, a common practice used to improve production levels [64]. Moreover, all constructs possessed C-terminal TEV protease-detachable GFP-His8-tags, enabling detection and affinity purification of the generated targets to facilitate downstream characterization [48,65]. Furthermore, the expression vector used here encompassed several important features, including the possibility to increase the plasmid copy number and an inducible promoter [42]. Importantly, our strategy involved also the employment of a modified *S. cerevisiae* strain that overexpresses the Gal4 transcriptional activator required for galactose induced transcription [66]. Finally, we took advantage of the ability of *S. cerevisiae* to perform homologous recombination to assemble the final constructs [67], a significant economical aspect of utilizing yeast.

The initial expression tests (Figure 3A,B) already indicated the power of our production strategy, as we were able to recover all 11 human TRP channels selected for this study, all with promising production yields reaching maximum 5.2 mg of accumulated protein per liter cell culture (Figure 3A). Moreover, as evident from the in-gel GFP fluorescence signal, all targets were synthesized as membrane-embedded full-length channels with only marginal signs of protein degradation (Figure 3B), yet another important advantage of the utilized yeast platform. Moreover, for one target, namely TRPM8, we observed indications of protein glycosylation (Figure 3B). It has been previously reported that N-glycosylation is important for the function and regulation of TRP channels, including TRPA [68], TRPC [69] and TRPM [70,71] subfamilies, respectively. *S. cerevisiae* PAP1500 strain utilized here is capable of glycosylating the heterologously expressed human membrane proteins [49,61]. Of importance, *S. cerevisiae* has been shown to hyper-glycosylate proteins [36] with a detrimental impact on expression levels [37,51]. Thus, additional optimization of employed constructs by engineering glycosylation site(s) could be beneficial to further enhance the TRP channel production yields and activity, however, it was not attempted here.

The initial expression tests (Figure 3A,B) already indicated the power of our production strategy, as we were able to recover all 11 human TRP channels selected for this study, all with promising production yields reaching maximum 5.2 mg of accumulated protein per liter cell culture (Figure 3A). Moreover, as evident from the in-gel GFP fluorescence signal, all targets were synthesized as membrane-embedded full-length channels with only marginal signs of protein degradation (Figure 3B), yet another important advantage of the utilized yeast platform. Moreover, for one target, namely TRPM8, we observed indications of protein glycosylation (Figure 3B). It has been previously reported that N-glycosylation is important for the function and regulation of TRP channels, including TRPA [68], TRPC [69] and TRPM [70,71] subfamilies, respectively. *S. cerevisiae* PAP1500 strain utilized here is capable of glycosylating the heterologously expressed human membrane proteins [49,61]. Of importance, *S. cerevisiae* has been shown to hyper-glycosylate proteins [36] with a detrimental impact on expression levels [37,51]. Thus, additional optimization of employed constructs by engineering glycosylation site(s) could be beneficial to further enhance the TRP channel production yields and activity, however, it was not attempted here.

Mammalian TRP channels are known to differ in subcellular localization and, in addition to the plasma membrane, can localize to intracellular membranes [72]. For four selected TRP channels, we also observed differences in localization in the *S. cerevisiae* cells (Figure 3C), with TRPV3 and TRPM8 accumulating mainly intracellularly. In accordance, intracellular membrane localization has previously been observed for these two targets also in human cells [72,73].

To enable successful TRP channel production, suitable detergents for membrane extraction and maintaining protein stability were identified. The initial choice of detergents for solubilization was based on our previous large-scale analysis, which compared the efficacy of different compounds for extracting overproduced human aquaporins using the same expression platform [61]. In the solubilization screen presented here, we discovered that harsher zwitterionic detergents of the fos-choline family displayed stronger extraction properties of human TRP channels from the *S. cerevisiae* membranes as compared to milder non-ionic maltosides (Figure 4A, Supplementary Table S2). Indeed, similar observations have also been reported for other membrane protein classes overexpressed in the same host [74]. In general, all 4 targets tested here were rather resistant to solubilization, with only TRPM8 channel demonstrating extraction efficacy in FC-16 exceeding 80%. Moreover, when using FC-16, we observed slightly higher solubilization efficacy of the two targets accumulating in the intracellular membranes (i.e., TRPV3 and TRPM8) as compared to TRPC3 and TRPML2 that localized to the plasma membrane. A similar trend was previously reported for the human aquaporin family produced using the same platform [61]. Fos-choline-solubilized material exhibited moderately more symmetric F-SEC profiles, however, the mono-dispersity of the maltoside-extracted material was also relatively high (Figure 4B–E), indicating that milder detergents are promising for isolation of human TRP channels from crude *S. cerevisiae* membranes. This is also in agreement with the two above-mentioned structural reports of human TRPV channels that were overproduced in *S. cerevisiae* cells and solubilized in maltosides [15,18].

Affinity-based protein purification yielded milligram amounts of relatively pure samples already following a single chromatography round (Figure 5A–D). Removal of GFP-His8-tag by TEV protease cleavage followed by reverse affinity purification was successful for two out of four targets. However, optimization of neither sequences of employed constructs nor cleavage conditions were attempted here. The quality of (reverse) affinity-purified samples was evaluated by SEC performed with the primary detergent, i.e., the respective detergent used for solubilization and affinity purification for each target, respectively. Strikingly, all tested protein samples, including human TRPML2 isolated using harsh FC-16, exhibited encouraging SEC profiles (Figure 6A–D).

In our final quality control test, we assessed whether human TRP channels produced using the described overproduction approach preserved functionality, an important checkpoint for any heterologous expression platform. DDM-solubilized human TRPM8 was selected as a representative medically relevant target, with the aim to compare its conductance with permeation properties of

TRPM8 isolated from other hosts. The slope conductance of TRPM8 reconstituted in lipid bilayers was 56.9 ± 3.2 pS (Figure 7C). Similar conductance (55 ± 3.9 pS) was found for TRPM8 from *R. norvegicus* expressed in *Xenopus laevis* oocytes [75]. Moreover, a study employing human kidney cells reported mean TRPM8 conductance of 72 ± 12 pS for outward currents, 42 ± 6 pS for inward currents, respectively, and sub-conductance burst openings at 30 ± 3 pS, suggesting that the channel has a strong outward rectification [76]. Thus, our functional data obtained for human TRPM8 isolated from *S. cerevisiae* are in accordance with the conductance of both rat and human channels expressed in higher eukaryotic heterologous systems, with subtle quantitative differences that likely are attributed to variations of the experimental conditions.

All-in-all, obtained results establish our *S. cerevisiae*-based platform as a cost-effective and high-throughput approach to produce milligram quantities of stable and functional human TRP channels. Thus, the approach can be applied in functional, pharmacological and structural studies of this important family of ion-conducting proteins.

Supplementary Materials: The following are available online at http://www.mdpi.com/2073-4409/8/2/148/s1, Table S1: Sequences of primers used to obtain recombinant transient receptor potential (TRP) channel constructs included in the study, Table S2: Solubilization of selected human TRP channels.

Author Contributions: L.Z. performed protein expression, purification and biochemical characterization from cell material provided by P.A.P. P.A.P. supplied the expression vector and yeast strain. K.W. cloned all the expression constructs. D.A.K., L.L. and K.C. performed activity measurements on TRPM8 sample provided by L.Z. K.W., P.G. and K.G. designed the project. L.Z.Y., P.G. and K.G. wrote the paper with contribution from all authors.

Funding: L.Z. was funded by China Scholarships Council through PhD scholarship. K.W. is supported by post-doc scholarships from The Independent Research Fund Denmark and Lundbeck foundation. P.G. is supported by the following Foundations: Lundbeck, Knut and Alice Wallenberg, Carlsberg, Novo-Nordisk, Brødrene Hartmann, Agnes og Poul Friis, Augustinus, Crafoord, as well as The Per-Eric and Ulla Schyberg. Funding is also obtained from The Independent Research Fund Denmark, the Swedish Research Council and through a Michaelsen scholarship. K.G. is supported by the Independent Research Fund Denmark and the Lundbeck Foundation.

Acknowledgments: We are thankful to David Soerensen for technical assistance.

Conflicts of Interest: The authors declare no conflict of interest.

References

1. Fernandes, E.S.; Fernandes, M.A.; Keeble, J.E. The functions of TRPA1 and TRPV1: Moving away from sensory nerves. *Br. J. Pharmacol.* **2012**, *166*, 510–521. [CrossRef] [PubMed]
2. Gees, M.; Colsoul, B.; Nilius, B. The Role of Transient Receptor Potential Cation Channels in Ca2+ Signaling. *Cold Spring Harb. Perspect. Biol.* **2010**, *2*, a003962. [CrossRef] [PubMed]
3. Brauchi, S. A Hot-Sensing Cold Receptor: C-Terminal Domain Determines Thermosensation in Transient Receptor Potential Channels. *J. Neurosci.* **2006**, *26*, 4830–4840. [CrossRef] [PubMed]
4. Levine, J.D.; Alessandri-Haber, N. TRP channels: Targets for the relief of pain. *Biochim. Biophys. Acta Mol. Basis Dis.* **2007**, *1772*, 989–1003. [CrossRef] [PubMed]
5. Philippaert, K.; Pironet, A.; Mesuere, M.; Sones, W.; Vermeiren, L.; Kerselaers, S.; Pinto, S.; Segal, A.; Antoine, N.; Gysemans, C.; et al. Steviol glycosides enhance pancreatic beta-cell function and taste sensation by potentiation of TRPM5 channel activity. *Nat. Commun.* **2017**. [CrossRef] [PubMed]
6. Eccles, R. Nasal physiology and disease with reference to asthma. *Agents Actions Suppl.* **1989**, *28*, 249–261. [PubMed]
7. Nilius, B. TRP channels in disease. *Biochim. Biophys. Acta (BBA) Mol. Basis Dis.* **2007**, *1772*, 805–812. [CrossRef]
8. Moran, M.M. TRP Channels as Potential Drug Targets. *Annu. Rev. Pharmacol. Toxicol.* **2018**, *58*, 309–330. [CrossRef]
9. Hellmich, U.A.; Gaudet, R. Structural biology of TRP channels. *Handb. Exp. Pharmacol.* **2014**, *223*, 963–990. [CrossRef]
10. Vriens, J.; Owsianik, G.; Voets, T.; Droogmans, G.; Nilius, B. Invertebrate TRP proteins as functional models for mammalian channels. *Pflugers Arch. Eur. J. Physiol.* **2004**, *449*, 213–226. [CrossRef]

11. Paulsen, C.E.; Armache, J.P.; Gao, Y.; Cheng, Y.; Julius, D. Structure of the TRPA1 ion channel suggests regulatory mechanisms. *Nature* **2015**, *520*, 511–517. [CrossRef] [PubMed]

12. Wilkes, M.; Madej, M.G.; Kreuter, L.; Rhinow, D.; Heinz, V.; De Sanctis, S.; Ruppel, S.; Richter, R.M.; Joos, F.; Grieben, M.; et al. Molecular insights into lipid-assisted Ca2+ regulation of the TRP channel Polycystin-2. *Nat. Struct. Mol. Biol.* **2017**, *24*, 123–130. [CrossRef] [PubMed]

13. Hulse, R.E.; Li, Z.; Huang, R.K.; Zhang, J.; Clapham, D.E. Cryo-EM structure of the polycystin 2-l1 ion channel. *eLife* **2018**, *7*, e36931. [CrossRef] [PubMed]

14. Gao, Y.; Cao, E.; Julius, D.; Cheng, Y. TRPV1 structures in nanodiscs reveal mechanisms of ligand and lipid action. *Nature* **2016**, *534*, 347–351. [CrossRef] [PubMed]

15. Huynh, K.W.; Cohen, M.R.; Jiang, J.; Samanta, A.; Lodowski, D.T.; Zhou, Z.H.; Moiseenkova-Bell, V.Y. Structure of the full-length TRPV2 channel by cryo-EM. *Nat. Commun.* **2016**, *7*, 11130. [CrossRef] [PubMed]

16. Singh, A.K.; McGoldrick, L.L.; Sobolevsky, A.I. Structure and gating mechanism of the transient receptor potential channel TRPV3. *Nat. Struct. Mol. Biol.* **2018**, *25*, 805–813. [CrossRef] [PubMed]

17. Deng, Z.; Paknejad, N.; Maksaev, G.; Sala-Rabanal, M.; Nichols, C.G.; Hite, R.K.; Yuan, P. Cryo-EM and X-ray structures of TRPV4 reveal insight into ion permeation and gating mechanisms. *Nat. Struct. Mol. Biol.* **2018**, *25*, 252–260. [CrossRef] [PubMed]

18. Hughes, T.E.T.; Pumroy, R.A.; Yazici, A.T.; Kasimova, M.A.; Fluck, E.C.; Huynh, K.W.; Samanta, A.; Molugu, S.K.; Zhou, Z.H.; Carnevale, V.; et al. Structural insights on TRPV5 gating by endogenous modulators. *Nat. Commun.* **2018**, *9*, 4198. [CrossRef] [PubMed]

19. Singh, A.K.; Saotome, K.; McGoldrick, L.L.; Sobolevsky, A.I. Structural bases of TRP channel TRPV6 allosteric modulation by 2-APB. *Nat. Commun.* **2018**, *9*, 2465. [CrossRef] [PubMed]

20. Fan, C.; Choi, W.; Sun, W.; Du, J.; Lu, W. Structure of the human lipid-gated cation channel TRPC3. *eLife* **2018**, *7*, e36852. [CrossRef] [PubMed]

21. Tang, Q.; Guo, W.; Zheng, L.; Wu, J.X.; Liu, M.; Zhou, X.; Zhang, X.; Chen, L. Structure of the receptor-activated human TRPC6 and TRPC3 ion channels. *Cell Res.* **2018**, *28*, 746–755. [CrossRef] [PubMed]

22. Duan, J.; Li, J.; Zeng, B.; Chen, G.L.; Peng, X.; Zhang, Y.; Wang, J.; Clapham, D.E.; Li, Z.; Zhang, J. Structure of the mouse TRPC4 ion channel. *Nat. Commun.* **2018**, *9*, 3102. [CrossRef] [PubMed]

23. Duan, J.; Li, J.; Chen, G.-L.; Zeng, B.; Clapham, D.; Li, Z.; Zhang, J. Cryo-EM structure of the receptor-activated TRPC5 ion channel at 2.9 angstrom resolution. *bioRxiv* **2018**, 467969. [CrossRef]

24. Azumaya, C.M.; Sierra-Valdez, F.; Cordero-Morales, J.F.; Nakagawa, T. Cryo-EM structure of the cytoplasmic domain of murine transient receptor potential cation channel subfamily C member 6 (TRPC6). *J. Biol. Chem.* **2018**, *293*, 10381–10391. [CrossRef] [PubMed]

25. Schmiege, P.; Fine, M.; Blobel, G.; Li, X. Human TRPML1 channel structures in open and closed conformations. *Nature* **2017**, *550*, 366–370. [CrossRef] [PubMed]

26. Hirschi, M.; Herzik, M.A.; Wie, J.; Suo, Y.; Borschel, W.F.; Ren, D.; Lander, G.C.; Lee, S.Y. Cryo-electron microscopy structure of the lysosomal calcium-permeable channel TRPML3. *Nature* **2017**, *550*, 411–414. [CrossRef] [PubMed]

27. Zhang, Z.; Tóth, B.; Szollosi, A.; Chen, J.; Csanády, L. Structure of a TRPM2 channel in complex with Ca2+explains unique gating regulation. *eLife* **2018**, *7*, e36409. [CrossRef] [PubMed]

28. Guo, J.; She, J.; Zeng, W.; Chen, Q.; Bai, X.C.; Jiang, Y. Structures of the calcium-activated, non-selective cation channel TRPM4. *Nature* **2017**, *552*, 205–209. [CrossRef] [PubMed]

29. Duan, J.; Li, Z.; Li, J.; Hulse, R.E.; Santa-Cruz, A.; Valinsky, W.C.; Abiria, S.A.; Krapivinsky, G.; Zhang, J.; Clapham, D.E. Structure of the mammalian TRPM7, a magnesium channel required during embryonic development. *Proc. Natl. Acad. Sci. USA* **2018**, *115*, E8201–E8210. [CrossRef]

30. Yin, Y.; Wu, M.; Zubcevic, L.; Borschel, W.F.; Lander, G.C.; Lee, S.-Y. Structure of the cold- and menthol-sensing ion channel TRPM8. *Science* **2018**, *359*, 237–241. [CrossRef]

31. Madej, M.G.; Ziegler, C.M. Dawning of a new era in TRP channel structural biology by cryo-electron microscopy. *Pflug. Arch. Eur. J. Physiol.* **2018**, *470*, 213–225. [CrossRef] [PubMed]

32. Carnevale, V.; Rohacs, T. TRPV1: A target for rational drug design. *Pharmaceuticals* **2016**, *9*, pii:E52. [CrossRef] [PubMed]

33. Kol, S.; Braun, C.; Thiel, G.; Doyle, D.A.; Sundström, M.; Gourdon, P.; Nissen, P. Heterologous expression and purification of an active human TRPV3 ion channel. *FEBS J.* **2013**, *280*, 6010–6021. [CrossRef] [PubMed]

34. Jia, B.; Jeon, C.O. High-throughput recombinant protein expression in *Escherichia coli*: Current status and future perspectives. *Open Biol.* **2016**, *6*, 160196. [CrossRef] [PubMed]

35. Pandey, A.; Shin, K.; Patterson, R.E.; Liu, X.-Q.; Rainey, J.K. Current strategies for protein production and purification enabling membrane protein structural biology. *Biochem. Cell Biol.* **2016**, *94*, 507–527. [CrossRef] [PubMed]

36. Gomes, A.R.; Byregowda, S.M.; Veeregowda, B.M.; Vinayagamurthy, B. An Overview of Heterologous Expression Host Systems for the Production of Recombinant Proteins. *Adv. Anim. Vet. Sci.* **2016**, *52*, 85–105. [CrossRef]

37. Liu, Z.; Tyo, K.E.J.; Martínez, J.L.; Petranovic, D.; Nielsen, J. Different expression systems for production of recombinant proteins in Saccharomyces cerevisiae. *Biotechnol. Bioeng.* **2012**, *109*, 1259–1268. [CrossRef] [PubMed]

38. Hou, J.; Tyo, K.E.J.; Liu, Z.; Petranovic, D.; Nielsen, J. Metabolic engineering of recombinant protein secretion by Saccharomyces cerevisiae. *FEMS Yeast Res.* **2012**, *12*, 491–510. [CrossRef] [PubMed]

39. Xing, H.; Ling, J.X.; Chen, M.; Johnson, R.D.; Tominaga, M.; Wang, C.Y.; Gu, J. TRPM8 mechanism of autonomic nerve response to cold in respiratory airway. *Mol. Pain* **2008**, *4*, 22. [CrossRef] [PubMed]

40. Zhang, L.; Barritt, G.J. Evidence that TRPM8 is an androgen-dependent Ca2+channel required for the survival of prostate cancer cells. *Cancer Res.* **2004**, *64*, 8365–8373. [CrossRef] [PubMed]

41. Bahk, J.D.; Kioka, N.; Sakai, H.; Komano, T. A runaway-replication plasmid pSY343 contains two *ssi* signals. *Plasmid* **1988**, *20*, 266–270. [CrossRef]

42. Cesareni, G.; Murray, J.A.H. Plasmid vectors carrying the replication origin of filamentous single-stranded phages. In *Genetic Engineering*; Springer: Boston, MA, USA, 1987; pp. 135–154.

43. Pedersen, P.A.; Rasmussen, J.H.; Jørgensen, P.L. Expression in high yield of pig α1β1 Na,K-ATPase and inactive mutants D369N and D807N in Saccharomyces cerevisiae. *J. Biol. Chem.* **1996**. [CrossRef]

44. Sherman, F. Getting Started with Yeast. *Methods Enzymol.* **1991**, *194*, 3–21. [CrossRef]

45. Scharff-Poulsen, P.; Pedersen, P.A. Saccharomyces cerevisiae-Based Platform for Rapid Production and Evaluation of Eukaryotic Nutrient Transporters and Transceptors for Biochemical Studies and Crystallography. *PLoS ONE* **2013**, *8*, e76851. [CrossRef]

46. Klaerke, D.A.; Tejada, M.L.A.; Christensen, V.G.; Lassen, M.; Pedersen, P.A.; Calloe, K. Reconstitution and Electrophysiological Characterization of Ion Channels in Lipid Bilayers. *Curr. Protoc. Pharmacol.* **2018**, *81*, e37. [CrossRef]

47. Erhart, E.; Hollenberg, C.P. The presence of a defective LEU2 gene on 2 mu DNA recombinant plasmids of Saccharomyces cerevisiae is responsible for curing and high copy number. *J. Bacteriol.* **1983**, *156*, 625–635. [CrossRef]

48. Drew, D.; Newstead, S.; Sonoda, Y.; Kim, H.; von Heijne, G.; Iwata, S. GFP-based optimization scheme for the overexpression and purification of eukaryotic membrane proteins in Saccharomyces cerevisiae. *Nat. Protoc.* **2008**, *3*, 784–798. [CrossRef]

49. Molbaek, K.; Scharff-Poulsen, P.; Helix-Nielsen, C.; Klaerke, D.A.; Pedersen, A.A. High yield purification of full-length functional hERG K+channels produced in Saccharomyces cerevisiae. *Microb. Cell Fact.* **2015**, *14*, 15. [CrossRef]

50. Ulăreanu, R.; Chirițoiu, G.; Cojocaru, F.; Deftu, A.; Ristoiu, V.; Stănică, L.; Mihăilescu, D.F.; Cucu, D. N-glycosylation of the transient receptor potential melastatin 8 channel is altered in pancreatic cancer cells. *Tumor Biol.* **2017**, *39*, 1010428317720940. [CrossRef]

51. Tang, H.; Wang, S.; Wang, J.; Song, M.; Xu, M.; Zhang, M.; Shen, Y.; Hou, J.; Bao, X. N-hypermannose glycosylation disruption enhances recombinant protein production by regulating secretory pathway and cell wall integrity in Saccharomyces cerevisiae. *Sci. Rep.* **2016**, *6*, 25654. [CrossRef]

52. Moiseenkova, V.Y.; Hellmich, H.L.; Christensen, B.N. Overexpression and purification of the vanilloid receptor in yeast (*Saccharomyces cerevisiae*). *Biochem. Biophys. Res. Commun.* **2003**, *310*, 196–201. [CrossRef]

53. Bomholt, J.; Hélix-Nielsen, C.; Scharff-Poulsen, P.; Pedersen, P.A. Recombinant Production of Human Aquaporin-1 to an Exceptional High Membrane Density in Saccharomyces cerevisiae. *PLoS ONE* **2013**, *8*, e56431. [CrossRef]

54. Arachea, B.T.; Sun, Z.; Potente, N.; Malik, R.; Isailovic, D.; Viola, R.E. Detergent selection for enhanced extraction of membrane proteins. *Protein Expr. Purif.* **2012**, *86*, 12–20. [CrossRef]
55. Kawate, T.; Gouaux, E. Fluorescence-Detection Size-Exclusion Chromatography for Precrystallization Screening of Integral Membrane Proteins. *Structure* **2006**, *14*, 673–681. [CrossRef]
56. Geertsma, E.R.; Groeneveld, M.; Slotboom, D.-J.; Poolman, B. Quality control of overexpressed membrane proteins. *Proc. Natl. Acad. Sci. USA* **2008**, *105*, 5722–5727. [CrossRef]
57. Stetsenko, A.; Guskov, A. An Overview of the Top Ten Detergents Used for Membrane Protein Crystallization. *Crystals* **2017**, *7*, 197. [CrossRef]
58. Almeida, J.G.; Preto, A.J.; Koukos, P.I.; Bonvin, A.M.J.J.; Moreira, I.S. Membrane proteins structures: A review on computational modeling tools. *Biochim. Biophys. Acta Biomembr.* **2017**, *1859*, 2021–2039. [CrossRef]
59. Audagnotto, M.; Dal Peraro, M. Protein post-translational modifications: In silico prediction tools and molecular modeling. *Comput. Struct. Biotechnol. J.* **2017**, *15*, 307–319. [CrossRef]
60. Luby, C.J.; Coughlin, B.P.; MacE, C.R. Enrichment and Recovery of Mammalian Cells from Contaminated Cultures Using Aqueous Two-Phase Systems. *Anal. Chem.* **2018**, *90*, 2103–2110. [CrossRef]
61. Bjørkskov, F.B.; Krabbe, S.L.; Nurup, C.N.; Missel, J.W.; Spulber, M.; Bomholt, J.; Molbaek, K.; Helix-Nielsen, C.; Gotfryd, K.; Gourdon, P.; et al. Purification and functional comparison of nine human Aquaporins produced in Saccharomyces cerevisiae for the purpose of biophysical characterization. *Sci. Rep.* **2017**, *7*, 1–21. [CrossRef]
62. Gotfryd, K.; Mósca, A.F.; Missel, J.W.; Truelsen, S.F. Human adipose glycerol flux is regulated by a pH gate in AQP10. *Nat. Commun.* **2018**, *9*, 4749. [CrossRef]
63. Edavettal, S.C.; Hunter, M.J.; Swanson, R.V. Genetic construct design and recombinant protein expression for structural biology. *Methods Mol. Biol.* **2012**, *841*, 29–47. [CrossRef]
64. Lanza, A.M.; Curran, K.A.; Rey, L.G.; Alper, H.S. A condition-specific codon optimization approach for improved heterologous gene expression in Saccharomyces cerevisiae. *BMC Syst. Biol.* **2014**, *8*, 33. [CrossRef]
65. Drew, D.; Lerch, M.; Kunji, E.; Slotboom, D.J.; de Gier, J.W. Optimization of membrane protein overexpression and purification using GFP fusions. *Nat. Methods* **2006**, *3*, 303–313. [CrossRef]
66. Schultz, L.D.; Hofmann, K.J.; Mylin, L.M.; Montgomery, D.L.; Ellis, R.W.; Hopper, J.E. Regulated overproduction of the GAL4 gene product greatly increases expression from galactose-inducible promoters on multi-copy expression vectors in yeast. *Gene* **1987**, *61*, 123–133. [CrossRef]
67. Wang, J.M.; Partoens, P.M.; Callebaut, D.P.; Coen, E.P.; Martin, J.J.; De Potter, W.P. Phenotype plasticity and immunocytochemical evidence for ChAT and DβH co-localization in fetal pig superior cervical ganglion cells. *Dev. Brain Res.* **1995**, *90*, 17–23. [CrossRef]
68. Egan, T.J.; Acuna, M.A.; Zenobi-Wong, M.; Zeilhofer, H.U.; Urech, D. Effects of N-glycosylation of the human cation channel TRPA1 on agonist-sensitivity. *Biosci. Rep.* **2016**, pii:BSR20160149. [CrossRef]
69. Dietrich, A.; Mederos Y Schnitzler, M.; Emmel, J.; Kalwa, H.; Hofmann, T.; Gudermann, T. N-Linked Protein Glycosylation Is a Major Determinant for Basal TRPC3 and TRPC6 Channel Activity. *J. Biol. Chem.* **2003**, *278*, 47842–47852. [CrossRef]
70. Pertusa, M.; Madrid, R.; Morenilla-Palao, C.; Belmonte, C.; Viana, F. N-glycosylation of TRPM8 ion channels modulates temperature sensitivity of cold thermoreceptor neurons. *J. Biol. Chem.* **2012**, *287*, 18218–18229. [CrossRef]
71. Woo, S.K.; Kwon, M.S.; Ivanov, A.; Geng, Z.; Gerzanich, V.; Simard, J.M. Complex n-Glycosylation stabilizes surface expression of transient receptor potential melastatin 4b protein. *J. Biol. Chem.* **2013**, *288*, 36409–36417. [CrossRef]
72. Dong, X.P.; Wang, X.; Xu, H. TRP channels of intracellular membranes. *J. Neurochem.* **2010**, *113*, 313–328. [CrossRef]
73. Wen, W.; Que, K.; Zang, C.; Wen, J.; Sun, G.; Zhao, Z.; Li, Y. Expression and distribution of three transient receptor potential vanilloid(TRPV) channel proteins in human odontoblast-like cells. *J. Mol. Histol.* **2017**, *48*, 367–377. [CrossRef]
74. Newstead, S.; Kim, H.; von Heijne, G.; Iwata, S.; Drew, D. High-throughput fluorescent-based optimization of eukaryotic membrane protein overexpression and purification in Saccharomyces cerevisiae. *Proc. Natl. Acad. Sci. USA* **2007**, *104*, 13936–13941. [CrossRef]

75. Raddatz, N.; Castillo, J.P.; Gonzalez, C.; Alvarez, O.; Latorre, R. Temperature and voltage coupling to channel opening in transient receptor potential melastatin 8 (TRPM8). *J. Biol. Chem.* **2014**, *289*, 35438–35454. [CrossRef]
76. Zakharian, E.; Thyagarajan, B.; French, R.J.; Pavlov, E.; Rohacs, T. Inorganic polyphosphate modulates TRPM8 channels. *PLoS ONE* **2009**, *4*, e5404. [CrossRef]

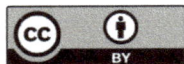

© 2019 by the authors. Licensee MDPI, Basel, Switzerland. This article is an open access article distributed under the terms and conditions of the Creative Commons Attribution (CC BY) license (http://creativecommons.org/licenses/by/4.0/).

cells

MDPI

Article

Manganese Suppresses the Haploinsufficiency of Heterozygous *trpy1Δ/TRPY1* *Saccharomyces cerevisiae* Cells and Stimulates the TRPY1-Dependent Release of Vacuolar Ca^{2+} under H$_2$O$_2$ Stress

Lavinia L. Ruta, Ioana Nicolau, Claudia V. Popa and Ileana C. Farcasanu *

Department of Organic Chemistry, Biochemistry and Catalysis, Faculty of Chemistry, University of Bucharest, Sos. Panduri 90-92, 050663 Bucharest, Romania; lavinia.ruta@chimie.unibuc.ro (L.L.R.), ioana.nicolau@chimie.unibuc.ro (I.N.), valentina.popa@chimie.unibuc.ro (C.V.P.)
* Correspondence: ileana.farcasanu@chimie.unibuc.ro; Tel.: +40-721-067-169

Received: 17 December 2018; Accepted: 18 January 2019; Published: 22 January 2019

Abstract: Transient potential receptor (TRP) channels are conserved cation channels found in most eukaryotes, known to sense a variety of chemical, thermal or mechanical stimuli. The *Saccharomyces cerevisiae* TRPY1 is a TRP channel with vacuolar localization involved in the cellular response to hyperosmotic shock and oxidative stress. In this study, we found that *S. cerevisiae* diploid cells with heterozygous deletion in *TRPY1* gene are haploinsufficient when grown in synthetic media deficient in essential metal ions and that this growth defect is alleviated by non-toxic Mn^{2+} surplus. Using cells expressing the Ca^{2+}-sensitive photoprotein aequorin we found that Mn^{2+} augmented the Ca^{2+} flux into the cytosol under oxidative stress, but not under hyperosmotic shock, a trait that was absent in the diploid cells with homozygous deletion of *TRPY1* gene. TRPY1 activation under oxidative stress was diminished in cells devoid of Smf1 (the Mn^{2+}-high-affinity plasma membrane transporter) but it was clearly augmented in cells lacking Pmr1 (the endoplasmic reticulum (ER)/Golgi located ATPase responsible for Mn^{2+} detoxification via excretory pathway). Taken together, these observations lead to the conclusion that increased levels of intracytosolic Mn^{2+} activate TRPY1 in the response to oxidative stress.

Keywords: TRP channel; TRPY1; *Saccharomyces cerevisiae*; calcium; manganese; oxidative stress

---

1. Introduction

Living cells are continuously exposed to various changes that threaten the dynamic equilibrium associated with the steady state of homeostatic balance. Such changes—often induced by stress agents—need to be sensed and signaled by cell components which belong to intricate networks responsible for homeostatic regulation. Calcium is a secondary messenger used by all eukaryotes—animal, plants, microorganisms—to connect various stimuli or stresses to their corresponding cellular responders. The budding yeast *Saccharomyces cerevisiae* has been constantly used as a model eukaryote to study the calcium-dependent response to various types of external stresses, which include salt [1], hypotonic [2,3], hypertonic [1,4,5], salicylate [6], alkaline [7], cold [8], ethanol [9,10], drugs [11] antifungals [12–16], electric [17] oxidative [18–20] or heavy metal [8,20–22] insults. The *S. cerevisiae* cells respond to such stresses by a sudden increase in cytosolic Ca^{2+}—denoted henceforth [Ca^{2+}]$_{cyt}$—following the stimulus-dependent opening of Ca^{2+} channels situated in the plasma membrane and/or in internal compartments. Abrupt increase in [Ca^{2+}]$_{cyt}$ represents a versatile and universally used mechanism which triggers either cell survival/adaptation or cell death [23].

In *S. cerevisiae* the stress-dependent rise in $[Ca^{2+}]_{cyt}$ can be a consequence of Ca^{2+} influx via the Cch1/Mid1 channel on the plasma membrane [1,2] release of vacuolar Ca^{2+} into the cytosol through the vacuole-located Ca^{2+} channel TRPY1 [4,24], or both [19,20]. After delivering the message, the normal very low level of $[Ca^{2+}]_{cyt}$ is restored through the action of Ca^{2+} pumps and exchangers [25]. Thus, the Ca^{2+}-ATPase Pmc1 [26] and a vacuolar Ca^{2+}/H^{+} exchanger Vcx1 [27,28] independently transport $[Ca^{2+}]_{cyt}$ into the vacuole, while Pmr1, the secretory Ca^{2+}-ATPase, pumps $[Ca^{2+}]_{cyt}$ into endoplasmic reticulum (ER) and Golgi along with Ca^{2+} extrusion from the cell [29,30].

In *S. cerevisiae*, TRPY1 is almost exclusively localized at the vacuolar membrane [4], playing an important role in adaptation to environmental stresses [4,19–21]. Initially named Yvc1, TRPY1 is encoded by *TRPY1* gene (systematic gene name, *YOR087W*) and it is the only member of the TRP (Transient Receptor Potential) superfamily of cationic channels expressed in *S. cerevisiae* [31]. TRP channels are conserved cation channels found in most eukaryotes, known to sense chemical, thermal, or mechanical stimuli in animals [32]. In yeast, TRPY1 is the main channel responsible for of $[Ca^{2+}]_{cyt}$ elevation under hyperosmotic shock [4,31], when calcium accrues predominantly from vacuolar stores [4]. This behavior can be explained by the mechano-sensitive traits of TRPY1: under hypertonic conditions water evacuates passively from the cytoplasm and then from the vacuole causing deformation of the vacuolar membrane and consequently the opening of the TRPY1 channel, with the release of vacuolar Ca^{2+} [5,33]. In contrast, under alkaline stress, the elevated $[Ca^{2+}]_{cyt}$ has its origin exclusively from the cell's exterior, with the Cch1/Mid1 channel solely responsible for the majority of Ca^{2+} entry, and with no contribution of vacuolar Ca^{2+} [7]. In between these two situations, oxidative stress triggers $[Ca^{2+}]_{cyt}$ waves which pool both external and vacuolar Ca^{2+} [19]. TRPY1 is necessary for attaining a maximum level of $[Ca^{2+}]_{cyt}$ under oxidative stress and TRPY1 depends on $[Ca^{2+}]_{cyt}$ elevation for maximal gating, in a process known as Ca^{2+}-induced Ca^{2+} release [34].

TRPY1 gene is not essential for survival and the knockout mutant cells *trpy1Δ* have no clear growth defects under various stresses. Rather, it was shown that *trpy1Δ* cells are slightly more resistant to the oxidative stress imposed by exogenous hydrogen peroxide or tert-butylhydroperoxide [19] and Cu^{2+} [20] but also less fit under high Cd^{2+} [21] or tunicamycin-induced ER-stress in Ca^{2+}-depleted medium [31]. In contrast, cells overexpressing the *TRPY1* gene are hypersensitive to surplus Ca^{2+} [4] or oxidative stress [19]. Also, it was revealed in a wide-scale survey that heterozygous *trpy1Δ/TRPY1* diploid cells are less fit under nutrient limiting conditions than the wild-type *TRPY1/TRPY1* ([35], Supplementary material). Haploinsufficiency occurs when the heterozygous mutation of a gene in a diploid organism results in a reduction of the corresponding gene product which can be correlated with negative alterations of the wild-type phenotype. In this study, we performed a chemical screen and found that non-toxic concentrations of Mn^{2+} alleviated the *trpy1Δ/TRPY1* haploinsufficiency observed by us in minimal growth medium containing half of the recommended amount of essential metal ions, probably by stimulating the TRPY1-mediated Ca^{2+} release into the cytosol.

2. Materials and Methods

2.1. Yeast Strains and Growth Media

The *S. cerevisiae* diploid strains used in this study were isogenic with the "wild-type" (WT) parental strain BY4743 (*MATa/α; his3Δ1/his3Δ1; leu2Δ0/leu2Δ0; met15Δ0/MET15; LYS2/lys2Δ0; ura3Δ0/ura3Δ0*), a S288C-based yeast strain [36]. The strains harbored either heterozygous (BY4732, *orf::kanMX4/ORF*) or homozygous (BY4732, *orf::kanMX4/orf::kanMX4*) knockout mutations of individual gene open reading frames (ORF). The heterozygous knockout mutants are referred to in the text as *orfΔ/ORF* and were *cch1Δ/CCH1, mid1Δ/MID1, pmc1Δ/PMC1, pmr1Δ/PMR1, vcx1Δ/VCX1, trpy1Δ/TRPY1*. The homozygous knockout mutants are referred to in the text as *orfΔ/orfΔ* and were *trpy1Δ/trpy1Δ, smf1Δ/smf1Δ*, and *pmr1Δ/pmr1Δ*. The strains were obtained from EUROSCARF (European *S. cerevisiae* Archive for Functional Analysis, www.euroscarf.de) and were propagated, grown, and maintained in YPD medium (1% yeast extract, 2% polypeptone, 2% glucose) or SD

(0.17% yeast nitrogen base without amino acids, 0.5% $(NH_4)_2SO_4$, 2% glucose, supplemented with the necessary amino acids) [37]. The strains transformed with the plasmids harboring apo-aequorin cDNA [38] were selected and maintained on SD lacking uracil (SD-Ura). Minimal defined media (MM) were prepared adding individual components as described [37] using ultrapure reagents (Merck, Darmstadt, Germany) and contained 1 mM Ca^{2+}, 0.25 μM Cu^{2+}, 2 μM Mn^{2+}, 2 μM Fe^{3+} and 2 μM Zn^{2+}. Low-metal minimal defined medium (LMeMM) had 0.5 mM Ca^{2+}, 0.1 μM Cu^{2+}, 1 μM Mn^{2+}, 1 μM Fe^{3+} and 1 μM Zn^{2+}, corresponding roughly to half of the amount of essential metals recommended [37]. The concentrations of metals in MM and LMeMM were confirmed by inductively coupled plasma with mass spectrometry (ICP-MS, Perkin-Elmer ELAN DRC-e, Concord, ON, Canada) against Multielement ICP Calibration Standard 3, matrix 5% HNO_3 (Perkin-Elmer Pure Plus, Shelton, CT, USA). All synthetic media had their pH adjusted to 6.5. For solid media, 2% agar was used. For growth improvement, all the synthetic media were supplemented with an extra 20 mg/L leucine [39]. All chemicals, including media reagents were from Merck (Darmstadt, Germany),

2.2. Plasmid and Yeast Transformation

For heterologous expression of aequorin, yeast cells were transformed with the multicopy *URA3*-based plasmid pYX212-*cytAEQ* harboring the apo-aequorin cDNA under the control of the strong *TPI* (triosephosphate isomerase) yeast promoter [40]. Plasmid pYX212-*cytAEQ* was a generous gift from Martegani and Tisi (University of Milano-Bicocca, Milan, Italy). Yeast transformation [41] was performed using S.c. EasyComp™ Transformation Kit (Invitrogen, Carlsbad, CA, USA) following manufacturer's indications.

2.3. Yeast Cell Growth Assay

2.3.1. Growth in Liquid Media

Unless otherwise specified, cells were incubated at 30 °C under agitation (200 rpm). Yeast strains were pre-grown overnight in MM then diluted (1/20) in fresh MM and grown for 2 h. Cells were harvested by centrifugation, washed with ice-cold water, and resuspended in liquid LMeMM at density which corresponded to optical density measured at 600 nm (OD_{600}) = 0.05. Strain growth in liquid LMeMM was monitored in time by measuring OD_{600} recorded in a plate reader equipped with thermostat and shaker (Varioskan, Thermo Fisher Scientific, Vantaa, Finland). Relative growth was expressed as the ratio between OD_{600} recorded at time *t* and OD_{600} recorded at time 0. For screening of chemicals against *trpy1Δ/TRPY1* haploinsufficiency (HIP), cells shifted to LMeMM (OD_{600} = 0.05) were incubated for 2 h before chemicals were added from concentrated sterile stocks. Cell growth (%) was determined 24 h from chemical addition and calculated relatively to growth (OD_{600}) of WT strain, no added chemicals. Chemicals used were $CuCl_2$, $FeCl_2$, $MnCl_2$, $ZnCl_2$, ascorbate, ethylene glycol-bis(2-aminoethylether)-*N,N,N′,N′*-tetraacetic acid (EGTA), $GdCl_3$, glutathione (GSH), indole and were all of high-grade purity.

2.3.2. Growth on Solid Media

For dilution plate assay, exponentially growing cells were 10-fold serially diluted in a 48-well microtiter plate and stamped on agar plates using a pin replicator (approximately 4 μL/spot). Plates were photographed after incubation at 30 °C for 3 days.

2.4. TRPY1 Gene Expression by Quantitative Reverse Transcriptase-Polymerase Chain Reaction (qRT-PCR)

Wild-type cells BY4743 (*TRPY1/TRPY1*), heterozygous (*trpy1Δ/TRPY1*), and homozygous (*trpy1Δ/trpy1Δ*) diploid cells from overnight pre-cultures were inoculated at OD_{600} = 0.1 in MM or LMeMM and grown to OD_{600} = 0.5 before Mn^{2+} was added to final concentration 10 μM, then incubated for 2 additional hours before being harvested for total ribonucleic acid (RNA) isolation. Total RNA was isolated using the RiboPure™ RNA Purification Kit for yeast (Ambion™, Thermo Fischer

Scientific, Vilnius, Lithuania) following the manufacturer's instructions. Approximately 500 ng of total RNA was transcribed into cDNA using GoScript™ Reverse Transcription System (Promega, Madison, WI, USA). Finally, a total of 10 ng cDNA was used for each qRT-PCR done with the GoTaq® qPCR Master Mix (Promega). Each reaction was performed in triplicate using MyiQ Single-Color Real-Time PCR Detection System (BioRad, Hercules, CA, USA). Expression of *TRPY1* mRNA was normalized to the relative expression of *ACT1* in each sample. The qRT-PCR cycling conditions were 95 °C for 1 min, and 40 cycles of 95 °C for 10 s, 59 °C for 10 s, 72 °C for 12 s. The primers used for amplification of cDNA were: TRPY1-F: 5′-AGATTCTCAG GGTTACGTTA, TRPY1-R: 5′-CAATATGGAATACCACTCAC; ACT1-F: 5′-GGTTGCTGCTTTGGTTATTG, ACT1-R: 5′-CAATTGGGTAACGTAAAGTC.

2.5. Assay of Cell Mn^{2+}

Measurements of cell total manganese content were done on cells grown in LMeMM medium to an OD_{600} of 1.0. Cells were harvested in triplicate samples, washed two times in ice-cold 10 mM 2-(*N*-morpholino) ethanesulfonic acid (MES)-Tris buffer (pH 6.0). Cells were finally suspended in deionized water (OD_{600} = 10) and used for manganese and cell protein assay. Manganese analysis was done by ICP-MS after digestion of cells with 65% ultrapure HNO_3 (Merck, Darmstadt, Germany). The metal cellular content was normalized to total cellular proteins, as described [42]. Total cellular manganese was expressed as nanomoles of metal per mg cell protein.

2.6. Detection of $[Ca^{2+}]_{cyt}$ by Aequorin Bioluminescence Assay

Cells transformed with pYX212-*cytAEQ* were maintained on SD-Ura selective medium and prepared for Ca^{2+} dependent luminescence detection as described [43] with slight modifications. Overnight pre-cultures of cells expressing apo-aequorin were washed and suspended (OD_{600} = 0.5) in LMeMM-Ura then incubated to late exponential phase (OD_{600} = 1, 4–6 h). For pre-incubation with Mn^{2+}, $MnCl_2$ was added to the desired concentration and cells were grown for an additional 2 h. Cells were harvested by centrifugation and resuspened (to OD_{600} = 10) in LMeMM-Ura in which the corresponding Mn^{2+} concentration was maintained. To reconstitute functional aequorin, native coelenterazine was added to the cell suspension (from a methanol stock, 20 µM final concentration) and the cells were incubated for 2 h at 30 °C in the dark. The excess coelenterazine was removed by centrifugation. The cells (approximately 10^7 cells/determination) were finally resuspended in LMeMM-Ura with corresponding Mn^{2+} concentration and transferred to the luminometer tube. A cellular luminescence baseline was determined for each strain by approximately one minute of recordings at 1/s intervals. After ensuring a stable signal, chemicals tested were injected from sterile stocks to give the final concentrations indicated, and the Ca^{2+}-dependent light emission was monitored in a single tube luminometer (Turner Biosystems, 20^n/20, Sunnyvale, CA, USA). The light emission was measured at 1 s intervals and expressed as relative luminescence units (RLU). To ensure that the total reconstituted aequorin was not limiting in our assay, at the end of each experiment aequorin activity was checked by lysing cells with 1% Triton X-100 with 5 mM $CaCl_2$ and only the cells with considerable residual luminescence were considered. Relative luminescence emission was normalized to an aequorin content giving a total light emission of 10^6 RLUs in 10 min after lysing cells with 1% Triton X-100. The relative luminescence maximum (RLM) was the average of the RLUs flanking the maximum value minus the average luminescence baseline recorded before cells were exposed to the stimulus (10 values on each side), all normalized as described above.

2.7. Statistics

All experiments were repeated, independently, in three biological replicates at least. For each individual experiment, values were expressed as the mean ± standard error of the mean (SEM). For aequorin luminescence determinations, traces represent the mean ± SEM from three independent transformants. The numerical data were examined by Student *t* test or by analysis of variance with multiple comparisons (ANOVA) using the statistical software Prism version 6.05 for Windows

(GraphPad Software, La Jolla, CA, USA). The differences were considered to be significant when $p < 0.05$. One sample t test was used for the statistical analysis of each strain/condition compared with a strain/condition considered as reference. Asterisks indicate the level of significance: * $p < 0.05$, ** $p < 0.01$, and *** $p < 0.001$.

3. Results

3.1. Haploinsufficiency of Yeast Strain Heterozyous for TRPY1 Is Alleviated by Mn^{2+}

To highlight new aspects related to TRPY1 function in yeast cells, the main target of our study was to identify conditions which interfere with TRPY1 activity. In this direction, haploinsufficiency is a genetic trait which can be very useful in the attempts to identify small molecules which influence the behavior of functional proteins [44]. A genome-wide survey had already pinpointed the heterozygous *trpy1Δ/TRPY1* as possibly less fit under nutrient limiting conditions ([35], Supplementary material). We noticed that the growth of the heterozygous *trpy1Δ/TRPY1* diploid mutant was not significantly different from the growth of the wild-type diploid when the two strains were incubated in YPD, SD (data not shown) or MM medium (Figure 1a), but *trpy1Δ/TRPY1* cells exhibited somehow slower growth ($p < 0.001$) in minimal synthetic medium LMeMM which had approximately half of the amount of essential metals recommended [37] (Figure 1b).

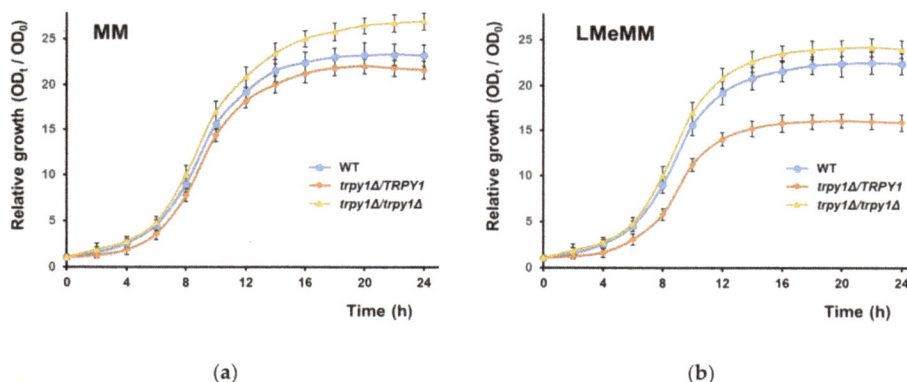

Figure 1. Growth of heterozygous *trpy1Δ/TRPY1*. Isogenic diploid strains WT (BY4743, *TRPY1/TRPY1*), *trpy1Δ/TRPY1* and *trpy1Δ/trpy1Δ* were shifted at time 0 to (**a**) minimal medium, MM or (**b**) minimum medium with low metal content, LMeMM, as described in Materials and Methods section. Growth was determined spectrophotometrically at 600 nm as the ratio between OD_{600} at time t and OD_{600} at time 0 for each individual strain.

The haploinsufficiency in LMeMM was noted only for *TRPY1*; no similar phenotype was recorded for heterozygous strains with mutations in the genes which encode the other transporters known to participate in regulating $[Ca^{2+}]_{cyt}$, e.g., *CCH1*, *MID1*, *PMC1* or *VCX1* (Figure 2a, dark blue bars).

To identify compounds which potentially interact with TRPY1 activity we screened for conditions which may alleviate or augment the haploinsufficient phenotype observed. The tested substances are presented in Table 1. These substances were added to the LMeMM at the point where the heterozygous *trpy1Δ/TRPY1* diploid cells were in the early log phase of growth ($OD_{600} = 0.1$) and the effect on growth was determined 24 h after chemical addition. We tested the effect of adding physiological concentrations of the metals initially depleted in LMeMM (i.e., Ca^{2+}, Cu^{2+}, Fe^{3+}, Mn^{2+}, Zn^{2+}) but also of glutathione and indole, which had been reported to interact with TRPY1 [45,46]. As glutathione is a universal intracellular antioxidant, we also tested an exogenous antioxidant, i.e., ascorbate. EGTA was chosen as a chelator of Ca^{2+} in the growth medium, while Gd^{3+} was tested as a blocker of the Ca^{2+}

channels. The results showing the effect of the tested compounds on *trpy1Δ/TRPY1* haploinsufficiency in LMeMM are included in Supplementary Files, Figure S1.

Table 1. Substances screened for the capacity to alleviate *trpy1Δ/TRPY1* haploinsufficiency in LMeMM.

Substance Tested [1]	Concentration Range	Effect on *trpy1Δ/TRPY1* Haploinsufficiency
$CaCl_2$	2–10 mM	No
$CuCl_2$	0.5–50 μM	No
$FeCl_3$	1–50 μM	No
$MnCl_2$	1–50 μM	Alleviation
$ZnCl_2$	1–50 μM	No
EGTA	0.1–2 mM	Augmentation
$GdCl_3$	0.1–1 mM	Augmentation
Ascorbate	1–10 mM	No
Glutathione [2]	1–10 mM	No
Indole [3]	1–10 mM	No

[1] The quantitative results are presented in Supplementary Files, Figure S1. [2] Glutathione depletion leads to TRPY1 activation [45]. [3] Indole activates TRPY1 under hyperosmotic stress [46].

Out of the compounds tested, only Mn^{2+} alleviated the *trpy1Δ/TRPY1* haploinsufficiency observed in LMeMM. In contrast, EGTA and Gd^{2+} augmented the LMeMM-associated growth defect (Figure 2a). The level of *TRPY1* gene expression was lower in *trpy1Δ/TRPY1* compared with wild-type, but this level was not significantly influenced by surplus Mn^{2+} (Figure 2b), suggesting that Mn^{2+} acts—directly or indirectly—by activating the TRPY1 channel. The *trpy1Δ/TRPY1* haploinsufficiency was also noted on solid LMeMM. In contrast, the *trpy1Δ/trpy1Δ* growth was not affected (Figure 2c).

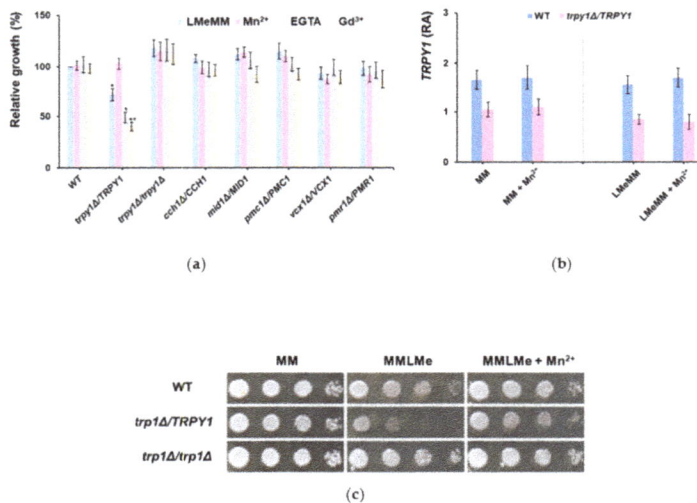

(a)

(b)

(c)

Figure 2. Haploinsufficiency of heterozygous *trpy1Δ/TRPY1*. (a) Mn^{2+} alleviates *trpy1Δ/TRPY1* haploinsufficiency in LMeMM. Diploid strains were shifted to LMeMM (final OD_{600} = 0.05) and grown for 2 h before $MnCl_2$ (10 μM), EGTA (0.5 mM) or $GdCl_3$ (50 μM) were added from concentrated stocks. Cell growth was recorded spectrophotometrically 24 h after the addition of the chemicals and normalized (%) to the growth of WT in the absence of chemicals. One sample *t* test compared WT in the absence of chemicals. * $p < 0.05$; ** $p < 0.01$. (b) Relative abundance (RA) of *TRPY1* mRNA in WT (*TRPY1/TRPY1*) and heterozygous *trpy1Δ/TRPY1*. Analysis of transcript abundance was done by qRT-PCR as described in Materials and Methods section. Expression of *TRPY1* mRNA was normalized to the relative expression of *ACT1* in each sample. (c) Heterozygous *trpy1Δ/TRPY1* exhibits haploinsufficiency in LMeMM, but not in normal MM. Cells in log phase (OD_{600} ~ 0.5) were 10-fold serially diluted (left to right) in a 48-well microtiter plate and stamped on the agar plates using a pin replicator (approximately 4 μL/spot). Plates were photographed after 3 days' incubation at 30 °C.

3.2. Mn^{2+} Potentiates the Increase of $[Ca^{2+}]_{cyt}$ under Oxidative Stress in Strain trpy1Δ/TRPY1

The observation that both EGTA (calcium chelator) and Gd^{3+} (inhibitor of Ca^{2+} transport across plasma membrane) augmented the LMeMM-related haploinsufficiency of the *trpy1Δ/TRPY1* strain prompted the idea that preventing Ca^{2+} entry into the cell is deleterious to *trpy1Δ/TRPY1*, while the observed opposite action of Mn^{2+} may be the result of Mn^{2+}-related activation of the extant TRPY1 that would compensate the heterozygous loss of *TRPY1*. To check this possibility, we used cells expressing aequorin, a system suitable for detecting transient modifications in the $[Ca^{2+}]_{cyt}$ [38]. For this purpose, *trpy1Δ/TRPY1* cells were transformed with a plasmid harboring the cDNA of the luminescent Ca^{2+} reporter apo-aequorin under the control of a constitutive promoter, which afforded abundant transgenic protein within the cytosol [40]. The cells expressing apo-aequorin were pre-treated with the cofactor coelenterazine to reconstitute the functional aequorin, and then the cells were exposed to various stimuli directly in the luminometer tube. It was noted that while Mn^{2+} alone failed to induce any increase in the luminescence of the reconstituted aequorin (data not shown), cell pre-incubation with 10 μM Mn^{2+} significantly increased the $[Ca^{2+}]_{cyt}$ elevation induced by H_2O_2 exposure (Figure 3a). Remarkably, pre-incubation with Mn^{2+} did not augment the cell luminescence when aequorin-expressing *trpy1Δ/TRPY1* cells were exposed to hyperosmotic shock (HOS, Figure 3b,c). Surplus Mn^{2+} reached maximum stimulating activity on *trpy1Δ/TRPY1* cells exposed to H_2O_2 at 10 μM (Figure 3c), a non-toxic concentration to both WT and *trpy1* mutants.

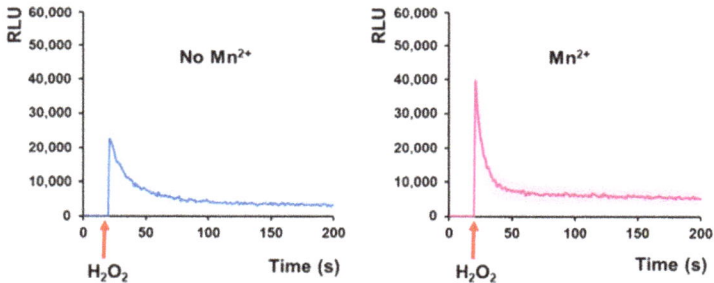

(a)

Figure 3. *Cont.*

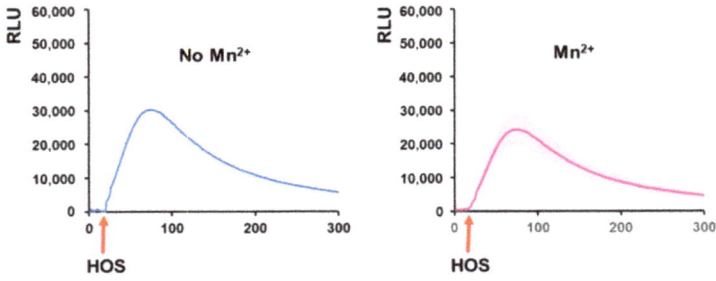

(b)

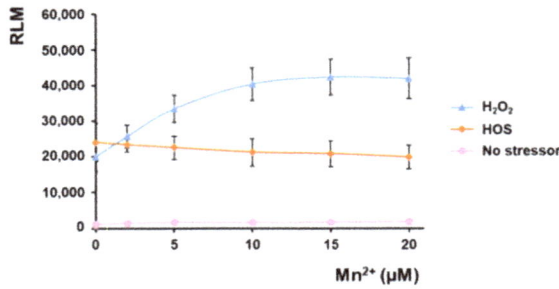

(c)

Figure 3. In *trpy1Δ/TRPY1* cells, Mn^{2+} pre-incubation stimulates the increase of $[Ca^{2+}]_{cyt}$ under H_2O_2 stress but not under hyperosmotic shock. Heterozygous *trpy1Δ/TRPY1* cells expressing reconstituted aequorin were pre-grown in LMeMM-Ura without or with 10 μM surplus Mn^{2+} before being exposed to (**a**) oxidative stress (5 mM H_2O_2) or (**b**) hyperosmotic stress (HOS, 0.8 M NaCl). $[Ca^{2+}]_{cyt}$-dependent aequorin luminescence was recorded on samples of approximately 10^7 cells. The arrow indicates the time when the stressor was added. The luminescence traces represent the mean ± SEM from 3 independent transformants. RLU, relative luminescence units. (**c**) Effect of pre-incubation with various concentrations of Mn^{2+} on the maximum intensity of the Ca^{2+}-dependent aequorin luminescence recorded under 5 mM H_2O_2, or 0.8 M NaCl (HOS). The relative maximum luminescence (RLM) was calculated as described in Materials and Methods. Bars represent the mean ± SEM from 3 independent transformants.

3.3. Mn^{2+} Stimulates TRPY1 to Release Ca^{2+} into the Cytosol under H_2O_2 Stress

Furthermore, we wondered whether Mn^{2+} influence on elevating $[Ca^{2+}]_{cyt}$ under H_2O_2 was the result of TRPY1 stimulation by Mn^{2+}. To test this possibility, we determined the effect of Mn^{2+} on the Ca^{2+}-mediated response to H_2O_2 of cells completely lacking TRPY1. It was noticed that in WT cells expressing reconstituted aequorin, the H_2O_2-induced Ca^{2+}-dependent luminescence was significantly increased by cell pre-incubation with 10 μM Mn^{2+}, indicating that in the case of WT cells too, Mn^{2+} potentiates the Ca^{2+}-dependent response to oxidative stress (Figure 4a). In contrast, homozygous knockout mutant *trpy1Δ/trpy1Δ* exhibited much lower H_2O_2-luminescence (Figure 4b, left), which was not altered by pre-incubation with 10 μM Mn^{2+} (Figure 4b, right). This observation suggested that Mn^{2+} augments the H_2O_2-induced $[Ca^{2+}]_{cyt}$ elevation by activating TRPY1, a phenotype clearly absent in the *trpy1Δ/trpy1Δ* homozygous knockout mutant (Figure 4b).

If Mn^{2+} were required for TRPY1 activation under oxidative stress, it would be expected that cells with low cytosolic Mn^{2+} would be less responsive in terms of increasing the $[Ca^{2+}]_{cyt}$ under oxidative stress. Mn^{2+} is an essential metal which is carried into the yeast cell by the divalent metal ion transporter Smf1, known to have high affinity for Mn^{2+} [47]. It was noted indeed that the homozygous knockout mutant *smf1Δ/smf1Δ* expressing reconstituted aequorin exhibited a significantly lower luminescence trace when exposed to H_2O_2 than WT (Figure 4c). In this line of evidence, the *pmr1Δ/pmr1Δ* cells expressing reconstituted aequorin responded strongly to H_2O_2 (in media not supplemented with Mn^{2+}) with a luminescence curve (Figure 4d) which was not significantly different from that obtained from WT cells preincubated with 10 µM Mn^{2+} (Figure 4a, right). *PMR1* encodes the major Golgi/ER membrane P-type ATPase ion pump responsible for transporting Ca^{2+} and Mn^{2+} into the Golgi apparatus [48] providing a major route for cellular detoxification of Mn^{2+} via the secretory pathway vesicles [49]. It was shown that cells knockout for *PMR1* gene have the intracellular Mn^{2+} levels considerably higher than the WT cells [50], a fact that may account for the stronger response of *pmr1Δ/pmr1Δ* cells (Figure 4d) compared to WT (Figure 4a, left). In this line of evidence, we found that *pmr1Δ/pmr1Δ* cells had significantly ($p < 0.05$) more cellular Mn^{2+} than the WT, while *smf1Δ/smf1Δ* cell had significantly ($p < 0.05$) less cellular Mn^{2+} than the WT (Table 2).

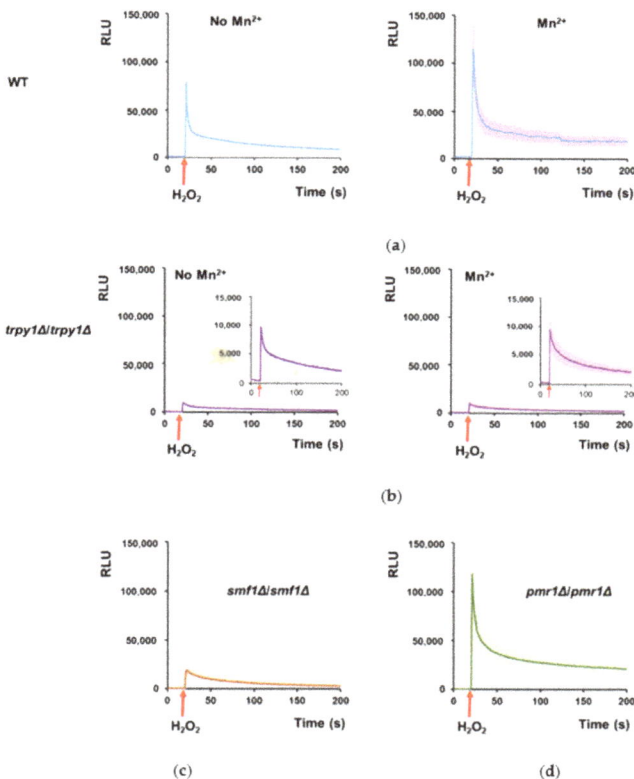

Figure 4. Variation of $[Ca^{2+}]_{cyt}$ in response to H_2O_2 exposure depends on Mn^{2+} cellular load. Diploid cells expressing reconstituted aequorin were pre-grown in LMeMM-Ura with or without 10 µM surplus Mn^{2+} before being exposed to oxidative stress (5 mM H_2O_2) as described in Materials and Methods. $[Ca^{2+}]_{cyt}$-dependent aequorin luminescence was recorded on samples of approximately 10^7 cells. The arrow indicates the time when the stressor (H_2O_2) was added. The luminescence traces represent the mean ± SEM from 3 independent transformants. (**a**) WT (BY4743). (**b**) *trpy1Δ/trpy1Δ*; insets: same representation at lower scale. (**c**) *smf1Δ/smf1Δ*. (**d**) *pmr1Δ/pmr1Δ*. RLU, relative luminescence units.

The influence of Mn^{2+} on the RLM recorded under oxidative stress for various strains which expressed reconstituted aequorin was also determined (Figure 5), revealing that Mn^{2+} significantly increased the RLM of WT cells exposed to H_2O_2. RLM determined for $trpy1\Delta/trpy1\Delta$ was significantly low and was not augmented by Mn^{2+}, indicating the necessity of functional TRPY1 for Mn^{2+} action. RLM for $smf1\Delta/smf1\Delta$ cells expressing reconstituted aequorin was also low under H_2O_2 exposure, indicating that the lack of the high-affinity Mn^{2+} transporter is associated with cytosolic Mn^{2+} concentration (Table2) which is too low for an efficient activation of TRPY1. In fact, $smf1\Delta/smf1\Delta$ attained responses similar to WT only at higher Mn^{2+} supplementation (Figure 5, grey line), when Mn^{2+} cell content was high enough (Table 2) for efficient TRPY1 activation. In contrast to $smf1\Delta/smf1\Delta$ strain, $pmr1\Delta/pmr1\Delta$ expressing reconstituted aequorin attained high RLM upon H_2O_2 exposure which was not significantly augmented by surplus Mn^{2+}, suggesting that the intrinsic high level of cytosolic Mn^{2+} associated with $PMR1$ knockout [50] is sufficient for attaining efficient activation of TRPY1 (Table2). Moreover, it was noted that when applying Mn^{2+} concentrations higher than 20 μM the maximum response of $pmr1\Delta/pmr1\Delta$ to H_2O_2 started to decline (Figure 5, yellow line) probably due to the hypersensitivity of this strain to Mn^{2+} [50].

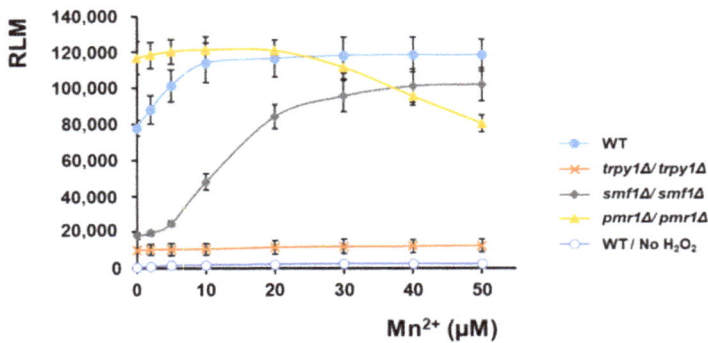

Figure 5. Effect of Mn^{2+} pre-incubation on the maximum intensity of the Ca^{2+}-dependent aequorin luminescence recorded for various strains under H_2O_2 stress. The relative maximum luminescence (RLM) was calculated as described in Materials and Methods. Diploid cells expressing reconstituted aequorin were pre-grown in LMeMM-Ura with or without surplus Mn^{2+} before being exposed to oxidative stress (5 mM H_2O_2) directly in the luminometer tube. $[Ca^{2+}]_{cyt}$-dependent aequorin luminescence was recorded on samples of approximately 10^7 cells. Bars represent the mean ± SEM from 3 independent transformants.

Table 2. Manganese content (pmoles/mg cell protein) of diploid yeast cells grown in LMeMM supplemented or not with Mn^{2+}.

Strain	Surplus Mn^{2+}		
	0	10 μM	50 μM
WT	0.12 ± 0.12	0.64 ± 0.2	0.92 ± 0.3
$trpy1\Delta/TRPY1$	0.11 ± 0.14	0.72 ± 0.1	0.98 ± 0.2
$trpy1\Delta/trpy1\Delta$	0.12 ± 0.2	0.7 ± 0.2	0.84 ± 0.2
$smf1\Delta/smf1\Delta$	0.01 ± 0.014	0.1 ± 0.2	0.72 ± 0.2
$pmr1\Delta/pmr1\Delta$	0.7 ± 0.22	0.84 ± 0.2	8.4 ± 1.2

4. Discussion

TRPY1 of *S. cerevisiae* is a key component in releasing vacuolar Ca^{2+} into the cytosol for the Ca^{2+}-dependent activation of mechanisms involved in the cell response to hyperosmotic [4] and oxidative stress [19]. Starting from the observation that Mn^{2+} alleviated the haploinsufficiency exhibited by the heterozygous *trpy1Δ/TRPY1* strain in synthetic media deficient in essential metals (LMeMM) we found that Mn^{2+} differentially stimulated TRPY1 to release Ca^{2+} from the vacuole under H_2O_2 exposure, but not under hyperosmotic shock. Mn^{2+} alone does not induce $[Ca^{2+}]_{cyt}$ elevation—neither under low (0.05–1 mM) nor under high (2–10 mM, lethal) surplus [21, unpublished observations]. The Mn^{2+} concentrations found to augment the H_2O_2-induced stimulation of TRPY1 were within the physiological limits (10–50 μM) and far below the concentration that would induce a hyperosmotic shock, explaining why the TRPY1 was not extra stimulated by Mn^{2+} under hyperosmotic stress (Figure 3b). It was shown that the release of vacuolar Ca^{2+} via TRPY1 can be stimulated by Ca^{2+} from outside the cell as well as that released from the vacuole by TRPY1 itself in a positive feedback, a process known as Ca^{2+}-induced Ca^{2+} release [34,51]. In this regard, Mn^{2+} surplus could stimulate TRPY1 similarly to Ca^{2+}. Mn^{2+} is an essential cation which strongly resembles Ca^{2+} not only in ionic radius but also in its affinity to oxygen-containing ligands, a trait which sometimes makes Mn^{2+} a good substitute of Ca^{2+} [52]; this would explain why other essential cations tested (Cu^{2+}, Fe^{3+}, Zn^{2+}) failed to alleviate the haploinsufficiency showed by *trpy1Δ/TRPY1* strain. That *TRPY1* haploinsufficiency in LMeMM is rescued by Mn^{2+} can be explained in three ways: (1) the supplemental Mn^{2+} simply counteracts the deficiency of essential metals of the LMeMM, providing the necessary amount of cations (albeit surrogate in certain cases) that support cell fitness; (2) Mn^{2+} stimulates TRPY1 activity by increasing the Ca^{2+} release to the cytososl, and consequently by stimulating other components involved in maintaining the cell fitness; (3) Mn^{2+} generates reactive oxygen species (ROS) by a Fenton-like reaction augmenting the oxidative stress and indirectly stimulating TRPY1. The fact that surplus Mn^{2+} augments the TRPY1-related increase in $[Ca^{2+}]_{cyt}$ under oxidative stress clearly correlates with the Mn^{2+} cytosolic level, as the strain lacking the high-affinity plasma membrane Mn^{2+} transporter Smf1 exhibited only a modest increase in $[Ca^{2+}]_{cyt}$ under H_2O_2, when compared with WT (Figure 4c). In this line of evidence, it was shown that a haploid *smf1Δ* was sensitive to H_2O_2 [20] probably by not attaining the optimum TRPY1 activation for adaptation to oxidative stress. On the other hand, it had been shown that deletion of *PMR1*—which leads to increased cytosolic Mn^{2+}—suppresses the sensitivity of superoxide dismutase (SOD) mutants to superoxide-generating drugs due to the Mn^{2+} capacity to scavenge superoxide ions [50]. In the light of our findings, it is also possible that the high cytosolic Mn^{2+} in cells devoid of Pmr1 rescue the SOD mutants from ROS attack not due to the scavenger traits of Mn^{2+}, but through TRPY1 activation. Whether Mn^{2+} rescues the haploinsufficient *trpy1Δ/TRPY1* by neutralizing ROS or by directly stimulating TRPY1 are issues to be addressed in the future; nevertheless, the observation that well-known antioxidants such as ascorbate or glutathione did not rescue the *trpy1Δ/TRPY1* haploinsufficiency rather supports the latter hypothesis. An open question remains: why is the homozygous *trpy1Δ/trpy1Δ* apparently more fit than the heterozygous *trpy1Δ/TRPY1*. The calcium-mediated responses to environmental insults are diverse: depending on the intensity or duration of the $[Ca^{2+}]_{cyt}$ waves, the cell can be led towards adaptation, survival (sometimes with growth arrest or slow growth) or death [19–21,23]. The *trpy1Δ/trpy1Δ* cells are probably more fit because they are never "bothered" by periodic nuisance caused by Ca^{2+} release from the vacuole; on the other hand, *trpy1Δ/TRPY1* cells need to find the right balance in Ca^{2+} gating while depending on only one gene copy, and sometimes extra help—external Ca^{2+} carried by Cch1/Mid1, mechanical force [34,51] or even surplus Mn^{2+}—may contribute to find the most suitable path to be followed.

Supplementary Materials: The following are available online. Figure S1: Effect of various substances on the haploinsufficiency of the heterozygous *trpy1Δ/TRPY1*.

Author Contributions: Conceptualization, I.C.F.; methodology, L.L.R., C.V.P. and I.C.F.; validation, L.L.R., C.V.P. and I.C.F.; formal analysis, I.N. and I.C.F.; investigation, L.L.R., C.V.P. and I.N.; resources, I.C.F.; data curation, L.L.R. and I.C.F.; writing—original draft preparation, I.C.F.; writing—review and editing, I.C.F.; supervision, I.C.F.; project administration, L.L.R.; funding acquisition, I.C.F.

Funding: This research was funded by the EEA Financial Mechanism 2009-2014, grant number 21 SEE/30.06.2014.

Acknowledgments: We thank Enzo Martegani and Renata Tisi (from University of Milano-Bicocca, Milan, Italy) for providing the plasmid pYX212-*cytAEQ* and Andrei F. Danet for technical support. We thank Aurora D. Neagoe for ICP-MS analysis.

Conflicts of Interest: The authors declare no conflict of interest.

References

1. Matsumoto, T.K.; Ellsmore, A.J.; Cessna, S.G.; Low, P.S.; Pardo, J.M.; Bressan, R.A.; Hasegawa, P.M. An osmotically induced cytosolic Ca^{2+} transient activates calcineurin signaling to mediate ion homeostasis and salt tolerance of *Saccharomyces cerevisiae*. *J. Biol. Chem.* **2002**, *277*, 33075–33080. [CrossRef] [PubMed]

2. Batiza, A.F.; Schulz, T.; Masson, P.H. Yeast respond to hypotonic shock with a calcium pulse. *J. Biol. Chem.* **1996**, *271*, 23357–23362. [CrossRef] [PubMed]

3. Rigamonti, M.; Groppi, S.; Belotti, F.; Ambrosini, R.; Filippi, G.; Martegani, E.; Tisi, R. Hypotonic stress-induced calcium signaling in Saccharomyces cerevisiae involves TRP-like transporters on the endoplasmic reticulum membrane. *Cell Calcium* **2015**, *57*, 57–68. [CrossRef] [PubMed]

4. Denis, V.; Cyert, M.S. Internal Ca^{2+} release in yeast is triggered by hypertonic shock and mediated by a TRP channel homologue. *J. Cell Biol.* **2002**, *156*, 29–34. [CrossRef] [PubMed]

5. Loukin, S.; Zhou, X.; Kung, C. Saimi, Y. A genome-wide survey suggests an osmoprotective role for vacuolar Ca^{2+} release in cell wall-compromised yeast. *FASEB J.* **2008**, *22*, 2405–2415. [CrossRef] [PubMed]

6. Mori, I.C.; Iida, H.; Tsuji, F.I.; Isobe, M.; Uozumi, N.; Muto, S. Salicylic acid induces a cytosolic Ca^{2+} elevation in yeast. *Biosci. Biotechnol. Biochem.* **1998**, *62*, 986–989. [CrossRef]

7. Viladevall, L.; Serrano, R.; Ruiz, A.; Domenech, G.; Giraldo, J.; Barcelo, A.; Arino, J. Characterization of the calcium-mediated response to alkaline stress in *Saccharomyces cerevisiae*. *J. Biol. Chem.* **2004**, *279*, 43614–43624. [CrossRef]

8. Peiter, E.; Fischer, M.; Sidaway, K.; Roberts, S.K.; Sanders, D. The *Saccharomyces cerevisiae* Ca^{2+} channel Cch1pMid1p is essential for tolerance to cold stress and iron toxicity. *FEBS Lett.* **2005**, *579*, 5697–5703. [CrossRef]

9. Araki, Y.; Wu, H.; Kitagaki, H.; Akao, T.; Takagi, H.; Shimoi, H. Ethanol stress stimulates the Ca^{2+}-mediated calcineurin/Crz1 pathway in *Saccharomyces cerevisiae*. *J. Biosci. Bioeng.* **2009**, *107*, 1–6. [CrossRef]

10. Courchesne, W.E.; Vlasek, C.; Klukovich, R.; Coffee, S. Ethanol induces calcium influx via the Cch1-Mid1 transporter in *Saccharomyces cerevisiae*. *Arch. Microbiol.* **2011**, *193*, 323–334. [CrossRef]

11. Gupta, S.S.; Ton, V.K.; Beaudry, V.; Rulli, S.; Cunningham, K.; Rao, R. Antifungal activity of amiodarone is mediated by disruption of calcium homeostasis. *J. Biol. Chem.* **2003**, *278*, 28831–28839. [CrossRef] [PubMed]

12. Rao, A.; Zhang, Y.Q.; Muend, S.; Rao, R. Mechanism of antifungal activity of terpenoid phenols resembles calcium stress and inhibition of the TOR pathway. *Antimicrob. Agents Chemother.* **2010**, *54*, 5062–5069. [CrossRef]

13. Hejchman, E.; Ostrowska, K.; Maciejewska, D.; Kossakowski, J.; Courchesne, W.E. Synthesis and antifungal activity of derivatives of 2- and 3-benzofurancarboxylic acids. *J. Pharmacol. Exp. Ther.* **2012**, *343*, 380–388. [CrossRef]

14. Roberts, S.K.; McAinsh, M.; Widdicks, L. Cch1p mediates Ca^{2+} influx to protect *Saccharomyces cerevisiae* against eugenol toxicity. *PLoS ONE* **2012**, *7*, e43989. [CrossRef] [PubMed]

15. Roberts, S.K.; McAinsh, M.; Cantopher, H.; Sandison, S. Calcium dependence of eugenol tolerance and toxicity in *Saccharomyces cerevisiae*. *PLoS ONE* **2014**, *9*, e102712. [CrossRef] [PubMed]

16. Popa, C.V.; Lungu, L.; Cristache, L.F.; Ciuculescu, C.; Danet, A.F.; Farcasanu, I.C. Heat shock, visible light or high calcium augment the cytotoxic effects of Ailanthus altissima (Swingle) leaf extracts against Saccharomyces cerevisiae cells. *Nat. Prod. Res.* **2015**, *29*, 1744–1747. [CrossRef]

17. Vilanova, C.; Hueso, A.; Palanca, C.; Marco, G.; Pitarch, M.; Otero, E.; Crespo, J.; Szablowski, J.; Rivera, S.; Domínguez-Escribà, L.; et al. Aequorin-expressing yeast emits light under electric control. *J. Biotechnol.* **2011**, *152*, 93–95. [CrossRef] [PubMed]

18. Pinontoan, R.; Krystofova, S.; Kawano, T.; Mori, I.C.; Tsuji, F.I.; Iida, H.; Muto, S. Phenylethylamine induces an increase in cytosolic Ca^{2+} in yeast. *Biosci. Biotechnol. Biosci.* **2002**, *66*, 1069–1074. [CrossRef]

19. Popa, C.V.; Dumitru, I.; Ruta, L.L.; Danet, A.F.; Farcasanu, I.C. Exogenous oxidative stress induces Ca^{2+} release in the yeast *Saccharomyces cerevisiae*. *FEBS J.* **2010**, *277*, 4027–4038. [CrossRef]

20. Ruta, L.L.; Popa, C.V.; Nicolau, I.; Farcasanu, I.C. Calcium signaling and copper toxicity in *Saccharomyces cerevisiae* cells. *Environ. Sci. Pollut. Res. Int.* **2016**, *23*, 24514–24526. [CrossRef]

21. Ruta, L.L.; Popa, V.C.; Nicolau, I.; Danet, A.F.; Iordache, V.; Neagoe, A.D.; Farcasanu, I.C. Calcium signaling mediates the response to cadmium toxicity in *Saccharomyces cerevisiae* cells. *FEBS Lett.* **2014**, *588*, 3202–3212. [CrossRef] [PubMed]

22. Ene, C.D.; Ruta, L.L.; Nicolau, I.; Popa, C.V.; Iordache, V.; Neagoe, A.D.; Farcasanu, I.C. Interaction between lanthanide ions and *Saccharomyces cerevisiae* cells. *J. Biol. Inorg. Chem.* **2015**, *20*, 1097–1107. [CrossRef]

23. Bootman, M.D.; Berridge, M.J.; Putney, J.W.; Llewelyn Roderick, H. *Calcium Signaling*; Cold Spring Harbor Laboratory Press: Cold Spring Harbor, NY, USA, 2011; 449p, ISBN 978-0-87969-903-1.

24. Palmer, C.P.; Zhou, X.; Lin, J.; Loukin, S.H.; Kung, C.; Saimi, Y. A TRP homolog in *Saccharomyces cerevisiae* forms an intracellular Ca^{2+}-permeable channel in the yeast vacuolar membrane. *Proc. Natl. Acad. Sci. USA* **2001**, *98*, 7801–7805. [CrossRef] [PubMed]

25. Cunningham, K.W. Acidic calcium stores of *Saccharomyces cerevisiae*. *Cell Calcium* **2011**, *50*, 129–138. [CrossRef] [PubMed]

26. Cunningham, K.W.; Fink, G.R. Calcineurin-dependent growth control in *Saccharomyces cerevisiae* mutants lacking *PMC1*, a homolog of plasma membrane Ca^{2+} ATPases. *J. Cell Biol.* **1994**, *124*, 351–363. [CrossRef]

27. Cunningham, K.W.; Fink, G.R. Calcineurin inhibits VCX1-dependent H^+/Ca^{2+} exchange and induces Ca^{2+} ATPases in *Saccharomyces cerevisiae*. *Mol. Cell Biol.* **1996**, *16*, 2226–2237. [CrossRef]

28. Miseta, A.; Kellermayer, R.; Aiello, D.P.; Fu, L.; Bedwell, D.M. The vacuolar Ca^{2+}/H^+ exchanger Vcx1p/Hum1p tightly controls cytosolic Ca^{2+} levels in *S. cerevisiae*. *FEBS Lett.* **1999**, *451*, 132–136. [CrossRef]

29. Sorin, A.; Rosas, G.; Rao, R. PMR1, a Ca^{2+}-ATPase in yeast Golgi, has properties distinct from sarco/endoplasmic reticulum and plasma membrane calcium pumps. *J. Biol. Chem.* **1997**, *272*, 9895–9901. [CrossRef]

30. Strayle, J.; Pozzan, T.; Rudolph, H.K. Steady-state free Ca^{2+} in the yeast endoplasmic reticulum reaches only 10 mM and is mainly controlled by the secretory pathway pump Pmr1. *EMBO J.* **1999**, *18*, 4733–4743. [CrossRef]

31. Hamamoto, S.; Mori, Y.; Yabe, I.; Uozumi, N. In vitro and in vivo characterization of modulation of the vacuolar cation channel TRPY1 from *Saccharomyces cerevisiae*. *FEBS J.* **2018**, *285*, 1146–1161. [CrossRef]

32. Clapham, D.E. TRP channels as cellular sensors. *Nature* **2003**, *426*, 517–524. [CrossRef] [PubMed]

33. Zhou, X.L.; Batiza, A.F.; Loukin, S.H.; Palmer, C.P.; Kung, C.; Saimi, Y. The transient receptor potential channel on the yeast vacuole is mechanosensitive. *Proc. Natl. Acad. Sci. USA* **2003**, *100*, 7105–7110. [CrossRef] [PubMed]

34. Chang, Y.; Schlenstedt, G.; Flockerzi, V.; Beck, A. Properties of the intracellular transient receptor potential (TRP) channel in yeast, Yvc1. *FEBS Lett.* **2010**, *584*, 2028–2032. [CrossRef] [PubMed]

35. Pir, P.; Gutteridge, A.; Wu, J.; Rash, B.; Kell, D.B.; Zhang, N.; Oliver, S.G. The genetic control of growth rate: A systems biology study in yeast. *BMC Syst. Biol.* **2012**, *6*, 4. [CrossRef] [PubMed]

36. Brachmann, C.B.; Davies, A.; Cost, G.J.; Caputo, E.; Li, J.; Hieter, P.; Boeke, J.D. Designer deletion strains derived from *Saccharomyces* cerevisiae S288C: A useful set of strains and plasmids for PCR-mediated gene disruption and other applications. *Yeast* **1998**, *14*, 115–132. [CrossRef]

37. Sherman, F. Getting started with yeast. *Methods Enzymol.* **2002**, *350*, 3–41. [PubMed]

38. Nakajima-Shimada, J.; Iida, H.; Tsuji, F.I.; Anraku, Y. Monitoring of intracellular calcium in *Saccharomyces cerevisiae* with an apoaequorine cDNA expression system. *Proc. Natl. Acad. Sci. USA* **1991**, *88*, 6878–6882. [CrossRef] [PubMed]

39. Cohen, R.; Engelberg, D. Commonly used *Saccharomyces cerevisiae* strains (e.g. BY4741, W303) are growth sensitive on synthetic complete medium due to poor leucine uptake. *FEMS Microbiol. Lett.* **2007**, *273*, 239–243. [CrossRef] [PubMed]

40. Tisi, R.; Baldassa, S.; Belotti, F.; Martegani, E. Phospholipase C is required for glucose-induced calcium influx in budding yeast. *FEBS Lett.* **2002**, *520*, 133–138. [CrossRef]

41. Dohmen, R.J.; Strasser, A.W.M.; Honer, C.B.; Hollenberg, C.P. An efficient transformation procedure enabling long-term storage of competent cells of various yeast genera. *Yeast* **1991**, *7*, 691–692. [CrossRef]

42. Ruta, L.L.; Kissen, R.; Nicolau, I.; Neagoe, A.D.; Petrescu, A.J.; Bones, A.M.; Farcasanu, I.C. Heavy metal accumulation by *Saccharomyces cerevisiae* cells armed with metal binding hexapeptides targeted to the inner face of the plasma membrane. *Appl. Microbiol. Biotechnol.* **2017**, *101*, 5749–5763. [CrossRef] [PubMed]

43. Tisi, R.; Martegani, E.; Brandão, R.L. Monitoring yeast intracellular Ca^{2+} levels using an in vivo bioluminescence assay. *Cold Spring Harb. Protoc.* **2015**, *2015*, 210–213. [CrossRef] [PubMed]

44. Petrovic, K.; Pfeifer, M.; Parker, C.N.; Schuierer, S.; Tallarico, J.; Hoepfner, D.; Movva, N.R.; Scheel, G.; Helliwell, S.B. Two low complexity ultra-high throughput methods to identify diverse chemically bioactive molecules using Saccharomyces cerevisiae. *Microbiol. Res.* **2017**, *199*, 10–18. [CrossRef] [PubMed]

45. Chandel, A.; Das, K.K.; Bachhawat, A.K. Glutathione depletion activates the yeast vacuolar transient receptor potential channel, Yvc1p, by reversible glutathionylation of specific cysteines. *Mol. Biol. Cell* **2016**, *27*, 3913–3925. [CrossRef] [PubMed]

46. John Haynes, W.; Zhou, X.L.; Su, Z.W.; Loukin, S.H.; Saimi, Y.; Kung, C. Indole and other aromatic compounds activate the yeast TRPY1channel. *FEBS Lett.* **2008**, *582*, 1514–1518. [CrossRef] [PubMed]

47. Supek, F.; Supekova, L.; Nelson, H.; Nelson, N. A yeast manganese transporter related to the macrophage protein involved in conferring resistance to mycobacteria. *Proc. Natl. Acad. Sci. USA* **1996**, *93*, 5105–5110. [CrossRef] [PubMed]

48. Dürr, G.; Strayle, J.; Plemper, R.; Elbs, S.; Klee, S.K.; Catty, P.; Wolf, D.H.; Rudolph, H.K. The medial-Golgi ion pump Pmr1 supplies the yeast secretory pathway with Ca^{2+} and Mn^{2+} required for glycosylation, sorting, and endoplasmic reticulum-associated protein degradation. *Mol. Biol. Cell* **1998**, *9*, 1149–1162. [CrossRef]

49. Mandal, D.; Woolf, T.B.; Rao, R. Manganese selectivity of Pmr1, the yeast secretory pathway ion pump, is defined by residue Gln783 in transmembrane segment 6. Residue Asp778 is essential for cation transport. *J. Biol. Chem.* **2000**, *275*, 23933–23938. [CrossRef]

50. Lapinskas, P.J.; Cunningham, K.W.; Liu, X.F.; Fink, G.R.; Culotta, V.C. Mutations in *PMR1* suppress oxidative damage in yeast cells lacking superoxide dismutase. *Mol. Cell. Biol.* **1995**, *15*, 1382–1388. [CrossRef]

51. Su, Z.; Zhou, X.; Loukin, S.H.; Saimi, Y.; Kung, C. Mechanical force and cytoplasmic Ca^{2+} activate yeast TRPY1 in parallel. *J. Membr. Biol.* **2009**, *227*, 141–150. [CrossRef]

52. Loukin, S.; Kung, C. Manganese effectively supports yeast cell-cycle progression in place of calcium. *J. Cell Biol.* **1995**, *131*, 1025–1037. [CrossRef] [PubMed]

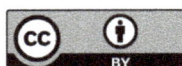

© 2019 by the authors. Licensee MDPI, Basel, Switzerland. This article is an open access article distributed under the terms and conditions of the Creative Commons Attribution (CC BY) license (http://creativecommons.org/licenses/by/4.0/).

![cells logo]

Review

MDPI

TRPs in Tox: Involvement of Transient Receptor Potential-Channels in Chemical-Induced Organ Toxicity—A Structured Review

Dirk Steinritz [1,2,*], Bernhard Stenger [1], Alexander Dietrich [2], Thomas Gudermann [2] and Tanja Popp [1,2]

[1]   Bundeswehr Institute of Pharmacology and Toxicology, 80937 Munich, Germany; bernhard.stenger@gmx.de (B.S.); tjjpopp@outlook.de (T.P.)

[2]   Walther-Straub-Institute of Pharmacology and Toxicology, Ludwig-Maximilians-Universität Munich, 80336 Munich, Germany; alexander.dietrich@lrz.uni-muenchen.de (A.D.); thomas.gudermann@lrz.uni-muenchen.de (T.G.)

*   Correspondence: dirk.steinritz@lrz.uni-muenchen.de or dr.dirk.steinritz@gmail.com; Tel.: +49-89-992692-2304

Received: 29 May 2018; Accepted: 31 July 2018; Published: 7 August 2018

Abstract: Chemicals can exhibit significant toxic properties. While for most compounds, unspecific cell damaging processes are assumed, a plethora of chemicals exhibit characteristic odors, suggesting a more specific interaction with the human body. During the last few years, G-protein-coupled receptors and especially chemosensory ion channels of the transient receptor potential family (TRP channels) were identified as defined targets for several chemicals. In some cases, TRP channels were suggested as being causal for toxicity. Therefore, these channels have moved into the spotlight of toxicological research. In this review, we screened available literature in PubMed that deals with the role of chemical-sensing TRP channels in specific organ systems. TRPA1, TRPM and TRPV channels were identified as essential chemosensors in the nervous system, the upper and lower airways, colon, pancreas, bladder, skin, the cardiovascular system, and the eyes. Regarding TRP channel subtypes, A1, M8, and V1 were found most frequently associated with toxicity. They are followed by V4, while other TRP channels (C1, C4, M5) are only less abundantly expressed in this context. Moreover, TRPA1, M8, V1 are co-expressed in most organs. This review summarizes organ-specific toxicological roles of TRP channels.

Keywords: toxicology; TRP channels; organ toxicity; chemicals; pollutants; chemosensor

---

1. Introduction

Most compounds originating from chemical industry, either as main products, intermediates, or as pollutants, frequently exhibit toxic properties. Exposure can result in severe adverse health effects or even death. Although health and safety measures are mandatorily introduced, at least in industrial nations, accidents may occur at any time [1,2]. One example is the Bhopal incident in India on 3 December 1984, when more than 40 t of methyl isocyanate, a precursor in pesticide production, was released, killing at least 2500 people [3]. Another is the accidental release of butene from a cut gas-pipeline which then became inflamed, and resulted in the explosion of an adjacent ethylene pipeline at BASF Ludwigshafen Germany in October 2017 [1]. Other omnipresent chemicals are phosgene and chlorine, which are essential for a broad range of chemical products. Approximately 15 million tons of chlorine are produced annually only in the US [4]. In addition to the unintended release of such chemicals, a systematic misuse of chemicals in warfare or terror attacks occurred in the recent past [5]. The most common route of exposure is through inhalation. Ingestion, dermal, and ocular absorption represent other possible entry routes, but account only for a smaller proportion. Chemicals can exhibit characteristic odors like "rotten eggs" in the case of thiol-containing compounds, but also pleasant smells like the flower-scented Lewisite, a chemical warfare agent from World War I. Some chemicals are irritants that trigger protective reflexes such as burning sensations, lacrimation, or cough. These findings clearly indicate that chemicals do interact with the human sensory system. As defense mechanisms are regarded to be uniform, a close correlation to the chemical structure of the causing compound was not suggested. Thus, it was also assumed that the molecular processes regarding chemical sensing were also rather unspecific. However, research in recent years has clearly demonstrated that distinct G-protein-coupled taste and olfactory receptors as well as chemosensory ion channels of the transient receptor potential family (TRP channels)—are fundamentally involved in the molecular (patho)physiology with regard to chemical perception [6–10]. Especially, TRPA1 channels were found to be activated by various compounds of different origins, and at least for some chemicals, certain TRP channels were identified as molecular targets that mediate toxicity. Although the precise molecular mechanism of TRP channel activation has not been unraveled in all cases, these channels represent promising therapeutic targets to counteract chemical-induced toxicity. Therefore, it is not surprising that chemosensing TRP channels are regarded as central players, and are in the spotlight of today's experimental, but also clinical pharmacological research [7,11].

In this review we provide a synopsis of published literature dealing with the role of TRP channels in chemical toxicity. A NCBI PubMed search was performed using the search term "(trp channel) AND (toxic * OR chemical)", which returned 579 hits. All abstracts were screened in detail by the authors according to the scheme provided in Figure 1. Finally, 139 publications were considered for this review and are listed in the reference section.

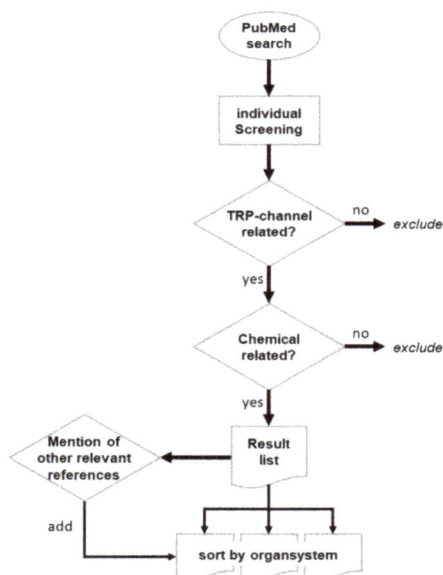

Figure 1. Search algorithm for the identification of relevant literature. The PubMed database was searched using "(trp channel) AND (toxic * OR chemical)" as a search term. The resulting 579 hits were screened. Literature not related to the topic of this review was excluded. If selected literature pointed to other references that were initially not identified in the PubMed search, these were also screened and included.

2. TRP Channels: General Structure and Function

TRP channels were first described in 1969 when Cosens and Manning noticed a distinct behavior of "a mutant strain of *Drosophila melanogaster* which, though behaving phototactically positive in a T-maze under low ambient light, is visually impaired and behaves as though blind" [12]. Electroretinograms identified the ion channel that was named after its electrophysiological function as transient receptor potential ion channel [13]. Montell and Rubin investigated the underlying biology in more detail using a *Drosophila* visual transduction mutant in which Ca^{2+}-dependent adaptation to light was impaired [14]. The physiological function of the channel was further characterized by Minke in 1992 [15]. These milestones were the beginning of modern TRP channel research in mammals. Today, 28 mammalian TRP proteins are known, belonging to the TRP channel gene superfamily (Figure 2), and they represent one of the largest superfamilies of ion channels in the human genome [16–20]. The TRP channel family can be phylogenetically subdivided into six subspecies (TRPA1, TRPP, TRPC, TRPM, TRPML, and TRPV4 (Figure 2) [18,21], and its members are highly conserved between species, thus allowing a good translation of interspecies experiments in general [22].

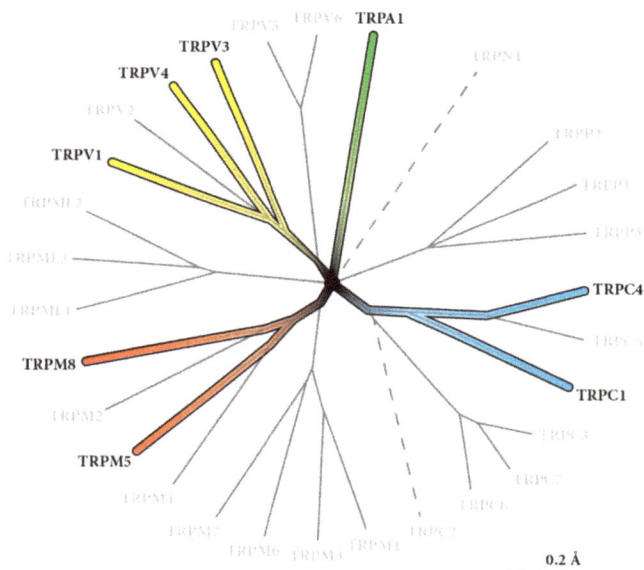

Figure 2. Phylogenetic tree of the transient receptor potential (TRP) channel family. In total, 28 human TRP channels have been identified so far. TRPN1 is expressed in insects and fish, but not in mammals, and TRPC2 is a pseudogene in humans. TRP channels that have been reported to be involved in chemosensing or that are affected by toxic chemicals are indicated by different colors ([20] modified).

TRP channels form homo- or heterotetramers of single TRP proteins. Every protein consists of six helices, the transmembrane domains (TMs), which resemble the biggest part of the channel (Figure 3) [23]. TM 5 and 6 form the pore region, while the pore itself is semi-selective for the corresponding ion [23]. The function of helices 1 to 4 is not fully understood but seems to contain important channel modulatory binding moieties (e.g., the capsaicin-binding site is located in the TM2 and TM3 region) and is considered as the "sensor" part of the channel [24]. TRP channels are permeable to monovalent Na^+, K^+, and bivalent Ca^{2+} or Mg^{2+} cations [24]. Most members of the TRPV family are described as being rather nonselective in this context, with a preference of TRPV5 and TRPV6 for Ca^{2+} [25] while TRPM4 and TRPM5 are reported to be impermeable for Ca^{2+} [26,27]. The C-

and N-termini are both located in the cytosol, and differ significantly between families, as they contain divergent binding motifs and reactive amino acids that modulate the channel function (e.g., the TRPA1 ligand allylisothiocyanate (AITC) has been described to activate the channel by binding to cysteine residues in the cytosolic ankyrin repeat sequence) [28] (Figure 3). However, it is important to note that also moieties at the C-terminal end and in the transmembrane parts themselves seem to have channel modulatory functions [29,30].

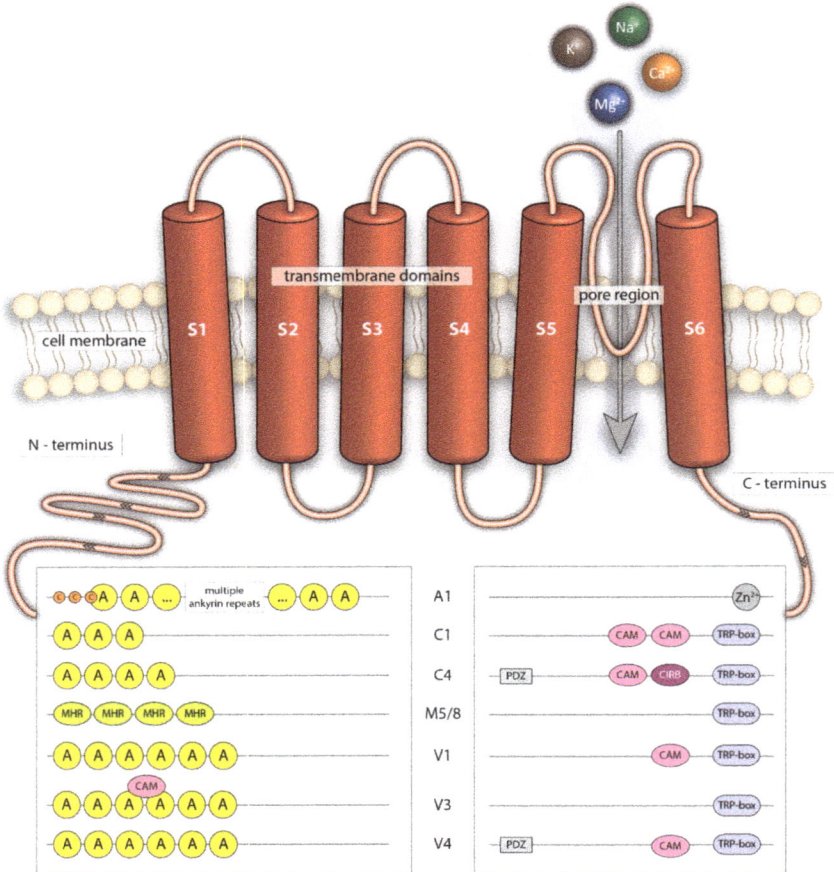

Figure 3. Schematic overview of TRP channel structure. "S1–S6" indicates the different segments of the transmembrane domains. "A" represents ankyrin repeats with reactive cysteines ("C"). "CAV1" is the caveolin interaction region, "MHR" represents the melastatin family channel homology region, "PDZ" symbolizes anchoring domain functions, "CAM" stands for calmodulin, "TRP box" is the motif containing the invariant EWKFAR sequence, "Zn^{2+}" indicates a zinc-binding site, and "CIRB" is the calmodulin/IP$_3$receptor-binding motif. The complete structure of some TRP channels are not known in detail. Synopsis from the following references: A1 [6,19,23,31,32], C1 [19,23,33], C4 [6,19,23], M5 [19,23,34], M8 [6,19,23,34,35], V1 [6,19,23,34], V3 [36–39], and V4 [6,19,23,34].

TRPA1 is the only member of the TRPA family, and it possesses multiple characteristic ankyrin repeat domains in the N-terminus. Other TRP channels, e.g., TRPV or TRPC, do also exhibit ankyrin repeat domains at their respective N-terminus, but to a lesser number compared to TRPA1. Another major difference is the lack of the so-called TRP-box, the sequence of the amino acids EWKFAR, which can be found in all TRP channels except TRPA1 [40]. TRPA1 is described to act as a chemo- or nociceptor [41]. The channel can be activated by pungent substances and plant ingredients like allicin from garlic, AITC from mustard oil, cinnamaldehyde from cinnamon oil, or gingerols from ginger [41–43]. Expression of TRPA1 is often found in neuronal structures, building heterotetramers with TRPV1 [44]. Here, TRPA1 is responsible for pain sensation, e.g., after consuming spicy mustard. In addition to the chemo-nociceptor function, TRPA1 was described to be sensitive to cold, which correlates well with the coexpression of TRPV1, as the latter is activated upon noxious heat [44–46].

The vanilloid TRP channel family (TRPV) consists of six members. TRPV1–4 show a closer phylogenetic relationship compared to TRPV5 and TRPV6 [20]. All TRPV channels contain ankyrin repeat domains at their N-terminus, as well as the TRP-box on the C-terminus. In contrast to other members of the family, TRPV1 carries a calmodulin-binding site at the C-terminus. TRPV channels can be activated by a plethora of different chemicals. TRPV1 is known to be sensitive to capsaicin or resiniferatoxin, and for some TRPA1 agonists, but to a lesser extent. Furthermore, the channel acts as a nociceptor for heat above 43 °C, and is involved in inflammatory pathways [47]. TRPV4, in contrast, is not known to be activated by plant-derived chemicals, although synthetic agonist like 4α-PDD or GSK1016790A were found to open the ion channel [48–50]. Functions of TRPV4 are related to controlling osmotic, chemical, and mechanical pressures, as well as sensing temperature [51].

Canonical TRP channels (TRPC) have also ankyrin repeat sequences at the N-terminus, and a TRP-box at the C-terminal site. As in TRPV channels, they contain a calmodulin-binding site [52]. In case of TRPC4, a PDZ binding site can be found downstream of the calmodulin binding site, which is lacking in the TRPC1 protein [52]. In general, all TRPC channels, with the exception of TRPC1, can be activated by phospholipase C stimulation via diacylglycerol [53,54].

Unlike TRPA, TRPV, or TRPC, TRPM channels do not possess ankyrin repeats at the N-terminus, but contain a distinct TRPM homology region [23]. A coiled-coil domain is located downstream of the TRP-specific TRP-box at the C-terminal end [55]. This coiled-coil domain is usually found in structural proteins like laminins, myosins, or fibrins. TRPM7 presents a kinase activity at its C-terminus, which is unique for that channel [56]. The physiological meaning is still not clearly understood, but is obviously related to mineral homeostasis [56].

3. Organ-Specific Expression of Chemosensing and Sensory TRP Channels

TRP channels are ubiquitously expressed. While basic pharmacological channel functions are well-understood, many organ-specific functions are still elusive in mammals. Screening of the current literature revealed that TRPA1, TRPM, and TRPV seem to be important for chemical sensing or organ-specific responses to chemical compounds. TRPA1, TRPM8, and TRPV1 are the most frequently involved TRP channels in the considered organs regardless of the different cell types present in the respective tissue. They are followed by V4 while other TRP channels (C1, C4, M5, and V3) are of minor importance with regard to chemical sensing. Moreover, TRPA1, M8, and V1 are co-expressed in most organs. Figures 4 and 5 summarize results of the screened literature.

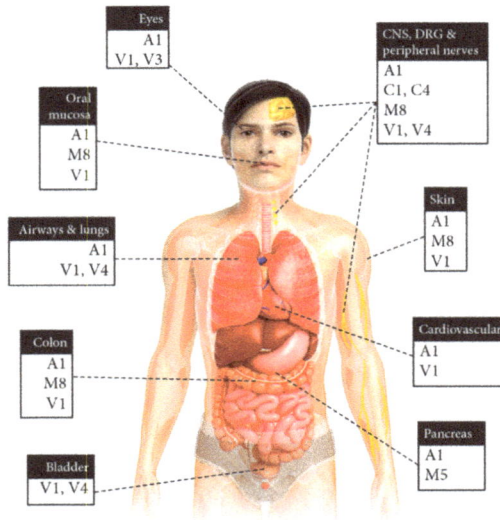

Figure 4. Schematic overview of chemical-sensitive or sensory TRP channel expression in different mammalian organs. Only TRP channels are illustrated that are discussed to be involved in chemical toxicity and are mentioned in this review.

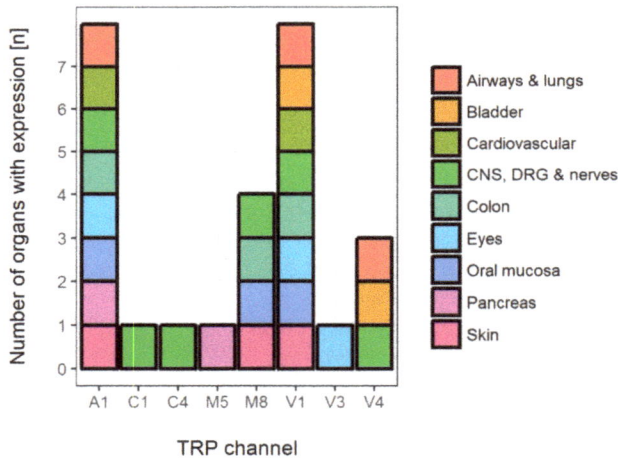

Figure 5. Overall numbers and subtypes of TRP channel expression with chemosensory properties. According to the considered literature in this review, TRPA1, TRPM8, and TRPV1 were identified as the most abundant channels. Colors represent organ-related expression.

3.1. Neuronal TRP Channels

In principle, the human nervous system can be divided into two parts: (i) the central nervous system (CNS) consisting of the brain and spinal cord; and (ii) the peripheral nervous system (PNS), originating from the dorsal root ganglia (DRG) with the peripheral nerve trajectories. TRP channels play a major role in both parts. They are involved in sensing stimuli in the PNS, transferring signals via DRGs to the CNS, and regulating neuronal network function in the brain. In the respective tissues, TRPs can be activated by endogenous neurotransmitters and signaling molecules, e.g., diacylglycerol (DAG) or substance P, but also by mechanical stimuli like pressure or temperature, as well as chemicals from natural or synthetic origin [40,57,58].

3.1.1. TRP Channels in the PNS and DRG

TRP channels were identified as key players in DRG, which link the peripheral nerve endings with the CNS. In DRG, TRPA1, and TRPV1 channels that are involved in nociception are found to be highly expressed, while TRPM8 or TRPV4 are expressed to a lesser extent. TRP channels do not serve exclusively as sensors of noxious stimuli. They are additionally affected by anesthetics, which are frequently used in clinical settings to minimize CNS function, or when locally applied, to block PNS signal initiation and transduction. TRP channels are highly expressed in all nervous tissue. Thus, it is not surprising that interaction of these channels with local anesthetics and central-acting narcotics influences analgesia and narcosis. A good example is the substantia gelantinosa, which plays a crucial role in pain reception. Here, neuronal cells respond with spontaneous L-glutamate release, which is mediated by TRPV1 and TRPA1 channels [59]. Moreover, induction of activating transcription factor 3 (ATF3), a reliable marker of nerve injury, was also found to rely on TRPV1 channels [60]. Wild type mice injected with capsaicin, mustard oil, formalin, or menthol into the hind-paw revealed increased ATF3 expression in distinct subpopulations of sensory neurons, whereas TRPV1 deficient mice did not [60]. Remarkably, only capsaicin-activated TRPV1 channels were required, while neither TRPA1, activated by mustard oil or formalin, nor TRPM8, activated by menthol or icilin, were necessary to increase ATF3 levels [60]. These findings clearly point to an essential role of especially TRPA1 and TRPV channels in nociception. Thus, it would be feasible to assume that analgesics and anesthetics should block these channels to prevent pain. However, some studies revealed that some general anesthetics surprisingly activate TRPA1 or TRPV1 channels. Eilers et al. found that inhalation of anesthetics with irritant properties indeed activate TRPA1, thereby inducing mechanical hyperalgesia and bronchial constriction [61]. Non-irritant anesthetics in contrast did not activate TRPA1, and provided no evidence for induction of hyperalgesia or bronchial constriction [61]. Other volatile anesthetics, i.e., isoflurane and the now obsolete chloroform, act as agonists of TRPV1 and TRPM8, while TRPA1 channels are inhibited [62]. These results are not completely in line with Eilers et al., who described increased sensitization of TRPA1 as a reason for hyperalgesia [62]. Lidocaine is another local anesthetic and anti-arrhythmic drug, which inhibits fast Na$^+$-channels. Leffler et al. further described the activation of TRPV1, and in parts of TRPA1, by lidocaine [63]. Interestingly, the vanilloid binding domain is required for an activation by lidocaine, but not for sensitization of the channel as induced by other agonists [63]. To prove TRPV1 specificity, known antagonists like capsazepine or *N*-(4-t-butylphenyl)-4-(3-chloropyridin-2-yl) tetrahydro-pryazine-1(2*H*)-carboxamide (BCTC) were successfully applied in patch-clamp experiments using DRG or HEK293 cells [63]. Beside their narcotic and analgesic effects, anesthetics activate TRPA1, TRPV1 and TRPM8 channels, which are ubiquitous present in neuronal structures. Since the modulation of TRPV1 for analgesia seems very promising, investigations of new compounds are ongoing. Marwaha et al. examined niflumic acids as potential TRPV1 blockers to treat neuropathic pain [64]. For the experiments, they used an animal pain model in which stavudine induces TRPV1-mediated pain sensations. Here, TRPV1 protein expression in the CNS increased after stavudine exposure [64]. Remarkably, treatment with niflumic acid not only reduced pain, which was measured after different time points with different behavioral tests for mechanical hyperalgesia, tactile allodynia, motor coordination, heat and cold, but also reduced nitrosative stress [64].

Bang et al. have elucidated the mechanism of the anesthetic butamben, which has been used as a topical anesthetic since the early 1960s. It was suggested that voltage gated channels are inhibited by this compound, and this was confirmed by their study [65]. Additionally, butamben was shown to act as an inhibitor of TRPA1 as well as TRPV4, but not as an antagonist of TRPV1 [65].

Other naturally derived compounds may work in a similar way. Pellitorine, an extract of *Tradium daniellii*, was recently described as a new antagonist of TRPV1 [66]. A study by Olah and colleagues focused on pellitorine as a new anesthetic and pain killer. Although the chemical structure of pellitorine exhibited a relationship to capsaicin, a widely known TRPV1 agonist, the isolated pellitorine inhibited TRPV1 with an IC_{50} of 0.69 mM in TRPV1-transfected HaCaT cells after stimulation with 2 µM capsaicin [66].

Another substance found in species of *Artemisia*, *Blumea*, and *Kaempferia* is borneol. It was shown that this naturally derived compound antagonizes TRPA1 in a dose-dependent manner [67]. Borneol is already used in traditional medicine against bronchitis, rheumatic disease, or cell swelling [67].

Many other compounds, drugs, and chemicals are thought to interact with TRP channels. Based on TRPA1-induced hyperalgesia, Nozadze et al. investigated nonsteroidal anti-inflammatory drugs with regard to their potential to counteract TRPA1-induced side-effects [68]. In the in vivo study, diclofenac, ketorolac, and xefocam have proven to diminish AITC-induced TRPA1 activation, and hyperalgesia was mitigated [68].

Patients receiving anti-cancer treatment with oxiplatin frequently complain about neuropathy and hyperalgesia [69]. After treatment with oxaliplatin increased levels of cyclic adenosine monophosphate (cAMP) can be detected, which are able to sensitize TRPA1 as well as TRPV1 channels [69]. The study of Anand et al. measured increasing calcium responses after oxaliplatin treatment, which might cause hyperalgesia [69]. It is suggested that antagonist for TRPA1 and TRPV1 might be able to countermeasure oxaliplatin side effects [69]. A different study was able to confirm these results, as calcium signaling was altered after prolonged oxaliplatin treatment, and led to phosphoinositide-induced increases in intracellular calcium levels compared to the control group [70].

Paclitaxel, another chemotherapeutic drug, acts in a comparable manner. During chemotherapy patients suffer from neuropathic pain. It can be observed that protease-activated receptor 2 (PAR2, involved in inflammatory responses), as well as both kinases PKA and PKC are upregulated [71]. The upregulation of these proteins is described to sensitize TRPV1, TRPV4 as well as TRPA1 [71]. Thus, it is comprehensible that application of respective antagonists did attenuate observed pain responses in mice [71].

Pain relieving cannabinoids are currently in the spotlight of research. In case of the synthetic compounds R-(+)-(2,3-dihydro-5-methyl-3-[(4-morpholinyl)methyl]pyrol-[1,2,3-de]-1,4-benzoxazin-6-yl)-(1-naphthalenyl) methanone mesylate and (R,S)-3-(2-iodo-5-nitrobenzoyl)-1-(1-methyl-2-piperidinylmethyl)-1 hindole, it is reported that these substances activate TRPA1 and TRPV1 channels, but also desensitize these channels for other agonists like capsaicin or mustard oil [69,72].

Camphor, among other monoterpenes, is another agonist for TRPA1, which is like the above-mentioned cannabinoids, in that it effectively desensitizes the channel for more harmful activators [73].

In a comparable manner, it was shown that nitro-oleic acid desensitizes both TRPA1 and TRPV1. The inhibition was observed in cells expressing TRPA1 homomers, as well as TRPA1-TRPV1 heteromers [64]. Furthermore, pain reactions in test animals were counteracted by the substance and might be useful in a clinical environment to prevent unwanted TRPA1/TRPV1-induced hypersensitivities [64].

These studies have proven that TRP channels play a crucial role in the peripheral nervous system, as many anesthetics interact with TRP channels, whereas other substances, like many natural derived compounds, have a more beneficial effect on the body after interacting with a TRP channel. With increasing knowledge about pain signaling pathways, as well as inflammation, these ion channels can already be considered as promising pharmacological targets, yet many important crosstalks are still unknown and need further investigation.

3.1.2. TRP Channels in the CNS and Cranial Nerves

Besides TRPA1 and TRPV1, which are known to be involved in pain sensation, TRPC, TRPV4, and TRPM8 are essential for signal transmission from the PNS or DRG to the CNS. Regarding physiological functions, TRPV4 channels are described to be involved in cell swelling and nociception [74]. TRPC1 and TRPC4 are expressed in the corticolimbic regions in the brain, controlling vasodilation and neurotransmitter release [75]. TRPC channels are also essential in the endothelial part of the blood-brain-barrier. Balbuena et al. reported upregulation of TRPC1 and TRPC4 after organophosphorus malathion/oxon or lead exposures in rats [76]. One major symptom that can be observed after malthion/oxon intoxication is the permeabilization of the blood-brain-barrier (BBB). Balbuena et al. reported increasing levels of TRPC1 and TRPC4 channels after exposure, which might lead to abnormal depletion of calcium stores. Subsequently, calcium-dependent pathways are likely to be dysregulated, contributing to the disruption of the BBB [76].

Comparable results were found by Zhang and colleagues, who blocked TRPC1 expression via RNA interference, and measured a decrease in lead levels (Pb) in the CNS [77]. In addition, overexpression of TRPC1 results in even higher levels of Pb in the CNS. Interestingly, knockdown of stromal interaction molecule 1 (STIM1), which is known as an endoplasmic reticulum Ca^{2+} sensor and together with Orai1 orchestrates the store-operated calcium entry, attenuated Pb-acetate entry [77].

Even though not directly related to chemical exposures, involvement of TRP channels in the pathophysiology of headache is discussed. In case of TRPV4, it is suggested that TRPV4 may lead to cell swelling in the brain, thereby causing headache due to extended pressure [74]. Treatment with arachidonic acid, among others found in caraway, or different phorbol ester compounds, agonize the channel, thereby reducing the pain [74]. Other compounds, e.g., umbellulone (UMB, which can be found in the leaves of the so-called "headache tree") were also found to activate TRPA1 and TRPM8, thereby causing severe headaches and cold sensations [78,79]. Remarkably, UMB inhibited TRPA1 when applied in higher concentrations [79].

TRPA1 and TRPV1 are expressed in trigeminal nerves, and they may fulfill the role of sensing potential toxic substances or transmitting pain [80]. Despite the well-described activation of these channels by capsaicin, mustard oil, or allicin, a plethora of irritants affect these channels. Irritants like acetophenone, 2-ethylhexanol, hexyl isocyanate, isophorone, and trimethylcyclohexanol are channel agonists, and they were shown to decrease respiratory rates in vivo, which might be caused by direct interaction with TRPs [81,82].

Clotrimazole represents another potent agonist of those two channels in the trigeminal nerve [81,83]. Patients often complain about a burning sensation and irritated skin after topical treatment with the drugs. It was shown by Meseguer et al. that the activation of TRPV1 and TRPA1 might be responsible for this observed adverse effect [83].

Two studies of Kunkler et al. described the activation of TRPA1 as a cause for environmental-irritant-induced headaches [84,85]. Substances like formaldehyde or acrolein activated the ion channel, thereby releasing calcitonin gene-related peptide (CGRP) and substance P, which further resulted in neurogenic inflammation [84]. Additionally, it was reported that the meningeal blood flow increased after TRPA1 activation, which is in correlation to the increase of substance P, as the process can be inhibited by the application of CGRP [84].

In this context it is important to note that TRPA1 is most commonly co-expressed with TRPV1. Kunkler et al. further suggested that the therapy with resiniferatoxin might result in a decreased expression of TRPV1, which then may also attenuate co-expressed TRPA1 ion channels, thereby decreasing the amount of released CGRP and substance P. As a result, the blood flow should stabilize. Thus, resiniferatoxin might be a potential countermeasure against environmental irritant-induced headaches [84].

3.2. Upper Respiratory System, Airways and Lungs

Expression of TRPC, TRPM, TRPV, and TRPA1 has been described in the respiratory system. TRPA1 was found mainly in sensory nerves [10] and to some extent, also in the lung epithelia [86].

Stimulation of A549 cells, a human lung cancer epithelial cell line endogenously expressing TRPA1, with the TRPA1-specific agonist AITC, resulted in the increase of intracellular calcium ($[Ca^{2+}]_i$) and subsequent activation of MAP kinases [86], providing evidence for a functional role of TRPA1 in non-neuronal lung tissue.

Eilers et al. reported that the pungent general anesthetic isoflurane is able to activate TRPA1 and induce TRPA1-mediated contraction of guinea pig bronchi [61]. In addition, desensitization of sensory nerves due to high concentration of the TRPV1 agonist capsaicin prevented isoflurane-induced bronchoconstriction. However, a TRPV1-specific antagonist alone had no effect on isoflurane-induced narrowing of the airways [61]. The authors proposed a TRPA1-dependent neurogenic mechanism for isoflurane-induced bronchoconstriction [61]. Animals also suffered from hyperalgesia after intraplantar injection of isoflurane, underlining the agonistic effect on TRPA1 channels [61]. These results are in line with the observed co-expression of TRPA1 and TRPV1 in a subset of C-fiber neurons [87]. Response of C-fibers towards chemical irritants was diminished in the nasal mucosa after pretreatment with capsaicin and/or AITC [88]. These findings point to a close interaction of TRPA1 and TRPV1 channels. In general, activation of neuronal TRPA1 and TRPV1 channels seems to initiate warning and defense reflexes, thereby attributing "protective" actions to the channel. In vitro experiments revealed that activation of TRPA1 by highly toxic alkylating compounds has a direct negative impact on cell viability [89]. This is in line with results published by Achanta et al., who suggested that TRPA1 and neurogenic inflammation contribute to the deleterious effects of alkylating compounds in vivo, activated either directly by alkylation, or indirectly, by reactive intermediates or pro-inflammatory mediators [90]. In contrast, zinc, a compound used in smoke screens, also activates TRPA1 [91] and induces lung cell injury [92], but not directly through TRPA1 [93]. Reactive oxygen species (ROS) as well as hypochlorite (OCl^-), the oxidizing mediator of chlorine, activated Ca^{2+} influx and membrane currents in an oxidant-sensitive subpopulation of chemosensory neurons, which were identified as TRPA1-expressing cells [94]. TRPA1-mediated Ca^{2+} influx was also activated by chloramine-T, a widely used chlorine-releasing chemical disinfectant which is a strong respiratory irritant [94]. TRPA1-deficient ($TRPA1^{-/-}$) mice were protected from OCl^--induced respiratory depression. In this study, response to other chemical stimuli remained unchanged in $TRPA1^{-/-}$ mice, pointing to a certain selectivity of TRPA1 channels [94]. Toxic industrial isocyanates and tear gases, both known to cause severe pulmonary distress, were also found to activate TRPA1 channels [95]. Genetic ablation or pharmacological inhibition of TRPA1 dramatically reduced isocyanate- and tear gas-induced effects after both ocular and cutaneous exposures [95]. As demonstrated by Lehmann et al., in vivo sensory irritation due to 2-ethylhexanol, a potent human irritant, was dependent on both TRPA1 and TRPV1 channels [82]. Acrolein (2-propenal), a highly toxic and reactive compound present in tear gas, vehicle exhaust, and smoke from burning vegetation, including tobacco products, is also a very potent TRPA1 activator [96]. Responses were completely absent in cultures from TRPA1-deficient mice, demonstrating that TRPA1 is, indeed, an essential transducer of acrolein action [96]. Cells expressing TRPV1, TRPV2, or TRPM8 did not respond to acrolein [96]. Cigarette smoke-evoked cough was attenuated by a TRPA1-specific antagonist in guinea pigs [97] and unsaturated aldehydes in the cigarette smoke were identified as the main causative substances for TRPA1 activation [97].

Stimulation of airway epithelial cells with lipopolysaccharides (LPS), which is part of the wall of gram-negative bacteria and plays a crucial role in the immune response, resulted in an increase of $[Ca^{2+}]_i$ [98], which was found to be mediated by TRPV4 channels [98] that are abundantly expressed in these cells [99]. Upon LPS challenge, TRPV4-mediated ciliary beat frequently, and production of bactericidal nitric oxide increased, suggesting a protective role of TRPV4 [98]. In contrast to these findings, TRPV4 inhibition counteracts toxic lung edema and inflammation in vivo after chlorine exposures [100]. Here, chemical induced vascular leakage and airway hyperreactivity were suppressed, while blood oxygenation was significantly improved [100]. In vivo experiments conducted by Andres et al. point in the same direction: phosgene-induced pulmonary injury and lethality in mice were partially improved by post-exposure treatment with ruthenium red (RR), an unspecific TRP channel blocker [101]. Although the experimental design did not allow the identification of the distinct TRP channel, the authors speculate that TRPV4 may be one of the possible candidates.

Unspecific inhibition of TRP channels by intraperitoneal injection of RR attenuated adverse effects on cardiovascular function in vivo after pulmonary ultrafine nanoparticles exposures. Although the route of administration as well as the use of the broad and unspecific TRP channel inhibitor RR does not allow a precise correlation to a distinct TRP channel, the authors suggest a lung-nodose ganglia-regulated pathway via the activation of pulmonary TRP channels [102].

An involvement of TRPV1 channels in the pathophysiology of asthma triggered by inhalation of allergens and chemicals, was investigated by McGarvey et al. using pulmonary human tissue and cells derived thereof [103]. Remarkably, patients that did not respond to standard asthma therapy (i.e., corticosteroids) revealed a significant increase of bronchial TRPV1 expression compared to controls [103]. The authors suggest a role of TRPV1 channels especially in patients with severe, uncontrolled asthma. Both, TRPA1 and TRPV1, together with mast cells were found to play a major role in chemical-induced immune-mediated asthma after application of toluene-2,4-diisocyanate (TDI), a chemical with a large number of industrial applications [104]. Remarkably, TDI was unable to activate TRPV1 in that study, pointing again to a close cross-talk between TRPA1 and TRPV1.

3.3. Colon

Acute enteritis is a common and serious disease after food poisoning in human patients and animals. The immunological and microbiological aspects of the pathology of gastroenteric diseases including inflammatory bowel disease (IBD) are studied extensively [105,106]. However, the neural network is also known for its impact on observed hyperesthesia to various chemical stimuli. For instance, acetic acid and capsaicin were shown to provoke pelvic nerve activity in a rat model of inflammatory bowel disease induced by dextran sulfate sodium (DSS) [107]. The induced neural signaling by capsaicin was enhanced in rats with early stages of colitis, compared to healthy rats. The frequency of discharge was blocked by RR, an unspecific TRP channel inhibitor. It is assumed that the augmented nociception to TRPV1 agonists in the colitis model is associated with changes of inflammatory mediators that regulate the activity of nociceptors. One of these mediators is CGRP, a neuroinflammatory peptide which is expressed TRPV1-dependent in the colon. The expression of some, pro-inflammatory cytokines and chemokines like TNFα, IL-1, IL-6, CXCL10, MIP1 can be attenuated by treatment with icilin, a commonly used TRPM8 agonist [108]. TRPM8 is very prominent in human and mouse colon tissue. The expression of this TRP channel is upregulated in inflamed colon tissue from IBD patients, as well as in chemically induced colitis by DSS and 2,4,6-trinitrobenzenesulfonic acid (TNBS) in mice [108]. Administration of TRPM8 agonists in the colitis models inhibited TRPV1-dependent CGRP expression, reduced pro-inflammatory cytokines, and attenuated the common hallmarks of colitis such as bowel thickness and infiltration of granulocytes. These attenuating effects of icilin were not observed in TRPM8-deficient mice, which emphasizes the potency of TRPM8 as an anti-inflammatory therapeutic target.

The frequent contamination of wheat with the fungi *Fusarium* leads to food contamination by trichothecene mycotoxin deoxynivalenol (DON, vomitoxin) [109]. DON suppresses food intake and thereby affects energy balance, which is a major concern in human and animal health. The exocytosis of satiety hormones like cholecystokinin and peptide YY_{3-36} is induced by DON-activated calcium-sensing receptor (CaSR) and TRPA1-mediated Ca^{2+} entry into enteroendocrine cells [110]. Further analysis of the role of CaSR and TRPA1 in the observed anorexia and emesis will shed light on the underlying mechanisms, and can therefore serve as a model to understand comparable symptoms induced by other foodborne toxins, environmental toxicants and chemotherapeutic drugs [109].

3.4. Pancreas

Diabetes mellitus is one of the most common metabolic disorders in the industrialized western world. Both types of diabetes are diseases in which high blood sugar levels persist over a long time. Type II diabetes is characterized by the combination of insulin unresponsiveness in the target tissue and the failure of pancreatic beta cells to secrete sufficient insulin. Treatment options include glibenclamide, which blocks ATPase-sensitive K^+ channels forcing beta cells to secrete more insulin. In addition, the TRPA1 channel was identified in pancreatic beta cells to transduce cationic non-selective currents. New studies revealed that the glibenclamide-induced intracellular currents are TRPA1-dependent [111]. However, the contribution of TRPA1 to diabetes treatment and the glibenclamide-related side effects like hyperactive bladder or abdominal pain is highly discussed [112]. TRPA1 seems to be a secretagogue which may still induce insulin secretion when cells do not effectively respond to glibenclamide after long-term treatment [111]. However, TRPA1 also disrupts beta cell physiology since long-term stimulation with TRPA1 agonists reduce both the responsiveness of insulin-secreting cells and the expression of pancreatic and duodenal homeobox 1 (PDX1), which is a transcription factor for insulin expression [112]. Consequently, the definite contribution of TRPA1 to glibenclamide-associated effects in type II diabetes patients remains to be clarified. Besides TRPA1, TRPM5 is also often associated with type II diabetes. Its expression in diabetic patients is negatively correlated with blood glucose concentrations [113]. TRPM5 is expressed in beta cells mediating depolarizing currents after glucose stimulation. Additional stimulation with stevioside, one of the main glycosides of the plant *Stevia rebaudiana* and used as a sweetener and sugar substitute, potentiates glucose-induced currents by increasing the frequency of Ca^{2+}-oscillations, which triggers insulin response [114,115]. In wild type mice, treatment with stevioside reduced blood glucose significantly, but not in TRPM5-deficient mice. Moreover, stevioside protects mice on high fat diet from hyperglycemia. Therefore, stevioside, as TRPM5 modulator, is a promising therapeutic option in type II diabetes patients [114]. Chronic and acute pancreatitis have distinct histopathologies and etiologies, but are both accompanied by inflammatory events and pain [116]. Pain reflects the sensitization of pancreatic sensory neurons. The pancreatitis-associated pain was shown to be related to TRPA1 and TRPV1 expression, and it functioned in afferents in an experimental acute pancreatitis model in mouse [117]. The administration of specific TRP channel antagonists in early phases of recurrent bouts of acute pancreatitis significantly reduces inflammation. The combined antagonist treatment even ameliorates morphological changes in the pancreas [118]. Additional behavioral experiments demonstrated that both antagonists also attenuate pain and signs of discomfort. Therefore, targeting of TRPA1 and TRPV1 in patients with recurrent bouts of acute pancreatitis may inhibit the progression to chronic pancreatitis.

3.5. Bladder

TRP channels are widely expressed in the urinary tract, neuronal fibers innervating the bladder, and urethra and epithelial and mucosal layers of the bladder and urethral walls. Therefore, they are involved in many effects of toxicants, and are consequently an attractive pharmaceutical target for the treatment of (chemically-induced) disorders in the urinary tract.

It is reported that patients treated with cyclophosphamide suffer from cystitis accompanied by inflammation and bleeding. During treatment, the cyclophosphamide metabolite acrolein accumulates in the bladder and promotes inflammation [119]. In female Wistar rats with cyclophosphamide-induced bladder inflammation, a considerably high transcriptional plasticity of urinary bladder TRP channels were demonstrated. Chronic cystitis increased TRPA1 and TRPV4 transcripts in the (sub)urothelium of female rats, whereas in acute cystitis, TRPV1 and TRPV4 mRNA levels are decreased. However, TRPV1 and TRPV4 protein levels are increased in acute and chronic cystitis [120]. This lack of correlation between transcript and protein expression may reflect changes in posttranscriptional modifications. The observed TRPV1 increase is associated with bladder hyperreflexia [121]. In addition, antagonism of TRPV4 increased functional bladder capacity and reduced micturition frequency in mice and rats with acute cystitis, suggesting that chronic cystitis in human patients may improve with TRPV4 antagonist treatment [122].

In bladder transitional cell carcinoma TRPV1 expression declines with the increase of tumor grade [123]. Curcumin, a popular Indian food spice, is a very cytotoxic agent in bladder tumor cell lines. Since curcumin has a vanilloid structure with a vanilloid-like activity via a selective binding to TRPV1, TRPV1 activation by curcumin could be a possible mechanism to induce cell death and prevent tumor growth [124].

Patients with bladder overactivity are initially treated with *Botulinum* neurotoxin A (BoNT/A) to block the presynaptic release of acetylcholine from the efferent parasynapatic nerves, to paralyze the bladder temporarily [125]. However, BoNT/A also reduces TRPV1 expression on afferent nerves while the nerves remain intact. Therefore, BoNT/A affects bladder contractility by modulating the expression of TRPV1 on peripheral nerve fibers [124].

3.6. Skin

Phtalate esters are widely used as plasticizers for plastics, synthetic leather, vinyl flooring, wall coverings, paint, adhesive agents, and cosmetics. These esters are also commonly found in house dust and are associated with allergic diseases in children [126]. Dibutyl phthalate (DBP) directly activates TRPA1 in dorsal root ganglia isolated from mouse, as well as in cultured TRPA1-overexpressing cells [127,128]. Thereby both, DBP and also common TRPA1 agonists enhance skin sensitization to fluorescein isothiocyanate (FITC), which can be completely abrogated with the specific TRPA1 antagonist HC-030031. For TRPV1 a comparable contribution in such sensitization processes was shown, whereas TRPM8 is not involved in the enhancement of skin sensitization to FITC [129]. It is speculated that neuropeptides like CGRP are released from peripheral nerve endings via activation of TRPA1. In this context, it has already been described that CGRP triggers FITC-induced chronic hypersensitivity, while it suppresses trinitrobenzene-induced hypersensitivity. CGRP differently regulates the immunological contribution in form of T helper cell (T_H1 and T_H2) responses [130].

In cutaneous photosensitivity, it is widely accepted that the symptoms like pain and itching are based on the accumulation of porphyrins, which enhance the production of free radicals [131]. A common feature in patients suffering from porphyria or undergoing photodynamic therapy is the experience of strong pain from bright light. Classical photosensitizers like protoporphyrin IX, an intermediate in the heme biosynthesis pathway, transfer an electron to molecular oxygen-producing ROS. In photodynamic therapy, photosensitization is induced by excess levels of protoporphyrin IX, generating singlet oxygen to treat precancerous lesions [132]. The formation of ROS upon exposure to UV light, activates TRPA1 mediating the calcium entry into the cell. Mutation studies revealed that cysteine C633 and C651 are indispensable for disulfide bonds to mediate this UV-induced calcium influx. The activation of TRPA1 was abolished by the treatment with antioxidants acting as ROS scavenger, suggesting that oxidative processes are essential for UV-light-mediated TRPA1 activation. Protoporphyrin IX enhanced TRPA1 and TRPV1 activation. This activation in pain signaling nerve endings acts as cellular sensors to detect the oxidative stress produced by near-UV and visible blue light, which is enhanced in the presence of cellular or exogenous photosensitizers [131]. Therefore, selective antagonist may provide new therapeutic options for porphyria patients and for unlimited use of photodynamic therapy.

In the cosmetic industry chemical reagents are applied on the skin for rejuvenation. These procedures cause protein coagulation and tissue injury in various depth of the skin. Trichloroacetic acid (TCA), the most-widely used chemical peeler, exerts direct toxic effects on the skin. TRPV1 was indispensable for the expression of growth factors and cytokines after TCA treatment. TRPV1-deficient mice showed even more severe ulcerations compared to the wild type mice, suggesting that the modulation of TRPV1 can support rejuvenation treatments [133].

Clotrimazole (CLT) is a widely used antifungal for topical treatment of yeast infections of the skin, vagina, and mouth. CLT induced calcium influx in TRPV1-expressing cells, but not in closely related heat-activated TRPV2, TRPV3, and TRPV4 channels. In TRPV4-expressing cells, CLT even led to a reduction of basal calcium levels. HEK293 cells expressing TRPA1 clearly showed an intracellular calcium increase, though it was significantly slower than the influx in TRPV1 cells. In mouse experiments, the injection of CLT evokes noci-defensive behavior which could be attenuated by specific antagonist of TRPV1. Moreover, CLT shifts the voltage dependence towards a more negative voltage for TRPA1 and TRPV1, whereas for TRPM8 it shifts toward more positive voltages. Thus, CLT acts more as a gating modifier than a classical antagonist/agonist of these channels [83]. Due to its different effects on TRPA1 and TRPM8, CLT is a useful tool to discriminate between menthol-induced TRPA1 and TRPM8 responses in nociceptors, which are either potentiated by CLT in TRPA1-expressing cells or otherwise heavily repressed in TRPM8-expressing cells. CLT was identified as the most sensitive inhibitor of TRPM8 known so far. This opens up new possibilities as therapeutic agent against TRPM8-driven diseases like cold allodynia, and even certain types of malignancies [83].

Skin can itch for various reasons, including bacterial infections, insect bites, allergies, and different types of dermatitis. Itch is also a common side effect of drug treatment, such as in the case of the anti-malaria drug chloroquine (QC). In DRG a QC-induced calcium influx was shown to be TRP channel dependent. Knockout experiments in mice revealed that TRPA1 mediates the calcium flux, whereas TRPV1 was not involved [134]. In behavioral studies, wild type and TRPV1-deficient mice showed QC-induced scratching, whereas TRPA1$^{-/-}$ mice did not, which is evidence that TRPA1-expressing neurons are required for QC-induced non-histaminic itch [134]. Also in acute contact dermatitis, resembled by an oxazolone-induced model of dermatitis in mice, TRPA1 is the determining channel to transduce the histamine-independent inflammation and pruritus [135].

3.7. Oral Mucosa

In oral mucosa TRPA1, TRPV1, and TRPM8 channels are predominantly expressed as chemosensors for irritants contained in food, drinks, and cigarette smoke. Lipophilic irritants such as mustard oil, capsaicin, and menthol activate TRPA1, TRPV1, and TRPM8, respectively, in sensory nerves of the buccal mucosa mediating the release of CGRP. Nicotine as a toxic substance, is, however, completely ineffective to induce CGRP exocytosis when applied in low concentrations [136]. Higher concentrations that may be reached in individuals consuming oral tobacco products evoked only a low CGRP secretion at pH 7.4. However, when deprotonated, uncharged and lipophilic nicotine was applied at pH 9, a robust TRPA1- and TRPV1-dependent response was observed. More physiological relevant experiments with full cigarette smoke containing hydrophilic nicotine, applied by smoking machines, showed moderate effects that were likely mediated by TRPA1 [136,137].

3.8. Cardiovascular System

There are only a few studies that suggest a role of TRP channels in chemical-induced cardiovascular toxicity. A single exposure to diesel exhausts was shown to increase the sensitivity of the heart to triggered arrhythmias [138]. This effect seemed to be mediated via the pulmonary activation of TRPA1, with subsequent sympathetic modulation, and it could be prevented by pre-incubation with RR [138]. Administration of TRPA1 or TRPV1 blockers prevented the increase of QRS duration, and a decrease in ST segment length (both are indicators for beginning cardiac stress), which were caused by diesel exhaust [138]. The results point to some evidence that activation of pulmonary sensory TRPA1 channels, which are known to be particularly sensitive to inhaled irritants, are involved in sympathetic activation [138]. Related results were found after pulmonary exposure of rats to ultrafine titanium dioxide particles, which resulted in elevated mean and diastolic blood pressure in response to norepinephrine [102]. RR inhibited substance P synthesis in nodose ganglia and associated functional and biological changes in the cardiovascular system [102].

3.9. Eyes

The eyes are one of the most sensitive organs with regard to irritation by chemicals. Most of the effects have been attributed to neuronal and sensory TRP channels (see section "Neuronal TRP channels") like TRPA1. However, it was speculated that TRPV channels may play a role in a variety of cellular functions directly in the corneal epithelium [139]. TRPV1, V3, V4, and weakly V2 were detected by polymerase chain reaction (PCR) in a human corneal epithelial cell line [139]. Immunohistochemical stainings, together with PCR experiments and functional calcium measurements, revealed expression of TRPV3 in the murine cornea or primary corneal epithelial cells [139]. Carvacrol, the major component of plants such as oregano, savoy, clove and thyme is known as sensitizer and allergen, activates TRPV3 channels and directly affects cell viability [139]. Unfortunately, cytotoxicity after pre-incubation with TRP channel blockers and carvacrol exposure was not evaluated. Remarkably, low dose exposures with carvacrol, that did not result in a significant TRPV3 activation, were found to improve corneal wound healing in the scratch assay [139].

4. Closing Remarks

TRP channels are important actors in many physiological, but also pathophysiological processes. Over the last few years, they have come into focus as specific targets to counteract toxicity of certain chemical compounds. For some chemicals, e.g., acrolein, specific activation of TRP channels has been explicitly proven in vivo and in vitro, whereas for other compounds, the overall picture is less clear. As example for the latter, sulfur mustard has been clearly identified to activate TRPA1 channels in vitro [89]. However, contact to that agent seems not to induce acute pain or irritation symptoms. There are more examples pointing to a mismatch of in vitro results, and the clinical in vivo picture. Moreover, results obtained from rodent animal experiments do not necessarily reflect the human situation. This illustrates the need for further comprehensive investigations. Elucidation of the exact activation mechanisms, as well as the identification of the biological consequences of TRP channel activation through chemicals, should be in the focus of upcoming research.

Author Contributions: Conceptualization D.S., B.S. and T.P.; Writing—Original Draft Preparation D.S., B.S., T.P.; Writing—Review & Editing, A.D. and T.G.; Visualization D.S.; Supervision, D.S.

Funding: This research received no external funding.

Conflicts of Interest: The authors declare no conflict of interest.

References

1. BASF. Update: Fire at the North Harbor in Ludwigshafen. Available online: https://www.basf.com/en/company/news-and-media/news-releases/2016/10/p-16-359.html (accessed on 6 August 2018).
2. Varma, D.R.; Guest, I. The Bhopal accident and methyl isocyanate toxicity. *J. Toxicol. Environ. Health* **1993**, *40*, 513–529. [CrossRef] [PubMed]
3. Lorin, H.G.; Kulling, P.E. The Bhopal tragedy—What has Swedish disaster medicine planning learned from it? *J. Emerg. Med.* **1986**, *4*, 311–316. [CrossRef]
4. Samal, A.; Honovar, J.; White, C.R.; Patel, R.P. Potential for chlorine gas-induced injury in the extrapulmonary vasculature. *Proc. Am. Thorac. Soc.* **2010**, *7*, 290–293. [CrossRef] [PubMed]
5. John, H.; van der Schans, M.J.; Koller, M.; Spruit, H.E.T.; Worek, F.; Thiermann, H.; Noort, D. Fatal sarin poisoning in Syria 2013: Forensic verification within an international laboratory network. *Forensic Toxicol.* **2018**, *36*, 61–71. [CrossRef] [PubMed]
6. Dietrich, A.; Steinritz, D.; Gudermann, T. Transient receptor potential (TRP) channels as molecular targets in lung toxicology and associated diseases. *Cell Calcium* **2017**, *67*, 123–137. [CrossRef] [PubMed]
7. Buch, T.; Schafer, E.; Steinritz, D.; Dietrich, A.; Gudermann, T. Chemosensory TRP channels in the respiratory tract: Role in toxic lung injury and potential as "sweet spots" for targeted therapies. *Rev. Physiol. Biochem. Pharmacol.* **2013**, *165*, 31–65. [CrossRef] [PubMed]

8.   Banner, K.H.; Igney, F.; Poll, C. TRP channels: Emerging targets for respiratory disease. *Pharmacol. Ther.* **2011**, *130*, 371–384. [CrossRef] [PubMed]

9.   Bessac, B.F.; Jordt, S.-E. Breathtaking TRP channels: TRPA1 and TRPV1 in airway chemosensation and reflex control. *Physiology* **2008**, *23*, 360–370. [CrossRef] [PubMed]

10. Bessac, B.F.; Jordt, S.-E. Sensory detection and responses to toxic gases: Mechanisms, health effects, and countermeasures. *Proc. Am. Thorac. Soc.* **2010**, *7*, 269–277. [CrossRef] [PubMed]

11. Nilius, B.; Szallasi, A. Transient receptor potential channels as drug targets: From the science of basic research to the art of medicine. *Pharmacol. Rev.* **2014**, *66*, 676–814. [CrossRef] [PubMed]

12. Cosens, D.J.; Manning, A. Abnormal electroretinogram from a Drosophila mutant. *Nature* **1969**, *224*, 285–287. [CrossRef] [PubMed]

13. Minke, B.; Wu, C.; Pak, W.L. Induction of photoreceptor voltage noise in the dark in Drosophila mutant. *Nature* **1975**, *258*, 84–87. [CrossRef] [PubMed]

14. Montell, C.; Rubin, G.M. Molecular characterization of the Drosophila trp locus: A putative integral membrane protein required for phototransduction. *Neuron* **1989**, *2*, 1313–1323. [CrossRef]

15. Hardie, R.C.; Minke, B. The trp gene is essential for a light-activated Ca^{2+} channel in Drosophila photoreceptors. *Neuron* **1992**, *8*, 643–651. [CrossRef]

16. Clapham, D.E.; Runnels, L.W.; Strübing, C. The TRP ion channel family. *Nat. Rev. Neurosci.* **2001**, *2*, 387–396. [CrossRef] [PubMed]

17. Montell, C.; Birnbaumer, L.; Flockerzi, V. The TRP channels, a remarkably functional family. *Cell* **2002**, *108*, 595–598. [CrossRef]

18. Montell, C.; Birnbaumer, L.; Flockerzi, V.; Bindels, R.J.; Bruford, E.A.; Caterina, M.J.; Clapham, D.E.; Harteneck, C.; Heller, S.; Julius, D.; et al. A unified nomenclature for the superfamily of TRP cation channels. *Mol. Cell* **2002**, *9*, 229–231. [CrossRef]

19. Rosasco, M.G.; Gordon, S.E. TRP Channels: What Do They Look Like? In *Neurobiology of TRP Channels*, 2nd ed.; CRC Press: Boca Raton, FL, USA, 2017.

20. Nilius, B.; Owsianik, G. The transient receptor potential family of ion channels. *Genome Boil.* **2011**, *12*, 218. [CrossRef] [PubMed]

21. Montell, C. The TRP superfamily of cation channels. *Sci. STKE Signal Transduct. Knowl. Environ.* **2005**, *2005*, re3. [CrossRef] [PubMed]

22. Venkatachalam, K.; Luo, J.; Montell, C. Evolutionarily conserved, multitasking TRP channels: Lessons from worms and flies. *Handb. Exp. Pharmacol.* **2014**, *223*, 937–962. [CrossRef] [PubMed]

23. Hellmich, U.A.; Gaudet, R. Structural biology of TRP channels. *Handb. Exp. Pharmacol.* **2014**, *223*, 963–990. [CrossRef] [PubMed]

24. Gaudet, R. Structural Insights into the Function of TRP Channels. In *TRP Ion Channel Function in Sensory Transduction and Cellular Signaling Cascades*; CRC Press: Boca Raton, FL, USA, 2007.

25. Peng, J.-B. TRPV5 and TRPV6 in transcellular Ca(2+) transport: Regulation, gene duplication, and polymorphisms in African populations. *Adv. Exp. Med. Boil.* **2011**, *704*, 239–275. [CrossRef]

26. Hofmann, T.; Chubanov, V.; Gudermann, T.; Montell, C. TRPM5 is a voltage-modulated and Ca(2+)-activated monovalent selective cation channel. *Curr. Boil.* **2003**, *13*, 1153–1158. [CrossRef]

27. Launay, P.; Fleig, A.; Perraud, A.L.; Scharenberg, A.M.; Penner, R.; Kinet, J.P. TRPM4 is a Ca^{2+}-activated nonselective cation channel mediating cell membrane depolarization. *Cell* **2002**, *109*, 397–407. [CrossRef]

28. Macpherson, L.J.; Dubin, A.E.; Evans, M.J.; Marr, F.; Schultz, P.G.; Cravatt, B.F.; Patapoutian, A. Noxious compounds activate TRPA1 ion channels through covalent modification of cysteines. *Nature* **2007**, *445*, 541–545. [CrossRef] [PubMed]

29. Survery, S.; Moparthi, L.; Kjellbom, P.; Högestätt, E.D.; Zygmunt, P.M.; Johanson, U. The N-terminal Ankyrin Repeat Domain Is Not Required for Electrophile and Heat Activation of the Purified Mosquito TRPA1 Receptor. *J. Boil. Chem.* **2016**, *291*, 26899–26912. [CrossRef] [PubMed]

30. Klement, G.; Eisele, L.; Malinowsky, D.; Nolting, A.; Svensson, M.; Terp, G.; Weigelt, D.; Dabrowski, M. Characterization of a ligand binding site in the human transient receptor potential ankyrin 1 pore. *Biophys. J.* **2013**, *104*, 798–806. [CrossRef] [PubMed]

31. Paulsen, C.E.; Armache, J.-P.; Gao, Y.; Cheng, Y.; Julius, D. Structure of the TRPA1 ion channel suggests regulatory mechanisms. *Nature* **2015**, *520*, 511–517. [CrossRef] [PubMed]

32. Marsakova, L.; Barvik, I.; Zima, V.; Zimova, L.; Vlachova, V. The First Extracellular Linker Is Important for Several Aspects of the Gating Mechanism of Human TRPA1 Channel. *Front. Mol. Neurosci.* **2017**, *10*, 16. [CrossRef] [PubMed]

33. Rychkov, G.; Barritt, G.J. TRPC1 Ca(2+)-permeable channels in animal cells. *Handb. Exp. Pharmacol.* **2007**, 23–52. [CrossRef]

34. Nakashimo, Y.; Takumida, M.; Fukuiri, T.; Anniko, M.; Hirakawa, K. Expression of transient receptor potential channel vanilloid (TRPV) 1–4, melastin (TRPM) 5 and 8, and ankyrin (TRPA1) in the normal and methimazole-treated mouse olfactory epithelium. *Acta Oto-Laryngol.* **2010**, *130*, 1278–1286. [CrossRef] [PubMed]

35. Yin, Y.; Wu, M.; Zubcevic, L.; Borschel, W.F.; Lander, G.C.; Lee, S.-Y. Structure of the cold- and menthol-sensing ion channel TRPM8. *Science* **2018**, *359*, 237–241. [CrossRef] [PubMed]

36. Shi, D.-J.; Ye, S.; Cao, X.; Zhang, R.; Wang, K. Crystal structure of the N-terminal ankyrin repeat domain of TRPV3 reveals unique conformation of finger 3 loop critical for channel function. *Protein Cell* **2013**, *4*, 942–950. [CrossRef] [PubMed]

37. Saito, S.; Fukuta, N.; Shingai, R.; Tominaga, M. Evolution of vertebrate transient receptor potential vanilloid 3 channels: Opposite temperature sensitivity between mammals and western clawed frogs. *PLoS Genet.* **2011**, *7*, e1002041. [CrossRef] [PubMed]

38. Broad, L.M.; Mogg, A.J.; Eberle, E.; Tolley, M.; Li, D.L.; Knopp, K.L. TRPV3 in Drug Development. *Pharmaceuticals* **2016**, *9*, 55. [CrossRef] [PubMed]

39. Hu, H.; Grandl, J.; Bandell, M.; Petrus, M.; Patapoutian, A. Two amino acid residues determine 2-APB sensitivity of the ion channels TRPV3 and TRPV4. *Proc. Natl. Acad. Sci. USA* **2009**, *106*, 1626–1631. [CrossRef] [PubMed]

40. Clapham, D.E. TRP channels as cellular sensors. *Nature* **2003**, *426*, 517–524. [CrossRef] [PubMed]

41. Samanta, A.; Kiselar, J.; Pumroy, R.A.; Han, S.; Moiseenkova-Bell, V.Y. Structural insights into the molecular mechanism of mouse TRPA1 activation and inhibition. *J. Gen. Physiol.* **2018**, *150*, 751–762. [CrossRef] [PubMed]

42. Bautista, D.M.; Movahed, P.; Hinman, A.; Axelsson, H.E.; Sterner, O.; Högestätt, E.D.; Julius, D.; Jordt, S.-E.; Zygmunt, P.M. Pungent products from garlic activate the sensory ion channel TRPA1. *Proc. Natl. Acad. Sci. USA* **2005**, *102*, 12248–12252. [CrossRef] [PubMed]

43. Guimaraes, M.Z.P.; Jordt, S.-E. TRPA1: A Sensory Channel of Many Talents. In *TRP Ion Channel Function in Sensory Transduction and Cellular Signaling Cascades*; CRC Press: Boca Raton, FL, USA, 2007.

44. Fernandes, E.S.; Fernandes, M.A.; Keeble, J.E. The functions of TRPA1 and TRPV1: Moving away from sensory nerves. *Br. J. Pharmacol.* **2012**, *166*, 510–521. [CrossRef] [PubMed]

45. Patil, M.J.; Jeske, N.A.; Akopian, A.N. Transient receptor potential V1 regulates activation and modulation of transient receptor potential A1 by Ca^{2+}. *Neuroscience* **2010**, *171*, 1109–1119. [CrossRef] [PubMed]

46. Staruschenko, A.; Jeske, N.A.; Akopian, A.N. Contribution of TRPV1-TRPA1 interaction to the single channel properties of the TRPA1 channel. *J. Boil. Chem.* **2010**, *285*, 15167–15177. [CrossRef] [PubMed]

47. Vandewauw, I.; de Clercq, K.; Mulier, M.; Held, K.; Pinto, S.; van Ranst, N.; Segal, A.; Voet, T.; Vennekens, R.; Zimmermann, K.; et al. A TRP channel trio mediates acute noxious heat sensing. *Nature* **2018**, *555*, 662–666. [CrossRef] [PubMed]

48. Vriens, J.; Owsianik, G.; Janssens, A.; Voets, T.; Nilius, B. Determinants of 4 alpha-phorbol sensitivity in transmembrane domains 3 and 4 of the cation channel TRPV4. *J. Boil. Chem.* **2007**, *282*, 12796–12803. [CrossRef] [PubMed]

49. Willette, R.N.; Bao, W.; Nerurkar, S.; Yue, T.-L.; Doe, C.P.; Stankus, G.; Turner, G.H.; Ju, H.; Thomas, H.; Fishman, C.E.; et al. Systemic activation of the transient receptor potential vanilloid subtype 4 channel causes endothelial failure and circulatory collapse: Part 2. *J. Pharmacol. Exp. Ther.* **2008**, *326*, 443–452. [CrossRef] [PubMed]

50. Thorneloe, K.S.; Sulpizio, A.C.; Lin, Z.; Figueroa, D.J.; Clouse, A.K.; McCafferty, G.P.; Chendrimada, T.P.; Lashinger, E.S.R.; Gordon, E.; Evans, L.; et al. N-((1S)-1-{4-((2S)-2-{(2,4-dichlorophenyl)sulfonylamino}-3-hydroxypropanoyl)-1-piperazinylcarbonyl}-3-methylbutyl)-1-benzothiophene-2-carboxamide (GSK1016790A), a novel and potent transient receptor potential vanilloid 4 channel agonist induces urinary bladder contraction and hyperactivity: Part I. *J. Pharmacol. Exp. Ther.* **2008**, *326*, 432–442. [CrossRef] [PubMed]

51. Berrout, J.; Jin, M.; Mamenko, M.; Zaika, O.; Pochynyuk, O.; O'Neil, R.G. Function of transient receptor potential cation channel subfamily V member 4 (TRPV4) as a mechanical transducer in flow-sensitive segments of renal collecting duct system. *J. Boil. Chem.* **2012**, *287*, 8782–8791. [CrossRef] [PubMed]

52. Zhu, M.X.; Tang, J. TRPC channel interactions with calmodulin and IP3 receptors. *Novartis Found. Symp.* **2004**, *258*, 44–58, discussion 58–62, 98–102, 263–266. [PubMed]

53. Venkatachalam, K.; Zheng, F.; Gill, D.L. Regulation of canonical transient receptor potential (TRPC) channel function by diacylglycerol and protein kinase C. *J. Boil. Chem.* **2003**, *278*, 29031–29040. [CrossRef] [PubMed]

54. Storch, U.; Forst, A.-L.; Pardatscher, F.; Erdogmus, S.; Philipp, M.; Gregoritza, M.; Mederos Y Schnitzler, M.; Gudermann, T. Dynamic NHERF interaction with TRPC4/5 proteins is required for channel gating by diacylglycerol. *Proc. Natl. Acad. Sci. USA* **2017**, *114*, E37–E46. [CrossRef] [PubMed]

55. Tsuruda, P.R.; Julius, D.; Minor, D.L.J. Coiled coils direct assembly of a cold-activated TRP channel. *Neuron* **2006**, *51*, 201–212. [CrossRef] [PubMed]

56. Chubanov, V.; Mittermeier, L.; Gudermann, T. Role of kinase-coupled TRP channels in mineral homeostasis. *Pharmacol. Ther.* **2018**, *184*, 159–176. [CrossRef] [PubMed]

57. Delgado, R.; Muñoz, Y.; Peña-Cortés, H.; Giavalisco, P.; Bacigalupo, J. Diacylglycerol activates the light-dependent channel TRP in the photosensitive microvilli of Drosophila melanogaster photoreceptors. *J. Neurosci. Off. J. Soc. Neurosci.* **2014**, *34*, 6679–6686. [CrossRef] [PubMed]

58. Oh, E.J.; Gover, T.D.; Cordoba-Rodriguez, R.; Weinreich, D. Substance P evokes cation currents through TRP channels in HEK293 cells. *J. Neurophysiol.* **2003**, *90*, 2069–2073. [CrossRef] [PubMed]

59. Kumamoto, E.; Fujita, T.; Jiang, C.-Y. TRP Channels Involved in Spontaneous L-Glutamate Release Enhancement in the Adult Rat Spinal Substantia Gelatinosa. *Cells* **2014**, *3*, 331–362. [CrossRef] [PubMed]

60. Braz, J.M.; Basbaum, A.I. Differential ATF3 expression in dorsal root ganglion neurons reveals the profile of primary afferents engaged by diverse noxious chemical stimuli. *Pain* **2010**, *150*, 290–301. [CrossRef] [PubMed]

61. Eilers, H.; Cattaruzza, F.; Nassini, R.; Materazzi, S.; Andre, E.; Chu, C.; Cottrell, G.S.; Schumacher, M.; Geppetti, P.; Bunnett, N.W. Pungent general anesthetics activate transient receptor potential-A1 to produce hyperalgesia and neurogenic bronchoconstriction. *Anesthesiology* **2010**, *112*, 1452–1463. [CrossRef] [PubMed]

62. Kimball, C.; Luo, J.; Yin, S.; Hu, H.; Dhaka, A. The Pore Loop Domain of TRPV1 Is Required for Its Activation by the Volatile Anesthetics Chloroform and Isoflurane. *Mol. Pharmacol.* **2015**, *88*, 131–138. [CrossRef] [PubMed]

63. Leffler, A.; Fischer, M.J.; Rehner, D.; Kienel, S.; Kistner, K.; Sauer, S.K.; Gavva, N.R.; Reeh, P.W.; Nau, C. The vanilloid receptor TRPV1 is activated and sensitized by local anesthetics in rodent sensory neurons. *J. Clin. Investig.* **2008**, *118*, 763–776. [CrossRef] [PubMed]

64. Marwaha, L.; Bansal, Y.; Singh, R.; Saroj, P.; Sodhi, R.K.; Kuhad, A. Niflumic acid, a TRPV1 channel modulator, ameliorates stavudine-induced neuropathic pain. *Inflammopharmacology* **2016**, *24*, 319–334. [CrossRef] [PubMed]

65. Bang, S.; Yang, T.-J.; Yoo, S.; Heo, T.-H.; Hwang, S.W. Inhibition of sensory neuronal TRPs contributes to anti-nociception by butamben. *Neurosci. Lett.* **2012**, *506*, 297–302. [CrossRef] [PubMed]

66. Olah, Z.; Redei, D.; Pecze, L.; Vizler, C.; Josvay, K.; Forgo, P.; Winter, Z.; Dombi, G.; Szakonyi, G.; Hohmann, J. Pellitorine, an extract of Tetradium daniellii, is an antagonist of the ion channel TRPV1. *Phytomed. Int. J. Phytother. Phytopharm.* **2017**, *34*, 44–49. [CrossRef] [PubMed]

67. Sherkheli, M.A.; Schreiner, B.; Haq, R.; Werner, M.; Hatt, H. Borneol inhibits TRPA1, a proinflammatory and noxious pain-sensing cation channel. *Pak. J. Pharm. Sci.* **2015**, *28*, 1357–1363. [PubMed]

68. Nozadze, I.; Tsiklauri, N.; Gurtskaia, G.; Tsagareli, M.G. NSAIDs attenuate hyperalgesia induced by TRP channel activation. *Data Brief* **2016**, *6*, 668–673. [CrossRef] [PubMed]

69. Anand, U.; Otto, W.R.; Anand, P. Sensitization of capsaicin and icilin responses in oxaliplatin treated adult rat DRG neurons. *Mol. Pain* **2010**, *6*, 82. [CrossRef] [PubMed]

70. Schulze, C.; McGowan, M.; Jordt, S.-E.; Ehrlich, B.E. Prolonged oxaliplatin exposure alters intracellular calcium signaling: A new mechanism to explain oxaliplatin-associated peripheral neuropathy. *Clin. Color. Cancer* **2011**, *10*, 126–133. [CrossRef] [PubMed]

71. Chen, Y.; Yang, C.; Wang, Z.J. Proteinase-activated receptor 2 sensitizes transient receptor potential vanilloid 1, transient receptor potential vanilloid 4, and transient receptor potential ankyrin 1 in paclitaxel-induced neuropathic pain. *Neuroscience* **2011**, *193*, 440–451. [CrossRef] [PubMed]

72. Akopian, A.N.; Ruparel, N.B.; Patwardhan, A.; Hargreaves, K.M. Cannabinoids desensitize capsaicin and mustard oil responses in sensory neurons via TRPA1 activation. *J. Neurosci.* **2008**, *28*, 1064–1075. [CrossRef] [PubMed]

73. Xu, H.; Blair, N.T.; Clapham, D.E. Camphor activates and strongly desensitizes the transient receptor potential vanilloid subtype 1 channel in a vanilloid-independent mechanism. *J. Neurosci.* **2005**, *25*, 8924–8937. [CrossRef] [PubMed]

74. Vriens, J.; Watanabe, H.; Janssens, A.; Droogmans, G.; Voets, T.; Nilius, B. Cell swelling, heat, and chemical agonists use distinct pathways for the activation of the cation channel TRPV4. *Proc. Natl. Acad. Sci. USA* **2004**, *101*, 396–401. [CrossRef] [PubMed]

75. Fowler, M.A.; Sidiropoulou, K.; Ozkan, E.D.; Phillips, C.W.; Cooper, D.C. Corticolimbic expression of TRPC4 and TRPC5 channels in the rodent brain. *PLoS ONE* **2007**, *2*, e573. [CrossRef] [PubMed]

76. Balbuena, P.; Li, W.; Rzigalinski, B.A.; Ehrich, M. Malathion/oxon and lead acetate increase gene expression and protein levels of transient receptor potential canonical channel subunits TRPC1 and TRPC4 in rat endothelial cells of the blood-brain barrier. *Int. J. Toxicol.* **2012**, *31*, 238–249. [CrossRef] [PubMed]

77. Zhang, H.; Li, W.; Xue, Y.; Zou, F. TRPC1 is involved in Ca(2)(+) influx and cytotoxicity following Pb(2)(+) exposure in human embryonic kidney cells. *Toxicol. Lett.* **2014**, *229*, 52–58. [CrossRef] [PubMed]

78. Nassini, R.; Materazzi, S.; Vriens, J.; Prenen, J.; Benemei, S.; de Siena, G.; La Marca, G.; Andrè, E.; Preti, D.; Avonto, C.; et al. The 'headache tree' via umbellulone and TRPA1 activates the trigeminovascular system. *Brain A J. Neurol.* **2012**, *135*, 376–390. [CrossRef] [PubMed]

79. Zhong, J.; Minassi, A.; Prenen, J.; Taglialatela-Scafati, O.; Appendino, G.; Nilius, B. Umbellulone modulates TRP channels. *Pflugers Arch. Eur. J. Physiol.* **2011**, *462*, 861–870. [CrossRef] [PubMed]

80. Salas, M.M.; Hargreaves, K.M.; Akopian, A.N. TRPA1-mediated responses in trigeminal sensory neurons: Interaction between TRPA1 and TRPV1. *Eur. J. Neurosci.* **2009**, *29*, 1568–1578. [CrossRef] [PubMed]

81. Lehmann, R.; Hatt, H.; van Thriel, C. Alternative in vitro assays to assess the potency of sensory irritants-Is one TRP channel enough? *Neurotoxicology* **2017**, *60*, 178–186. [CrossRef] [PubMed]

82. Lehmann, R.; Schobel, N.; Hatt, H.; van Thriel, C. The involvement of TRP channels in sensory irritation: A mechanistic approach toward a better understanding of the biological effects of local irritants. *Arch. Toxicol.* **2016**, *90*, 1399–1413. [CrossRef] [PubMed]

83. Meseguer, V.; Karashima, Y.; Talavera, K.; D'Hoedt, D.; Donovan-Rodriguez, T.; Viana, F.; Nilius, B.; Voets, T. Transient receptor potential channels in sensory neurons are targets of the antimycotic agent clotrimazole. *J. Neurosci.* **2008**, *28*, 576–586. [CrossRef] [PubMed]

84. Kunkler, P.E.; Ballard, C.J.; Oxford, G.S.; Hurley, J.H. TRPA1 receptors mediate environmental irritant-induced meningeal vasodilatation. *Pain* **2011**, *152*, 38–44. [CrossRef] [PubMed]

85. Kunkler, P.E.; Ballard, C.J.; Pellman, J.J.; Zhang, L.; Oxford, G.S.; Hurley, J.H. Intraganglionic signaling as a novel nasal-meningeal pathway for TRPA1-dependent trigeminovascular activation by inhaled environmental irritants. *PLoS ONE* **2014**, *9*, e103086. [CrossRef] [PubMed]

86. Buch, T.R.H.; Schafer, E.A.M.; Demmel, M.-T.; Boekhoff, I.; Thiermann, H.; Gudermann, T.; Steinritz, D.; Schmidt, A. Functional expression of the transient receptor potential channel TRPA1, a sensor for toxic lung inhalants, in pulmonary epithelial cells. *Chem. Boil. Interact.* **2013**, *206*, 462–471. [CrossRef] [PubMed]

87. Inoue, T.; Bryant, B.P. Multiple types of sensory neurons respond to irritating volatile organic compounds (VOCs): Calcium fluorimetry of trigeminal ganglion neurons. *Pain* **2005**, *117*, 193–203. [CrossRef] [PubMed]

88. Brand, G.; Jacquot, L. Sensitization and desensitization to allyl isothiocyanate (mustard oil) in the nasal cavity. *Chem. Senses* **2002**, *27*, 593–598. [CrossRef] [PubMed]

89. Stenger, B.; Zehfuss, F.; Muckter, H.; Schmidt, A.; Balszuweit, F.; Schafer, E.; Buch, T.; Gudermann, T.; Thiermann, H.; Steinritz, D. Activation of the chemosensing transient receptor potential channel A1 (TRPA1) by alkylating agents. *Arch. Toxicol.* **2015**, *89*, 1631–1643. [CrossRef] [PubMed]

90. Achanta, S.; Chintagari, N.R.; Brackmann, M.; Balakrishna, S.; Jordt, S.-E. TRPA1 and CGRP antagonists counteract vesicant-induced skin injury and inflammation. *Toxicol. Lett.* **2018**, *293*, 140–148. [CrossRef] [PubMed]

91. Hu, H.; Bandell, M.; Petrus, M.J.; Zhu, M.X.; Patapoutian, A. Zinc activates damage-sensing TRPA1 ion channels. *Nat. Chem. Boil.* **2009**, *5*, 183–190. [CrossRef] [PubMed]

92. Adamson, I.Y.; Prieditis, H.; Hedgecock, C.; Vincent, R. Zinc is the toxic factor in the lung response to an atmospheric particulate sample. *Toxicol. Appl. Pharmacol.* **2000**, *166*, 111–119. [CrossRef] [PubMed]

93. Steinritz, D.; Zehfuß, F.; Stenger, B.; Schmidt, A.; Popp, T.; Kehe, K.; Mückter, H.; Thiermann, H.; Gudermann, T. Zinc chloride-induced TRPA1 activation does not contribute to toxicity in vitro. *Toxicol. Lett.* **2017**, *293*, 133–139. [CrossRef] [PubMed]

94. Bessac, B.F.; Sivula, M.; von Hehn, C.A.; Escalera, J.; Cohn, L.; Jordt, S.-E. TRPA1 is a major oxidant sensor in murine airway sensory neurons. *J. Clin. Investig.* **2008**, *118*, 1899–1910. [CrossRef] [PubMed]

95. Bessac, B.F.; Sivula, M.; von Hehn, C.A.; Caceres, A.I.; Escalera, J.; Jordt, S.-E. Transient receptor potential ankyrin 1 antagonists block the noxious effects of toxic industrial isocyanates and tear gases. *FASEB J.* **2009**, *23*, 1102–1114. [CrossRef] [PubMed]

96. Bautista, D.M.; Jordt, S.-E.; Nikai, T.; Tsuruda, P.R.; Read, A.J.; Poblete, J.; Yamoah, E.N.; Basbaum, A.I.; Julius, D. TRPA1 mediates the inflammatory actions of environmental irritants and proalgesic agents. *Cell* **2006**, *124*, 1269–1282. [CrossRef] [PubMed]

97. Andrè, E.; Campi, B.; Materazzi, S.; Trevisani, M.; Amadesi, S.; Massi, D.; Creminon, C.; Vaksman, N.; Nassini, R.; Civelli, M.; et al. Cigarette smoke-induced neurogenic inflammation is mediated by alpha,beta-unsaturated aldehydes and the TRPA1 receptor in rodents. *J. Clin. Investig.* **2008**, *118*, 2574–2582. [CrossRef] [PubMed]

98. Alpizar, Y.A.; Boonen, B.; Sanchez, A.; Jung, C.; López-Requena, A.; Naert, R.; Steelant, B.; Luyts, K.; Plata, C.; de Vooght, V.; et al. TRPV4 activation triggers protective responses to bacterial lipopolysaccharides in airway epithelial cells. *Nat. Commun.* **2017**, *8*, 1059. [CrossRef] [PubMed]

99. Alvarez, D.F.; King, J.A.; Weber, D.; Addison, E.; Liedtke, W.; Townsley, M.I. Transient receptor potential vanilloid 4-mediated disruption of the alveolar septal barrier: A novel mechanism of acute lung injury. *Circ. Res.* **2006**, *99*, 988–995. [CrossRef] [PubMed]

100. Balakrishna, S.; Song, W.; Achanta, S.; Doran, S.F.; Liu, B.; Kaelberer, M.M.; Yu, Z.; Sui, A.; Cheung, M.; Leishman, E.; et al. TRPV4 inhibition counteracts edema and inflammation and improves pulmonary function and oxygen saturation in chemically induced acute lung injury. *Am. J. Physiol. Lung Cell. Mol. Physiol.* **2014**, *307*, L158–L172. [CrossRef] [PubMed]

101. Andres, D.; Keyser, B.; Benton, B.; Melber, A.; Olivera, D.; Holmes, W.; Paradiso, D.; Anderson, D.; Ray, R. Transient receptor potential (TRP) channels as a therapeutic target for intervention of respiratory effects and lethality from phosgene. *Toxicol. Lett.* **2016**, *244*, 21–27. [CrossRef] [PubMed]

102. Kan, H.; Wu, Z.; Lin, Y.-C.; Chen, T.-H.; Cumpston, J.L.; Kashon, M.L.; Leonard, S.; Munson, A.E.; Castranova, V. The role of nodose ganglia in the regulation of cardiovascular function following pulmonary exposure to ultrafine titanium dioxide. *Nanotoxicology* **2014**, *8*, 447–454. [CrossRef] [PubMed]

103. McGarvey, L.P.; Butler, C.A.; Stokesberry, S.; Polley, L.; McQuaid, S.; Abdullah, H.; Ashraf, S.; McGahon, M.K.; Curtis, T.M.; Arron, J.; et al. Increased expression of bronchial epithelial transient receptor potential vanilloid 1 channels in patients with severe asthma. *J. Allergy Clin. Immunol.* **2014**, *133*, 704–712. [CrossRef] [PubMed]

104. Devos, F.C.; Boonen, B.; Alpizar, Y.A.; Maes, T.; Hox, V.; Seys, S.; Pollaris, L.; Liston, A.; Nemery, B.; Talavera, K.; et al. Neuro-immune interactions in chemical-induced airway hyperreactivity. *Eur. Respir. J.* **2016**, *48*, 380–392. [CrossRef] [PubMed]

105. Oliver, M.R.; Tan, D.T.; Kirk, D.R.; Rioux, K.P.; Scott, R.B. Colonic and jejunal motor disturbances after colonic antigen challenge of sensitized rat. *Gastroenterology* **1997**, *112*, 1996–2005. [CrossRef] [PubMed]

106. Jurjus, A.R.; Khoury, N.N.; Reimund, J.-M. Animal models of inflammatory bowel disease. *J. Pharmacol. Toxicol. Methods* **2004**, *50*, 81–92. [CrossRef] [PubMed]

107. Makimura, Y.; Ito, K.; Kuwahara, M.; Tsubone, H. Augmented activity of the pelvic nerve afferent mediated by TRP channels in dextran sulfate sodium (DSS)-induced colitis of rats. *J. Vet. Med. Sci.* **2012**, *74*, 1007–1013. [CrossRef] [PubMed]

108. Ramachandran, R.; Hyun, E.; Zhao, L.; Lapointe, T.K.; Chapman, K.; Hirota, C.L.; Ghosh, S.; McKemy, D.D.; Vergnolle, N.; Beck, P.L.; et al. TRPM8 activation attenuates inflammatory responses in mouse models of colitis. *Proc. Natl. Acad. Sci. USA* **2013**, *110*, 7476–7481. [CrossRef] [PubMed]

109. Wu, W.; Zhou, H.-R.; Pestka, J.J. Potential roles for calcium-sensing receptor (CaSR) and transient receptor potential ankyrin-1 (TRPA1) in murine anorectic response to deoxynivalenol (vomitoxin). *Arch. Toxicol.* **2017**, *91*, 495–507. [CrossRef] [PubMed]

110. Zhou, H.-R.; Pestka, J.J. Deoxynivalenol (Vomitoxin)-Induced Cholecystokinin and Glucagon-Like Peptide-1 Release in the STC-1 Enteroendocrine Cell Model Is Mediated by Calcium-Sensing Receptor and Transient Receptor Potential Ankyrin-1 Channel. *Toxicol. Sci.* **2015**, *145*, 407–417. [CrossRef] [PubMed]

111. Babes, A.; Fischer, M.J.M.; Filipovic, M.; Engel, M.A.; Flonta, M.-L.; Reeh, P.W. The anti-diabetic drug glibenclamide is an agonist of the transient receptor potential Ankyrin 1 (TRPA1) ion channel. *Eur. J. Pharmacol.* **2013**, *704*, 15–22. [CrossRef] [PubMed]

112. Diaz-Garcia, C.M. The TRPA1 channel and oral hypoglycemic agents: Is there complicity in beta-cell exhaustion? *Channels* **2013**, *7*, 420–422. [CrossRef] [PubMed]

113. Young, R.L.; Sutherland, K.; Pezos, N.; Brierley, S.M.; Horowitz, M.; Rayner, C.K.; Blackshaw, L.A. Expression of taste molecules in the upper gastrointestinal tract in humans with and without type 2 diabetes. *Gut* **2009**, *58*, 337–346. [CrossRef] [PubMed]

114. Philippaert, K.; Pironet, A.; Mesuere, M.; Sones, W.; Vermeiren, L.; Kerselaers, S.; Pinto, S.; Segal, A.; Antoine, N.; Gysemans, C.; et al. Steviol glycosides enhance pancreatic beta-cell function and taste sensation by potentiation of TRPM5 channel activity. *Nat. Commun.* **2017**, *8*, 14733. [CrossRef] [PubMed]

115. Pawar, R.S.; Krynitsky, A.J.; Rader, J.I. Sweeteners from plants–with emphasis on Stevia rebaudiana (Bertoni) and Siraitia grosvenorii (Swingle). *Anal. Bioanal. Chem.* **2013**, *405*, 4397–4407. [CrossRef] [PubMed]

116. Anaparthy, R.; Pasricha, P.J. Pain and chronic pancreatitis: Is it the plumbing or the wiring? *Curr. Gastroenterol. Rep.* **2008**, *10*, 101–106. [CrossRef] [PubMed]

117. Schwartz, E.S.; Christianson, J.A.; Chen, X.; La, J.-H.; Davis, B.M.; Albers, K.M.; Gebhart, G.F. Synergistic role of TRPV1 and TRPA1 in pancreatic pain and inflammation. *Gastroenterology* **2011**, *140*, 1283–1291. [CrossRef] [PubMed]

118. Schwartz, E.S.; La, J.-H.; Scheff, N.N.; Davis, B.M.; Albers, K.M.; Gebhart, G.F. TRPV1 and TRPA1 antagonists prevent the transition of acute to chronic inflammation and pain in chronic pancreatitis. *J. Neurosci.* **2013**, *33*, 5603–5611. [CrossRef] [PubMed]

119. Boudes, M.; Uvin, P.; de Ridder, D. TRPV4, new therapeutic target for urinary problems. *Med. Sci.* **2011**, *27*, 232–234. [CrossRef]

120. Merrill, L.; Girard, B.M.; May, V.; Vizzard, M.A. Transcriptional and translational plasticity in rodent urinary bladder TRP channels with urinary bladder inflammation, bladder dysfunction, or postnatal maturation. *J. Mol. Neurosci.* **2012**, *48*, 744–756. [CrossRef] [PubMed]

121. Nilius, B.; Owsianik, G.; Voets, T.; Peters, J.A. Transient receptor potential cation channels in disease. *Physiol. Rev.* **2007**, *87*, 165–217. [CrossRef] [PubMed]

122. Everaerts, W.; Zhen, X.; Ghosh, D.; Vriens, J.; Gevaert, T.; Gilbert, J.P.; Hayward, N.J.; McNamara, C.R.; Xue, F.; Moran, M.M.; et al. Inhibition of the cation channel TRPV4 improves bladder function in mice and rats with cyclophosphamide-induced cystitis. *Proc. Natl. Acad. Sci. USA* **2010**, *107*, 19084–19089. [CrossRef] [PubMed]

123. Lazzeri, M.; Vannucchi, M.G.; Spinelli, M.; Bizzoco, E.; Beneforti, P.; Turini, D.; Faussone-Pellegrini, M.-S. Transient receptor potential vanilloid type 1 (TRPV1) expression changes from normal urothelium to transitional cell carcinoma of human bladder. *Eur. Urol.* **2005**, *48*, 691–698. [CrossRef] [PubMed]

124. Everaerts, W.; Gevaert, T.; Nilius, B.; de Ridder, D. On the origin of bladder sensing: Tr(i)ps in urology. *Neurourol. Urodyn.* **2008**, *27*, 264–273. [CrossRef] [PubMed]

125. Schurch, B.; Stöhrer, M.; Kramer, G.; Schmid, D.M.; Gaul, G.; Hauri, D. Botulinum-A toxin for treating detrusor hyperreflexia in spinal cord injured patients: A new alternative to anticholinergic drugs? Preliminary results. *J. Urol.* **2000**, *164*, 692–697. [CrossRef]

126. Bornehag, C.-G.; Sundell, J.; Weschler, C.J.; Sigsgaard, T.; Lundgren, B.; Hasselgren, M.; Hägerhed Engman, L. The association between asthma and allergic symptoms in children and phthalates in house dust: A nested case-control study. *Environ. Health Perspect.* **2004**, *112*, 1393–1397. [CrossRef] [PubMed]

127. Imai, Y.; Kondo, A.; Iizuka, H.; Maruyama, T.; Kurohane, K. Effects of phthalate esters on the sensitization phase of contact hypersensitivity induced by fluorescein isothiocyanate. *Clin. Exp. Allergy J. Br. Soc. Allergy Clin. Immunol.* **2006**, *36*, 1462–1468. [CrossRef] [PubMed]

128. Shiba, T.; Maruyama, T.; Kurohane, K.; Iwasaki, Y.; Watanabe, T.; Imai, Y. TRPA1 and TRPV1 activation is a novel adjuvant effect mechanism in contact hypersensitivity. *J. Neuroimmunol.* **2009**, *207*, 66–74. [CrossRef] [PubMed]

129. Kurohane, K.; Sahara, Y.; Kimura, A.; Narukawa, M.; Watanabe, T.; Daimon, T.; Imai, Y. Lack of transient receptor potential melastatin 8 activation by phthalate esters that enhance contact hypersensitivity in mice. *Toxicol. Lett.* **2013**, *217*, 192–196. [CrossRef] [PubMed]

130. Mikami, N.; Matsushita, H.; Kato, T.; Kawasaki, R.; Sawazaki, T.; Kishimoto, T.; Ogitani, Y.; Watanabe, K.; Miyagi, Y.; Sueda, K.; et al. Calcitonin gene-related peptide is an important regulator of cutaneous immunity: Effect on dendritic cell and T cell functions. *J. Immunol.* **2011**, *186*, 6886–6893. [CrossRef] [PubMed]

131. Babes, A.; Sauer, S.K.; Moparthi, L.; Kichko, T.I.; Neacsu, C.; Namer, B.; Filipovic, M.; Zygmunt, P.M.; Reeh, P.W.; Fischer, M.J.M. Photosensitization in Porphyrias and Photodynamic Therapy Involves TRPA1 and TRPV1. *J. Neurosci.* **2016**, *36*, 5264–5278. [CrossRef] [PubMed]

132. Ishizuka, M.; Abe, F.; Sano, Y.; Takahashi, K.; Inoue, K.; Nakajima, M.; Kohda, T.; Komatsu, N.; Ogura, S.-I.; Tanaka, T. Novel development of 5-aminolevurinic acid (ALA) in cancer diagnoses and therapy. *Int. Immunopharmacol.* **2011**, *11*, 358–365. [CrossRef] [PubMed]

133. Li, H.-j.; Kanazawa, N.; Kimura, A.; Kaminaka, C.; Yonei, N.; Yamamoto, Y.; Furukawa, F. Severe ulceration with impaired induction of growth factors and cytokines in keratinocytes after trichloroacetic acid application on TRPV1-deficient mice. *Eur. J. Dermatol.* **2012**, *22*, 614–621. [CrossRef] [PubMed]

134. Kittaka, H.; Tominaga, M. The molecular and cellular mechanisms of itch and the involvement of TRP channels in the peripheral sensory nervous system and skin. *Allergol. Int.* **2017**, *66*, 22–30. [CrossRef] [PubMed]

135. Liu, B.; Escalera, J.; Balakrishna, S.; Fan, L.; Caceres, A.I.; Robinson, E.; Sui, A.; McKay, M.C.; McAlexander, M.A.; Herrick, C.A.; et al. TRPA1 controls inflammation and pruritogen responses in allergic contact dermatitis. *FASEB J.* **2013**, *27*, 3549–3563. [CrossRef] [PubMed]

136. Kichko, T.I.; Neuhuber, W.; Kobal, G.; Reeh, P.W. The roles of TRPV1, TRPA1 and TRPM8 channels in chemical and thermal sensitivity of the mouse oral mucosa. *Eur. J. Neurosci.* **2018**, *47*, 201–210. [CrossRef] [PubMed]

137. Kichko, T.I.; Kobal, G.; Reeh, P.W. Cigarette smoke has sensory effects through nicotinic and TRPA1 but not TRPV1 receptors on the isolated mouse trachea and larynx. *Am. J. Physiol. Lung Cell. Mol. Physiol.* **2015**, *309*, L812–L820. [CrossRef] [PubMed]

138. Hazari, M.S.; Haykal-Coates, N.; Winsett, D.W.; Krantz, Q.T.; King, C.; Costa, D.L.; Farraj, A.K. TRPA1 and sympathetic activation contribute to increased risk of triggered cardiac arrhythmias in hypertensive rats exposed to diesel exhaust. *Environ. Health Perspect.* **2011**, *119*, 951–957. [CrossRef] [PubMed]

139. Yamada, T.; Ueda, T.; Ugawa, S.; Ishida, Y.; Imayasu, M.; Koyama, S.; Shimada, S. Functional expression of transient receptor potential vanilloid 3 (TRPV3) in corneal epithelial cells: Involvement in thermosensation and wound healing. *Exp. Eye Res.* **2010**, *90*, 121–129. [CrossRef] [PubMed]

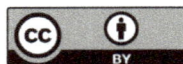

© 2018 by the authors. Licensee MDPI, Basel, Switzerland. This article is an open access article distributed under the terms and conditions of the Creative Commons Attribution (CC BY) license (http://creativecommons.org/licenses/by/4.0/).

MDPI
St. Alban-Anlage 66
4052 Basel
Switzerland
Tel. +41 61 683 77 34
Fax +41 61 302 89 18
www.mdpi.com

Cells Editorial Office
E-mail: cells@mdpi.com
www.mdpi.com/journal/cells

www.ingramcontent.com/pod-product-compliance
Lightning Source LLC
Chambersburg PA
CBHW051724210326
41597CB00032B/5592